Drug Information

A Guide to Current Resources
2nd edition

Bonnie Snow

Medical Library Association
and
The Scarecrow Press, Inc.
Lanham, Maryland, and London
1999

SCARECROW PRESS, INC.

Published in the United States of America
by Scarecrow Press, Inc.
4720 Boston Way
Lanham, Maryland 20706
http://www.scarecrowpress.com

4 Pleydell Gardens, Folkestone
Kent CT20 2DN, England

British Library Cataloguing in Publication Information Available

Library of Congress Cataloging-in-Publication Data

Snow, Bonnie.
    Drug information: a guide to current resources / Bonnie Snow — 2nd ed.
        p.   cm.
    Includes bibliographical references and index.
    ISBN 0-8108-3320-4 (cloth : alk paper).—ISBN 0-8108-3321-2
(pbk : alk. paper)
        1. Pharmacy Bibliography.   2. Pharmacy—Information resources Directories.
3. Drugs Bibliography.   4. Drugs—Information resources Directories.
5. Pharmaceutical libraries.   I. Title.
        [DNLM: 1. Pharmacology Bibliography.   2. Pharmacology Terminology—
English. 3. Drug Industry Bibliography.   4. Drug Industry Terminology—English.
5. Drug Information Services Bibliography.   6. Drug Information Services
Terminology—English.   7. Legislation, Drug Bibliography.   8. Pharmaceutical
Preparations Bibliography.   9. Pharmaceutical Preparations. ZQV 4 S674d 1999]
Z6675.P5S64   1999
[RS91]
016.615'1—dc21
DNLM/DLC for Library of Congress   99-31655
                                                                        CIP

∞ ™ The paper used in this publication meets the minimum requirements of
American National Standard for Information Sciences—Permanence of Paper for
Printed Library Materials, ANSI/NISO Z39.48–1992. Manufactured in the United
States of America.

Contents

PREFACE   vii

ACKNOWLEDGMENTS   xi

LIST OF FIGURES   xiii

CHAPTER ONE: Prescription for Using This Guide   1
    Indications for Use   1
    Recommended Regimen   2
    Special Instructions for Online, CD-ROM, and Internet Users   4
    Precautions   6

CHAPTER TWO: Drug Nomenclature and Its Relationship to Scientific
Communication   7
    Types of Drug Names   9
    Drug Classification   13
    Less Frequently Used Identifiers   14
    Other Nomenclature Issues   16
    Name Recognition and Effective Problem Solving   19

PRACTICUM 1   20

CHAPTER THREE: Drug Identification and Nomenclature Sources   21
    Official Compendia   22
    Commercial Sources   26
    Beyond the Basics: Expanding Drug Identification Capabilities   29

CHAPTER FOUR: Background on Drug and Device Laws and
Regulations   39
    History of Drug Regulation in the United States   39
    The New Drug Application Process Today   44
    Laws and Regulations Dealing with the Drug Lag   51
    Narcotic Drug Law   64

Regulatory Hot Topics and Frequently Asked Questions   66
Laws Governing the Practice of Pharmacy   80
Medical Device Regulation   88
Keeping Up-to-Date on Regulatory Developments   94
Summary: Implications for the Information Provider   98

CHAPTER FIVE: Evaluating Drug Information Sources and
Developing a Search Protocol   107
   Structure and Organization of the Literature: Scaling the
     Pyramid   109
   Source Evaluation Checklist   110
   Guides to the Literature   113
   Internet Pathfinders   122
   Guides to the Terminology of Pharmacy and Related
     Disciplines   130

CHAPTER SIX: Pharmacology and Therapeutics Reference Sources   139
   An International Compendium   139
   Core Collection for Access to U.S. Pharmacotherapeutic
     Information   142
   Alternative Selections and Additional Bibliography   149
   Drug Handbooks on the Internet   177

PRACTICUM 2   187

CHAPTER SEVEN: Side Effects: Sources of Adverse Drug Reactions
and Interactions Information   189
   Adverse Reactions Information Sources   191
   Reference Sources for Drug Interactions   194
   Specialized Adverse Effects Publications   197
   Parenteral Incompatibilities   202

CHAPTER EIGHT: Side Effects: Sources of Poisoning and Toxicology
Information   209
   Quick-Reference Sources for Poisoning Therapy   209
   Textbooks in Clinical Toxicology   214
   Sourcebooks in Analytical Toxicology   216
   Teratogenicity Information Sources   218
   Other Toxicology Reference Bibliography   224

PRACTICUM 3   236

CHAPTER NINE: Drug Information for the Consumer/Patient   237
   Recommended Core Collection   238
   Additional Selections   247
   Consumer Drug Information on the Internet   254
   Aids to Medication Counseling   269

CHAPTER TEN: Product Identification: Imprint Indexes and Foreign
Drug Sources 277
    Drug Identification from a Description or Observation of a Dosage
      Form 277
    Foreign Drug Identification Sources 283
    Multilingual Guides: Help for the Xenophobe 295

CHAPTER ELEVEN: Industrial Pharmacy 301
    Official Compendial Standards 304
    Biopharmaceutics Guides 308
    Resources to Support Formulation Development 309
    Sourcebooks in Pharmaceutical Technology 317

CHAPTER TWELVE: Special Topics 321
    Pharmacognosy: The Literature of Natural Drugs 321
    Veterinary Drugs 347
    Information on the History of Pharmacy 351

CHAPTER THIRTEEN: Business Directories and Statistical Data
Sources 361
    Resources to Determine U.S. Product Availability 361
    Company or Service Directories and Buyer's Guides 362
    Retail Trade Directories: Chain and Independent Pharmacies 370
    Sources of Drug Sales and Utilization Data 372
    Pharmacy Services, Operations, and Manpower Data 379
    Directories of Pharmacy Faculty and Educational Programs 380

PRACTICUM 4 385

CHAPTER FOURTEEN: Compiling a Bibliography with Online
Resources 387
    Pharmacology and Therapeutics Databases 389
    Influential Factors in Database Selection 409
    Databases to Answer Adverse Effects and Interactions
      Questions 426
    Drug Information for the Consumer or Patient 434
    Pharmaceutics and Pharmaceutical Technology Sources 437
    Pharmacognosy 439
    Drug Identification and Nomenclature Sources 440

CHAPTER FIFTEEN: Market Research and Competitive Intelligence
Online 447
    Drugs-in-Development Directories 447
    Tracking Pharmaceutical News Online 476

Probing the Internet for Health Economics and Outcomes
    Research 481
Exploring Licensing Opportunities 486
Investigating Line Extensions 488
Company and Product Directories 490
Statistical Sources: Market Share, Sales, and Epidemiological
    Data 496
Summary and Segue 506

CHAPTER SIXTEEN: Regulatory Sources Online   509
Finding Information on Product Approvals 510
Sources for Product Recall Notices 524
Checking a Device's Track Record of Adverse Experience
    Reports 527
Establishment Inspection Reports and Form 483s 529
Warning Letters as Competitive Intelligence Tools 531
FDA Guidelines and Regulations 533
The FDA Home Page on the Internet 535
Specialty Fee-Based CD-ROM Services 543
Verifying Patent Numbers, Expirations, and Extensions 545
The Importance of Regulatory Surveillance 561

PRACTICUM 5   564

APPENDIX A: The Core Drug Information Collection   567

APPENDIX B: Database Selection Aids and Additional Online
Resource Annotations   575

APPENDIX C: A Selection of Current Awareness Newsletters Available
in Full-Text Format Online   597

APPENDIX D: Professional and Trade Associations   603

APPENDIX E: Practicum Exercises: Suggested Answers   633

APPENDIX F: Directory of Internet Resources Cited in the Guide 657

APPENDIX G: Key to Abbreviations   673

GLOSSARY   689

INDEX   711

ABOUT THE AUTHOR   752

Preface

In the ten years that have elapsed since publication of the first edition of this book, much has changed and much has remained the same in the world of drug information. What has changed, as might be expected, is the number and types of resources available, which have been steadily increasing in hardcopy and have grown to such an extent online that just keeping pace with new developments is a major preoccupation. At the same time, what seems to remain immutable is the need for guidance in selecting the most appropriate sources and in using them effectively.

Drug Information: A Guide to Current Resources was written to address this need. It is designed for use as either a self-help manual for continuing education or as a course text to support more formal classroom instruction programs. There is, of course, no substitute for hands-on experience with the sources discussed and in-person advice on their use from seasoned colleagues. At best, this *Guide* is a stand-in for the latter, and as such is just as prone to bias based on past experience, good and bad, and personal preferences. The selection of materials covered necessarily reflects the author's selective judgment and should not be regarded as comprehensive. Guiding principles have been: What would I have benefited from most, when beginning a career as a pharmaceutical information specialist? And what types of questions do I encounter most often today, in working with drug and device industry personnel?

The answers to these questions have led to some major changes in the second edition of this book, compared to the first. Far more space is dedicated to providing background on regulatory issues and resources and to discussion of ways in which people use pharmaceutical information once it is obtained. The drug development and regulatory review process and its critical relationship to, and influence on, information availability and accessibility is a topic often neglected in introductions to the literature. The result is an understandable lack of confidence, and some gaps in competence, on the part of professionals who need to deal with the drug bibliography every day. Knowing what's likely to be available, when, where, and under what name is so closely linked with stages in drug development and government oversight that coverage of these issues has been greatly expanded in this edition, including an entire chapter dedicated to pertinent online sources and more material related to medical devices.

Extending the *Guide*'s discussion to highlighting possible applications arises from a growing perception that information mediators often don't know what to ask before beginning research in response to many questions they receive, because they lack this conceptual context. As a result, their efforts are sometimes wasted or severely undervalued, because they deliver data in a quantity or format inappropriate for the ultimate use intended. Gaining more perspective on the rationale behind some typical requests may promote better dialogue and pre-search preparation necessary to transform undifferentiated data into true solutions to problems clientele are confronting. Exploring the context is also important to information professionals who extend their duties to proactive promotion of their services, rather than confining themselves to a reactive role. The "rightsizing" reality of corporate life in the 1990s has prompted more of us to ask: Here's all this information—how can we, or should we, use it? Why isn't department X asking more questions? What kind of current awareness activities and tools will help us remain competitive, so that we'll all have a job five or ten years hence?

This edition of the *Guide* also features a new chapter (Chapter Eleven) on industrial pharmacy, offering an overview of compendial standards, biopharmaceutics guides, and resources to support formulation development and investigations related to pharmaceutical technology topics. Although Chapter Eleven's bibliography provides no more than a basic introduction, it can, hopefully, be used by nontechnical staff who need to know more about research requirements in this area. Also new in this edition is a chapter (Chapter Fifteen) devoted to market research and competitive intelligence sources online, augmenting Chapter Thirteen's examination of hardcopy business directories and statistical data sources. Here, too, more attention is devoted to providing a foundation on which non-information-specialist staff can build awareness of available resources and their applications. Sample records, tables, and other illustrative material interpolated throughout the book underscore its "applications" orientation.

More detailed annotations of individual resources, as well as evaluative commentary, have been included for information specialist readers with responsibilities for collection development and bibliographic instruction. A total of 467 publications are singled out for close examination. Feedback from users of the first edition and participants in the continuing education course based on this book indicated that "one collection" recommendations, in particular, would be useful. Again, it should be emphasized that "beauty is in the eye of the beholder" when applied to the bibliography, as much as to other matters of opinion. Evaluations of the relative utility of sources present some opportunities for disagreement and even controversy. Recognizing this, let me apologize in advance for any assessments that may offend; errors in judgment should be attributed to the author and not to the publishers.

A new appendix (Appendix B) offers database selection aids and additional database annotations. Core collection recommendations, introduced separately in chapters dedicated to resources designed to answer typical subject categories of questions, are assembled in one unified list in Appendix A. As in the previous edition, a glossary defines specialized pharmaceutical and information science terminology. Another portion replicated (and revised) is the Practicum. Developed to encourage self-evaluation and review, Practicum exercises illustrate typical quick-reference queries and suggested solutions, with an emphasis on systematic problem-solving.

The writing style exemplified in Practicum discussion has, in this second edition of the *Guide,* been extended to other portions of the text. It is intentionally more personal and colloquial. Conventional usage (regrettably) separates scholarship from everyday expression. The more generally accepted formality that characterizes much of the literature *about* literature often fails to convey the genuine excitement that learning to use it well can bring. Knowledge is, indeed, power, if the practical utility of assembled data is readily apparent. An unrelenting succession of dispassionate descriptions of sources cannot relay this fact with conviction. Seemingly dry-as-dust details about indexing and scope add up to answers only through skillful selection and application, a process that requires imagination, creativity, and no small measure of enthusiasm. These intangible ingredients are more easily demonstrated when drug information skills are learned working side-by-side with experienced peers. Translating that mentoring experience into the printed word sometimes calls for an equally personal approach. The style of direct address is also intended to decrease the distance between mastery of the bibliography and the ability to impart its benefits. Information professionals, to be effective, must be able to recognize and communicate the real-life rewards of their wares in language that clients can understand.

Acknowledgments

This book began as a syllabus for use in presenting a one-day continuing education course sponsored by the Medical Library Association. Since 1979, students in this course have contributed many ideas that have affected its rebirth as a monograph. Course participants in the United States, Canada, Japan, Australia, and New Zealand are due special thanks for their contributions. Thanks are also due to colleagues in the pharmaceutical industry who have included me in discussions of their day-to-day challenges and creative solutions during the past fifteen years. Insight gained from their experience and questions inspired many installments in the "Caduceus" series of columns for *Online* and *Database,* which, in turn, fostered additions to the searcher's portion of the *Guide.* I also wish to express my gratitude to the library staff of the Philadelphia College of Pharmacy and Science for welcoming me as a frequent visitor and permitting access to an outstanding reference collection.

Figures

2.1 The Drug Development Process and Scientific Communication/
    Publication   8
2.2 The Structural Formula for *ifetroban sodium*   15
4.1 Milestones in U.S. Drug and Device Law   40
4.2 FDA Drug Classification for INDs and NDAs   60
4.3 Regulatory Hot Topics and Frequently Asked Questions   74
4.4 Procedure for Promulgating Federal Regulations   75
4.5 Outline of the Medical Device Approval Process in the United
    States   90
4.6 Legal and Regulatory Specialty Sites on the Internet   99
5.1 Types of Drug Information Questions   108
5.2 Structure of the Scientific Literature   109
5.3 Checklist for Evaluating Drug Compendia and Basic Reference
    Sources   111
5.4 Best Bets among Internet Pathfinders   131
5.5 Free Glossaries on the Internet   134
6.1 Free Sources of Compounding Information on the Internet   165
6.2 Best Bets among Free Drug Ready-Reference Sources on the
    Internet—For Healthcare Professionals   180
7.1 Two Specialized Adverse Effects Publications on the Internet   198
8.1 FDA Pregnancy Categories Used in Package Inserts for Rx
    Drugs   220
8.2 Free Sources of Botanical Toxicity Information on the Internet   231
10.1 Two Non-English Sources of European Drug Information on the
    Internet   287
10.2 Subject Specialty Multilingual Guides on the Internet   288
12.1 Free Internet Sources of Veterinary Drug and Therapeutics
    Information   352
12.2 History of Pharmacy on the Internet   355
13.1 Resources to Determine U.S. Product Availability   362

13.2   A Selection of Specialized Company Directions on the Internet   368
13.3   URLs for a Selection of Drug Sales and Utilization Sources   376
13.4   Internet Directories of Pharmacy Schools and Continuing
       Education Sites   382
14.1   A Selection of MEDLINE Subheadings for the Pharmaceutical
       Searcher   391
14.2   EMBASE Link Terms   394
14.3   International Pharmaceutical Abstracts Section Headings and
       Scope Notes   400
14.4   MEDLINE Descriptors for Routes of Drug Administration   416
14.5   Sample IPA Record Showing Indexing/Abstract of a Brand Name
       Comparison   418
14.6   Sample MEDLINE Reference on DIALOG   419
14.7   Extracts from *Medical Subject Headings—Annotated Alphabetic
       List*   421
14.8   Extracts from *Medical Subject Headings—Tree Structures*   422
14.9   Extract from EMBASE Classification Scheme (EMTREE)   422
14.10 Extract from AHFS Pharmacological-Therapeutic Classification
       Scheme   423
14.11 Selected Publication/Document Types Identified in MEDLINE
       Indexing   426
14.12 TOXLINE Subfiles   429
15.1   Sample Pharmaprojects Record Online   449
15.2   Sample Record from IMSworld R&D Focus Drug Updates   456
15.3   Sample Online Record from ADIS R&D Insight   459
15.4   Sample Record from NME Express   462
15.5   Sample Record from Drug Data Report Online   464
15.6   Sample Record from Drugs of the Future Online   467
15.7   Sample Online Record from NDA Pipeline   471
15.8   Pharmaceutical and Health Technology Industry News Sources
       Online   482
15.9   A Selection of Market Research Report Databases Online   502
15.10 Subject Hubs to Locate Healthcare Statistics on the Internet   506
16.1   Sample Drug Approval Notice in F-D-C Reports Online   512
16.2   Sample ANDA Approvals in F-D-C Reports Online   513
16.3   Monthly Drug Approval Notices in Diogenes   514
16.4   Sample Entries from FDA's Quarterly New Drug List in
       Diogenes   515
16.5   Differences in Sources of U.S. Drug Approval Information
       Online in Diogenes   516
16.6   PMA Database Search Form on the FDA Web Site   517
16.7   Sample PMA Approval Notice from F-D-C Reports Online   518
16.8   Sample PMA Approval Notice from the Federal Register   519

16.9   Sample Diogenes Record from the FDA Quarterly PMA Listing   521
16.10 510K Database Search Form on the FDA Web Site   522
16.11 Sample 510K Record from Diogenes   522
16.12 Sample Records for Basis-of-Approval Documents (SBA, SSE)
         in Diogenes   524
16.13 Sample Product Recall Notice in Diogenes   526
16.14 Sample Action Item Record from Health Devices Alerts   528
16.15 Sample MDR Record from Diogenes   529
16.16 Sample Establishment Inspection Report and Form 483 Record
         in Diogenes   530
16.17 Warning Letter Search Form on the FDA Web Site   532
16.18 Useful FDA CDER Home Page Drug Info Options   537
16.19 Sample Record from IMSworld Patents International   551
16.20 Patent Extension Application Notice in the Federal Register
         Online   554
16.21 Indexing of Patent Extension Requests in F-D-C Reports Online 556
16.22 Sample Record for a Patent Extension in CLAIMS/RRX   556
16.23 Sample Record from Investigational Drug Patents Fast-Alert   561

1

Prescription for Using This Guide

This book is as much about the art and science of pharmaceutical information provision and applications as it is about sources available to help answer questions about drugs and medical devices. Although yet another annotated bibliography would, no doubt, assist truly dedicated readers determined to build or enhance a core collection of reference books, their efforts would not necessarily lead to quicker or more trustworthy answers. The *Guide*, by including background on specialized terminology, legal issues, and literature search protocols, makes the assumption that more effective use of drug information sources is the primary goal of the user group for which it was written.

Indications for Use

- You have a sound background in medical bibliography, but feel less confident about your knowledge of drug literature. You're already working with what you hope is a good, basic collection, but have wondered, when you have difficulty finding answers, if it's the collection—or you.
- Your usual method of finding out more about a drug or therapy of a particular disease is to do a *MEDLINE* search and check a few well-known reference books, such as the *PDR*. Yet, you suspect that there is important information you may be missing. What are the best choices to match the needs of your practice setting? How do they compare with what you're accustomed to using?
- In working with colleagues and customers in the pharmaceutical industry, you've realized that it would be beneficial to gain a better understanding of how different types of information can be used to increase productivity and profitability. For example, what sources should typically be monitored for current awareness? What data are needed by various departments, and why? What

is the significance of material requested and the meaning of terms frequently used? What are hot topics to anticipate, and why?

- Your academic course work on drug information and medical literature prepared you to evaluate clinical studies. But in day-to-day practice, you're finding it difficult to locate such studies. How can you retrieve an adequate representation of available information on which to base your critical assessment and solve therapeutic problems posed?

- You've just started a job where there's an outstanding, but bewilderingly large, collection of specialized pharmaceutical books, CD-ROMs, and online databases from which to choose whenever a question arises. You know that everything you need is there, because more experienced colleagues find their answers with ease. But you could use some guidance to ensure that you're making the most efficient use of your company's time and resources when conducting literature research.

An underlying factor in all of these descriptions is *problem solving.* Assembling (and learning) lists of sources that contain information on topics most likely to be the subject of drug queries is not enough. Effective drug information provision involves not only selecting the tools, but also determining the most efficient method and sequence for their use to get the job done. Accordingly, much of this *Guide* is devoted to identifying characteristics of individual resources that affect their applicability and potential utility in problem-solving. Practicum exercises and suggested answers emphasize systematic techniques to transform isolated data supplied in source annotations into integrated information solutions.

Recommended Regimen

There are at least four different ways to approach the subject matter in this book. One is to read each chapter in the sequence in which it is printed. Material is organized so that each section builds on background provided in previous discussion. The first five chapters, in particular, form a logical unit that can be regarded as preparatory material, defining terminology, outlining important regulatory issues, and generally paving the way to informed use of the bibliography. Introductory essays and transitional text in each subject-oriented section of subsequent chapters will also assist readers who may not need to delve deeply into the literature themselves, but who want to find out what information is available, how it can be applied in their work, and where its acquisition could offer competitive advantages.

Since this is not a "novel" and can hardly be regarded as recreational reading, many users will, no doubt, quickly survey the table of contents, then skip ahead to selected chapters of interest. If the objective is to learn more about how to answer certain types of drug information requests, turning directly to the pertinent portion of this *Guide* will be one way to start. Sources cited in Chapters Six through Thirteen are organized into broad subject categories of questions they are likely to answer. However, an *in medias res* approach to this volume calls for two caveats. One is that, although the drug reference literature lends itself to the applications-oriented arrangement employed in this book, sometimes individual publications defy strict compartmentalization. When a source could be helpful in answering many different types of inquiries, it is difficult to decide where it belongs. The solution used here is a compromise employed every day in organizing library collections: assign the source to one shelf location where it would logically belong and use cross references in the catalog to show its relationship to other areas of the bibliography. Accordingly, readers consulting one section of this *Guide* will, inevitably, be referred to titles in other sections. The format employed in cross references is to cite a title, often in shortened form, followed by a two-part number in parentheses: e.g., *Remington's* (6.52). The first part of the number designates the chapter where the source is discussed in more detail, and the second is the precise sequential locator within the chapter. Such references are intended to save readers a trip to the index in order to track down related sources.

The second caveat for the user intent on a highly focused foray into these pages is that discussion in a given section may assume familiarity with topics covered elsewhere. For example, an abbreviation may be used or a term cited (OBRA, schedule V, category 3) that is meaningless to you. A book on any specialized subject, when dipped into out of context, presents the same pitfalls. The best way to overcome the difficulty, should it occur, is to turn to the index for help. Cross references there will direct you to previous sections in the text where terms are introduced and their significance is explained. Consulting the back-of-the-book glossary is another option, but the definitions it contains often cannot supply solutions to terminology barriers that require background discussion for their conceptual relationships to be understood. In other words, the intended "quick dip" into an area of drug information featured in one section may, after all, require immersion in other material beyond that originally planned.

Ideally, when discussion focuses on reference tools to which you already have access in your library's collection, you will consult them in conjunction with the *Guide*'s annotations. There is no substitute for hands-on experience in using the literature. At the same time, without a healthy sample of ten to twenty real-life questions to work on when handling a book for the first time, it's easy to overlook its key characteristics. This is one reason why discussion of major resources is so detailed, to encourage critical assessment and comparison with counterparts. Completing the checklist for evaluation in Chapter Five (Figure 5.3) when reviewing a succession of complementary resources will make hands-on examination more meaningful, in the absence of a set of sample questions to answer.

Experienced information professionals may be tempted to skip descriptions of resources already employed. Yet, if less familiar reference tools are to be true enhancements to your problem-solving repertoire, you may find it helpful to turn back to the sources you've been using, in order to verify how each newly introduced book differs from those commonly consulted. Point-by-point comparisons often disclose characteristics in publications used every day that have not been fully exploited. Contrasts can uncover special features that, until viewed in the context of an expanded literature landscape, have gone unnoticed. The end result of detailed comparisons may be more efficient use of the collection you have, rather than acquisition of additional material.

A third anticipated use for this book is, in fact, library collection development. Readers with this responsibility will find that annotations attempt to address this need. The emphasis is on identifying access points and reviewing organization of material, because it is these factors that dispassionately delineate the relative value of reference resources with similar content and subject scope. The *Guide*'s evaluative commentary and recommendations for a "core" drug information collection (summarized in Appendix A) are, necessarily, subjective and must always be weighed against the specific needs and expectations of your own user community.

Finally, a fourth way to use this book is through the index. When you need to know where to find a list of grandfather drugs, controlled substances, state immunization requirements, or alcohol-free antidiarrheals, or when you want information on the bioequivalency ratings of specific products, their off-label indications, or even how to pronounce their names, index entries will help locate pertinent sources. Detailed keyword subject analysis of material embedded in annotations is designed to assist quick reference look-ups of this type. This *Guide* will not be the final source consulted for an answer, but it can serve as an aid to memory and as a temporary stand-in for an information professional, to help you navigate a direct course through unknown territory to facts needed.

Special Instructions for Online, CD-ROM, and Internet Users

"Integrated information solutions" is more than a slogan, it is rapidly becoming a reality in most healthcare settings. Answering drug information questions frequently involves use of both hardcopy (printed) publications and computerized databases. Yet, by segregating discussion of online resources into the final three chapters, the *Guide*'s organization may make their potential utility less evident than it should be. The problem is, again, one of subject classification. Many databases, like *MEDLINE*, are ecumenical in scope and could, conceivably, have been cited *ad nauseum* as additional sources of information throughout the book. More specialized electronic resources, had they been annotated side-by-side with related reference books, could well have become lost in the shuffle, their value obscured in the information overload first readings of the text are likely to induce.

The decision to isolate database annotations into separate chapters is, admittedly, another compromise. What it requires is for users to be forewarned that cross references to further resources available in machine-readable format (online or CD-ROM) are not incorporated into all sections where they are, in fact, relevant. In short, it would be a good idea to survey the contents of Chapters Fourteen through Sixteen as follow-up to consulting any other section of the *Guide*. Additional aids to database selection are included in Appendix B.

If you are expecting tips on navigating the 'Net to find pharmaceutical information, you may be disappointed. Although all online databases discussed in this volume are available on the Internet, the "information superhighway" is mentioned in this context simply as one of several telecommunication routes. Despite its exponential growth during the period when this book was being written, the Internet is still a supplement to (rather than substitute for) the core collection that is the focus of these pages. Data from a study described in Chapter Five (see 5.7) support this assessment. Out of 2,478 questions received at a large drug information center over a three-month period, only 10% clearly called for Internet usage. These findings paint an accurate picture of the relative value of the Web in reference service to professionals. Accordingly, notes about complementary Net resources have been incorporated into subject-oriented discussion throughout the *Guide*, but these citations have not been assigned separate reference numbers.

This policy is, in part, due to expendiency. From the time the manuscript was first submitted for peer review until completion of the final draft, many new Internet sources came online. Altogether this book has been in press for more than two years, so the large number of Web sites added during that time could not, from a practical point of view, be allowed to affect the already frequently revised numbering of other resources. Thus, a check of the index under "Internet" will show that coverage has been confined to a selection of World Wide Web sites. Many, many more were examined than those singled out for special mention. Criteria applied for inclusion here were: 1) subject specialty orientation, 2) breadth and depth of scope, 3) ease of accessibility (no or low fees, no restrictions to educational users or licensed practitioners only, reasonably user-friendly design), and 4) overall utility in problem-solving—as seen through the eyes of an (admittedly critical) information professional.

At the same time, it must be acknowledged that the Internet environment in the mid-1990s is sufficiently volatile to render any hardcopy guide to its sources immediately obsolete. Therefore, descriptions of home pages come with the caveat that their content and quality is especially mutable, meriting re-evaluation with each use. The *FDA Home Page*, for example, changed its options for finding product approval information four times during the fourteen-day period initially allocated to its appraisal (included in Chapter Sixteen). Lack of continuity and stability of Internet sources means that annotations and assessments included here have expiration dates implied, but unlike medication labeling, unexpressed.

Precautions

One-stop shopping is rare in information work. No single resource, no matter how encyclopedic in scope, can provide a complete answer. Information in one publication should generally be cross-checked and verified through consultation of other sources to ensure its accuracy, especially when patient care decisions depend upon the answer. Accuracy (and, incidentally, potential liability) is not the sole impetus for multi-source selection. Sometimes, data provided in the original request may be insufficient to approach publications likely to contain the answer. In such cases, it will be necessary to "flesh out" the "bare bones" of the query with information found in one set of sources before proceeding to those where the answer is located.

For example, you've been asked about possible interactions of *Os-Cal 500* with oral ciprofloxacin. The name *Os-Cal 500* is not indexed in any of the standard reference books that you check first. What next? "Translate" terminology used in this request to the language preferred in interactions publications with the answer. In other words, find out other names under which relevant literature might appear by consulting drug nomenclature sources, then return to interaction indexes armed with alternative names for look-up (e.g., calcium carbonate, antacids).

This example illustrates not only the commonly-encountered need to consult more than one source in order to find an answer, but also two fundamental areas of knowledge that information providers must master to be successful: (1) distinguishing among types of drug names used in requests and (2) matching them with individual resource capabilities. A book can be an astounding compendium of factual information but, nonetheless, remain on the shelf unused, unless its organization and indexing are known to be a good "fit" with questions posed. Since the starting point in most questions is product or substance name(s), gaining familiarity with types of drug name indexing offered in each resource available to you will be a key factor in selection and search sequencing to avoid backtracking. Therefore, the *Guide* begins with a review of nomenclature options likely to be encountered, and explores their relationship to scientific communication and publication. Names can be powerful predictors of how much you can expect to find, where you should look, and what else you may need to know before starting research.

2

Drug Nomenclature and Its Relationship to Scientific Communication

Figure 2.1 outlines basic steps in the drug development process and relates stages of development with publication sources and types of drug nomenclature. At the beginning of their life cycle, drugs are usually cited by codes, both for simplicity's sake and for security purposes. Chemical names can be long and cumbersome to use in speech or writing and have the added disadvantage, from the developing company's viewpoint, of revealing too much about a proprietary discovery's composition. Compounds that show enough therapeutic potential after initial screening to warrant animal testing are likely to be the subject of conference papers. If test results indicate that benefits outweigh risks, research will continue and communication of results become more widespread, being newsworthy in the scientific community and meriting journal publication.

The further along the research and development (R&D) pipeline that a drug progresses, the more scientists are engaged in testing and talking or writing about it. Code designations are awkward in speech and prone to errors in printed transcription, making it imperative at this point to coin a simplified, descriptive name for the drug to facilitate communication. A simplified name reinforces accuracy in references to the compound and encourages early name recognition, should the product eventually be introduced into the marketplace. The pioneer company or other organization responsible for the drug's discovery and further development will generally propose a nonproprietary name to a centralized agency responsible for promulgating nomenclature standards. Such agencies play an important role in scientific communication. They screen names to ensure uniformity in nomenclature practices and, ideally, eliminate or reduce confusion with other substances by avoiding similarities with proprietary names.

Brand name designation, often accomplished by trademark registration, usually comes fairly late in a product's development cycle. Once a drug is launched, it may acquire many different trade names to identify various dosage forms and strengths, and, after its patent protection expires, to distinguish it from competing companies' proprietary preparations.

Figure 2.1   The Drug Development Process and Scientific Communication/Publication

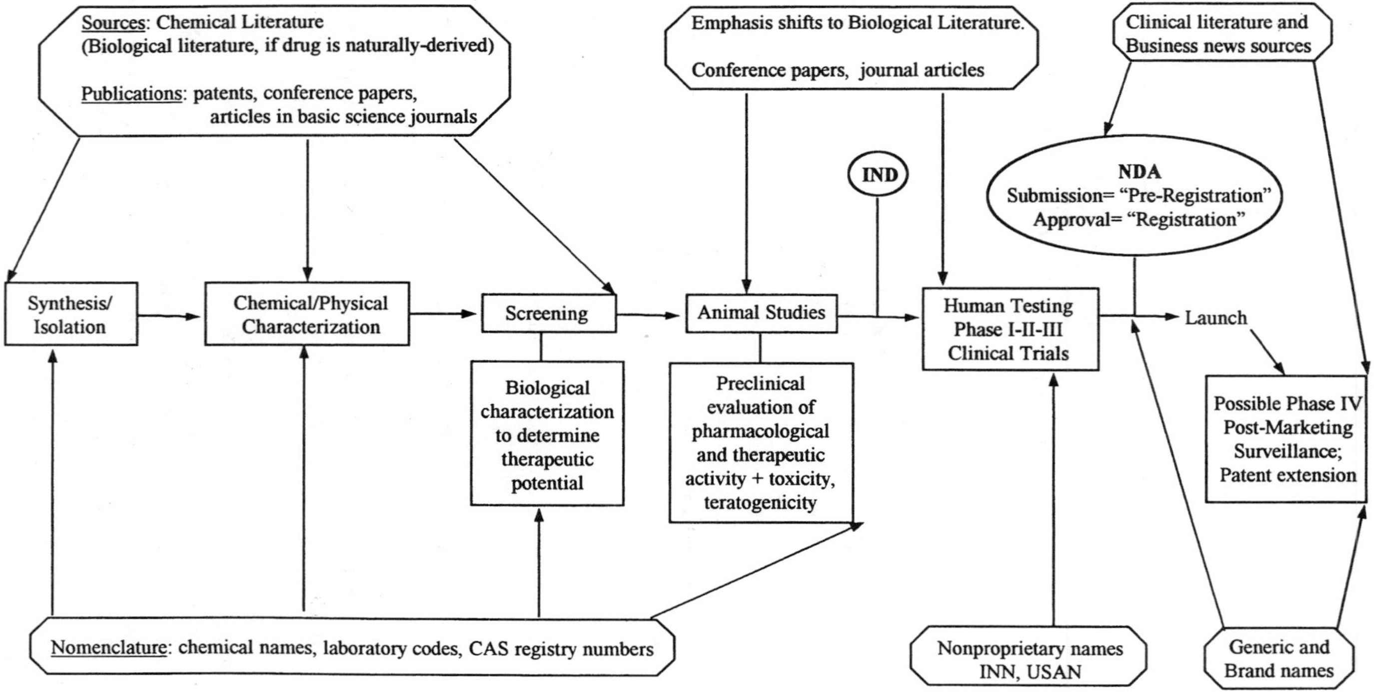

The evolution of a pharmaceutical compound from laboratory to launch covers an eight- to fifteen-year time period, during which a single substance may be referred to in the literature under at least seven different names. The implications for the information provider are obvious:

- Since there is no single, universal name for a chemical, different sources will use different types of names in indexing.
- To find information on a specific compound at various stages in its development cycle, it may be necessary to look under different names.

Types of Drug Names

Because understanding the diversity of nomenclature used in reference sources is essential for effective drug information retrieval, the following discussion provides examples of each type of drug name and offers guidelines in answering questions that cite them.

Chemical Name

Since all drugs consist of one or more chemical substances, a therapeutic agent will have at least one chemical name, once its identity is known. Such a name attempts to describe the quantitative elementary composition of a compound and its unique structural features. It is important to recognize that there are many ways of transcribing chemical names. Most standard reference tools that originate in the United States have adopted American Chemical Society (ACS) conventions for naming compounds. These conventions implement guidelines devised by the International Union of Pure and Applied Chemistry (IUPAC). However, even ACS-approved nomenclature may change. For example, the preferred name for *bretylium tosylate* in the eighth collective index period (8CI, 1972–1976) of *Chemical Abstracts* was *Ammonium, (o-bromobenzyl) ethyl dimethyl-, P-toluene-sulfonate*. In the ninth collective index (9CI, 1977–1981), the same compound was listed under *Benzenemethanaminium, 2-bromo-n-ethyl-n, n-dimethyl-, salt with 4-methylbenzen sulfonic acid*. Still another chemical name under which this drug has appeared in the literature is *bretylium P-toluenesulfonate*.

When a drug information question begins with a chemical name, it's a good idea to find alternative names before proceeding to literature indexes or reference books. Anticipate segmentation and permutation (rotation) of names in different ways, leading to alphabetization in widely separate places in hardcopy and online index displays. The examples cited illustrate the ACS convention of inverting chemical names, listing the "heading parent" compound first. Beware: relatively few reference sources prefer chemical names in indexing or systematically provide access using alternative entry formats.

Chemical Abstracts Service Registry Number (CAS® RN)

Since 1965, Chemical Abstracts Service (CAS) has been assigning numeric codes to chemicals described in the literature, in an attempt to transcend problems arising from inconsistencies in converting structures into unique descriptive names. Today, more than 16,000,000 chemicals have been assigned a registry number (RN). Recently, CAS also began registering chemicals cited from 1920–1964. However, most older compounds have already been assigned RNs, because they have been mentioned in the literature published since January 1965.

It should be noted that registry numbers are not derived from a classification scheme, do not bring together groups of similar chemicals in indexing, and do not imply a hierarchical relationship among substances with similar codes. The intent behind the registry system is simply to provide one unique code for each compound. However, because authors may describe the same substance in different ways, the same drug may, inadvertently, be assigned more than one registry number during its history. For example, the current RN for *prednisolone* is 50–24–8, replacing CAS registry numbers 8056–11–9 and 58201–11–9. When it became apparent that two separate articles with different compound descriptions (and thus different RN assignments) actually referred to the same substance, the new registry number was assigned to replace the others. This problem is not at all uncommon. Unfortunately, it is not feasible to re-index older bibliographic references to a substance cited under now superseded RNs. Hence, retrospective searches for journal literature require use of replaced, as well as current, codes, and consultation of nomenclature sources that contain all codes. This technique will be particularly important when preparing for online searching.

Relatively few hardcopy resources systematically index by RNs, but many include these numbers in their product descriptions as an additional aid to identification. Searchers should augment RNs with alternative nomenclature (laboratory codes, etc.) before beginning research.

Laboratory Code or Research Number

Originating companies or organizations typically assign codes to new products under investigation. These codes provide a convenient way of referring to substances without resorting to use of lengthy chemical names. Also, in contrast to chemical names, laboratory (lab) codes offer some security for a new drug discovery, revealing nothing about its composition. A research code is usually alphanumeric: the alphabetical portion designating the company (often mnemonic, such as SK for SmithKline), and the numeric portion serving as an internal control number, one digit perhaps identifying pharmacological activity or potential therapeutic class, and other digits delineating chronological placement in the company's research efforts in the class of compounds For example, *4–390* might designate the 390th drug discovered in class 4, beta blockers. More than one lab code may be assigned to the same substance. For example, *nifuraldezone* was referred to in early studies as *NSC-3184* (the National Service Center of the U.S. National Cancer Institute's research number), as well as the manufacturer's code number *NF-84* (Norwich Eaton). Another type of code encountered in the drug literature is a simple abbreviation based on chemical constituents or a common name, such as *CCNU* for *3 cyclohexyl chloroethylnitrosourea*, *AZT* for *azothymidine*, *TPA* for *tissue plasminogen activator*.

Of the three types of names used to refer to drugs early in their development cycle (chemical names, RNs, or research numbers), lab codes are the most consistently used in indexing. When a question begins with this type of name, bear in mind that it may appear in variant formats which will affect its alphabetic placement in indexing: e.g., SK 4–390 or SK 4390 or SK4390. Such variations will also affect online searching format.

Nonproprietary or Generic Name

Further along in its development cycle, when a drug is more frequently cited in the journal literature, a chemical substance will be identified with a simple name that may describe its pharmacological activity. This nonproprietary name is commonly referred to as a "generic" name, although the two terms are not, by definition, strictly synonymous. Doherty[1] explains the distinction well: "The generic name refers to a class (or genera) of drugs, e.g., the generic name Vitamin D includes several compounds whose nonproprietary names are: cholecalciferol, dihydrotachysterol, and ergocalciferol." A nonproprietary name, on the other hand, refers to a specific compound, rather than to a class of drugs. Nonetheless, the fact that many nonproprietary names contain syllables or word stems which are common to a group of drugs related in their mode of action (e.g., *-caine* for local anesthetics, *-pirdine* for cognition enhancers, *som-* for growth hormone derivatives) has, perhaps, led to nonproprietary names being referred to as "generic" names.

Determining the nonproprietary name for a drug is an important preliminary step in drug information provision, since nonproprietary names are preferred over all other types of nomenclature in the indexing of most reference sources. In the United States, an official nonproprietary name is assigned by the U.S. Adopted Names Council, a quasi-official agency sponsored by the American Medical Association, the American Pharmaceutical Association, and the U.S. Pharmacopeial Convention. When a company or other organization has developed a substance with therapeutic potential which may lead to its being approved for marketing in this country, a proposal for a U.S. Adopted Name (USAN) is submitted to, or invited by, the Council. This process "should be initiated preferably during the period of investigation when the substance is under clinical study in human and animal subjects, so that the adoption of the USAN will be complete by the time the relevant New Drug Application is filed."[2] The procedures for selecting a USAN, in addition to the philosophy and guiding principles underlying official name designation, are outlined in detail in the annually published, cumulative list of names (*USP Dictionary*, 3.1) discussed in the next chapter. The U.S. Food and Drug Administration (FDA) recognizes USANs as official designations and requires their use in regulatory documents, such as drug labeling.

Yet, the researcher should be aware that a drug may be indexed under more than one nonproprietary or generic name. Great Britain, France, Italy, Japan, and the Nordic countries also have official nomenclature agencies that may assign a different name to the same substance. Thus, the information seeker should look for sources which index not only USAN, but also possible variants, such as the BAN (British Approved Name), DCF (Dénomination Commune Française), JAN (Japanese Accepted Name), NFN (Nordiska Farmakopenamden), or the INN (International Nonproprietary Name) promulgated by the World Health Organization. For example, *acetaminophen* is a USAN, but the BAN and INN for the same substance is *paracetamol*. Use of both nonproprietary names when consulting reference tools would be wise.

Brand, Proprietary, Trade, or Trivial Name

Brand or proprietary drug names are selected and often registered as exclusive trademarks by the manufacturer to identify a specific product formulation and indication. Although in common parlance "trade name" and "brand name" are both used as synonyms for "proprietary," a "trade name" as defined in U.S. law is a company name (e.g., Bristol-Myers Squibb). Under this legal definition, trade names cannot become federally registered trademarks. However, when drug information sources (including this one) refer to "trade name indexing," they use the term as it is generally understood, i.e., providing access to brand names used in trade. Scope notes in some sources also use the term "trivial names" for drug nomenclature other than officially recognized nonproprietary names. This is a somewhat pejorative way of referring to brand names, laboratory codes, and other common usage.

Many products will have multiple trade names and may be marketed under different brand designations in different countries, even when manufactured by the same company. For example, Depakene is a U.S. trade name for *sodium valproate*. Brand names used in other countries for this product include *Depakine*, *Epilim*, *Ergenyl*, and *Labazene*. Comprehensive or systematic international brand name indexing is rare in most information sources.

When a question begins with a proprietary name, it's important to determine if the brand is relevant, or if the name has merely been used for convenience. For example, you might be asked to find references to the use of *Foscavir* versus *Cytovene* in the treatment of cytomegalovirus retinitis. An acceptable response would include any data comparing *foscarnet sodium* and *ganciclovir* for this indication, as both brand names are merely being used as synonyms for their generic constituents. But a query about the immediate physiologic effects on the neonate of *Exosurf* and *Survanta* would require proprietary name access to the literature, to locate studies comparing these two brand name pulmonary surfactants, particularly if relative bioavailability were the issue.

Drug Classification

There are three ways commonly used to categorize drugs: 1) by action, 2) by use, or 3) by chemical derivation or affiliation. Pharmaceutical information sources generally prefer the first two types of terminology when classifying drugs for broad category access.

Pharmacological Action

Pharmacological terms describe the mechanism of action of a drug (how it works). For example, *dimercaprol* and *penicillamine* are classified together in many reference sources as "chelating agents," because they selectively form soluble chelates with metal ions, such as lead or mercury, and promote the excretion of these metals in the body. *Levodopa*, *apomorphine*, and *amantidine* may be classified together as "dopaminergic agents," which replenish central dopamine or which themselves can act as dopamine receptors (dopamine agonists), and thus may alleviate symptoms of Parkinsonism, hyperprolactinemia, and related disorders. Drugs with a single pharmacological action can have several therapeutic applications.

Therapeutic/Diagnostic Use

Therapeutic terminology describes the desired effect, or medical application ("indication"), of a drug. Examples include *anthelmintics, anorectics, muscle relaxants, antineoplastics, antimalarials*, etc. Drugs with different pharmacological actions may have the same therapeutic use. For example, *diuretics, enzyme inhibitors, monoamine oxidase inhibitors*, and *beta-adrenoceptor blocking agents* can all be used as antihypertensive agents. The therapeutic class "dermatological agents" could include the pharmacological categories *antimicrobials, corticosteroids*, and *immunosuppressants*.

Chemical Derivation or Affiliation

A third type of general terminology sometimes used to index drugs is chemical affiliation, which groups compounds by origin or derivation. For example, *cefotetan, cefmetazole*, and *cefixime* could be classified together under the term "cephalosporins." *Phenobarbital, secobarbital*, and *eterobarb* might be indexed under "barbiturate acid derivatives." Chemically affiliated compounds tend to exhibit similar pharmacological actions, but may have different therapeutic uses.

Effect of Drug Classification on Information Retrieval

Often a single reference book or index to the journal literature will employ both pharmacological and therapeutic vocabulary, grouping entries regarding individual drugs under broad "action" or "use" terms. In such a classified arrangement, information about a specific product could appear in multiple places and, unless fully duplicated under each heading, lead the researcher on a merry chase before divulging all relevant data needed. Ideally, a back-of-the-book index will be provided to locate separate entries.

Another challenge that users must frequently cope with is a mixture of pharmacological and therapeutic vocabulary without adequate cross referencing to related groups of drugs. Furthermore, relatively few hardcopy compendia cite and use a standardized vocabulary. There is no single reference standard for pharmacological/therapeutic terminology. However, it's a good sign if the introduction to a source cites one of the following as its source for drug classification, because this fact will at least indicate that quality control through consistency is a goal.

MeSH Tree Structures Category D. Vocabulary compiled to index citations added to the online database *MEDLINE* (14.1) includes many terms to characterize pharmacological action and therapeutic use(s) of drugs. These terms are classified together in the "D" category of the hierarchical *Tree Structures* volume of *Medical Subject Headings* (*MeSH*, 14.3). Keywords or phrases derived from *MeSH* offer an extensive list of options to encompass most drugs, if adopted by a hardcopy indexing source (very few have done so).

AHFS Classification. Pharmacy reference sources often prefer section headings originally introduced in the *American Hospital Formulary Service* (*AHFS*, 6.4) as drug category terms. This vocabulary sometimes differs from *MeSH* (e.g., "trichomonicides" versus "antitrichomonal agents," "antidiabetic agents" versus "hypoglycemic agents"). Two online databases that prefer *AHFS* over *MeSH* are *International Pharmaceutical Abstracts* (14.8) and *Drug Information Fulltext* (14.18).

USP Categories. *United States Pharmacopeia* (11.8) terminology provides the basis for *BIOSIS Previews®* "drug affiliation" descriptors (14.6) and for *NDA Pipeline* (4.20, 15.8) and *Merck Index* (3.5) therapeutic category keywords.

EPhMRA Classification. *Pharmaprojects* (15.1) and IMS publications (e.g., 15.2, 15.18) both use an anatomical/therapeutic classification scheme developed by the European Pharmaceutical Market Research Association (EPhMRA), but each information provider has introduced modifications to the scheme.

Less Frequently Used Identifiers

Several other types of drug names will be found in the drug literature. None are prevalent enough in indexing or sufficiently unambiguous to serve as reliable starting points in requests for further information. When a question begins with any one of the following, the first step should be to find other, more consistently used, names for the same substance before proceeding to standard reference tools for an answer.

Molecular or Empirical Formula

Although a molecular or empirical formula is not a unique identifier, it does describe the components of a compound by atom count. For example, $C_{16}H_{21}NO_2$ is the molecular formula for both *propranolol* and *DL-propranolol* (racemic propranolol). Many publications index formulas or include them in product descriptions, so that having a formula for a substance on hand prior to initiating a literature search can be useful. But, because of a formula's possible ambiguity, other names are preferred starting points.

Chemical Structure, Structural Formula

An attempt to represent in two-dimensional print a structure that exists in three dimensions in nature, structural formulas are static pictures or diagrams of a compound which is in constant motion, rotating around axes, surrounded by an electron cloud (see Figure 2.2). Few hardcopy reference sources have attempted to index drugs by structural formula, but some product descriptions do include this type of "name" for more accurate identification. Some online search systems, most notably STN and ORBIT-QUESTEL, provide software capabilities for graphic structural retrieval.

Enzyme Commission Number

Assigned by the Enzyme Commission (EC) of the International Union of Pure and Applied Chemistry (IUPAC), EC numbers are derived from a decimal classification scheme, with the first digit representing one of six enzyme groups (oxidoreductases, transferases, hydrolases, lyases, isomerases, or ligases), and the re-

Figure 2.2   The Structural Formula for *ifetroban sodium*

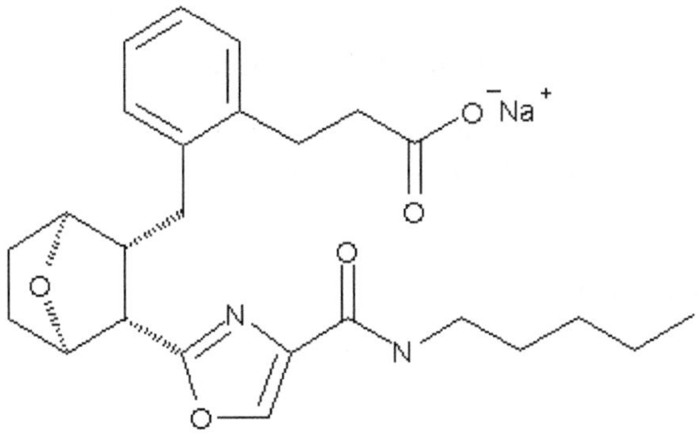

maining three levels of the number expressing refinements in the classification of these compounds. When used in the literature, the EC number functions as a substitute or synonym for an enzyme name, which is typically long and cumbersome to use in writing. Such numbers also help clarify author discussion where enzymes may be cited by a variety of ambiguous abbreviations (HGPRT, APRT, etc.)

Although more than 2,000 enzymes have been officially classified by IUPAC, the pharmaceutical researcher will also need other enzyme names to retrieve pertinent information, because very few published sources index compounds using these codes. For example, EC 1.1.1.4 is the Enzyme Commission Number for *d-butanediol dehydrogenase*, which may, however, be indexed instead under its current CAS RN 37250–09–2, its replaced RN 37250–12–7, or under common synonyms such as *butylene glycol dehydrogenase* or *diacetyl (acetoin) reductase*. *MEDLINE* (14.1) is the only online database that consistently adds EC numbers as access points to relevant literature. *BIOSIS Previews* (14.6) also indexes by EC codes, but includes them online only when they are cited by source authors.

National Drug Code

The National Drug Code (NDC) system was established by the FDA in 1969 to serve as a product identification scheme for drugs marketed in the United States. Ideally, each manufacturer, dosage form, strength, and package size is assigned a unique identification number under this system. Since 1976, the published codification (*NDC Directory*, 10.9) has largely been limited to human prescription and selected nonprescription drugs. Each company has a four-digit code, which sometimes appears on the dosage form itself (note that this may assist in physical identification queries—refer to Chapter Ten). The FDA requests, but does not require, that the entire ten-digit, three-part code appear on labels. This nomenclature system facilitates automated processing for inventory management and reimbursement. It is rarely used in indexing information sources.

An example of an NDC is 0004–0006–01 for *Valium*. The first four numbers, 0004, are the company code for Roche Laboratories; 0006 is the code for a specific strength, dosage form, and formulation, in this case representing *Valium* 10 mg. tablets; 01 stands for a 100-tablet package size.

Other Nomenclature Issues

Additional terms encountered in drug information queries originating from the patient population and popular media reveal other issues regarding nomenclature and resource coverage.

Synthetic versus Natural

The distinction between synthetic and "natural" drugs is one often mentioned by consumers, with the underlying implication that production by chemical synthesis in a laboratory is undesirable. The reality is that human metabolic processes cannot distinguish between molecules derived from synthetic versus natural sources; both are absorbed and used to the same extent. Most drugs marketed today are synthetic or semisynthetic, in order to meet quality control standards for strength and purity and to limit production costs. Isolating active constituents directly from biological sources, such as plants or animals, is expensive and often proves impractical on a large scale, due to depletion of natural resources. Practical considerations in preparing palatable dosage forms also influence product formulation. "Natural" vitamin preparations are frequently supplemented with synthetic forms. For example, rose hips cannot deliver desired labeled amounts of ascorbic acid without supplementation by synthetic vitamin C, or tablet size becomes unacceptably large.

Given the realities of modern pharmaceutical production, it's not surprising that most ready-reference drug compendia offer little information to help answer questions from consumers who request a natural, versus a synthetic, form of a drug. Preparations sold in health food stores are not well indexed, in part because they are marketed as dietary supplements rather than drugs, to avoid more stringent regulations imposed on products whose labels claim therapeutic efficacy in serious medical conditions. Homeopathic products, many of which are naturally derived, are somewhat more accessible through indexes that cover nonprescription preparations. Because many major drugstore chains now stock a selection of homeopathic remedies, publications that provide drug lists for retailers may prove helpful in identifying "natural" products (see *The Red Book*, 3.15).

Prescription versus Over-the-Counter

Printed reference tools often base coverage decisions on another consumer-oriented classification: Rx versus OTC. Relatively few information sources index over-the-counter (OTC) drugs, i.e., those that may be sold without a prescription. Instead, most publications concentrate on indexing prescription, Rx, or "legend" drugs. The terms are synonymous and refer to products which may be purchased only with a licensed practitioner's prescription. *Rx* is an abbreviation for *recipe*, the Latin word for "take them." The term "legend drugs" is derived from the fact that such products must bear a prescription "legend" on their labels: "Caution: federal law prohibits dispensing without prescription."

Surprisingly, this labeling requirement is not based solely upon the relative safety of a drug. The FDA's designation of prescription status is also influenced by whether adequate directions for safe and effective use can be written for the average layperson. If this is not found to be the case, prescription status is mandated, and directions intended for healthcare professionals only are prepared. Because this is also the audience targeted by most medical publishers, drug reference sources focus on practitioners' needs for information on prescription products.

"Ethical" as a Marketing Term

Other sources limit their coverage to "ethical" drugs. Ethical drugs can be either nonprescription or prescription, and are distinguished by the way they are marketed. Drugs marketed directly to physicians, hospitals, and other healthcare providers are designated "ethical," as opposed to those marketed through the mass media directly to the consumer. Although this distinction is disappearing, the term "ethical" is still found in introductions to some information sources when defining scope. It does not convey a moral connotation in the context of drug literature.

"Generic" as a Marketing Term

The consumer/patient's use of the term "generic drugs" should not be confused with its use to describe a type of drug name as previously defined in this chapter. All drugs are "generic" in this sense, but the consumer's and popular media's use of the term usually refers to a drug marketed in a particular manner. Pharmaceutical preparations whose patent or market exclusivity has expired may be manufactured by any company with FDA approval to do so. Many companies will sell these products labeled only with the generic or nonproprietary name and no brand name. These so-called "generic drugs" are often less expensive than brand name preparations, because less money has been spent on research and development or on promotion to the ethical market.

There has been some controversy over the substitution of generic drugs for brand name products. Generic substitution is controlled by law at the state level in the United States. Authorized substitution is usually limited to products listed in a state formulary or its designated equivalent. Further restrictions may apply under individual state laws as to who may authorize substitution of generic drugs (the physician, the pharmacist, or the patient). Another source of controversy lies in the concept of bioequivalency: do the generic and brand name drugs act in exactly the same manner in the body? Chemically equivalent generic entities are not necessarily also therapeutically equivalent. Factors in formulation and manufacture, such as fillers used, particle size, and tablet hardness or coating, can affect the bioavailability and efficacy of otherwise chemically equivalent products. The FDA classifies as "therapeutically equivalent" products that 1) display comparable bioavailability ($-20\% / +25\%$) and 2) are pharmaceutically equivalent, in that they contain the same amounts of the same active ingredients in the same dosage form, have the same route of administration, and they meet official compendial standards of strength, quality, purity, and identity. The agency does not recommend substitution between different dosage forms.

In other words, the controversy extends beyond the economic one the consumer may perceive. Information providers should be familiar with their state's substitution regulations and with the FDA's therapeutic equivalence evaluations published annually (see *Approved Drug Products*, 4.42).

Name Recognition and Effective Problem Solving

By this time, it should be apparent that there is no comprehensive index listing drugs by all the various forms of nomenclature discussed in this chapter. Names used in information requests may prove to be unreliable access points to reference sources that can provide the answer. Sources of alternative names will often need to be consulted before further research is attempted. The next chapter is devoted to this essential area of the bibliography.

Names can also provide critical clues to the stage of development of the product under investigation, which, in turn, can influence resource selection. Practicum 1 will serve as a learning check to test your drug name recognition skills and reinforce knowledge of their important relationship to the search process.

References

1. Doherty, P. Foreign drug information. *Drexel Libr Q* 1982 Spr;18(2):49.
2. *USP dictionary of USAN and international drug names 1995*. 32nd ed. Rockville, MD: The United States Pharmacopeial Convention, 1994:7.

Additional Sources of Information

Agency tightens up on booming homeopathic industry. *Wash Drug Letter* 1988 Jun 13;20(24):Diogenes accession no.206301.

Blake MI. Naming of drugs. *Pharm Tech* 1983 Jun;7:44,46,49–50.

Freimanis R, Schiffman DO. Drug nomenclature—United States Adopted Names. In: Gennaro AR, ed. *Remington's pharmaceutical sciences*. 19th ed. Easton, PA: Mack Publishing, 1995:413–424.

Halperin JA. Product selection, bioequivalence, and therapeutic equivalence: the generic drug market. *Drug Inf J* 1983;17:73–76.

Newgreen DB. Differences in English language generic drug nomenclature. *Am J Hosp Pharm* 1980 May;37:624.

Pizzorno JE. Availability, labeling & safety of 'natural therapeutics' still controversial; OTA group to help formulate policy. *Health News Rev* 1993 Fall;3(4):1–2.

Rubin M. Ethical OTCs, an endangered species. *Pharm Exec* 1985 Nov;5:62,64.

Sonnenreich MR, Menger JM. State substitution laws—A lawyer's view. *US Pharmacist* 1977 Apr;2:18–23.

Stehlin D. Harvesting drugs from plants. *FDA Consum* 1990 Oct;24(8):20–23.

Wehrli A. How to select generic names for drugs. *Pharm Int* 1982 Dec;3:405–408.

Practicum 1

This exercise will test your knowledge of drug nomenclature and how it relates to the R&D pipeline and literature retrieval process. Questions posed can be answered without actual reference to hardcopy sources. Suggested answers are included in Appendix E.

Directions: For each of the drug names listed below, answer the following questions:

a. What type of nomenclature does this name represent?

b. If an information query uses this name, what does that indicate to you about the stage of development of the compound under scrutiny? Where would you place the drug in the development process shown in Figure 2.1?

c. How reliable is this name likely to be as a candidate search term/access point to the literature? Rate on a scale of 1 to 5.

least reliable			most reliable	
1	2	3	4	5

1. calcipotriene
2. 112965–21–6
3. decaderm
4. MDL 73,945
5. (2) 9-[[hydroxy-1-(hydroxymethyl)ethoxy]methyl]guanine
6. $C_9H_{12}N_5NaO_4$
7. anxiolytic
8. angiotensin-converting enzyme inhibitor
9. antihypertensive
10. adrenocorticoid steroid

3

Drug Identification and Nomenclature Sources

In a chapter dedicated to identification and nomenclature sources, it's perhaps inevitable that discussion begins with clarifying terms and clearing the air of some familiar misnomers. There is a common misconception that pharmacopeias are the chief printed source of drug information today. This misunderstanding is underscored each time an interview begins with "Do you have the — pharmacopeia?" (where — represents a national jurisdiction, such as British, Polish, etc.). Further inquiry usually reveals that the questioner's goal is finding out more about a drug believed to originate in the named country. The best source to achieve that goal is unlikely to be a national pharmacopeia.

How has the widespread belief in the importance of pharmacopeias evolved? One probable explanation is that it was once true. The term "pharmacopeia" (alternatively spelled "pharmacopoeia") is a combination of two Greek words: *pharmakon* (drug) and *poiein* (to make). Books given this name, dating from the seventeenth century, were the earliest publications devoted to drug information. True to their name, they were intended to help compounders identify therapeutic substances, extract or derive them from natural sources, and formulate them into medications. This remains the primary purpose of pharmacopeias today: to establish standards of identity, strength, purity, and quality for drugs in general use in the issuing or sponsoring country. That being the case, notes on such publications appear in Chapter Eleven of the *Guide*.

One legacy of the *United States Pharmacopeia* (*USP*) and *National Formulary* (*NF*) that will, however, affect discussion here is one of vocabulary. Each entry in the USP-NF (11.8) is referred to as a "monograph." This specialized usage of a term generally reserved for separately published books on a single subject carries over into other references to the drug information literature, so that brief entries dedicated to a single substance in, for example, *The Merck Index* (3.5) or dosage handbooks are each also called "monographs."

Jargon has been described as shorthand between cognoscenti[1]. Admittedly, any introduction to a subject specialty like this one treads a fine line between being cryptic or pedantic. Yet, in the interest of clarity, still another definition is necessary to set down the precise boundaries in scope of books described here as identification sources. Unless a questioner plans to analyze or assay a drug to chemically identify it or test its purity, a pharmacopeia is not what's really needed. "Identification" in the context of most drug-related inquiries is not the kind performed in a laboratory, but requires, instead, the means to establish identity through words and verbal description. Many sources are dedicated to the latter form of drug identification, and they are the topic of this chapter.

Official Compendia

Although the 1962 Kefauver-Harris Amendments to the Food, Drug and Cosmetic Act authorized the U.S. government to designate official names for drugs, this privilege is rarely exercised. Regulations issued in 1984 clarify FDA policies and, in effect, abdicate responsibility to a nongovernment agency.

> The Food and Drug Administration will not routinely designate official names. . . . Interested persons, in the absence of the designation . . . may rely on as the established name for any drug . . . the USAN adopted name listed in *USAN and the USP Dictionary of Drug Names.* . . .[2]

The United States Adopted Name Program, begun in 1961, is an organized effort to produce simple nonproprietary names for drugs and related agents (e.g., pharmaceutic aids, surgical materials) for the purpose of facilitating communication. A cumulative list of names adopted has been published each year since 1963 and should be part of any core collection of drug information sources.

3.1 Fleeger CA, ed. *USP Dictionary of USAN and International Drug Names.* Rockville, MD: United States Pharmacopeial Convention, 1995–. Annual (publication suspended in 1998).

The title of this publication changed with the 1995 edition, but it still incorporates the text previously known as *USAN and the USP Dictionary of Drug Names*, superseding all earlier volumes in the series (1963–1994). Entries are arranged alphabetically and include not only all USANs assigned since 1961 (3,361 names through January, 1997—the cut-off date for the 1998 volume), but also briefer monographs for all International Nonproprietary Names (INN) published by the World Health Organization from the beginning of the INN program in 1953 through 1996. A total of 8,713 nonproprietary name entries appear in the 1998 edition, supplemented with more than 4,115 brand names, 4,051 code designations, and more than 9,599 CAS registry numbers.

Full USAN monographs begin with the generic name in boldface, followed by year of adoption, a key to pronunciation, and a compendial status indicator (if applicable, e.g., USP or NF). Identification information routinely supplied includes empirical formula and molecular weight, INN and other nonproprietary names (BAN or JAN), chemical name(s), CAS RN(s), pharmacological or therapeutic category, U.S. brand names, manufacturers, and laboratory codes. Graphic, structural formulas also accompany 6,983 entries. Meticulous attention to detail is evident in several special features: 1) agencies responsible for alternative nomenclature are clearly linked with each name; 2) variant forms of chemical names (inverted/uninverted) and registry numbers (both current and replaced) for related compounds (e.g., anhydrous forms, parent RN for salts) are always given; and 3) former brand names are identified as such, as are companies no longer associated with the product. All brand, code, and alternate generic names embedded in monographs are also used as separate access points in the alphabetical dictionary arrangement, cross referenced to relevant monograph entries. For example:

ACC-9089. Code designation for Flestolol Sulfate.
Accupril. Parke-Davis brand of Quinapril Hydrochloride.
Acinitrazole (BAN)—See Nithiamide.
Aminitrozole (INN)—See Nithiamide.

Entries for INNs with no USAN counterpart consist of abbreviated monographs, with the INN followed by the molecular formula and weight, chemical name, CAS RN, and name authority (e.g., INN, JAN). Structural formulas are included for many, but not all, non-USAN generic entries. The main dictionary portion of the volume is followed by a listing of USAN names by category of activity (either pharmacological or therapeutic), drawing terminology from a number of different classification schemes. Separate indexes offer access by CAS RN, by NSC number (390 in all), or by empirical formula. Appendices include a name-and-address directory of "domestic firms concerned with articles for which USAN have been selected" and a cumulative list, by generic name, of orphan product designations and approvals from 1983 through 1996. Chemical and brand names are provided in this list, as well as indication, the date orphan status was granted, date of approval (when applicable), and name and address of sponsoring firms. (Refer to Chapter Four for more information about orphan products.)

In May 1998, the Pharmacopeial Convention announced that it was suspending annual publication of the *USP Dictionary* in print. This makes the 1998 (35ᵗʰ) edition a landmark volume destined for retention long past its imprint date. Henceforward, users will need to consult other sources for updates (USANs added from February 1997 forward) and somehow integrate—into the last cumulative volume—the approximately 70 new official names designated each year. Probably the easiest way to do this is to construct a running list on diskette, using a word processing program to re-sort entries alphabetically and produce updated printed lists. A digital scanner could also be used to capture new entries. Where will they appear? New USANs are announced in monthly updates to *USP Dispensing Information* (6.5) and in bimonthly issues of the *Pharmacopeial Forum* (11.9) *Unlisted Drugs* (3.8) also systematically indexes newly adopted official names (both USAN and INN). Hopefully, the online version of the *USP Dictionary* (available on Dialog and STN) will be maintained as an alternative up-to-date source.

3.2 *International Nonproprietary Names (INN) for Pharmaceutical Substances: Cumulative List.* Geneva: World Health Organization, 1976–.

Given that the *USP Dictionary* (3.1) includes INNs retrospective to 1953, purchase of WHO's separately published list is unnecessary except for libraries striving for comprehensive coverage. *International Nonproprietary Names* is neither more up-to-date nor more complete than the combined USAN and INN compilation published by the U.S. Pharmacopeial Convention. Moreover, this cumulative list is difficult to use. It presents names in a hard-to-read tabular format, beginning with Latin on the left, as the primary access point, followed by English, French, Russian, and Spanish equivalents. Although English-language drug names are alphabetically close to Latin forms (e.g., bromocriptine and bromocriptinum), it is necessary to remember that F is nearly always preferred to PH in Latin (clorofenum, rather than clorophene), T supplants TH (tiabendazolum, versus thiabendazole), E replaces AE or OE, and I is substituted for Y (politefum, rather than polytef). Entries for the 6,085 INNs compiled in the 1992 WHO list (superseding the previous 1988 edition) each include a CAS registry number, molecular formula, and references to other national nonproprietary names. Cited alternatives include USAN, BAN, DCF, JAN, and DCIT (Denominazione commune italiana). Between editions, newly designated International Nonproprietary Names are published in *WHO Drug Information*.

Three special features could add to the value, for subject specialty users, of *International Nonproprietary Names*. First, entries indicate if a drug is on the "List of Narcotic Drugs under International Control." The 1992 edition cites the United Nations list of March 1990 as its authority, so information may be somewhat dated. Second, a special symbol flags names of substances that have not reached the market and whose development has been abandoned. Another symbol identifies substances once marketed (either in a single-entity preparation or a composite product), but no longer in trade. About 1,000 INN entries bear one or the other marker, based on information supplied by manufacturers. Third, cross references also indicate whether the named INN substance is recognized as an International Biological Standard or Reference Preparation, an International Chemical Reference Substance, or an ISO reference name (International Standards Organization common names for pesticides and other agrochemicals).

3.3 British Pharmacopoeia Commission. *British Approved Names 1994*. London: HMSO, 1994.

Published approximately every four years, each cumulative edition of *British Approved Names* incorporates names published in supplements issued periodically between consolidated updates. Molecular formulas were added to each entry, beginning with the 1990 edition, along with a separate formula index, and the reintroduction of a cross reference list linking brand names to generic counterparts, an index omitted in the 1986 edition. (Unlike the *USP Dictionary*, such cross references are not embedded in the main portion of the text.)

BAN entries provide a CAS registry number, empirical formula, pronunciation key, brand names, notes regarding proposed or granted INNs or USANs that differ significantly from the BAN, and an indication of drug activity. Therapeutic use terminology and pharmacological vocabulary follows the standard established in the *British National Formulary* (10.22). The cumulative list includes both current and abandoned/discontinued names, making distinctions in typeface between the two. Appendices include graphic structural formulas and "Guidelines for the Construction of Pharmaceutical Trade Marks."

3.4 Society of Japanese Pharmacopoeia. *Japanese Accepted Names for Pharmaceuticals*. Tokyo: Yakuji Nippon, 1992.

Publication of *Japanese Accepted Names for Pharmaceuticals* represents the latest revision and enlargement of a cumulative list of JAN, incorporating twelve annual supplements. Arranged by generic name, monographs in the 1992 listing include chemical name, identification of pharmacopeias where the compound has been recognized, molecular formula and weight, CAS registry number, structural formula, and therapeutic category. Indexes provide cross references from trademarks (in both Japanese and English) and non-JAN designations, and also offer access by CAS RN, empirical formula, and pharmacotherapeutic category. A directory of manufacturers, including addresses and telephone numbers, completes the volume.

An important distinction to bear in mind when using identification information located in any of these official compendia is that named substances are not necessarily available commercially, even when brand names accompany entries. Proprietary names are often adopted by manufacturers long before approval and launch. Also, brand names may refer to products on the market abroad, but not yet approved in the United States. Conversely, omission of a brand name does not indicate unapproved status. Official compendia make no attempt to supply exhaustive listings of products in trade. Furthermore, when multiple proprietary names are given, do not assume equivalency or interchangability. Products cited may be available in entirely different dosage forms and strengths and may well be intended for unrelated indications.

Remember that the single-entity approach to indexing that is prevalent in nonproprietary name listings automatically limits their scope to individual ingredients, rather than products. This practice also undercuts their utility in identifying combination preparations characteristically found on the OTC market. There are, of course, exceptions. The *USP Dictionary* (3.1), for example, does offer cross references from a number of brand names in current use in the United States for multi-ingredient products: e.g., "Demulen. Searle brand of combination product; *See* Ethinyl Estradiol; Ethynodiol Diacetate." *USAN* monographs for individual substances also note when the compound is a component in combinations, citing them by brand and manufacturer.

The introduction to *British Approved Names* (3.3) mentions that some combination products have been assigned a generic name, a practice influenced by evolving National Health Service regulations regarding prescribing. The *USP Dictionary* also includes "generic" entries of this type, not as officially recognized USANs, but as "PEN" names offered for convenience when full titles of the components in common combinations would be cumbersome to use. A Pharmacy Equivalent Name (PEN) is generally devised by combining portions of official names for ingredients and is almost invariably preceded by the prefix CO; for example, *co-trimoxazole* is the PEN for *sulfamethoxazole* and *trimethoprim*. Reliance on official compendia for more than very selective indexing of drug products, versus substances, would severely limit a core collection's capabilities in helping answer identification inquiries.

Commercial Sources

The term "commercial" has acquired a negative connotation, the implication being that if something is done for sale or profit, it is somehow tainted with regard to its honesty and integrity and, therefore, less likely to adhere to standards of quality. In the context of drug information, such assumptions would condemn, undeservedly, a very large number of excellent sources known for their rigorous scholarship and praiseworthy scope, without which good reference service would be impossible. Competition in the marketplace may, in fact, account for their steadily improving quality and ever-increasing breadth, when compared to government-sponsored or not-for-profit publishing efforts. For example, no drug information collection would be complete without *The Merck Index*, the product of a major pharmaceutical company.

3.5 Budavari S, ed. *The Merck Index*. 12th ed. Whitehouse Station, NJ: Merck & Co, 1996.

Tracing its origins to a simple 170-page catalog of chemicals sold by Merck, first published in 1889, this encyclopedic reference work long ago sloughed off its "commercial" chrysalis to emerge as a leading ready-reference source for identifying chemicals, drugs, and biologics. It accomplishes this task by compiling all types of nomenclature, including generic, brand, and chemical names, as well as CAS RN, empirical formula, and a graphic depiction of molecular structure. Any of these names, save the latter, can be used as starting points when approaching the 2,600-page volume, which includes a comprehensive "Cross Index of Names" (more than 60,000 synonyms) to lead the user to one of the more than 10,300 monographs. Index entries cite specific monograph numbers, rather than page. Formulas and registry numbers are accessible in separate indexes.

Information professionals soon learn never to trust a request for help prefaced by the assertion: "I've already looked in *The Merck Index* and can't find this drug." Tact usually dictates waiting to recheck *Merck* in the absence of the requester, but such a step is, nevertheless, recommended to save time and frustration. Why? The alphabetic arrangement tempts many readers to dip directly into the dictionary-like listing, simply examining names used to label monographs and ignoring the warning printed at the bottom of each page: "Consult the cross-index before using this section." Entries for many compounds can easily be missed if monograph labels alone are relied upon.

Once the relevant *Merck* entry is reached, uninformed struggles to locate it are soon forgotten, due to the wealth of information provided. Physical data include color, odor, boiling or flash point, solubility, and LD_{50}. Another bonus, beyond nomenclature and physical data, is bibliographic references to the isolation and preparation/synthesis of the compound, structural studies, patent information (number, nation, assignee, date), and, when relevant, citations to the literature describing pharmacology, toxicology, activity of derivatives, and a review of clinical studies. Entries also identify biological activity, therapeutic category, or other uses (e.g., insecticide, nematocide). Therapeutic vocabulary matches that used in the *USP Dictionary* (3.1), except when that source lists only a mechanism of action. *The Merck Index* prefers "indication" terms and has been enhanced with a separate therapeutic category and biological activity index, newly added in the 1989 (11th) edition. Although its coverage is limited to single entities, *Merck* includes not only human medicinals, but also chemicals used in household products, industrial and agricultural substances, laboratory reagents, naturally occurring (e.g., plant-derived) compounds, and veterinary pharmaceuticals (a definite plus).

Drug nomenclature in monographs does, however, tend to be delivered in a slightly unpalatable mixture, lumping together alternate nonproprietary names and a stream of proprietary names, without identifying official nomenclature as such (no USAN or INN notations) or affiliating brand names with companies. Brand names can be distinguished from generic designations by the fact that brands are capitalized. Curiously, companies associated with specific trademarks are supplied in the Cross Index, but not in the body of *Merck* monographs. (Note for online searchers: *The Merck Index* database does link brands with companies in its monographs.)

Reference material at the back of the volume includes a listing of selected acronyms for combination cancer chemotherapy regimens (e.g., FAC = fluorouracil
+ doxorubicin + cyclophosphamide), a key to initial code letters used by companies for their investigational drugs, and a guide to prescription notations that
translates apothecary symbols for weight and volume and lists abbreviations for
Latin terms and their meaning. Another back-of-the-book gem is information on
organic name reactions, last appended in the tenth (1983) edition and reintro-
duced in 1996. A Company Register with locations (not full mailing addresses)
is also provided.

Needless to say, each new edition of *The Merck Index* is eagerly awaited. The
drawback of lengthy intervals between printed volumes (eight to ten years) can
be overcome by consulting the online version of *Merck*, updated semiannually
both with revisions to current monographs and with additions for new substances.

3.6 Billups NF, ed. *American Drug Index*. St. Louis: Facts & Comparisons, 1950–. Annual, with quarterly updates.

A third "must-have" selection for the drug information provider's collection
is the *American Drug Index*. *ADI*'s inclusion of combination products and OTC
drugs, often listing inactive ingredients as well as active components, along with
its nearly comprehensive coverage of single-entity drugs currently on the market
in the United States, makes it a valuable complement to the *USP Dictionary* (3.1)
and *Merck* (3.5). Some investigational, as well as discontinued, products are identified.

The basic dictionary arrangement is easy to use, requiring no reminders to consult extra indexes. More than 20,000 entries are arranged alphabetically in one
list, integrating monographs for both nonproprietary and brand names, with cross
references from selected chemical and other nomenclature. Pertinent data supplied with the brand name under which a product is marketed include manufacturer, generic or chemical name(s), composition and strength, pharmaceutical
forms available, package size, and use. USAN nomenclature predominates, but
BANs and Veterinary British Approved Names are also cited. Generic name
monographs refer to relevant brands, which aids in finding drug combinations
where only one major ingredient is known. Therapeutic and pharmacological
class terms can also be used as access points. Status indicators (e.g., Rx, OTC,
c–v), when applicable, are added to product monographs (commencing with the
1996 edition). Marginal bullets now also highlight officially designated names
(i.e., *USP* or *USAN*), and upper/lower case distinctions differentiate between
brand and generic names. Pronunciations of generic names were added to the
hardcopy edition in 1997. (*ADI* on CD-ROM includes 3,300 audio pronunciations of generic drug names.)

Current appendices to the *American Drug Index* list common abbreviations
used in medical orders, normal laboratory values for frequently requested tests,
container and storage requirements for USP and sterile drugs (e.g., when light-

resistant, tamper-proof, glass, or plastic are advised), oral dosage forms that should not be crushed or chewed, drug names that look alike and sound alike, and equivalents/conversion factors for weights and measures encountered in pharmacy practice. The latter are intended to assist in calculating dosages in metric, apothecary, and avoirdupois systems. A table summarizing vaccination recommendations and schedules for childhood immunizations was added in 1997. A Trademark Glossary focuses on identifying trademarked dosage forms and package types. Two company directories conclude the volume, one a quick-reference index to companies by their NDC designations and a second, traditional alphabetic guide to mailing addresses, usefully augmented with telephone numbers and NDCs. The company directory in the *American Drug Index* is a hidden treasure, because it identifies many smaller generic firms not easily located elsewhere.

Beyond the Basics: Expanding Drug Identification Capabilities

If you already have the *USP Dictionary* (3.1), *Merck Index* (3.5), and *American Drug Index* (3.6) and are fully exploiting their potential, chances are that there are still identification problems that you're unable to solve. Acquisition of one or more publications listed in this section will expand a basic reference collection to support information service when inquiries frequently involve drugs still under investigation or those originating abroad.

3.7 Swiss Pharmaceutical Society. *Index Nominum. International Drug Directory.* 17th ed. Stuttgart: Medpharm Scientific Publishers, 1997. Biennial.

Index Nominum is a wise choice for information centers faced with a large number of foreign drug identification requests. Similar in format to the *USP Dictionary* (3.1), it includes nomenclature for a larger number of non-U.S. drugs, both investigational and approved, but is, for the most part, limited to single-entity preparations. More than 7,000 nonproprietary name entries identify products from any of thirty-eight countries in the 1997 edition, which also includes cross references from more than 28,000 trademarks and 15,200 other synonyms.

INNs are the preferred nomenclature in main entries, followed by therapeutic class, chemical name and formula, official and unofficial synonyms, monograph titles in various pharmacopeias, and an alphabetical list of trademarks with their corresponding manufacturers. Following the first English-language edition of *Index Nominum* in 1990, therapeutic terminology, formerly given only in French, is now translated into English, with all categories listed at the front of the volume. Structural formulas and CAS registry numbers accompany main entries, but not those for derivatives or related compounds, such as sodium salts, sulfates, etc. Official synonyms (marked OS) supplied in this biennial directory's brief monographs include USAN, BAN, and DCF. Investigational drug codes predominate among listings of other alternative names, flagged as IS for "inofficial" [sic] synonyms. Geographic locations (in parentheses) follow most, but not all, companies cited in monographs, with selections and omissions unexplained (and undeducible). However, this problem is somewhat mitigated with the addition of a new appendix in 1995, consisting of an alphabetical listing of more than 4,000 manufacturers, accompanied by full address information.

3.8 *Unlisted Drugs*. Chatham, NJ: Pharmaco Medical Documentation, 1949–. Monthly.

Indispensable for identifying drug investigational codes, *Unlisted Drugs* (*ULD*) also indexes new generic and brand names the first time they appear in the literature, citing sources ranging from patents and journal articles to advertisements and manufacturer's notices. Coverage encompasses all names not previously cited in *Unlisted Drugs* and not found in current or previous editions of other major drug compendia, including *American Drug Index* (3.6), *Merck Index* (3.5), *Martindale* (6.1), the French *Dictionnaire Vidal* (10.12), and the German *Rote Liste* (10.10). Lab codes are always considered "unlisted," "because coverage of this important class of investigational drug designations is particularly poor and unsystematic"[3] in other information sources. Given that supplying more information about compounds identified by codes is a special focus of this directory, it is unfortunate that its index arrangement is somewhat difficult to use. Research codes are sorted by number, without regard to preceding or intervening letters or punctuation. This policy produces some daunting sequences, such as the following:

```
GAT-3
HP-DO3A-Gd
ALK 7
BE-8
FIX
reM10
PB1.3
WBCT20
```

However, once located, an *Unlisted Drugs* monograph presents information in an easy-to-use format, listing alternative nomenclature, therapeutic/pharmacological class, a citation to the original source of the name, and cross references to previous entries in *ULD*, when applicable. Many entries are also accompanied by a structural formula. Subscribers can choose to receive monographs and references for individual substances on 3″ × 5″ cards or paperbound in monthly journal issues.

The card option requires higher maintenance (accurate filing of 200+ cards/

month and guarding against loss or incorrect re-filing), but has the advantages of 1) automatic creation of a running cumulative index, 2) ability to arrange lab code entries in a more conventional letter-by-letter sequence, and 3) option of integrating them, if desired, into one master file encompassing all types of names in alphabetic order. (Monthly journal issues separate research code entries from monographs documenting other types of drug names.) On the other hand, card service recipients miss the broad-ranging, descriptive book reviews included in each issue of the paperbound journal. These reviews cover sources rarely surveyed elsewhere and are particularly valuable in alerting users to the availability of new editions of international drug directories and other specialized reference sources. All books reviewed can also be ordered from Pharmaco Medical Documentation, the publishers of *ULD*. For ongoing collection development, the review section of *Unlisted Drugs* is invaluable.

Users receiving monthly journal issues are sent an interim cumulative name/ number index in June, covering entries from January forward, and a final cumulative index for the year in December. To overcome the tedium of consulting a succession of separate annual indexes, long-term subscribers can purchase multi-year cumulative indexes, published periodically.

3.9 *Unlisted Drugs Index-Guide/10*. Chatham, NJ: Pharmaco Medical Documentation, 1995.

This tenth edition of the *Index-Guide* cumulates indexing to *Unlisted Drugs* from 1949 through 1994, cross referencing entries for more than 240,000 drug names and 25,000 lab codes. Each name entry is followed by synonyms, linked with company/organization, and a reference to the *Unlisted Drugs* issue containing the original monograph for each alternative name. Users will find brand names listed under generic entries and pointers to products where the generic entity is part of a composite formulation. Under brand names for combination products, each active ingredient is identified. The *Index-Guide*'s two lists of manufacturers/originating organizations offer access by mnemonic codes used in ULD entries and by full company/institution name (8,800 in the tenth edition), accompanied by addresses. In addition to cumulative drug name indexing, this volume compiles the full text of all book reviews into one easy-to-consult section, covering reviews published in the 1984–1994 volumes of *ULD*.

The sole drawback (beyond a hefty list price) is that the *Index-Guide* offers only a few category terms, such as Extracts (botanical, mammalian) and Vaccines. The *Pharm-AID* (3.10) directory must be purchased separately if comprehensive drug category access is needed.

3.10 *Pharmaceutical Activities Index-Directory/93*. 4th ed. Chatham, NJ: Pharmaco Medical Documentation, 1994.

Usually referred to by its short title *Pharm-AID*, the *Pharmaceutical Activities Index-Directory* provides cross references from both pharmacological and thera-

peutic activity terms (e.g., vasodilator, gynecologic) to individual drug name/
number monograph citations located in *Unlisted Drugs* (3.8) and to manufacturers associated with each (indicated by codes). Subdivisions under "activity"
headings are generic names of active ingredients, followed by entries that refer
to brand names and their location in previous *ULD* issues. When the named compound is part of a combination preparation, the brand name index entry also
shows the total number of ingredients. For example, under Antihypertensives,
entries for the nonproprietary name atenolol include:

i/Igroseles 2i, 35:178N
i/Kalten 3i, 37:213N

The first index entry shown above indicates that atenolol is an active ingredient
in Igroseles, that this brand name preparation contains a total of two active ingredients (of which atenolol is one), and that a monograph summarizing more information about the product will be found in volume 35 of *Unlisted Drugs* on page
178 at location N. Letter locators in indexing greatly facilitate rapid follow up in
monthly issues, where densely printed pages include referenced alphabetic characters in their margins. The fourth (1994) edition of *Pharm-AID* cumulates indexing for the time period January 1972 through December 1993.

Most drugs in *Pharm-AID* are indexed under several broad class terms. Category assignment is based on terminology used to describe the drug in the original
reference cited in *Unlisted Drugs*. The introduction to the volume lists all activity
category terms, corresponding mnemonic abbreviations used in subsequent drug
class index entries (e.g., anti-inflammatory drugs, steroids = INFLS), and the
starting page in the directory where each coded category listing begins. A separate section in the introduction offers an index to preferred category terms, listing
alternative drug class names that *ULD* editors anticipate readers might use, and
cross referencing them to preferred codes. For example, under corticosteroids,
the reader is referred to INFLS. However, to find the starting page for INFLS,
it's still necessary to return to the first, preferred category list, which is annoying.

Indeed, the prevalence of codes in *Pharm-AID* is an impediment to efficient
use. The separate set of codes created for manufacturers requires consultation of
yet another section in the directory in order to translate them into full names.
Because company codes are only somewhat mnemonic, this look-up process demands careful concentration. Users endowed with less-than-perfect memories
often need to retrace their steps when they find themselves confronted with the
fine print of the manufacturer listing and many distressingly similar codes. Since
the starting point in many inquiries leading to consultation of *Unlisted Drugs* is
a drug number, finding still more codes to deal with in order to use this cumulative index detracts from its value.

A partial (in terms of years covered) solution to problems encountered in this
printed index is available to online searchers, who can access the *Unlisted Drugs*

database from 1988 forward in machine-readable format. Any keywords present in monographs can be used to locate pertinent entries, including activity terms, company names, and drug names/numbers. Special software features also offer users the capability of extracting individual data elements from separate monographs and compiling them into tables.[4]

Whether searched online or in hardcopy format, *Unlisted Drugs'* chief advantage is its truly ecumenical scope. It is one of very few sources that indexes 1) both combination and single-entity products, 2) Rx and OTC medications, 3) investigational, as well as approved, drug formulations, and that provides global access to identification information for 4) herbal, homeopathic, dietary, and other preparations marketed with therapeutic claims. Products launched by very small companies, clinics and health spas, or individual practitioners are indexed side-by-side with formulations under investigation by major pharmaceutical firms, independent laboratories, or academic institutions. Thorough cross referencing among *ULD* issues enables users to track products throughout their development cycle, linking name changes with dates and companies. When a generic name compound is the starting point, cumulative indexes facilitate identification of all preparations in which it is an active ingredient, along with their manufacturers. When these special features are considered in conjunction with historical coverage that predates most other identification sources and timely monthly updates, *Unlisted Drugs* stands out as a strong contender for core collection status in larger libraries and drug information centers.

3.11 Elks J, Ganellin CR, eds. *Dictionary of Drugs.* London: Chapman and Hall, 1990.

In an ambitious description of scope, the editors of the *Dictionary of Drugs* state their intent to cover drugs currently in use or in late stages of development worldwide, as well as discontinued products and plant derivatives used as remedies in folk medicine. At the time of its publication in 1990, the *Dictionary* included monographs for all USANs through 1989, INNs through 1988, and BANs through 1986, Supplement 6. Arranged alphabetically by generic name, entries include physical property data derived from patent literature and cross references to works providing further pharmacological and clinical information, such as *Martindale: The Extra Pharmacopoeia* (6.1).

Alternative nomenclature, compiled in individual monographs and accessible in separate indexes, includes molecular formulas, CAS registry numbers, alternate generic names, pharmacological activity terms, and structures. A triangle flags generic names in the index whose monographs include toxicity information. Bibliographic citations incorporated into each entry are drawn from a survey of patents and other primary literature through July 1989. Such references help users quickly identify sources for isolation and properties data, pharmacology, and toxicity. In this way, drug monographs are comparable to those found in *The Merck Index* (3.5), but no attempt is made to compile extensive lists of brand names characteristic of more commercially-oriented identification sources. Subtitled "Chemical Data, Structures and Bibliographies," the *Dictionary of Drugs* is intended for medicinal and pharmaceutical chemists as an aid in research, not as a guide to prescription or use of drugs.

3.12 Negwer M. *Organic-Chemical Drugs and Their Synonyms.* 7th ed. 4 v. Berlin: Akademie-Verlag, 1994.

Another reference tool intended for chemists is a four-volume set generally referred to as *Negwer*. This well-known source is arranged by empirical formulas in Hill notation. Entries include structural formulas and alternative names (INN, BAN, DCF, USAN) for each substance, plus CAS registry numbers. No attempt is made to identify manufacturers or provide comprehensive trade information. In addition to an index by CAS RNs, volume 4 also contains a Group Index by more than 2,200 "catchwords." Terminology emphasizes chemical categories of compounds (e.g., acridines, antibiotics), rather than potential therapeutic applications. Pharmacological vocabulary is also used sparingly (no access by beta blockers, etc.). Nonetheless, its unique organization by formula, Group Index access to chemically related compounds, and undoubtedly extensive scope, encompassing 12,111 drug compounds and more than 80,000 synonyms, have earned *Negwer* a guaranteed place on most academic library's reference shelves.

3.13 Marler EEJ. *Pharmacological and Chemical Synonyms.* 10th ed. Amsterdam: Elsevier Science Publishers, 1994.

Also known by its editor/compiler's name, *Marler* includes listings for drugs, pesticides, and other compounds cited in the medical literature. Entries identify chemical and nonproprietary names, research codes, and a selection of brand names. To conserve space, monographs for well-established drugs sometimes omit compilations of proprietary nomenclature, but the extensive index to this volume does supply cross references from many relevant brand names. INNs are preferred access points to drugs in the main dictionary portion of *Marler*. Although other generic names may be listed in monographs and used as access points in indexing, these nonproprietary alternatives to INN are not separately identified as either BAN, USAN, DCF, or NFN. Instead, an asterisk is simply used to flag names officially recognized by nomenclature authorities other than WHO and can designate any of the options listed here. For pesticides, International Standards Organization (ISO) terminology is preferred.

The focus of this work is on identifying single-entity compounds. Entries for combination preparations (dubbed "multiple products" by *Marler*) are rarely included, unless the drugs are commonly used in the form of mixtures (e.g., co-trimoxazole). Monographs for the few combinations that are covered list only active ingredients and not their proportions or quantities. With coverage of more than 10,000 drugs and chemicals and access to 50,000 synonyms used internationally, *Marler* nonetheless does not claim any attempt to provide comprehensive brand name indexing. Once considered an essential drug reference source, *Pharmacological and Chemical Synonyms* is now less valuable, due to its infrequent update schedule and extensive overlap with other sources cited previously.

3.14 Glasby JS. *Encyclopedia of Antibiotics*. 3rd ed. Chichester, England: John Wiley & Sons, 1992.

Designed to identify compounds by generic name, the *Encyclopedia of Antibiotics* provides empirical formulas and broad "action" statements ("active against yeast," "against fungi," "antitumor activity") in each of its monographs, some of which also supply structural formulas. References to the patent literature accompany many entries, as well as citations to journal articles describing synthesis or derivation. The *Encyclopedia* is not a guide to trade names, research codes, or companies, but aims, instead, to assist users in locating pertinent structure and synthesis information. Rapid access to these hard-to-find data is its strength, along with a scope encompassing more than 3,000 compounds of natural, semisynthetic, or wholly synthetic origin.

3.15 *The Red Book*. Montvale, NJ: Medical Economics, 1879–. Annual.

The Red Book is intended for use in community pharmacies, with the primary purpose of providing pricing and package size information. Checking this retail compendium is one way of confirming that a product is on the market in the United States. It can also expand your product identification capabilities by encompassing a larger number of OTC preparations. *The Red Book* includes, for example, many nutritional supplements, dietary products, health foods, and natural products not always listed in other sources because, lacking therapeutic claims, such products are not necessarily classified as drugs. It also offers assistance in locating suppliers of ingredients that may be needed for compounding medicinals in-house, such as flavoring agents, emulsifiers, etc. This publication is, however, unabashedly commercial. Liberally peppered with advertisements and nearly devoid of cross references, the large paperbound volume is, from an information professional's point of view, somewhat awkwardly arranged.

Issued by the publishers of the *PDR* (6.10), *The Red Book* lists more than 100,000 drug and healthcare products sold in the United States. It includes average wholesale and direct prices, as well as government ratings of bioequivalency (*Orange Book* codes, 4.42). The two main sections segregate prescription drug entries from OTC and nondrug listings. Products are arranged alphabetically in each section by brand name. Generic name entries list drugs marketed under that name, as well as cross references to branded products and manufacturers. Absent are indications and any other identification data beyond name, company, active ingredients, available forms/strengths/package sizes, NDC code, and price. *The Red Book* also includes an aid to visual identification of commonly prescribed drug products in the form of color photographs of more than 1,000 dosage forms and packages. Separate lists show drugs approved by the FDA during the previous year (giving "months at FDA"), products with patent expirations due before the end of the calendar year, and the top 200 medications dispensed in the United States, based on the IMS National Prescription Audit. Another bonus is an extensive directory of manufacturers, augmented in 1995 with listings for wholesalers.

Other quick-reference material added to enhance the utility of *The Red Book* in retail pharmacies includes tables for pharmacy calculations, an Emergency Information Section, with a poison antidote chart, a national poison information center directory, and a directory of drug information centers available for telephone service to health science professionals. A Clinical Reference Section compiles listings of drugs that should not be crushed or chewed, sugar-free products (arranged by therapeutic class), alcohol-free medications, sulfite-containing products, drugs that can induce photosensitivity, and drugs excreted in breast milk. A drug/food interactions guide added in 1994 was supplemented with a drug/alcohol and drug/tobacco interactions guide in 1995.

A section on Medicaid includes prices; a directory of federal government offices, state Medicaid administrators, and third-party administrators; and a chart summarizing officially mandated patient counseling requirements. A Pharmaceutical Care Reference Section offers a series of summary charts on home test kits for blood glucose monitoring, pregnancy determination, and ovulation prediction. This section concludes with translations of safe medication use instructions into Spanish. *The Red Book*'s Pharmacy Organizations Section lists national and state professional and trade groups, state boards of pharmacy, state drug utilization offices, state licensure requirements, and an industry events calendar.

New features added in 1998 include tables comparing herbal products and vitamins and a guide to alternative medicines. A directory of pharmacy buying and benefits management groups has also been introduced, along with a list of the top 200 generics, based on domestic prescriptions during the previous year.

Other Drug Identification Sources

Many sources cited in other sections of this *Guide* can assist in product identification. For example, Chapter Ten includes discussion of foreign drug compendia and of resources designed to assist in identification based on descriptions or observations of dosage forms. Chapter Eleven annotates references that cover food, drug, and cosmetic excipients and raw materials used in manufacturing pharmaceuticals. Nomenclature databases available online are identified in Chapter Fourteen. In addition, many pharmacology and therapeutics publications, the topic of Chapter Six, supply identification and nomenclature information, along with data regarding indications and precautions.

References

1. Bowman WC, Bowman A, Bowman A. *Dictionary of pharmacology*. Oxford: Blackwell Scientific Publications, 1986: vi.

2. *21CFR* 299.4.

3. What is an "unlisted" drug? *Unlisted Drugs* 1967 Jul;19:87.

4. Snow B. Unlisted Drugs: A new drug identification resource online. *Online* 1994 Mar;18:97–103.

Additional Sources of Information

International Union of Biochemists and Molecular Biologists. *Enzyme nomenclature 1992*. New York: Academic Press, 1992.

Schomburg D, Salzmann M, eds. *Enzyme handbook 4*. Berlin: Springer-Verlag, 1991.

4

Background on Drug and Device Laws and Regulations

A fundamental issue in defining the scope of most drug information sources is whether products and uses covered include investigational, as well as officially approved, preparations. Furthermore, as discussion in Chapter Two has indicated, nomenclature needed to conduct a successful search of the literature is closely linked with the stage in a drug's development when the information being sought was made available. Laws governing the testing and marketing of drugs also control, to a large extent, the availability of published data. Because of their impact and interrelationship with disclosure and access to information, government regulations concerning drugs and medical devices are a topic that must be addressed in any introduction to pharmaceutical publications.

Language used in regulatory requests is rife with cryptic references to government agencies, forms, and procedures. Mastery of basic terminology is critical to effective communication with clientele and their perception of your credibility as an information intermediary and professional peer. Accordingly, identifying and defining important "buzzwords" and abbreviations is an underlying objective in discussion here, backed up by the quick-reference key to abbreviations compiled in Appendix G and the Glossary included at the back of this book. Other core competencies addressed in this chapter are familiarity with issues likely to be the topic of inquiries (and why), as well as potential applications of answers to these inquiries.

History of Drug Regulation in the United States

The first consumer products to be covered by U.S. government regulation were drugs. Yet, major legislation governing these products was not enacted until the twentieth century (see Figure 4.1). Although the Drug Importation Act of 1848 addressed the safety and quality of drugs entering the country from overseas, most histories of federal regulation cite the 1906 Pure Foods and Drug Act as the starting point in government efforts to control medicinal products. The 1906 Act was promulgated in response to concerns regarding harmful or inferior substances being introduced into commerce, brought to public attention through investigations lead by Dr. Harvey Wiley, chief chemist at the Department of Agriculture. Health problems associated with the patent medicines then in widespread use, as well as Upton Sinclair's exposé of the food industry in *The Jungle*, pointed to the need for government intervention. Accordingly, the 1906 law defined "adulterated" or "misbranded" foods and drugs and prohibited their shipment across state lines. The 1911 Sherley Amendment extended its scope to regulate false and fraudulent curative or therapeutic labeling claims. Because no premarket clearance was mandated, these original laws were difficult to enforce. The onus was on the government to prove that a promoter had intended to defraud, and a drug could be seized only after it was already available to the public.

Figure 4.1   Milestones in U.S. Drug and Device Law

1902		Biologics Control Act
1906		Pure Foods and Drug Act (the Wiley Bill)
1911		Sherley Amendment to Pure Foods and Drug Act
1915		Harrison Narcotics Act
1938	✧	Food, Drug, and Cosmetic Act (FDC, the Copeland Bill)
1944		Public Health Service Act
1951		Durham-Humphrey Amendment to FDC
1962	✧	Kefauver-Harris Amendments to FDC
1970		Comprehensive Drug Abuse Prevention and Control Act
1976	✧	Medical Device Amendments to FDC
1977		Medicare-Medicaid AntiFraud and Abuse Amendments
1983		Orphan Drug Act
1984	✧	Drug Price Competition and Patent Term Restoration Act
1984		Comprehensive Crime Control Act (Emergency Scheduling Act)
1986		Controlled Substances Analogue Enforcement Act (Designer Drug Bill)
1986		Drug Export Amendments to FDC
1987		Prescription Drug Marketing Act (PDMA)
1988		Generic Animal Drug and Patent Term Restoration Act
1990		Anabolic Steroids Control Act
1990		Omnibus Budget Reconciliation Act (OBRA, Medicaid Drug Rebate Law)
1990	✧	Safe Medical Device Act (SMDA)
1992		Medical Device Amendments to SMDA
1992		Generic Drug Enforcement Act
1992	✧	Prescription Drug User Fee Act
1994		Dietary Supplement Health and Education Act
1997	✧	FDA Modernization Act

Federal oversight of the class of drugs known as biologics was also initiated in the first decade of this century. When ten children died after being treated with diphtheria antitoxin contaminated with tetanus in 1901, Congress addressed the complex issue of production problems likely to occur in processing infectious materials and toxins for therapeutic use. The Biologics Control Act of 1902 regulated facilities involved in manufacturing and preparation of vaccines and antitoxins by requiring a valid establishment license and periodic inspection. Preparation, rather than products, was the focus of this legislation; no premarket review or sanction of the biological preparations themselves was mandated. Later regulations, issued in 1919, drew on the authority of the 1902 Act to incorporate into government inspection rights the examination and approval of product samples before batch release.

Tragedy triggered the next regulatory milestone. In 1937, 107 deaths were associated with use of sulfonilamide elixir, a product whose labeled ingredient was dissolved in diethylene glycol. A recently discovered "miracle drug" in the treatment of bacterial diseases, sulfonilimide was, unfortunately, insoluble in water. When another vehicle was substituted for water, fatalities occurred when the glycol was metabolized to oxalic acid, which crystallized in the kidney and caused acute renal failure. This incident resulted in the first U.S. legislation specifically requiring proof of safety before a drug could be introduced into interstate commerce. The 1938 Food, Drug and Cosmetic Act (FDC, the Copeland Bill) stipulated that manufacturers submit a New Drug Application (NDA) to the Food and Drug Administration before a new medicinal product could be marketed. Three points about this legislation are noteworthy: 1) no proof of efficacy was required; 2) approvals automatically became effective within sixty days after NDA filing, in the absence of FDA objections; and 3) in order to prevent a new drug's introduction into trade, the FDA was required to prove that it was not safe.

Although the FDC Act also called for preparation of adequate directions for use and appropriate warnings, and attempted to restrict distribution to professional channels (physicians, dentists, veterinarians, etc.) of drugs deemed unsafe for unsupervised consumption, it was not until 1951 that prescription drugs were officially defined by law. The Durham-Humphrey Amendment based the distinction between prescription and over-the-counter (OTC) products on the "misbranding" section of the FDC Act. A drug dispensed without a prescription is deemed misbranded if it is habit-forming or if, because of its potentially harmful effects, it can be administered safely only under the supervision of a licensed practitioner. As mentioned in Chapter Two, an important delimiter for OTC status is a drug's capability of being labeled for appropriate use by the general public.

The Public Health Services Act of 1944 extended control of biologic drugs beyond the mandated licensing of manufacturing facilities that had been required since 1902. Sponsors of new biologics had to obtain a product license, in addition to an establishment license, prior to introducing their preparation into interstate commerce.

Birth defects linked to thalidomide provided strong impetus to further tighten regulatory controls. With the passage of the Kefauver-Harris Amendments in 1962, proof of both safety and efficacy was required before a drug could be approved for marketing. The 1962 law also extended the FDA's inspection rights, outlined good manufacturing practices, mandated informed consent of investigational drug study participants, and required that complete information regarding hazards and precautions become part of prescription drug packaging and sales literature distributed to practitioners. Most important, new, more stringent regulations shifted the burden of proof of safety and effectiveness onto manufacturers, stipulating formal approval by the FDA before marketing. For the first time, official authorization would be based on submission of substantial evidence, demonstrated by adequate, well-controlled clinical trials by qualified experts.

The FDA was then faced with the task of reevaluating drugs newly marketed between 1938 and 1962, for which no proof of efficacy had been required. To do this, the agency contracted with the National Academy of Sciences/National Research Council (NAS/NRC) to conduct the review, which commenced in 1966 under the title "Drug Efficacy Study Implementation" (DESI). The NRC reviewed data submitted on more than 3,400 prescription products with, collectively, 16,573 separate therapeutic claims. Only 12% of drugs examined under DESI were found to be effective for all claimed indications. Although 60% were judged to have proven at least one effective use, 60% of product efficacy claims were also rejected due to inadequate evidence.

It was not until 1972 that the FDA began its review of nonprescription drugs, mandated under legislation passed a decade earlier. Because more than 300,000 OTCs are estimated to be currently on the market, the agency is reviewing their active ingredients and labeling by therapeutic class, rather than examining claims of individual drug products. Nearly 1,000 ingredients and more than 1,500 indications have been identified. This review, still ongoing, has involved three stages: 1) advisory panels first examine available evidence and submit recommendations to the FDA, 2) the agency publishes its tentative conclusions (proposed rules) for public comment, and 3) final monographs will identify active ingredients recognized as safe and effective for OTC use and spell out labeling claims that may appear on products.

Only the first stage in the process is complete; advisory panel recommendations on more than eighty therapeutic categories had all been published in the *Federal Register* (4.24) by 1983, including classification of ingredients into one of three categories (category 1 = safe and effective for intended use, 2 = not safe or effective, 3 = more data needed). Proposed rules (stage 2) have subsequently been issued for many, but not all, drug classes, and final monographs (stage 3) are available for others. Once a final monograph for an OTC drug category has been issued (effective one year from date of publication), no premarketing clearance will be required for a product containing an active ingredient it authorizes, provided that recommended dosage falls within the approved range and that labeling is limited to indications specified in the monograph. If a manufacturer plans to use ingredients, dosage levels, recommended regimens, new formulations, alternative delivery technologies (e.g., timed-release), or claims not covered in OTC monograph standards, the product is subject to full New Drug Application requirements (see next section).

Even before completion, the review process has led to several products being recalled, reformulated, relabeled, or switched from prescription to OTC status. Nonprescription aphrodisiacs, hair growers, orally-administered insect repellents, topical hormones, and daytime sedatives have been banned entirely. More than 220 ingredients were removed from the FDA-accepted list by 1990 and an additional 400 + were crossed out in 1993. Another effect of OTC reviews has been a reduction in the number of combination products, because the safety and efficacy of each ingredient has had to be demonstrated separately, as well as its individual contribution to therapeutic mixtures, without negation of the effects of other ingredients or any significant increase in risks.

Controversy has surrounded the legality of products continuing on the market with ingredients classified as category 3 (more data needed) in panel recommendations or proposed rules, despite practical empirical evidence through long-term use that safety is not an issue. "Grandfather drugs" have provoked comparable criticism. Under the 1962 amendments, manufacturers of drugs introduced prior to the 1938 FDC legislation are not required to submit proof of safety or efficacy. Under the so-called "grandfather clause," their products will not be declared new drugs, subject to modern testing requirements, unless new information adversely affecting safety or efficacy claims is uncovered, or a variation in labeling, dosage form, or use is undertaken. See *Approved Drug Products and Legal Requirements* (4.42) for a complete list of grandfather drugs.

The widespread use of dietary supplements merited separate legislation, enacted by Congress in 1994, to ensure the continuing availability of this special category of OTC products. Its provisions exempt ingredients used in supplements from premarket safety evaluations required for other food ingredients, as long as no information is available that points to significant or unreasonable risks associated with their use as directed on the label or, lacking directions, under normal conditions of use. The Dietary Supplement Health and Education Act also broadened the legal definition of preparations covered beyond essential nutrients (i.e., vitamins, minerals) to include herbs and other natural substances, such as fish oils, enzymes, and glandular extracts. A dietary supplement is now formally defined as a product intended to augment (not replace) conventional food and marketed for ingestion in pill, capsule, tablet, or liquid form.

Stringent food additive regulations were not the only impediments to commercial availability that the 1994 Act was designed to overcome. Products making health claims had, traditionally, been subject to rigorous premarket review to establish proof of safety and efficacy. This requirement was, in many cases, forcing suppression of informative labeling on supplements, to avoid their classification as drugs. When claims went underground, the door was opened to potentially unsafe use of supplements by consumers exposed to nutritional advice disseminated through less regulated channels, such as the popular press. The Act established more realistic labeling standards in an effort to correct this problem. In the absence of formal approval as a drug, claims still cannot be made about a product's ability to diagnose, prevent, mitigate, treat, or cure a specific disease. However, labels can refer, when appropriate, to established facts about nutritional deficiencies, such as calcium's reducing the risk of osteoporosis. Manufacturers can also describe a supplement's effect on well-being or its possible influence on structure or function of the body, provided that statements can be substantiated and are not intended to be misleading. References to nutritional diseases must be accompanied by truthful disclosures of their prevalence in the United States.

It should be noted that FDA rules regarding dietary supplement health claims have subsequently been the subject of litigation. An Appeals Court decision in January 1999 instructed the agency to define its standard of "significant scientific agreement," a regulatory barrier that has heretofore blocked many claims from appearing on labels. Questioning the validity of FDA rules that had prohibited certain nutrient-disease relationship claims, the court endorsed use of disclaimers on labels, rather than suppression of all claims outright. Although the overall effect of this landmark litigation has yet to be realized, the general premise is that "more speech is better" in labeling.

Provisions of the 1994 Act have also increased the informational value of dietary supplement labeling in another important way: namely, clearer identification of ingredients. For example, labeling of products containing herbal or botanical ingredients must designate the part of the plant from which they are derived. Despite apparent relaxation of labeling standards regarding health claims, changes made possible by this legislation would be more accurately described as clarification of what can and cannot be stated. Neither this law nor the OTC drug reviews alter the definition of a drug (see Glossary) or modify rigorous requirements that must be met before a medication can be introduced into commerce in the United States.

The New Drug Application Process Today

Drugs newly marketed since 1962 must pass through a review process outlined below, beginning with step 5 (see also Figure 2.1). Stages in development (1–4) prior to officially defined steps are implied in the requirements for an Investigational New Drug (IND) application.

1. Synthesis, isolation, or fermentation
2. Chemical and physical characterization

3. Screening, biological characterization
4. Animal studies, preclinical evaluation
5. IND, Investigational New Drug Application to the FDA
6. Clinical trials
    Phase I human testing
    Phase II pilot efficacy studies
    Phase III extended clinical evaluation
7. New Drug Application (NDA) to FDA, "pre-registration"
8. NDA approval, "registration"
9. Launch, introduction into marketplace
10. Possible Phase IV, post-marketing surveillance

The initial screening process known as biological characterization (step 3) involves testing *in vivo* and *in vitro* to determine a drug's possible therapeutic activity before proceeding to more expensive animal studies. If preliminary screening indicates good therapeutic potential, lengthier systematic studies in animals are undertaken. Extensive preclinical testing (step 4) is required to determine: 1) acute, subacute, and chronic toxicity, including LD_{50} and teratogenicity; 2) therapeutic index, or the ratio of the effective dose for 50% of animals (ED_{50}) to the lethal dose for 50% of the population under investigation, expressed as LD_{50}/ED_{50}; and 3) pharmacological activity, including absorption, distribution, metabolism, and mechanism of action. By the time animal testing is completed, the potential new drug has typically been under investigation for three to six years. It has been estimated that out of every 5,000 compounds subjected to preclinical screening, only five emerge as candidates meriting testing in humans.

It is at this point that government regulations begin to play a major role in the drug development process. Before the product on trial can be administered to humans, its sponsor (manufacturer or potential marketer) must submit a "Notice of Claimed Investigational Exemption for a New Drug," commonly known as an IND (Investigational New Drug application). An IND documents results of preclinical investigations and describes protocols (detailed research plans) for further testing. If the IND is not disapproved by the FDA within thirty days, clinical trials can begin.

Phase I human testing focuses on pharmacological evaluation to determine the drug's metabolic pathways, kinetics, effects on target organ systems, and parameters for a safe dose range in humans, conducted on a limited number (20–80) of healthy volunteers. In Phase II, trials are initiated under a carefully controlled protocol involving 100–300 patients with the target disease or condition. Studies are designed to compare the effect of the drug in treated patients with the effect of a placebo or alternative therapy in a separate "control" group. Ideally, human subjects in the study are unaware of whether they number among the treatment or control group (a practice known as "blinding," in order to minimize bias). Results of Phase II trials will determine whether the drug is effective and represents sufficient therapeutic gain over other existing treatment(s) to have commercial potential.

Meanwhile, animal testing continues for evaluation of long-term (chronic) toxicity, with studies designed to match the contemplated duration of administration in humans, and animal species selection influenced by metabolic data obtained in Phase I. Serious or unexpected adverse effects, should they occur in either clinical or parallel nonclinical studies, must be reported to the FDA within ten days in a written IND Safety report, referred to as an "S-2 Report." A final dosage form will be selected by the end of successful Phase II clinical trials and formulation, as well as production, details will be determined. Wording for labeling (therapeutic claims) will also be proposed.

With few exceptions, a drug cannot be approved for marketing in the United States without submission of voluminous data gathered from extended clinical evaluation. Phase III studies are conducted on a large number of volunteer patients (usually 1,000–3,000) in both controlled and open trials. Studies are initiated at a variety of sites and by many investigators, in an effort to emulate conditions under which the drug would be administered, should it be approved for marketing. This final stage of testing should confirm efficacy, uncover most adverse effects, and provide additional information on contraindications and optimum dosage schedules in special population subgroups (e.g., patients where age, gender, or other medical conditions affect the form or severity of the targeted disease and its treatment). Proposed labeling will be altered to incorporate such information and reinforce safe prescribing practices.

After up to seven years of human testing, only one out of five candidate products remains in the R&D pipeline, ready to proceed to the final step: preregistration with regulatory authorities. In the United States, this stage begins with submission of a New Drug Application (NDA) by the sponsoring company to the Food and Drug Administration. Subsequent review of the application by the FDA can take as long as two to three years, involving careful evaluation of information on manufacturing specifications, stability and bioavailability data, proposed packaging and labeling, results of toxicology studies, and statistical analyses of safety and efficacy data from clinical trials. Meanwhile, clinical trials may continue (trials conducted after NDA submission, but prior to approval, are designated Phase IIIb). NDA approval ("registration") signals clearance for interstate marketing in the United States for specified indications and dosage forms. Any proposed alteration in dosage form, strength, or indications requires a "supplemental NDA," and labeling changes, such as the addition of newly identified adverse effects or extra precautions information, require a "supplemental labeling NDA."

Traditionally, the approval process for biologics has required simultaneous submission of both a Product License Application (PLA) and an Establishment License Application (ELA). This two-part approach reflects the importance of the manufacturing environment on products of this type, where facilities and production methods can have profound effects on safety and effectiveness. A PLA differs from an NDA in its greater emphasis on industrial processes, in addition to pharmacological and toxicological evaluation. Data presented to support the latter are also generally more limited than found in an NDA. Long-term toxicity testing is, for example, necessarily less rigorous for certain biologics, due to immunogenicity factors. Also, only one well-controlled human clinical trial may be sufficient to gain licensure for a biologic. Submission of product samples for validation testing by the FDA constitutes another critical segment in the PLA/ELA review process for approval of biologics. Legislation passed in 1997 eliminates certain requirements for batch certification of insulin and selected antibiotics and, in a further effort to minimize paperwork, condenses separate PLA and ELA authorization procedures into a single Biologic License Application (BLA).

Readers interested in acquiring additional background knowledge of drug development and related regulations will find that several excellent sources have been published on this topic. Shah and Goldstein[1] provide a useful introduction to "New Drug Applications" in the *Encyclopedia of Pharmaceutical Technology.* Edwards[2] adds an international perspective on the regulation of nonprescription drugs in the same volume, published in 1994.

4.1 Mathieu M. *New Drug Development: A Regulatory Overview*. 4th ed. Waltham, MA: Parexel International, 1998.

4.2 Mathieu M, ed. *Biologics Development: A Regulatory Overview*. 2nd ed. Waltham, MA: Parexel International, 1997.

4.3 Hamner CE, ed. *Drug Development*. 2nd ed. Boca Raton, FL: CRC Press, 1990.

Parexel publications authored and edited by Mathieu stand out as well-written and authoritative resources providing a detailed introduction to current and prospective regulations governing new drug and biologics development in the United States. Both volumes offer practical guidance on compliance and helpful insight into recent FDA reorganization. Discussion is backed up with numerous charts, figures, and tables summarizing agency actions. For example, a chapter on regulation of preclinical testing contains an analysis of Good Laboratory Practice (GLP) violations cited in FDA inspections, listing types of violations and numbers and percentage of labs found to be deficient in each. Illustrative materials in both Parexel publications include reduced, but readable, copies of important FDA forms. Brief bibliographies also accompany each chapter. Subject indexing is somewhat general, but both books are fairly easy to navigate, due to their logical organization and descriptive chapter and section headings.

CRC's publication *Drug Development*, edited by Hamner, also provides a good summary of the process, with chapters on such topics as screening compounds for pharmacological activity, the statistician in R&D, and legal aspects of product protection. Bibliographic references conclude each chapter here, as

well. This book could be used as an educational tool for nontechnical staff who
want to understand more about the industry.

4.4 O'Reilly JT. *Food and Drug Administration (Regulatory Manual Series)*. 2 v.
      Colorado Springs: Shepard's/McGraw-Hill, 1979–. Annual cumula-
      tive supplements.

The *Food and Drug Administration* installment in Shepard's *Regulatory Manual Series*, on the other hand, is intended to provide attorneys or regulatory affairs personnel with a guide to practices and procedures of the agency. Its format
in very thick looseleaf binders makes it nearly impossible to read without a table
and two hands to hold pages open, indicating that quick reference, rather than
leisurely study, is the anticipated use. However, with no informative tabs, even
the admirably detailed table of contents is difficult to locate quickly. The second
volume includes an index of cases cited, statutes cited, and regulations cited, plus
a subject index.

4.5 Burley DM, Clarke JM, Lasagna L, eds. *Pharmaceutical Medicine*. 2nd ed.
      Boston: Little, Brown, 1993.

The editors of *Pharmaceutical Medicine* explain that the discipline has much
in common with clinical pharmacology, but that its practitioners—physicians
working in the pharmaceutical industry—must also be familiar with other aspects
of their employers' drug discovery and development efforts. Accordingly, this
book provides insight into the social and legal aspects of medicines and related
regulatory controls. It includes chapters on how therapeutic compounds are discovered, preclinical toxicity testing, making drugs into medicines, clinical trials,
statistical considerations, post-marketing surveillance and adverse reactions, as
well as pharmacoepidemiology. Although strongly oriented toward readers in the
United Kingdom, discussion does incorporate information on the regulation of
medicines in Europe and the United States.

Anyone seeking to gain greater familiarity with industry practices (such as individuals marketing products and services to pharmaceutical companies) would
benefit from the content of *Pharmaceutical Medicine*. Its overview of emerging
issues is particularly useful, touching on a diverse group of topics such as economics in the pharmaceutical industry, the ethics of clinical research, product
liability and recent group litigation, second generation drug injury (e.g., DES),
consumer protection legislation, and drugs and crime.

Biopharmaceuticals, produced by recombinant DNA, monoclonal antibody, or
other biotechnological methodologies, present special challenges in regulatory
information provision. Two books from John Wiley & Sons and another from
Parexel are excellent sources for learning more about the industry and basic regulatory guidelines governing it.

4.6 Hoxsoll JF, ed. *Quality Assurance for Biopharmaceuticals*. New York: John
      Wiley & Sons, 1994.

4.7 Lubinieki AS, Vargo SA, eds. *Regulatory Practice for Biopharmaceutical Production.* New York: John Wiley & Sons, 1994.

4.8 Struck MM, Mathieu M, Okabe H. *Global Biotechnology Product Registration: E.U., U.S., and Japan.* Waltham, MA: Parexel International, 1997.

Quality Assurance for Biopharmaceuticals is a collection of articles by individual authors currently working in biotechnology companies. Their contributions each include background bibliography. Documentation, validation, analytical methods, sampling methodologies, data (as well as biochemical) analysis, environmental and occupational safety programs are among topics addressed, with the overall purpose of providing information to assist in compliance with Good Manufacturing Practice (GMP) guidelines. Discussion includes an introduction to regulatory issues in the United States, Japan, and Europe.

With chapters on licensing biotech facilities, contract manufacturing, and computerized systems validation, *Regulatory Practice for Biopharmaceutical Production* broadens its scope beyond GMP. Contributing authors offer insight into regulatory issues related to biotechnology processes, facilities, equipment, and products, once again extending coverage to include discussion of drug registration procedures in Europe and Japan, as well as the United States, illustrated with numerous case histories.

Global Biotechnology Product Registration will serve as an update on changes in the product approval process in three regions that together represent more than 75% of the worldwide market for biopharmaceuticals. Struck *et al.* outline the FDA's new single license scheme and centralized European Medicines Evaluation Agency (EMEA) procedures discussed later in this chapter.

4.9 Peterson GR, ed. *Understanding Biotechnology Law.* New York: Dekker, 1993.

Background on legal issues that are critical in earlier stages of a product's life cycle is the focus of *Understanding Biotechnology Law.* Subtitled "Protection, Licensing and Intellectual Property," this informative text addresses the needs of research scientists in evaluating and reporting innovative developments to employers, choosing a form of legal protection, preparing a patent application, engaging in research and consulting agreements, and participating in technology transfer and commercialization. Inventor and ownership rights in university and other research laboratory settings are discussed, along with conflict of interest, patent infringement, and intellectual property policies in general.

4.10 Cook T, Doyle C, Jabbari D. *Pharmaceuticals Biotechnology & The Law.* New York: Stockton Press, 1991.

Cook, Doyle, and Jabbari focus on the regulatory framework within England and Wales, the English court system, and the European Community. Their work complements that of Appelbe and Wingfield (see 4.39) by covering laws affecting industry, such as Good Laboratory Practice, genetic manipulation regulations, environmental protection, and controls on animal experimentation. Chapters related to patents and other intellectual property claims (e.g., copyright and gene sequences, trademarks) set this volume apart as highly recommended reading.

4.11 *Drug Registration Requirements in Japan.* 6th ed. Tokyo: Yakugyo Jiho, 1998.

The 1998 edition of *Drug Registration Requirements in Japan* updates information, in English, on guidelines and standards for clinical studies and new drug approval recently revised by government authorities. Special topics covered include the registration of dental drugs and guidelines for manufacturing when recombinant DNA technology is employed.

4.12 Chidmere EC. *Drug Regulation in African Countries.* Buffalo Grove, IL: Interpharm, 1991.

Chidmere, affiliated with the Federal Ministry of Health in Nigeria, provides an overview of drug legislation and registration procedures in African countries, with the stated intent of compiling information useful to other developing nations in the process of formulating their own national drug policies. Case studies describe implementation of such policies in Egypt, Mozambique, Mexico, and Bangladesh, with an emphasis on legal structures and procedures. Appendices include discussion of basic elements in drug legislation, country statistics, and an essential drug list.

Parexel, publisher of *New Drug Development* (4.1) and *Biologics Development* (4.2), began issuing a *Worldwide Pharmaceutical Regulation Series* in 1995, including separate volumes on new drug approval in the European Union, Japan, Germany, France, Italy, the United Kingdom, Spain, Canada, Brazil, South Korea, and the United States (the world's top pharmaceutical markets). Intended as guidebooks for regulatory personnel, these texts are structured to provide a step-by-step analysis of approval requirements. They cover special submission guidelines for foreign companies, ways in which clinical trials in the target country differ from those conducted elsewhere, and the relationship of the national review process to other regulatory authorities. Refer to Additional Sources of Information at the end of this chapter for specific titles. Parexel's Home Page on the Internet lists other useful titles, accompanied by descriptions and ordering instructions (http://www.parexel.com).

4.13 *CTFA International Regulatory/Resource Manual.* 4th ed. Washington, DC: Cosmetic, Toiletry, and Fragrance Association, 1995.

4.14 *CTFA Labeling Manual.* 6th ed. Washington, DC: Cosmetic, Toiletry, and Fragrance Association, 1997.

Another prolific publisher in an industry closely related to pharmaceuticals is the Cosmetic, Toiletry, and Fragrance Association (CTFA). The category of consumer goods known as personal care products includes many items regulated as OTC drugs or medical devices. Accordingly, the *CTFA International Regulatory/ Resource Manual* could be a useful complement to collections serving industry personnel. It provides detailed analyses of cosmetic and cosmetic-drug regulations in seventy countries, including South American, Eastern European, and Middle East nations. Chapters consist of point-by-point discussions intended to assist comparisons among countries. Product and establishment registration requirements, labeling rules, ingredient restrictions, testing standards, packaging issues, and environmental initiatives are among topics covered. These are supplemented with quick-reference tables summarizing licensing and labeling regulations worldwide. The 600-page *Resource Manual* also compiles a directory of important contact information for each country, with addresses, telephone, and fax numbers of government agencies, embassies, industry and professional groups, and publishers.

The scope of the *CTFA Labeling Manual* is limited to U.S. regulations. It includes the full text of the latest, revised OTC drug monographs for personal care products such as sunscreens, antimicrobials, antidandruff shampoos, and anticaries preparations. It also examines labeling requirements in depth in chapters devoted to ingredient identification, warning statements, net content declaration, and metric labeling. An advertising law section highlights recent developments in industry self-regulation, along with government-imposed restrictions. Issues in import law affecting cosmetics and OTC drugs are also covered, with details regarding U.S. customs and FDA procedures and jurisdiction. Discussion highlights new rules necessitated under NAFTA (North American Free Trade Agreement) and guidelines for country-of-origin labeling, such as "Made in USA" claims. Appendices reprint important FDC Act and Department of Commerce rule-making documents.

Both the *CTFA Labeling Manual* and the *International Regulatory/Resource Manual* are available on CD-ROM as part of a searchable database cross-linking related content from several additional CTFA publications (see also 8.37, 11.29–11.31).

Laws and Regulations Dealing with Drug Lag

Stringent regulatory standards can delay new product introductions. With total elapsed time from laboratory to launch averaging ten to fifteen years, a drug's shelf life under patent protection guaranteeing exclusive marketing rights to its developer is relatively short. This makes it difficult for companies to recover research costs without inflating prices. In response to public and industry concern over the "drug lag" postponing access to promising new therapies (with a perceived side effect of escalating costs to the consumer), legislators in recent years have focused reforms on accelerating the approval process. Concomitant goals are reducing prices, decreasing government oversight costs, and encouraging innovative research regardless of commercial potential.

The Drug Price Competition and Patent Term Restoration Act: Waxman-Hatch Amendments to FDC

U.S. legislation introduced by Senators Waxman and Hatch and enacted in 1984 was designed to facilitate "generic" product introductions, with the intended effect of lowering drug costs to consumers. It authorizes Abbreviated New Drug Applications (ANDAs) for copies of FDA-approved pioneer products after their patent protection expires. ANDAs need not contain full safety and efficacy test results of the type required in NDAs. Instead, documents submitted for evaluation focus on proof of bioequivalence to drugs already on the market.

By encouraging more competition through reduction of development costs to "me-too" companies and shortening the approval process for generic products, Waxman-Hatch proposals, when first introduced in Congress, sparked heated discussion. The pharmaceutical industry press had a lot to say about the burden placed on major corporations to assume the research and development costs for smaller firms that would also profit in the long run. As a result, the 1984 Act also contains provisions intended to help sustain new therapeutic advances by encouraging continuation of original drug research by innovator companies.

The incentives? Legislation permitted drug and device patent term extensions, to a maximum of five years beyond the then-statutory seventeen years. A product's regulatory review period (testing and approval phases) forms the basis for determining the length of extensions. Waxman-Hatch provisions also grant market exclusivity beyond patent term expiration, even without formal application for patent term extension, to products that meet stated "novelty" criteria. For drugs approved immediately prior to passage of the legislation (NDAs authorized from January 1982 through September 24, 1984), ten years of market exclusivity (no ANDAs permitted, regardless of patent life) were granted, provided that the active ingredients in these products had never before been approved. After passage of the Act, newly approved products meeting the same novelty criterion are granted five years of exclusivity. Freedom from submission of rival ANDAs extends to three years for products with an active ingredient previously approved, but whose NDA includes reports of new clinical investigations essential to approval, and conducted or sponsored by the applicant.

There are three exceptions to these market exclusivity provisions: 1) An ANDA for a product protected under the five-year extension may be submitted after four years if it can certify that the drug patent is not valid or will not be infringed by the proposed application. 2) Three-year exclusivity terms do not bar ANDAs to use the products for indications not covered at the time of approval.

3) No exclusivity is granted to antibiotics (subsequent legislation has modified this provision—see below). Furthermore, Waxman-Hatch provisions do not prevent the submission or approval of second, full New Drug Applications for me-too products.

For three years immediately following enactment of this legislation, the increasing number of off-patent generic drug introductions indicated that the Act was accomplishing its purpose of offering consumers lower cost options. Parallel legislation for veterinary products, the Generic Animal Drug and Patent Term Restoration Act, authorized abbreviated New Animal Drug Applications (NADAs), as well. Then, in 1988, illegal and unethical practices uncovered at the FDA and in the burgeoning generic drug industry nearly closed down the ANDA route to market. Investigations revealed that several FDA employees had accepted money and other bribes from industry representatives in exchange for privileged information and assistance in the approval process. Furthermore, some manufacturers were found to have submitted false or fraudulent data as part of their ANDAs, sometimes substituting brand name products for generics in bioequivalency comparisons, and thus ensuring favorable results. In addition, subsequent inspections showed below-standard manufacturing practices at more than half of the generic drug companies audited.

What has come to be known as the "generic drug scandal" resulted in the 1992 Generic Drug Enforcement Act, which gave the FDA authority to bar new product approvals and to reverse previous authorizations for companies convicted of fraudulent practices with regard to new drug application submissions. A side effect of the scandal was a pending ANDA list of crisis proportions in 1990; 660 preregistrations languished in agency limbo by November of that year. However, this backlog has since been reduced, enabling effective measurement of the relative success of the original 1984 legislation in accomplishing its overall objectives. Average review time for ANDAs submitted 1990–1993 was approximately twenty-four months.[3] Median approval time was reduced to 19.3 months by 1997. Total generic drug approvals have risen from the 1990 low of 80, to 193 in 1991, 302 in 1995, and 431 in 1997.

4.15 Beers DO. *Generic and Innovator Drugs: A Guide to FDA Approval Requirements.* 4th ed. Englewood Cliffs, NJ: Aspen Law & Business, 1995.

A book that focuses on explanation of Waxman-Hatch legislation and its implementation, *Generic and Innovator Drugs* covers the evolution of the FDA's position regarding the definition of a new drug and other legal issues. It is illustrated, when applicable, with case law. Chapters cover: approval requirements, content and procedures for filing full NDAs, abbreviated New Drug Applications and "Paper NDAs," delaying approval of competitive products, public availability of NDA data, potential for government compensation of innovators, FDA fraud policy, and debarment of individuals and corporations. Extensive appendices reproduce pertinent extracts of the *U.S. Code*, including the statute implementing GATT (General Agreement on Tariffs and Trade), and a table of cases. A detailed table of contents and tabbed section arrangement make the 1,294-page volume easy to use. A back-of-book subject index is also provided, with entries offering more detailed access to specific topics covered in each section.

4.16 *Drugs Under Patent*. Rockville, MD: FOI Services, 1989–. Annual.

This book provides a complete list (as of its issue date each year) of drugs affected by the 1984 Act, offering indexes by company name, brand and generic names, patent expiration date, dosage form, exclusivity code, patent number, and NDA number. Information is based on patent information now required as part of NDA filings. This includes any patent that claims either the drug covered by the application or a method of using the drug could form the basis for a reasonable patent infringement claim, if a generic copy were marketed. Patents cited by applicants may be those claiming intellectual property rights over active ingredients, product composition, or formulation, but exclude claims on method of manufacture. Because patent protection is a complex issue, data presented in this volume should be regarded only as a starting point when investigating ownership rights for legal, potential investment, licensing, or other competitive purposes. It is chiefly valuable as a quick-reference guide to exclusivity expirations. The online database *Diogenes* (16.1) includes the same information and can be used to derive a more up-to-date list. Refer to Chapter Sixteen for other sources to verify patent expirations and extensions. *The Orange Book* (4.42) also includes a patent and exclusivity information addendum, updated monthly.

Questions regarding U.S. patent expirations and possible extensions can be difficult to resolve, because legislation signed into law in December 1994 redefined terms of patent protection. Following adoption of the General Agreement on Tariffs and Trade (GATT), it was necessary for the United States to switch from a seventeen-year patent term (dating from issue) to the more common European standard of a twenty-year term, commencing on the date a patent application is submitted. The legislation, known as the Uruguay Round Agreements Act or URAA, affects all drugs with a patent effective on June 8, 1995. URAA does not necessarily translate into an automatic extension of three years beyond the original expiration date. The length of time from the date of patent application to issuance must be subtracted from the three-year extension.

Whether existing Waxman-Hatch extensions can be added to GATT-adjusted patent terms has been a point hotly disputed. Although the U.S. Patent and Trademark Office (PTO) determined, in June 1995, that companies must choose between Waxman-Hatch extensions and the twenty-year patent term, this PTO decision was overruled in a subsequent federal court decision. Patents whose original seventeen-year term was in force when the URAA change took effect are entitled to add Waxman-Hatch restoration extensions to the twenty-year-from-filing term. However, drug patents in force on June 8, 1995 solely due to an extension cannot benefit from prolonged patent life possible under GATT adjustments. The fact that, in many cases, the coveted time period amounted to only a few months of extended exclusivity is a clear indicator of the revenue potential of brand name monopoly in the U.S. market for drugs with widespread applicability. When that applicability is perceived to be relatively limited, as in the case of treatments for rare diseases, further inducements to encourage innovations may be needed.

Orphan Drug Act of 1983

Developing a new molecular entity (NME) requires a substantial financial invest-ment, especially when costs of the estimated four out of five products that un-dergo clinical testing without reaching the marketplace are taken into account. Mossinghoff,[4] in testimony at a Congressional hearing in 1996, estimated the price tag for developing a new molecular entity to be $500 million, citing a study conducted by the Boston Consulting Group on behalf of the Pharmaceutical Re-search and Manufacturers of America (PhRMA). Therapeutic merit alone does not guarantee commercial success and consequent return on investment. Demo-graphics also play a major role. Thus, patients with relatively rare diseases or conditions become therapeutic "orphans" in a highly competitive, free trade en-vironment.

To mitigate this problem in the United States, the Orphan Drug Act of 1983 provides incentives for manufacturers to develop and market drugs intended to treat or prevent medical conditions that affect fewer than 200,000 citizens. Incen-tives include seven-year market exclusivity (regardless of patentability or nov-elty), tax credits on overall firm profits amounting to 50% of funds spent on or-phan drug clinical development, protocol assistance in the form of written recommendations for preclinical and human studies needed for approval, and ap-propriations for grants or contracts to support development and testing.

Officially-designated orphan drugs are also accorded a higher priority for FDA review when they reach the NDA submission stage. The result is an accelerated assessment cycle and decreased time to approval. Designated drugs introduced into commerce during the ten-year period following implementation of the Or-phan Drug Act (1984–1994) show an average of thirteen months for NDA re-view, versus twenty-three months for non-orphans. Further evidence of the suc-cess of this legislation can be found simply by adding up pre- and post-Act NDA approvals. Ten drugs targeting orphan indications entered the U.S. market in the decade preceding enactment, compared to 108 products approved for patient pop-ulations under 200,000 during the fourteen years following passage.

Moreover, orphan drug legislation has subsequently been introduced in other countries. Since 1993, Japan has offered special incentives to developers of drugs intended to treat or prevent conditions affecting fewer than 50,000 patients. Pro-posals endorsed by the European Commission (EC) in mid-1997, and expected to go into effect in the year 2000, would grant orphan designation to diseases with a prevalence in the total EC population of less than 5 per 10,000 (compared to the U.S. rate of 7.5 per 10,000 or Japan's epidemiological threshold of 4 per 10,000). Another difference in EC measures is that market exclusivity would be granted for 10 years (versus seven in the United States).

Asbury[5] describes circumstances leading to orphan drug legislation in a well-written introductory essay published in the *Encyclopedia of Pharmaceutical Technology* in 1995. Haffner[6] compiles statistical data cited here as a measure of its impact. For a complete list of FDA-designated orphan drugs, see the *USP Dictionary* (3.1), *NDA Pipeline* (4.20, 15.8), or *USP DI Volume 1* (6.5).

Prescription Drug User Fee Act of 1992

Despite earlier amendments intended to reduce drug lag, the growing backlog of New Drug Applications at the FDA, and consequent delays in approvals spurred another landmark law in 1992, the Prescription Drug User Fee Act (PDUFA). In return for annual fees assessed on all domestic and foreign prescription drug manufacturing establishments and on each strength and dosage form of all approved prescription drug products, as well as payments to be required as part of NDA filing, the FDA committed to review drug applications on a much more timely basis than in the past. First phased in during the government fiscal year 1994, accelerated review goals were fully implemented by 1997, when agency action on 90% of NDAs submitted began within six to twelve months of filing. (Note: "action" is not necessarily equivalent to approval.) Nourished by an estimated $325 million in user-fee revenues from 1993 through 1997, the FDA's efforts to streamline the drug approval process divided expenditure among hiring additional staff, expanding office space, and extending use of computer technology.

PDUFA measures have proved effective. The average time from application submission to initial FDA action was 8.4 months for NDAs handled during its five-year term. More importantly, the median time from filing to final approval (rather than first action) was shortened to 12.2 months for NDAs. This figure represents a 40% reduction from performance levels experienced prior to User Fee mandates. Congress renewed PDUFA late in 1997, extending its provisions through the year 2002.

The Food and Drug Administration Modernization Act of 1997

The U.S. Congress reauthorized prescription drug user fees through the year 2002 as part of major legislation approved in November 1997, known as the FDA Modernization Act (FDAMA). Many other provisions of this law address the drug lag problem. For example, FDAMA extends market exclusivity by six months for new pediatric indications on drugs. Every year, more than half of medications approved for marketing lack pediatric labeling information. By providing an economic incentive in the form of increased market exclusivity, the law encourages manufacturers to compile and submit scientific evidence in support of specific dosing information for safe use of their products in children.

The Modernization Act also authorizes a new mechanism for fast track approval of drugs for serious or life-threatening conditions. It expands access to investigational therapies for these conditions by underwriting a public databank of clinical trial information. Thus, the NIH clinical trials databases currently available on the Internet are expected to expand to include private sector trials by the year 2000.

Lag time in biologic drug approvals is targeted in several provisions of FDAMA. As mentioned earlier in this chapter, previous requirements for separate product and establishment license applications (PLA/ELA) have been condensed into a single BLA. The agency can contract for outside expert review of BLAs to supplement limited in-house staff, when needed. Batch certification of insulin and selected antibiotics has been waived under FDAMA, which also grants sponsors of biologics the right to apply for market exclusivity under Waxman-Hatch provisions previously denied them.

The 1997 legislation relaxes restrictions on pharmacy compounding, permitting qualified practitioners to manufacture, at a local level and on a limited scale, products not commercially available. The Act mandates compilation of a list of substances that can, and cannot, be used in extemporaneous preparation of such products (in response to a legal prescription order for an identified individual). Substances already approved as components in marketed products or covered by *USP/NF* (11.8) monographs are automatically included. In addition, twenty bulk drug substances historically used in compounding are currently under consideration as qualified additions to the list. By the end of 1998, the FDA had also published a list of products not to compound, including sixty drugs previously withdrawn from the market (1960 forward) for safety reasons. The goal of this list making is, again, expanding access, via pharmacy compounding, to products not commercially available.

The most controversial segment of FDAMA deals with information dissemination. The new law tackles the thorny issue of off-label uses of drugs approved for other indications. Prior to its passage, manufacturers were prohibited from distributing information on these uses, except in response to specific requests from licensed practitioners. As a result, communication of research into further legitimate uses was, in effect, driven underground. To close the gap thus created between actual medical practice and official validation of new drug uses, the Modernization Act permits manufacturers to distribute peer-reviewed journal articles on off-label uses, provided that they first agree to file Supplemental New Drug Applications to bring underground practices into the mainstream. In this way, legislators hoped, once again, to accelerate the availability of promising therapies, at the same time ensuring public safety through validation of scientific evidence by regulatory authorities.

Treatment INDs, Surrogate Endpoints, and Parallel Track Testing

The AIDS crisis has quickened the pace of regulatory reform aimed at streamlining drug approval and increasing accessibility to new treatments desperately needed. For example, in 1987, final rules legalized a much broader form of "treatment INDs," whereby drugs still under investigation could be made more widely available to seriously ill patients outside the regular, but limited, route of formal participation in clinical trials.

The FDA followed up this extension of what had formerly been referred to as Compassionate INDs with "Interim Rules on Procedures for Drugs Intended to Treat Life-Threatening or Severely Debilitating Illnesses," issued in 1988. Also known as Subpart E, these rules permitted, for the first time, departures from standard drug testing procedures, including compression of Phase III clinical trials into Phase II studies, after which an NDA would be accepted.

Another significant alteration in the standard path to drug approval was recognition that surrogate endpoints could be accepted as proof of efficacy in trials of designated products. Under regulations referred to as Subpart H, issued at the end of 1992, the FDA may grant marketing approval based on a drug's effect on observable clinical data other than survival or irreversible morbidity. Surrogate endpoints are measurable factors that are reasonably likely, based on epidemiological, therapeutic, pathophysiological, or other evidence, to predict clinical benefit. For example, drugs for hypertension have been approved based on blood pressure measurements, rather than survival or stroke rates.

The year 1992 also ushered in a further dramatic departure from established procedures with official recognition of "parallel track" testing, permitting AIDS drugs to be made available following completion of Phase I studies. Qualified patients can be granted access to new therapies, even when efficacy data do not meet the requirements necessary for a treatment IND. More recently, streamlined investigational drug accessibility and approval procedures, first implemented in 1987 rulings applied to AIDS therapies, have been officially extended to cancer drugs. New guidelines announced in April 1996[7] allow for acceptance of surrogate markers in judging the approvability of antineoplastic agents. Partial, and possibly transient, responses, such as tumor shrinkage, can be used as indicators for prolonged patient survival and enhanced quality of life. Justification for early cancer drug release for use in experimental programs in the United States can also now be supported by the *de facto* evidence of approvals in any of twenty-six other countries, rather than requiring lengthy clinical testing within U.S. boundaries.

FDA Classification of Drugs for Priority Review

The FDA employs a classification system to govern the review priority accorded an NDA submission, based on the proposed product's chemical novelty and therapeutic significance. This two-part coding scheme was revised in late 1992 to incorporate new categories necessitated by orphan drug, AIDS, and Interim Rule Subpart E provisions (see Figure 4.2). The first digit, representing a drug's chemical classification, designates the product's relationship to other active moieties already marketed in the United States. Letters refer to the agency's assessment of the candidate drug's therapeutic value, dictating the priority given its NDA review and consequent lag time in the preregistration stage. Priority drugs (Type P) offer a therapeutic gain over existing alternatives either by targeting a disease heretofore not adequately treated or diagnosed, by improving therapy by greater effectiveness or safety, by reducing annoying (not necessarily serious) side effects, or by extending treatment to a subpopulation not well covered in previously approved products' indications (e.g., pediatric or geriatric patients or those exhibiting intolerance). NDAs classified as Type S are accorded standard (slower) review, being substantially equivalent to drugs already available.

Phase IV Clinical Studies

Accelerated approvals raise concerns over product safety. It is not uncommon for a new product showing great therapeutic potential to be approved before clinical data sufficient to uncover serious adverse effects are available and before chronic toxicity studies in animals are complete. Standard post-approval regulatory controls require ongoing submission of reports of adverse experiences. They also subject manufacturers to unannounced FDA inspections, with the purpose of monitoring quality control in production, distribution, and recordkeeping.

When circumstances warrant it, the FDA has, in recent years, also requested further, post-marketing clinical studies as a contingency to approval for selected products. Although this practice has not been formally defined in existing federal regulations, Phase IV post-marketing surveillance is likely to become an increasingly important factor in ensuring public safety without compromising other FDA commitments to accelerate approvals and accessibility. Phase IV studies are usually conducted on a much broader scale than premarketing trials and may be less rigorously controlled. They can be, nonetheless, an effective means, compared to the voluntary adverse event reporting system, to gather information on long-term effects, interactions, and subpopulation risks. Manufacturers may also initiate Phase IV studies on their own authority, without FDA instigation (but with agency authorization still required), to test different dosage regimens, use in special patient groups not represented in preapproval trials, or to develop pharmacoeconomic (cost-effectiveness) data to support marketing strategies against competing therapies.

CANDAs and NDA Days

Although only about thirty drug companies have submitted Computer-Assisted New Drug Applications (CANDAs), first filings of this type began more than ten

Figure 4.2   FDA Drug Classification for INDs and NDAs

By Chemical Type:

1	New Molecular Entity	The active moiety is not yet marketed in the United States by any drug manufacturer, either as a single entity or as part of a combination product.
2	New Ester, Salt, or Other Noncovalent Derivative	The active moiety is marketed by the same or another manufacturer, but the salt, ester, or derivative is not yet marketed in the United States.
3	New Formulation	The compound is marketed in the United States by the same or another company, but the particular dosage form or formulation is not.
4	New Combination	Drug contains two or more compounds not previously marketed together in a drug product in the United States.
5	New Manufacturer	A "me-too" drug that duplicates an active moiety, salt, formulation, or combination already marketed by another firm.
6	New Indication	Duplicates a product already approved or marketed by the same or another firm, except that it provides for a new indication (use).
7	Marketed drug without an approved NDA	First application for a drug marketed prior to 1938, i.e., "grandfather drug," or a DESI-related product marketed between 1938 and 1962 without an NDA. Indication may be the same as, or different from, the already marketed product.

By Therapeutic Potential:

P	Priority review	Therapeutic gain over existing alternatives (replaced "A" or "B" ranking in 1992).
S	Standard review	Substantially equivalent to existing therapies (replaced "C" ranking in 1992).
AA	Priority for AIDS drug	Important therapeutic gain among drugs indicated for AIDS.
E	Drug for severely debilitating or life-threatening illness	Under provisions of FDA Interim rules introduced in 1988, known as Subpart E procedures.
H	Accelerated approval	Under provisions of 21CFR 314 Subpart H.
V	Orphan Drug	Drug has received official orphan designation.
A	Significant therapeutic gain	Replaced by "P" in 1992.
B	Modest therapeutic gain	Replaced by "P" in 1992.
C	Little or no therapeutic gain	Replaced by "S" in 1992.

years ago and had reached a total of seventy by 1992. Regulations permit the use of "electronic signatures" and are intended to protect security in electronic transfers of agency and industry documents. These innovations will accommodate increased usage of automated systems and paperless electronic recordkeeping.

Computer technology has assisted in yet another initiative at the FDA to reduce the drug lag. Inaugurated in 1988, an "NDA Day" involves convening representatives from both the drug sponsor and the agency for an intensive one- or two-day working session late in the approval evaluation process, to expedite resolution of remaining issues. Compared to the alternative of separate meetings and intermittent discussions typically stretched over many months, this approach has led to rapid problem resolution and definitely speeded approval of targeted drugs. Use of dedicated computer databases and telefacsimile (fax) of responses from the remote sponsor site have facilitated NDA Days, as have, more recently, direct computer links between FDA local area networks and company headquarters' computers.

International Cooperative Efforts: EMEA, ICH, Harmonization, and Drug Export Amendments

Drug lag is by no means a problem limited to the United States. Multinational corporations face similar, but separate, drug registration requirements in other nations before gaining access to lucrative markets in Europe, Asia, and Latin America. Data from clinical trials conducted onsite in target countries are often required before approval. Preclinical testing standards sometimes differ, necessitating expensive, and partially redundant, repetition of procedures to comply with local laws. Lack of standardization undoubtedly adds to delays in the introduction of promising new therapies. But several recent developments in the form of treaties and other covenants show a trend toward international cooperation with a common goal of reducing regulatory impediments to scientific advances.

The European Community (EC), formed with the intent of creating a single market without trade barriers, is focusing efforts on "harmonization" of drug approval regulatory requirements, including reciprocity in accepting data. The first official step toward EC marketing authorizations in Europe was a procedure known as "concertation," established in 1987 and effective through 1994. Under this EC directive, a manufacturer's application could be submitted to one EC member state, designated the "rapporteur," whose authorities would review and assess the data it contained. The application then proceeded to the Committee for Proprietary Medical Products (CPMP), where representatives from all member states reviewed its merits. A favorable opinion by CPMP endorsed (but did not mandate) marketing authorization in any nation to which the company would submit preregistration documents.

Concertation eventually evolved into the drug approval process in place today, one that employs a choice of two new mechanisms: 1) centralized registration or

2) mutual recognition. A new EC administrative entity, the European Medicines Evaluation Agency (EMEA), was created to oversee the process. The EMEA opened its doors in London in January 1995, with a stated mission of coordinating the work of evaluation and supervision of medicinal products at the national level in member states, in an effort to avoid duplication of effort.

Under the centralized system for the evaluation of new drug applications, manufacturers of medicines produced by biotechnology or of veterinary products designed to boost animal production are required to submit preregistration documents directly to the EMEA, if they wish to market their drugs across the European Community. The centralized procedure differs from the former concertation approval process in two important ways: 1) the CPMP, rather than the applicant, chooses the rapporteur (although the company's preference is taken into account), to distribute the workload equitably among member states' regulatory authorities; and 2) final marketing authorization by CPMP is now binding on all member states, resulting in mandatory and automatic approval for commercial introduction throughout the EC.

For all other nonbiotech/high tech medical products, manufacturers have a choice of submission to the central agency or to individual countries. Although companies could continue applying for market authorization in a succession of separate European nations under existing arrangements until 1998, they also now have the option to seek multistate clearance after just one EC member approves their product. A system of mutual recognition of national marketing authorizations is the underlying mechanism for multistate approvals, a decentralized procedure that became the only alternative to EMEA centralized registration from 1998 forward. If disagreement arises under mutual recognition protocols, the EMEA is charged with the responsibility to step in and supervise binding arbitration at the Community level.

Under both the centralized and decentralized (mutual recognition) European Community initiatives, it is now possible for an innovator company to achieve registration through submission of documents meeting a single set of requirements (versus differing, but somewhat duplicative and redundant, regulations of fifteen individual nations in any of eleven languages). For example, only one Summary of Product Characteristics (SPC) and draft Patient Information Leaflet (PIL) need be filed under the decentralized mutual recognition procedure. In fact, many companies have chosen the centralized method of authorization in preference to decentralized mutual recognition.

The EMEA issues a European Public Assessment Report (EPAR) for each product it approves, outlining the scientific basis on which the drug was authorized and background information used in evaluating its safety, quality, and efficacy. The EMEA Web site offers the full text of all EPARs, as well as agency guidelines and standard operating procedures, a calendar of forthcoming meetings, and a directory of personnel (see http://www.eudra.org/emea/emea.html).

In 1999, several central and eastern European countries will also implement a simplified procedure for recognizing marketing authorizations granted under the EC centralized approval option. Nations participating in CADREAC (Collaboration Agreement of Drug Regulatory Authorities in European Union Associated Countries) include Bulgaria, the Czech Republic, Estonia, Hungary, Latvia, Lithuania, Poland, Romania, and Slovakia. This and other changes outlined here should certainly serve to reduce the drug lag in reaching a market of 365 million people with an estimated worth of $70 billion in medical product revenue.

Another source of delays in worldwide product introductions has been widely divergent national policies regarding drug standards and test methodologies. When officials of the U.S., Japanese, and European pharmacopeias formed a voluntary alliance in 1989, harmonization in the critical area of quality control in manufacturing began in earnest. Excipients were chosen by the Pharmacopeial Discussion Group as the initial focus of their consensus-building efforts. These efforts are aimed at reducing impediments to registration, manufacture, and shipping of drug products around the world, rather than trying to implement complete unification or mandate identical monograph requirements. Chowhan[8] reports on the process employed in pharmacopeial harmonization.

Initiated in 1991 after pharmacopeial tripartite coordination had begun, biennial International Conferences on Harmonization (ICH) have also brought together officials from the EC, Japan, and the United States. ICH focuses on development of mutually acceptable guidelines addressing technical requirements for registration and R&D procedures which, when adopted, could reduce drug lag. By the adjournment of the Fourth International Conference on Harmonization (ICH4) held in Brussels in 1997, thirty-six of the thirty-eight topics originally selected for harmonization had either been incorporated into domestic regulations or recommended for adoption. ICH recommendations for acute toxicity studies, the duration of chronic toxicity testing in rodents, and reproductive toxicity testing were the first guidelines adopted by the FDA.

Another ICH initiative (dubbed M1) addresses the development of a standardized vocabulary of terminology for use in regulatory affairs worldwide (e.g., product labeling, electronic data systems for adverse event reporting, descriptions of health effects). The FDA has already adopted MEDDRA (the Medical Dictionary for Drug Regulatory Affairs) in its coding of adverse effects. ICH also hopes to greet the new millennium with completion of a Common Technical Document: a core technical information package specifying a uniform format and content that could be submitted in all three regions for approval of a new medication.

A further example of international cooperation to reduce drug lag is joint NDA appraisals by both U.S. and Canadian authorities. The FDA and Canada's Health Protection Branch (HPB) have already completed joint reviews of at least five AIDS-related drugs. The advantage of such cooperative efforts is the ability to bring needed therapies to market sooner, facilitated by pooled information and shared evaluation of clinical data. A further important step toward cross-border coordination was a November 1993 regulation that authorized sharing of confidential information with foreign regulators.

Another significant milestone was passage of the Drug Export Amendments to FDC in 1986, which loosened restrictions on shipment of drugs not yet approved for marketing in the United States. Unapproved U.S. products are eligible for export to any of twenty-one designated countries if 1) they are approved in the importing country and are actively under investigation in the United States (authorized IND holders), or 2) their sole intended use is clinical trial investigations.

Conversely, the FDA has promulgated regulations covering importation of foreign drugs by individual U.S. citizens for their own use, legalizing therapies for serious conditions when 1) no effective domestic counterpart is available, 2) no unreasonable risk is involved, 3) no commercialization or promotion is intended, and 4) treatment is under the supervision of a licensed practitioner. A three-month supply is generally the maximum permitted under current policy.

Narcotic Drug Law

With the exception of laws prohibiting the import of specific addictive or otherwise harmful substances (e.g., a ban on opium in 1886), the Harrison Narcotics Act of 1915 was the first federal legislation specifically directed at control of substances with potential for abuse. The method used was taxation under Internal Revenue regulations, although it was soon bolstered by a narcotics import and export Act. Subsequently, Drug Abuse Control Amendments to the 1938 Food, Drug, and Cosmetic Act were repealed and superseded by the Comprehensive Drug Abuse Prevention and Control Act of 1970. Enforcement of the 1970 Act is the responsibility of the Drug Enforcement Administration (DEA) of the U.S. Department of Justice.

The law established five "schedules" of controlled substances, based on their potential for abuse. The schedule into which a drug falls affects its availability and the degree of regulation governing its dispensing, such as the number of prescription refills permitted, the quantity dispensed at one time, whether identification of the patient is required, special inventory recordkeeping procedures and reporting, and official registration of dispensing agents. The lower the schedule number, the higher the degree of control stipulated for listed drugs.

Schedule I drugs have no acceptable, official medicinal use in this country; examples are mescaline, peyote, heroin, LSD, and dihydromorphine. Schedule II drugs, formerly known as "Class A narcotics," have a high potential for abuse, but also have accepted and proven medical utility. Amphetamine, codeine, cocaine, morphine, and secobarbital are examples of drugs in this category. Schedule III drugs were once called "Class B narcotics." Their abuse can lead to moderate, rather than severe, dependence. Codeine-containing combinations, such as acetaminophen with codeine, as well as some nonnarcotic drugs, are listed on

Schedule III. Schedule IV drugs, such as chloral hydrate or phenobarbital, and Schedule V drugs have, successively, lower abuse potentials and contain smaller quantities of substances known to cause at least limited dependence.

The escalating problem of drug abuse has spawned a recent flurry of additional legislation dealing with substances not included within the scope of the original schedules. The 1984 Comprehensive Crime Control Act provides a section commonly known as the Emergency Scheduling Act, with the means to regulate "designer" drugs: new analogs or variations of existing controlled substances. In 1986, the Controlled Substance Analogue Enforcement Act (the "designer drug bill") bolstered enforcement powers by permitting prosecution for trafficking with unscheduled drugs when they are analogous either in structure or action to scheduled substances and intended for use in humans. Notoriety of specialty substance abuse in athletes added steroids to the lengthening list of controlled substances, with passage of the Anabolic Steroids Control Act in 1990.

Although a controlled substance is not necessarily a narcotic, the term "scheduled drug" is often used as a synonym for narcotic drugs. Nor is a scheduled drug necessarily a prescription product. Some OTC preparations are listed on Schedule V, such as cough syrups with low levels of codeine and antidiarrheals containing small amounts of opium. Under federal law, these products can be sold without a prescription, but only by a registered pharmacist.

Several publications discussed elsewhere in this volume include lists of controlled substances, but the following sources offer additional background information.

4.17 Shulgin AT. *The Controlled Substances Act: A Resource Manual of the Current Status of the Federal Drug Laws*. Lafayette, CA: Alexander T. Shulgin, 1988.

4.18 *Controlled Substances Quarterly*. Arlington, VA: Government Information Services, 1971–.

Shulgin includes three forewords in his *Resource Manual*: "for the lawyers," "for the criminalists," and "for the scientists." Separate chapters on scheduled drugs follow, providing common synonyms, CAS Registry Numbers for many (but not all) substances, chemical structures, controlled substances code numbers used by the DEA for import/export permits and registration purposes, and classification of drug activity as stated in the law and in *Merck Index*, when applicable. Because there are drug names in the original 1970 Public Law list for which there are no entries in *The Merck Index* (3.5), *USAN* (3.1), or the *U.S. Pharmacopeia* (11.8), additional identification data compiled by Shulgin could be a useful adjunct to reference collections aiming for comprehensive coverage. The *Manual* also outlines the history of relevant drug law and includes an empirical formula index. Note: not all scheduled drugs have DEA codes (only when brought under legal consideration), and not all DEA-coded substances represent scheduled drugs.

The Controlled Substances Quarterly, published in January, April, July, and October, is intended to keep subscribers up-to-date on the latest regulatory actions by the DEA and to update other lists of scheduled drugs, which are typically issued annually.

Regulatory Hot Topics and Frequently Asked Questions

Information on FDA regulatory activities has implications beyond compliance. The competitive intelligence value of monitoring new drug approvals, patent extensions, product recalls, drug export applications, and official warning letters is recognized by a growing number of individuals involved in market research, investment, advertising, insurance, and the media. Yet, despite increased recognition of the potential commercial significance of regulatory information, few courses on medical bibliography or printed guides to the literature cover this challenging area of information provision. Perhaps as a result, few areas are more misunderstood or downright avoided. Misconceptions and confusion most often arise from incomplete understanding of so-called "sunshine laws" dealing with freedom of information, of distinctions between legislation and regulation, and of issues related to federal versus state jurisdiction. Refer to Figure 4.3.

Freedom of Information and Effects on Answers Available

Despite its title, the Freedom of Information Act (FOI) of 1966 does not authorize *carte blanche* communication of federal documents. The Food and Drug Administration must take precautions to protect trade secrets and patient confidentiality revealed in NDAs, for example, such as details regarding manufacturing, excipients or inactive ingredients used in formulations, investigative site locations, and study participant names. Such data are routinely purged (literally blacked out) in documents obtained under FOI provisions and the necessity to do so can delay their release, often requiring review by a toxicologist, chemist, or other scientific expert. Full NDA filings are unobtainable, but Summary Basis of Approval (SBA or SBOA) documents or their equivalents are available upon request, usually no sooner than one to two years following launch.

Protection of trade secrets explains why all ingredients in prescription drug products need not be disclosed. Naive consumers are often outraged at this lack of full disclosure, applicable until recently even to OTC products. Yet, sober reflection should suggest that much of the selling value of a preparation that may set it apart from competitors derives from the unique formulation, including flavors, colorants, and other additives. If the reason behind a request for all ingredients is hypersensitivity to a commonly used dye or other unlabeled substance, manufacturers will respond with a simple affirmative or negative to a telephone request from a health science professional querying the presence of a specific substance in their formulation of a named drug. The good news is that, under 1997 FDA Modernization Act provisions, labels for OTC products must now disclose names of all inactive, as well as active, ingredients.

Another set of questions that bump against Freedom of Information provisions would be: Has company X applied for an NDA on product Y yet? Is this drug in clinical trials? When did human studies start on compound ABC? Announcement by the FDA of the mere fact of an IND or NDA filing is prohibited, since it would destroy competitive advantages gained by discretion on the part of applicant companies. If the innovators themselves choose to announce news about drugs under development, information will be available about products still under investigation from sources other than the FDA. However, preapproval publicity is closely monitored by the FDA, which must enforce policies against premarketing promotion. Ironically, regulation of the pharmaceutical industry by another federal agency, the Securities and Exchange Commission (SEC), sometimes leads to conflict. The SEC requires public disclosure by companies of all information relevant to their business in stock-offering prospectuses. Hence, some of the best sources of information on drugs in the pipeline are investment analysts' and brokers' reports and commentary in the financial press and trade journals. If you are asked to find out about IND or NDA filings, rely on business sources and never guarantee success (refer to Chapter Fifteen for drugs-in-development directories).

Medical literature databases limited to journal coverage, such as *MEDLINE* (14.1) and *EMBASE* (*Excerpta Medica* online, 14.4), tend to pick up references to clinical trials fairly late in the development process. This delay is due to lag time imposed by peer review before traditional scientific journal publication, as well as by innovator companies delaying public release of results for competitive reasons. Online databases that include conference proceedings and separately issued symposia in their scope, such as *BIOSIS Previews* (14.6), *CA Search* (14.37), and *Conference Papers Index*, often cite clinical trial results presented at meetings as much as two years in advance of journal publication. Activities of major companies and news of potential therapeutic blockbusters are more likely to be traceable than small firms, me-too products, or line extensions (variations on previously approved drugs).

Drug Approvals

Drug approvals (NDAs already authorized) are, on the other hand, fairly easy to locate. FOI Services has published a complete retrospective compilation of basic identification information for all drugs approved by the FDA since FDC Act provisions became effective in September 1938.

4.19 *FDA Approved Drugs*. Gaithersburg, MD: FOI Services, 1998. Annual.

Previously published in hardcopy as *The NDA Book*, this CD-ROM compendium lists more than 28,000 products. Entries for approved and/or discontinued/

withdrawn drugs are accessible by brand name, company, approval or withdrawal dates, nonproprietary names of active ingredients, and dosage form and route. Information is current up to the calendar year of issue. More recent NDA approvals can be found in the FOI database *Diogenes* (16.1), from which the CD-ROM *FDA Approved Drugs* file is derived, or by consulting F-D-C Reports' *Pharmaceutical Approvals Monthly*. Refer to Chapter Sixteen for a comparison of online sources, including the *FDA Home Page* on the Internet.

4.20 *NDA Pipeline.* Chevy Chase, MD: F-D-C Development, 1983–. Annual.

Both new drug/biologic approvals and monitoring products on the road to U.S. approval are the focus of *NDA Pipeline*. Eight sections present information in tabular format, with each annual edition offering a complete listing of the previous year's original NDAs grouped by the FDA's classification system (e.g., 1P, 3S). Another table arranges NDAs alphabetically by generic name. Company name access is provided in a third section, which includes both new approvals and a status summary of drugs in research. It lists brand name (when available), generic name, a brief description of pharmacological action and probable therapeutic application, and a stage indicator (e.g., Phase I, IND filing planned, supplemental NDA submitted). The same drugs-in-research information is extracted from the separate company-by-company listing and compiled in another section, arranged by generic name, lab code, or product category when no name is available. This information is derived from a weekly newsletter published by F-D-C, known as *The Pink Sheet* (4.49, 15.10).

NDA Pipeline also provides a cumulative list of all FDA-designated orphan drugs, including products previously approved, as well as those still undergoing clinical investigation. Another section summarizes FDA Advisory Committee activities during the preceding year, with membership rosters, meeting agendas, and an index to all products discussed. Section VII charts ANDA Suitability Petition activity, including both petitions filed during the previous year and those still pending. Following FDA approval of their petitions, companies planning me-too generic products can begin preparation of Abbreviated New Drug Applications. (ANDA Suitability Petitions are also tracked in *The Orange Book*, 4.42.) The volume concludes with a current address and telephone listing of companies featured in the book.

For a retrospective annual review of drugs in development aiming for U.S. marketing authorization and of new drug approvals, there is no better choice than *NDA Pipeline*, which should be part of any sizable medical library's core collection. Perhaps its only flaw is omission of an overall subject/name index. The introduction of this valuable resource online in 1994 offers users the capability of access by any keyword included in the text, plus the advantage of monthly updates (see 15.8).

4.21 *Pharmaceutical Approvals Monthly.* Chevy Chase, MD: F-D-C Reports, 1995–. Monthly.

The most up-to-date hardcopy source for new drug approvals is *Pharmaceutical Approvals Monthly*. It presents information on original, supplemental, supplemental labeling, and abbreviated NDA authorization announcements in tabular format. It also includes biologic PLAs cleared for marketing and a listing of "approvables" and those pending. All announcements are also made available through e-mail or fax to subscribers immediately following their release by the FDA.

In addition, each issue of F-D-C's monthly newsletter identifies NDAs/PLAs recommended for approval, cross-referenced to FDA advisory committee meeting dates. A section entitled Drug Development Profiles contains substantive, evaluative discussions of significant new approvals. Here, clinical evidence and FDA reviewer commentary are extensively reported. Profiles conclude with complete descriptions of pivotal trials and investigators, identify FDA reviewers and their areas of responsibility. Profiles also compile an itemized, annotated IND and NDA timeline for each drug.

The Clinical Trial Updates section in each issue provides detailed summaries of Phase I, II, and III company-sponsored studies. A 1995 spin-off of *The Pink Sheet* (4.49), *Pharmaceutical Approvals Monthly* continues the Trademark Watch previously included in its parent newsletter. For retrospective coverage of new drug approvals and trademarks, consult the *F-D-C Reports* (15.10) database online.

Gauging Length of Time to Market: IND/NDA Chronology

Another recurring regulatory hot topic is locating dates of INDs and of subsequent NDAs for representatives of an entire class of products. Often, the reason behind this type of information request is an effort to gauge the average length of time to market. It is asked by companies new to the drug category, who are attempting to predict development costs, the profitability window after introduction, and the probability of return on investment. Such information is also needed in benchmarking with competitors. Your answer? This is not publicly available information, except at the discretion of individual applicants, so comprehensive research is not possible and can be extremely time-consuming and expensive.

The FDA does publish annual score card information about the number of NDAs approved against the number under review and the average length of review time for newly authorized products.[9, 10] Such reports are extensively analyzed from an historical perspective in the pharmaceutical press, most notably in *The Pink Sheet* (4.49, 15.10). Examination of FDA determinations on patent term extensions published in the *Federal Register* (4.24) will provide IND and NDA filing dates for a selection of products. Analysis of these data could be used as a basis for extrapolation of average length of time to market (see Chapter Sixteen). The *Pharmaceutical Approvals Monthly* newsletter (4.21), in its Drug Development Profiles section, features detailed, annotated IND and NDA chronologies for a selection of products approved since September 1995. Remember, also, that *The Red Book*'s (3.15) annual listing of drugs approved during the previous year indicates "months at FDA."

Legal Drug Use and Off-Label Indications

Somewhat less elusive, but nonetheless sometimes challenging to find, is information about unapproved indications and dosage. A fact not well understood by the general public and popular press is that when a drug is approved for marketing in the United States, its use is officially authorized only for specified uses and at dosage levels indicated in labeling prepared for prescribers. Drug ready-reference sources typically base their content on information provided in package inserts. These are composed by manufacturers under strict FDA guidelines, which ensure that directions for use comply with conditions approved by the agency after careful review of safety and efficacy data. Consumers (or their information intermediaries), when consulting such sources to find out more about medications they have been prescribed, sometimes assume that any use or dosage regimen that departs from what is described in official package inserts is incorrect, possibly harmful, and probably illegal.

This assumption is not true. Licensed practitioners may legally exercise their professional judgment in treating patients by prescribing drugs for "off-label" uses, provided that such discretionary practices are not directly contraindicated in labeling. In fact, questions about unapproved uses originate not only from consumers, but also from health science professionals, who may need to verify acceptable dosage for unlabeled indications or may ask for authoritative references to alternative therapies. Therefore, to be even minimally adequate, a medical reference book collection should include sources that go beyond official labeling information. Since not all drug compendia offer this extended scope, annotations in the *Guide* will highlight coverage of off-label uses, when applicable (see Chapter Six).

The status quo regarding correct or legal drug use is undoubtedly confusing. For example, the *U.S. Pharmacopeia Dispensing Information* (*USP DI*, 6.5, 14.19), recognized under federal law as a basis for Medicaid reimbursement, cites uses deemed "unofficial" under FDA regulations. In a recent study, Beales[11] found that such indications appeared in the *USP DI*, on average, 2.5 years before they were approved by the FDA. Reasons most often cited for this form of drug lag (the gap between accepted medical practice and official recognition of that practice in product labeling) are 1) the high costs of clinical trials, 2) lengthy testing requirements companies must complete to support applications for new uses, and 3) delays in processing supplemental NDAs at the FDA.

Anticipated revenues from extended labeling must exceed costs if manufacturers are to invest further time and money in studies for supplemental submissions. The relatively poor track record for timely reviews of these submissions has to be added into the equation for calculating return on investment, basically deducting time from commercial shelf-life remaining before exclusivity expiration. Data show that the mean regulatory review time for new chemical entities (NCEs) with supplemental indications approved during 1989–1994 was 28.3 months. That's 3.7 months longer than the mean review time for their original indications. This disproves the reasonable assumption that when concerns over safety and toxicity (which preoccupy initial NDA assessments) are presumably less acute for products already on the market, evaluations should be easier. Review times for supplemental uses were, on average, ten months longer than those for originally approved indications during 1963–1988.[12] The Prescription Drug User Fee Act, by setting stringent goals for more timely performance by the FDA, has helped to reduce efficacy supplement lag times. Median elapsed time from SNDA submission to authorization dropped to 19 months in 1993 and 11.9 months in 1997. However, median approval time for original NDAs in 1997 was still less, at 11.5 months, than for efficacy supplements.

Statistics such as these represent powerful disincentives to companies contemplating pursuit of additional labeling claims. Furthermore, the User Fee Act disallows bundling of multiple indications into either original or supplemental NDAs, instead requiring separate applications for each proposed use. However, the FDA Modernization Act of 1997 provides yet another stimulus to increase SNDA filings for off-label uses. Manufacturers who agree to submit SNDAs can now proactively disseminate to medical practitioners peer-reviewed journal articles about as yet unapproved indications, provided that materials are clearly marked as documenting unofficial uses and that oral communication promoting them does not accompany dissemination. What effect this incentive will have on the overall legislative intent of expediting access by patients to new therapies remains to be seen. Meanwhile, both healthcare and information professionals must cope with the dichotomy between what is acceptable medical practice and what is legally recognized as such in product labeling. Bridging the gap between the two can lead to many reference inquiries.

Line Extensions

Difficulties in answering questions about other types of "line extensions" are imposed less by freedom of information than by benign neglect in the published literature. Historically, the practice of marketing new product variations under an established brand name was a way to build on consumer trust and recognition, thereby lengthening a drug's commercial shelf life. Recent regulatory changes, as well as unofficial healthcare reforms, have provided new impetus for line extensions, which may mean that they will receive more attention in future indexing by reference resources. Provisions of the 1984 generic drug law offer market exclusivity beyond patent expiration to any drug product that has a unique feature recognized as new and improved therapy. Thus, for example, by introducing a transdermal form of a drug originally approved as a tablet, a manufacturer can earn additional exclusivity for the new dosage form, whether patented or not, provided that it is distinguishable from current therapy.

Furthermore, even when government-sanctioned exclusivity has expired, a product's new mode of drug delivery can, in itself, serve as a barrier to multi-sourcing. Line extensions involving controlled-release dosage forms are, for example, more difficult for would-be competitors to duplicate, in terms of bioavailability. Delayed-action preparations necessitate measurements over a longer period following administration, during which drug blood levels are more likely to show variability from the standard established by the innovator product. The greater time investment required to establish comparable bioavailability (necessary to qualify for generic substitution) will, in effect, prolong this type of line extension's market monopoly.

Another trend, unofficial control of prescribing by managed care organizations (insurers) that limit reimbursement to selected drugs to control costs, also encourages development of more drug delivery options. Changes in dosage form, route of administration, and overall regimen that improve patient compliance, reduce side effects, or otherwise decrease overall healthcare costs are powerful persuaders used in marketing to managed care. When safety and efficacy are not at issue, a convenient administration schedule compared to competitive products can tip the balance in reimbursable drug list decisions. For example, a line extension that enables less frequent or at-home administration of a traditionally hospital-based product can reduce an insurer's total hospital admissions and duration-of-stay statistics. In addition, marketing companies can often offer drug delivery line extensions at a lower price, because their R&D costs are relatively low and development times shorter than those associated with new chemical entities.

Accordingly, questions about line extensions often originate from market researchers. For U.S. pharmaceuticals, line extensions are documented in supplemental NDAs and as such are indexed thoroughly in *Diogenes* (16.1) online. Comprehensive coverage of line extensions in the international marketplace is the objective of the *IMSworld Product Monographs* database (15.19), which features country-by-country product entries documenting date of change and other details. More selective indexing of line extensions worldwide is also offered in *Drug News and Perspectives* (15.13).

Discontinued Products

Both marketing and legal investigators may ask for a list of discontinued products. *FDA Approved Drugs* (4.19) is a good place to start. It compiles information on both approved and withdrawn products from September 1938 forward. Two publications from Facts and Comparisons are designed to answer such inquiries.

4.22 *Quick Reference to Discontinued Drugs.* St. Louis: Facts and Comparisons, 1988.

4.23 *D-List.* St. Louis: Facts and Comparisons, 1989–1991. Annual.

The *Quick Reference to Discontinued Drugs* is a cumulative compilation of information on products withdrawn from the U.S. market from 1976 through 1987, accessible by brand name. Dosage form, ingredients, and strength will assist physicians and pharmacists, who may need basic information on a formulation in order to find a contemporary counterpart. Entries also identify distributors and date of discontinuation. The names, addresses, and telephone numbers of all manufacturers cited are included.

Subsequent editions of the *D-List*™ from the same publisher update the *Quick Reference* compilation, but annual issues appear to have ceased with the 1991 list (covers 1990). The *Diogenes* database online (16.1) offers the easiest answer to questions requiring lists of discontinued products. Its retrospective coverage is identical to that of *FDA Approved Drugs* (4.19), commencing with passage of the FDC Act and continuing to the present (product discontinuations are updated quarterly online). When more than company, active ingredients, dosage form, strength, and route of administration are needed, back volumes of several sources discussed in Chapter Six of this *Guide* will supply needed information, such as approved indications, labeling precautions, and known adverse effects. Such details are often required in contemplated malpractice or product liability litigation.

Distinguishing among Laws, Regulations, Enforcement, and Implementation Documents

When information is requested about "drug law"—e.g., approvals, recalls, good manufacturing practice, investigator qualifications and guidelines, acceptable ingredients, and similar legal issues—it's important to bear in mind the distinction between legislation and regulation. Laws or Acts passed by Congress are usually rather general in wording, leaving room for interpretation. Thus, the text of the drug laws themselves, compiled chronologically in the *United States Statutes at Large* and consolidated and classified by subject ("codified") in the *United States Code*, will generally not be of much interest or use to pharmaceutical information providers or their clientele. Instead, most "drug law" questions actually require consultation of regulations, rather than legislation.

An Act of Congress usually creates an agency to administer the law or assigns this duty to an existing agency. To fulfill its mandate, the agency then develops regulations or standards, which represent government-sanctioned interpretations, expansions, and detailed elaboration of the enabling legislation. Figure 4.4 outlines the process for promulgating federal regulations and identifies government publications where information will be available at each stage in the process.

Figure 4.3   Regulatory Hot Topics and Frequently Asked Questions

- [ ] I want a full list of this product's ingredients.
- [ ] I have a prescription a doctor wrote for me while I was on vacation. Can I get it refilled here?
- [ ] Is it okay to substitute this brand for that one?
- [ ] I need to know the patent number for this drug.
- [ ] Has an NDA been filed for this product?
- [ ] Has this medical device or similar models been the subject of adverse event reports or recalls in the past?
- [ ] Is this drug in clinical trials?
- [ ] Is this a prescription drug?
- [ ] What should I do if I think my pharmacist dispensed the wrong drug?
- [ ] When did this drug change its formulation?
- [ ] I need to find the IND and NDA filing dates for these products.

- [ ] What drugs have been granted orphan status?
- [ ] What dyes are permissible in contact lenses?
- [ ] What states have mandatory patient medication counseling laws?
- [ ] Has anyone ever tried marketing this kind of drug in a patch?
- [ ] When was this drug officially approved by the FDA?
- [ ] Compile a list of discontinued drugs in 1978–1979.
- [ ] When did this product come out in capsule, as well as tablet, form?
- [ ] What new antiarthritics were approved last year, worldwide?
- [ ] When did human studies begin for this compound?

- [ ] Has company Z applied for a patent extension on their new drug? What was the outcome?
- [ ] Has this clinical investigator ever failed an FDA inspection in the past?
- [ ] Isn't my consent required before a generic drug can be substituted for the one my doctor prescribed?
- [ ] How many drug recalls has this company experienced in the past five years?
- [ ] What data were submitted to substantiate bioequivalence of this product compared to drug Y?
- [ ] How many drugs have been approved with this active ingredient in this dosage form?
- [ ] I'd like data to construct a graph comparing the number of new drug approvals for each of these companies in each of the past ten years.

Regulations are usually quite precise and spell out what in the original law may be only intent. Their content is nearly always subjected to advance public review and comment before official adoption. Both proposed and final drafts of these agency documents are published in the *Federal Register*, the U.S. government's daily newspaper issued Monday through Friday, excluding holidays. Once finalized, new regulations effected each year are subsequently incorporated into the next annual issue of the *Code of Federal Regulations* (*CFR*).

Figure 4.4 Procedure for Promulgating Federal Regulations

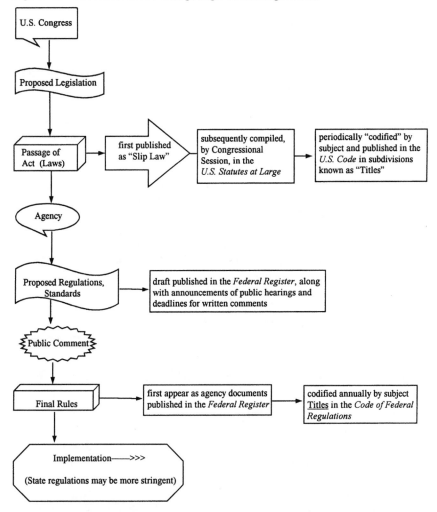

4.24 *Federal Register*. Washington, DC: Office of the Federal Register, National Archives and Records Service, General Services Administration, 1936–. Daily.

4.25 *Code of Federal Regulations*. Washington, DC: Office of the Federal Register, National Archives and Records Service, General Services Administration, 1936–. Annual.

The *CFR*, like the *U.S. Code*, consolidates legal reference material and classifies it by subject in separately-issued subdivisions known as "titles." Title 21 of the *CFR* (usually cited as *21CFR*) contains most government regulations regarding foods, drugs, and cosmetics. The promulgating and enforcing agencies are the FDA and the Drug Enforcement Administration (DEA). A *21CFR* annual issue consists of several volumes, each with a distressingly general and relatively uninformative table of contents and no detailed subject indexing.

For this reason, experienced information professionals will consult only computerized versions of *21CFR*. Good online or CD-ROM editions of the database will enhance access by locating user-entered keywords in the full text of regulations and enable selective display of relevant sections and parts. In this way, the problem of limited access by the general, barely descriptive, subject headings used in the printed document is circumvented, and pertinent regulations can be identified quickly and cost effectively.

What is important to remember, however, is that when asked to find information likely to be part of official regulations, you will need to consult not only the annual edition of *CFR*, but also subsequent issues of the *Federal Register*. The latter step is necessary to check for additions or changes published between Title 21 yearly editions. Fortunately, the *Federal Register* provides an index to *CFR* Sections Affected, so that relevant Title, Section, Part, and Paragraph numbers can be used as starting points when consulting issues. Once again, computerized versions of the *Federal Register* augment access by offering keyword, as well as section number, search capabilities. Online or CD-ROM databases are far more practical to use in day-to-day regulatory information problem-solving than struggling with voluminous printed issues. (Refer to Chapter Sixteen for online sources.)

4.26 *Food Drug Cosmetic Law Reports. Rx ed.* Chicago: Commerce Clearing House, 1938–. Weekly.

Once a relevant item is located, researchers may also find interpretation of written regulations somewhat daunting, due to their language and style. Commerce Clearing House offers a valuable (and expensive) looseleaf service which not only indexes *CFR* and *Federal Register* material in detail and depth, but also paraphrases regulations for greater clarity. *Food Drug Cosmetic Law Reports* adds useful commentary and informed explanations.

Information requesters often unintentionally short circuit the research process by imprecisely describing their needs or omitting their desired goal. For example, a question may be stated as: What's the law about informed consent in clinical investigations? Further inquiry may disclose that your institution's review board is wondering what its precise responsibilities are overseeing a clinical trial about to commence onsite. What is actually needed is not "law." Distinguishing between law and regulation is obviously an important first step in answering such a question.

Resource selection will also be influenced by your ability to distinguish between "regulation" and "implementation" inquiries. For example, further investigation may fail to uncover actual examples of acceptable patient consent forms or precise recordkeeping requirements for institutional review boards (IRBs). Official FDA regulations cannot solve all regulatory information problems. You may need to look, instead, for quasi-official guidelines published by the agency. If none are found on the topic in question, the text of enforcement documents may reveal current FDA interpretations of acceptable practice not yet codified in other agency publications.

The agency uses a bewildering number of communication mechanisms to define policy. For example, "Guidance" documents are often preferred over "Guidelines," because the latter must be developed under a standardized (and slow) process requiring multiple drafts and time allocation for public comment. To remain responsive to change, regulators frequently use their own working documents as underground vehicles to convey their current expectations. Thus, locating Warning Letters and Establishment Inspection Reports is frequently the only answer to many regulatory questions. For example, what kinds of methods validation will be required by the FDA for specific manufacturing processes? Which responsibilities of IRBs are most open to criticism during FDA inspections and could lead to possible withdrawal of approval? Both of these inquiries require review of implementation and enforcement documents, rather than regulations in *21CFR* (see Chapter Sixteen).

Another form of enforcement is litigation. In common with other industries supplying products to consumers, pharmaceutical manufacturers are vulnerable to product liability class action suits, as well as individual claims of injury associated with drug use. McMann[13] provides an excellent introduction to liability aspects of drugs and devices in the *Encyclopedia of Pharmaceutical Technology*. Most liability cases involving drugs are based on the manufacturer's failure to warn of side effects or risks. In some instances, companies have also failed to report known side effects to the FDA and to file a supplemental labeling NDA to reflect new warnings. The legal online services WESTLAW and LEXIS, both commonly in use in law firms and graduate law libraries in the United States, offer the most information to answer questions related to drug litigation. Two hardcopy ready-reference sources can assist in preliminary research within the context of the medical or pharmacy school library.

4.27 Dixon MG, ed. *Drug Product Liability Reporter*. 3 v. New York: Matthew Bender, 1987–.

This looseleaf service, updated periodically as needed, addresses concepts and relationships needed to evaluate and understand injuries associated with drugs and medical devices. The subject index includes terms enabling access by product class (e.g., beta blockers, adrenergic agents, pacemakers), as well as other topics likely to be the subject of inquiry, such as package inserts. The brand name locator and generic name locator are, unfortunately, two separate indexes. A fourth way of approaching these volumes is through the Table of Cases. One curious feature is a chapter dedicated to Drugs in the Medical Literature, which offers synopses on a selection of drugs. Although this chapter is marginally useful, at best, the remainder of *Drug Product Liability* provides a solid platform from which to launch further investigation.

4.28   Patterson RM, ed. *Drugs in Litigation: Damage Awards Involving Pre-scription and Nonprescription Drugs.* Charlottesville, VA: The Michie Company, 1995.

Arranged by U.S. generic name, from acetaminophen to zomepirac sodium, entries in *Drugs in Litigation* include summaries of appellate, trial court, and jury verdict drug decisions. The volume includes an index to cases by case name (e.g., Needham v. Mead Johnson) and a general subject index. Sample entries from the latter illustrate its broad scope: cataracts, choice of proper drug, as well as some drug class names, such as hypoglycemic agents. Monographs attempt to provide a brief technical introduction to each drug and its relevant adverse reactions. They recommend use of *Goodman and Gilman* (6.51), *USP DI* (6.5), the *Physicians' Desk Reference* (6.10), *The Orange Book* (4.42), and *The Medical Letter* (6.17), from which their technical information is derived. *Drugs in Litigation* is a good beginning reference source for legal researchers, and one that many medical and public libraries may want to have on hand.

The bottom line in handling regulatory hot topics and frequently asked questions is the importance of cultivating skills in classifying information requests. Specific resources to answer each type of query will be the focus of a separate chapter dedicated to online retrieval of regulatory information. Consult Chapter Sixteen when you need to find answers to such questions as: What new anti-arthritics were approved last year? Has the clinical director we propose to use as our principle investigator in this Phase III trial ever been cited for alleged violations of FDA regulations in past studies for which he has been responsible? Has this pacemaker or similar models been the subject of adverse experience reports or recalls in the past? What data were submitted to substantiate bioequivalence of this product compared to brand name Y? What kinds of stability studies and data analysis are generally included in NDAs for products of this type?

Federal versus State Control

The phrase "introduced into interstate commerce" has appeared before in this chapter. Federal laws outlined here apply only to those products making thera-peutic claims and intended for marketing across state lines. The laetrile contro-versy and local clinic or individual practitioner introductions of other drugs with-out federal approval have brought this important issue into the limelight. People asked: How could this happen? Isn't that against the law? The answer is: Only if it could be proven that interstate marketing was intended and that misleading or false therapeutic claims were made.

A reminder of where the line is, literally, crossed from state to federal jurisdiction is present in the often overlooked official title of an IND: "Notice of Claimed Investigational Exemption for a New Drug." It originates in the regulatory requirement that drugs shipped across state lines must be the subject of an approved NDA or PLA. Because the sponsor will probably need to transport the product to clinical investigators in several states, exemption from the approval requirement must be requested. The application for exemption, at the same time, provides sufficient information for the FDA to judge whether clinical trials should proceed.

A frequently asked question is one regarding prescription versus nonprescription status. A little-known fact is that a state may restrict a drug to prescription-only status even if it has been granted nonprescription status under federal law. This occurs most frequently with OTCs in Schedule V, so it's a good idea to probe for more information when such questions arise. It's fairly easy to determine federal status, as it is included in NDA approval announcements and standard reference compendia. Further local constraints on distribution are the province of the State Board of Pharmacy (a telephone number to keep on hand).

States may tighten, but not loosen, federal controls. Several recent developments have raised "the specter of a balkanized regulatory system"[14] that free exercise of states' authority could mean not only to the pharmaceutical industry, but also to information seekers and providers. California has proposed additional labeling of products regarding health risk factors (Proposition 65). Newly introduced measures in New York state would require special OTC label warnings for the elderly. Texas legislators would mandate the inclusion of bittering agents in topical OTCs. Another controversial practice is creation of a third class of drugs beyond Rx and OTC: those available only from a pharmacist. Florida has already authorized this category, and other states are considering similar measures. Again, the State Board of Pharmacy is the best source of information on restrictions of this type. It should be noted that the FDA Modernization Act of 1997 attempts to counteract "balkanization" by saying that states cannot impose more stringent requirements than the Federal government, except by petition.

A related issue is: Who may prescribe drugs? The Durham-Humphrey Amendments, perhaps because they were sponsored by two Congressmen-pharmacists, refer only to "licensed practitioners," leaving the door open to states to define precisely which practitioners qualify. In addition to physicians, some states permit prescribing by licensed physicians' assistants, nurse practitioners, optometrists, pharmacists, emergency medical technicians, nurse midwives, naturopaths, homeopaths, etc. Even where authority is granted only to MDs, questions may arise about the legality of filling out-of-state (and foreign) prescriptions. Physicians are licensed by individual states; reciprocity licensing agreements between certain states, but not others, can make finding answers difficult unless your collection includes a good source on pharmacy law.

Laws Governing the Practice of Pharmacy

Regulation of the practice of pharmacy is a function of the states, not of the federal government. In most states, the original laws that effectively defined American pharmacy for the first time and delineated its practice were adopted between 1870 and 1900, influenced by recommendations from the newly founded American Pharmaceutical Association (APhA), formed in Philadelphia in 1852. More recent legislation has benefited from a Model State Pharmacy Act first published in the late 1960s by the APhA and reinforced today by standards promulgated by the National Association of Boards of Pharmacy (NABP).

4.29 *Model State Pharmacy Act and Model Rules of the National Association of Boards of Pharmacy*. Park Ridge, IL: NABP, 1992.

This NABP publication is now available on computer diskette, updated and supplemented as needed. It provides expert legal commentary on each section of the Model Act, offering prototype language and useful definitions of relevant terminology. It also points out where controversy may arise in implementation of state laws. Model Rules in the current edition cover institutional pharmacy practice, nuclear/radiologic pharmacy, sterile pharmaceuticals, and licensure of wholesale distributors. Guidelines for the regulation of pharmacy interns and pharmaceutical care are included. Appendices offer a Model Inspection Form for Nuclear Pharmacies and suggested Computerized Compliance Reports, including controlled substance audits and a sample patient profile record format. A third appendix covers good compounding practices. While pharmacy laws vary from state to state, they are in agreement on a number of points.

- No one may practice pharmacy without a license.
- Periodic relicensing is required, often contingent on evidence of continuing education.
- Practical experience is a prerequisite to licensure in every state. Pharmacy college curricula integrate this practical experience into professional degree requirements as "externship," "practicum," or "preceptorship" programs.
- Reciprocity in licensing is common from state to state, enabling dispensing under prescription orders from licensed practitioners in contiguous states.
- Laws typically distinguish between prescribing authority and dispensing authority, designating specific groups of licensed healthcare professionals who may legally issue prescription drug orders, versus those who may fill such orders.
- Drug product selection and conditions under which generic substitution is permissible are addressed in all state pharmacy laws.
- Requirements for patient counseling by dispensing pharmacists may also be mandated at the state level. N.B.: The Omnibus Budget Reconciliation Act

of 1990 (OBRA) dictates patient counseling for all recipients of the federally funded Medicare and Medicaid programs.

- Administration of the law is usually delegated to a state board of pharmacy (to which all suspected infringements should be reported).
- Minimum standards are established for professional and technical equipment, including printed information sources.

"Society regulates the practice of pharmacy more than it does any other health care profession."[15] Medical information professionals can, therefore, anticipate numerous inquiries related to this highly specialized area of government regulation. Simonsmeier and Fink[16] have crafted an eminently readable introduction to laws governing pharmacy in *Remington's Pharmaceutical Sciences*.

4.30 Fink JL, Marquardt KW, Simonsmeier LM, eds. *Pharmacy Law Digest*. St. Louis: Facts and Comparisons, 1985–.

A core collection to support effective reference service should include, at minimum, the *Pharmacy Law Digest*. Tables compiling information on specific issues in pharmacy practice across fifty states make this resource a veritable gold mine of regulatory data. State licensure requirements, continuing education for accreditation, status of pharmacy technicians, patient counseling mandates, prescribing authority, and dispensing authority are among topics addressed in tables. The *Digest* can help answer such questions as: Where can a Doctor of Homeopathy prescribe medications in the United States? Can podiatrists legally dispense drugs in Minnesota? Does our state law specify that patients be counseled in person, face-to-face, when presenting prescription orders for fulfillment? How many states impose patient age restrictions on the sale of anorectic agents? Where are electronically transmitted prescriptions permitted, such as telefacsimiles? Do some states prohibit prescriber ownership of pharmacies? Can penalties be imposed on pharmacists for the sale of drug paraphernalia? Is patient consent required before a generic drug can be substituted for a brand name product prescribed?

In addition, the *Pharmacy Law Digest* includes textual discussion sections dedicated to laws governing controlled substances, pharmacy inspection, civil liability, and business practices. Another section on Court Cases provides synopses of important lawsuits pertaining to pharmacy practice. Useful bibliographies conclude each section, and a detailed index enhances access to the entire looseleaf volume, which is updated periodically, as needed. Appendices include a glossary of terms, the United States Constitution, and a name-and-address directory of State Boards of Pharmacy.

4.31 *Survey of Pharmacy Law*. Washington, DC: National Association of Boards of Pharmacy, 1942–. Annual.

The NABP's annual *Survey of Pharmacy Law* compiles information in four sections dedicated to organizational law, licensing law, drug law, and census data.

It includes summary data about important issues such as prescribing and dispensing authority, pharmacy technicians, facsimile and electronic transmission of prescriptions, and patient counseling requirements. Tables and charts assist cross-state comparisons. The *Pharmacy Law Digest*, with its more detailed explanations and broader scope, is, however, a better candidate for a core drug information collection.

4.32 *NABLAW*. Washington, DC: National Association of Boards of Pharmacy. Annual.

NABLAW® is a databank of state pharmacy laws and regulations issued on CD-ROM by NABP. Annual subscriptions include two interim updates and can accommodate site licensing for multi-user access, if desired.

4.33 *Special State Supplement: Approved Drug Products and Legal Requirements. Supplement to Vol. 3 of U.S. Pharmacopeia Dispensing Information*. Rockville, MD: United States Pharmacopeial Convention, 1989–. Annual.

Included as part of a subscription to Volume 3 of *USP DI* (4.43), the *Special State Supplement* reproduces selected portions of the subscriber's state pharmacy practice act and regulations affecting dispensing, including product selection and generic substitution guidelines.

Liability in alleged cases of dispensing errors is likely to be the subject of many questions directed to drug information specialists. What happens when the wrong drug is dispensed? Or if the correct medication is delivered, but in an incorrect strength or with inappropriate directions? Where can a pharmacist, or lawyer, find out more about such potential malpractice issues?

4.34 Brushwood DB. *Medical Malpractice Pharmacy Law*. Colorado Springs, CO: Shepard's/McGraw-Hill, 1986. Cumulative supplements issued annually.

"Too often I have seen cases involving pharmacists in which attorneys are well intentioned but do not understand the pharmacy profession." Following up this statement of purpose in his introduction to *Medical Malpractice Pharmacy Law*, Brushwood offers an informative overview of facts to remedy the situation. Part One covers the practice of pharmacy, outlining education, organizations, settings and types of practice, and the nature of the literature. Part Two addresses drug control law, Part Three reviews pharmacist professional liability, Part Four discusses medication errors and adverse reactions, and Part Five examines use of scientific principles in drug-related litigation. An excellent book for pharmacists and lawyers alike, Brushwood's volume offers clear, concisely written summaries of key issues, with frequent reference to relevant court decisions affecting questions such as patient confidentiality and generic substitution.

Textbooks commonly used in U.S. pharmaceutical education can also provide an excellent foundation on which to build better-informed information services to pharmacists.

4.35　DeMarco C. *Pharmacy and the Law*. 2nd ed. Germantown, MD: Aspen Systems, 1984.
4.36　Wetherbee H, White BD. *Pharmacy Law Cases and Materials*. St. Paul, MN: West Publishing, 1980.
4.37　Nielsen JR. *Handbook of Federal Drug Law*. 2nd ed. Philadelphia: Lea & Febiger, 1992.
4.38　Strauss S. *The Pharmacist and The Law*. Baltimore: Williams & Wilkins, 1980.

Readable and well-organized, DeMarco's *Pharmacy and the Law* is generally considered a classic text. Part I explains the nature of the law, discussing public versus private and criminal law, legal resources, government organization and function, as well as the adjudicatory process. Part II, dedicated to legal issues in professional practice, addresses licensure, rational drug use, and generic substitution. Parts III–V cover drug laws, controlled substances, and professional liabilities, respectively. An informative table of contents, concluding subject index, and good bibliography help explain this book's continuing stature as required reading in pharmacy school curricula.

One noticeable omission in DeMarco's work is substantive discussion of pertinent business or commercial law. Wetherbee and White, therefore, can be used to supplement DeMarco with their section on business law principles for pharmacists and a chapter on Commercial Paper. Intended for both students and practitioners, Nielson's *Handbook of Federal Drug Law* updates DeMarco and is also designed for use as a course text. One particularly useful feature is self-study examination questions and suggested answers. Finally, despite its 1980 imprint date, Strauss' collection of reprints of monthly columns originally published in *U.S. Pharmacist* will complement textbook coverage. It includes articles on diverse special topics, such as prescribing by veterinarians, legalities in filling out-of-state prescriptions, recommended recordkeeping, and more.

4.39　Appelbe GE, Wingfield J. *Pharmacy Law and Ethics*. 6th ed. London: The Pharmaceutical Press, 1997.

Appelbe and Wingfield provide an outline of laws affecting pharmacy practice in the United Kingdom, including contemporary British regulations related to medicines and poisons. The bulk of their text is devoted to explanation of extensive provisions in the Medicines Act of 1968, with supplementary chapters on the Misuse of Drugs Act of 1971 and the British Poisons Act. Discussion also covers the National Health Service, the Access to Health Records Act, pharmacopeias and other publications, and the impact of the European Community. A chapter on legal decisions affecting pharmacy in the United Kingdom will, no doubt, prove to be useful, since litigation is evidently on the rise following the removal of Crown immunity from National Health Service hospitals in 1991. Also, because of greater official recognition of homeopathic and herbal remedies in Great Britain (compared to the United States), separate sections are devoted to these classes of medicinals. Published in a convenient softbound handbook format, the value of this ready-reference source is enhanced by a very detailed table of contents and an excellent index. A new companion volume, *Practical Exercises in Pharmacy Law and Ethics*, supplies sample problems designed to increase student readers' understanding of key issues.

4.40 Spivey RN, Wertheimer AI, Rucker TD, eds. *International Pharmaceutical Services*. Binghamton, NY: Pharmaceutical Product Press, 1992.

International Pharmaceutical Services outlines pharmacy practice in twenty-three countries, encompassing dispensing, recordkeeping, formularies, reimbursement, and patient education. Coverage includes an industry overview for each country, with discussion of drug patents, licensing, and regulations governing product approvals, advertising and promotion, pricing, competition, imports, and exports. Healthcare systems descriptions for each nation highlight historical developments, the social, political, and economic environment, as well as facilities and manpower demographics. Strengths, weaknesses, and trends are assessed in this context. When applicable, contributing authors from each country also discuss use of traditional (indigenous, non-Western) remedies and healing systems. Each chapter offers numerous graphs, figures, and tables, accompanied by references and selected readings. Extensive subject indexing and the expert evaluations of individuals contributing to this ambitious work make it a recommended text for pharmacy collections and drug industry analysts and strategists.

The American Society of Consultant Pharmacists has contributed an outstanding resource for practitioners in U.S. nursing homes and other long-term care facilities.

4.41 *Pharmacy Legislation Regulations Guidelines for Long-Term Care*. Arlington, VA: American Society of Consultant Pharmacists, 1992.

After summarizing the main provisions of the Medicaid Drug Rebate Law (OBRA '90) and the Medicare-Medicaid AntiFraud and Abuse Amendments of 1977, this ASCP publication discusses, in plain language, business and payment practices that would not be treated as criminal offenses (known as "safe harbors") and those which would raise red flags among enforcement personnel as indicators of potential abuse. This information-packed source also covers DEA regulations for filling prescription orders and filing reports on schedule II drugs, as well as destruction of controlled substances. With repackaging increasingly common in this type of pharmacy practice, liabilities associated with packaging and repackaging are outlined, with particular attention to labeling for expiration dating. What are the consultant pharmacist's responsibilities in federally mandated nursing home resident assessments? Practical guidance is, once again, available for fulfilling these requirements, accompanied by discussion on auditing patient drug regimens to prevent/detect overprescribing, abuse, or medication errors. Unusually thorough treatment is also accorded Occupational Safety and Health Administration regulations, including applicability of, and exemptions from, OSHA's Hazard Communication Standards and OSHA rules regarding bloodborne pathogens.

OSHA Hazard Communication Standards and MSDS

OSHA standards may, of course, be the topic of inquiry outside long-term care settings. They migrated from the manufacturing sector to healthcare delivery sites in 1990 and require employers, including pharmacies, to inform workers about chemical hazards to which they may be exposed. OSHA-mandated hazard communication programs rely on container labeling, material safety data sheets (MSDS), and training to warn workers of potential health effects. Although both prescription and OTC drugs packaged for sale to consumers in a retail setting are exempt from MSDS requirements, those used for compounding or extemporaneous formulation onsite are not. This distinction means that employees involved in preparation of parenterals or of antineoplastic mixtures for use in chemotherapy are entitled to a data sheet and hazard training. As a result, hospital pharmacies are most likely to be impacted by OSHA requirements. Fortunately, solid drug dosage forms ready for administration to patients, whether packaged or not, are exempt, as are medications in unit-dose containers, both solid and liquid, and biologics, such as vaccines.

Apart from these broad guidelines, it is often difficult for pharmacists to determine when an MSDS must be supplied to employees and "downstream users," e.g., nursing facilities to which medications are dispensed. Drug manufacturers have tended to provide material safety data sheets with their products, whether needed or not. Which of these should actually be backed up by pharmacist employers with full hazard communication program compliance procedures is, therefore, sometimes in question. The general rule of thumb is to consult the package insert for a drug, checking for statements about potential topical irritation, sensitization, mutagenicity, carcinogenicity, or organ system damage after repeated topical or airborne exposure. All of these effects are indicators that the product may fall within the definition of a hazardous chemical subject to OSHA communication standards. When an MSDS is available (these may be requested from drug manufacturers or wholesalers, if not automatically supplied), the physical and health hazards section will identify if a product should actually be considered a hazardous chemical. Many pharmacists simply retain every MSDS supplied. This practice does not ensure inspection-proof compliance, because it does not fulfill additional OSHA program requirements for training, special labeling, and dissemination of data sheets, when appropriate, to downstream users.

Feinberg[17] offers succinct and practical advice on compliance in pharmacy settings, although her summary does not refer to commercial sources of generic (rather than manufacturer-specific) material safety data sheets, such as the *CHEMTOX Online* (14.30) database or *OHS MSDS* (14.31). These can be extremely helpful when checking the status of hazardous chemicals, including information on state and other federal regulations that may apply to specific substances. Other sources identified in the appendix to the official standard[18] as means to evaluate the hazards of chemicals include *The Merck Index* (3.5) and several publications discussed in Chapter Eight, such as *Clinical Toxicology of Commercial Products* (8.8), *Casarett and Doull's Toxicology* (8.12), *RTECS* (8.33, 14.28), *IARC Monographs* (8.39), and *Threshold Limit Values* (8.45) issued by the American Conference of Governmental Industrial Hygienists.

OBRA and PDMA

Among other federal regulations affecting pharmacy practice in the United States, OBRA has had, perhaps, the broadest impact, due to its mandate for patient counseling of Medicare and Medicaid recipients. The American Pharmaceutical Association's *Patient Counseling Handbook* (9.42) specifically addresses OBRA requirements and includes a checklist to assist the pharmacist in this process. Provisions of the Prescription Drug Marketing Act of 1987 (PDMA) may also be the topic of information requests. Its intent was to reduce public health risks that occur when approved drugs are diverted from legitimate commercial channels. States must license wholesale distributors and enforce minimum standards for storage, handling, and recordkeeping. PDMA bans the sale, trade, or purchase of drug samples and trafficking in discount drug coupons.

Changes in pharmacy practice at the local level have also been accelerated by the Drug Price Competition and Patent Term Restoration Act of 1984. Previous discussion of this landmark legislation focused on its effects on the approval process and reducing drug lag. However, in the context of pharmacy law, its primary influence has been in the controversial area of generic substitution.

Generic Substitution

Generic drugs now account for 45% of prescriptions filled, compared to 14% in 1985.[19] All fifty states have enacted laws governing drug product selection and use a formulary as the basis for allowable substitution of generics for brand name preparations. Laws differ only on points such as whether prior notification or consent of the prescriber or patient is required for substitution and how that consent is conveyed (e.g., "no substitution" box on prescription form). The *Pharmacy Law Digest* (4.30) provides a quick-reference table covering details of substitution laws in specific states.

Formularies were originally "recipe books" compiled to provide information needed to compound, or formulate, drug preparations and to establish standards of quality and strength. With extemporaneous compounding largely outmoded by modern mass production of pharmaceuticals, formularies began to play a different role in pharmacy practice dating from the late 1940s. Hospitals frequently developed their own formularies to influence prescribing practices. Pharmacy and Therapeutics (P&T) committees at individual institutions evaluated available alternatives to treat conditions most commonly encountered in patients admitted. They then selected preferred products to be stocked in their pharmacy, and compiled professional package insert information into their own hospital formulary. It was felt that such publications encouraged rational prescribing practice and helped control costs through limiting in-house drug inventories and permitting bulk purchases at discount of commonly used medications through predetermination of branded products.

Passage of the Drug Price Competition and Patent Term Restoration Act in 1984 and the advent of new third-party reimbursement plans such as Health Maintenance Organizations (HMOs) and Preferred Provider Organizations (PPOs) have rapidly transformed the product selection process in the past decade. Insurance coverage of prescription drug costs began to be limited to formularies developed by HMOs and PPOs, rather than hospital P&T committees. Therapeutic decisions and product selection responsibilities have gradually shifted from individual prescribers and dispensers to managed care organizations and, in the case of Medicaid, to state government authorities. The new generation of formularies are far removed from their origins as aids in formulation, having evolved simply into lists of allowable (reimbursable) products.

Because the following FDA publication is used as a basis for formulary selection decisions by states, it should be considered a core reference for any drug information collection.

4.42 *Approved Drug Products with Therapeutic Equivalence Evaluations.* Rockville, MD: U.S. Food and Drug Administration, 1985–. Annual, with monthly supplements.

Known as *The Orange Book*, this resource identifies drugs on the market that have been approved on the basis of safety and efficacy requirements instituted in 1962. It omits drugs approved only on the basis of safety (i.e., covered by the ongoing Drug Efficacy Study review) and also excludes grandfathered pre-1938 products. Its primary purpose is to provide information to states regarding generic drugs acceptable as candidates for substitution formularies. Equivalence evaluations (positive = A or negative = B) are included for all multisource approved drug products. It's important to remember, however, that *Orange Book* bioequivalence ratings are not binding under generic substitution laws, in that they do not preempt state decisions regarding formulary inclusion. Lobbying of state formulary boards by brand name companies can be influential in excluding *Orange Book* A-rated products as acceptable for substitution.

The basic arrangement of *The Orange Book* is alphabetic by nonproprietary

(USAN) name of active ingredients, but the list is divided into separate sections for Rx, OTC, biologics, and discontinued drugs. Fortunately, a single index offers integrated access to the more than 9,000 products via brand names cross referenced to generic names. Also included is a product nonproprietary name list arranged by applicant (manufacturer). Product entries in each section list active ingredients, dosage forms, route of administration, strengths, product names, application holders, approval application numbers, and approval date (1982 forward). A separate listing identifies ANDA Suitability Petitions approved and denied.

Appendices include a cumulative list of products and indications granted orphan status, with full sponsor addresses. An Addendum identifies drugs that qualify for market exclusivity as mandated under the provisions of the 1984 Drug Price Competition and Patent Term Restoration Act, including a compilation of patent numbers and expiration dates. Unfortunately, although monthly updating is scheduled for *The Orange Book*, a three- to four-month lag time makes this a poor source for up-to-date information on product approvals. (Refer to the discussion of regulatory sources online in Chapter Sixteen for comprehensive access to approved drug products.)

The latest edition of *The Orange Book* and its cumulative supplements is among options offered under the Human Drugs icon on the *FDA Home Page* (http://www.fda.gov/cder).

4.43 *Approved Drug Products and Legal Requirements. Vol. 3 of U.S. Pharmacopeia Dispensing Information.* Rockville, MD: United States Pharmacopeial Convention, 1989–. Annual, with monthly updates.

Contents of *The Orange Book* are also integrated into volume 3 of *USP DI* (see also 6.5), where information is augmented with a separate listing of B-rated drugs, a list of pre-1938 grandfathered products, and selections from *USP-NF* (11.8) monographs related to requirements for labeling, packaging, and quality. This volume also reprints portions of federal regulations regarding controlled substances, good manufacturing practice for finished pharmaceuticals, and the Poison Prevention Packaging Act. Monthly updates include cumulative *Orange Book* supplements, as well as six-month cumulative lists of drug product recalls and new USAN designations. Parts of each state's pharmacy practice act and regulations for dispensing, including product selection guidelines, are issued in a separate supplement to subscribers in that state (4.33).

Medical Device Regulation

Many pharmaceutical companies are engaged in the manufacture of medical devices, as well as drugs, and pharmacists are involved in the distribution and sale of certain types of devices. It follows that information professionals serving both groups are likely to be asked to help answer questions about devices. Szycher[20] supplies an excellent introductory overview of medical devices in the *Encyclopedia of Pharmaceutical Technology*.

What is a medical device? It is defined in U.S. law as an instrument, apparatus, implement, machine, implant, *in vitro* reagent, or other "contrivance" used in health care that is not dependent upon being metabolized to achieve its intended purpose. This definition covers an incredibly diverse group of therapeutic and diagnostic aids, including artificial organs and other prostheses, infusion pumps, respiratory therapy equipment, wound dressings, home test kits, renal dialysis machines, dental anesthetic needles, intravenous fluid pouches, and stethoscopes. New drug delivery systems, such as subcutaneous controlled-release implants, combine a device component with chemical action in the body, blurring the thin dividing line between drugs and devices drawn for regulatory purposes.

The distinction between the two has not always been so narrow. Although the 1938 Food, Drug, and Cosmetic Act (FDC) included devices in its coverage, subjecting them to the same adulteration and misbranding standards as drugs, when devices were omitted from regulatory requirements for premarketing submission of proof of safety, this first law ostensibly governing devices established a broad boundary between the two forms of therapy. Kefauver-Harris Amendments tightened drug regulations in 1962, but, once again, did not extend more stringent controls to include device premarket clearance procedures.

As more and more consumers came into contact with the contributions of engineering to biomedicine and were exposed to new biomaterials made possible with the introduction of synthetic polymers, problems inevitable in a largely unregulated industry began to surface. The National Heart and Lung Institute issued a report in 1970 that cited more than 10,000 injuries caused by medical devices and documented in the literature. In 1973 and 1975, several Congressional hearings gathered evidence to gauge the extent of regulatory control needed. Possible hazards associated with intrauterine devices, pacemakers, indwelling catheters, and dental devices mentioned in witness testimony drew widespread press coverage and resulted in renewed efforts to pass legislation languishing in committee since its proposal in 1971. The outcome was enactment of the Medical Device Amendments to FDC in 1976.

These Amendments established a three-tiered system for regulating device introductions to the marketplace (pre-1976 grandfathered devices are exempt). Class I devices, judged to be low risk (e.g., thermometers, nebulizers, periodontal syringes), are subject only to general control requirements, including registration of manufacturing sites, product listing with the FDA, and adherence to good manufacturing practices. Class II devices are those for which general controls are deemed insufficient to assure safety and efficacy, based on the potential risk to health posed by their use. The FDA develops mandatory performance standards as additional special controls for regulating Class II devices, which include items

such as x-ray machines, hearing aids, gastrointestinal irrigation systems, electro-
cardiographs, and percutaneous catheters.

To obtain authorization to market across state lines in the United States, manufacturers of Class I and II devices that are substantially equivalent to those on the
market prior to 1976 need submit only a "premarket notification" (PMN) describing device specifications and characteristics. This notification, dubbed a
510k after the relevant section of the 1976 law, is usually reviewed and passed
by the FDA within 120–180 days of filing.

Much more stringent regulations apply to Class III devices. These products,
which include life-supporting, implanted, and other devices with a potential for
significant risk to users, are subject to a premarket application (PMA) process
comparable to that required for new drugs (see Figure 4.5). PMA submissions
must include proof of safety and efficacy demonstrated in clinical trials. Before
testing in humans can commence, manufacturers of Class III devices must submit
an application for Investigational Device Exemption (IDE), a procedure similar
to the IND requirement for drug clinical trial authorization.

The 1976 Amendments also authorized the FDA to institute a mandatory adverse event reporting system, but regulations establishing such a system were not

Figure 4.5   Outline of the Medical Device Approval Process in the United States

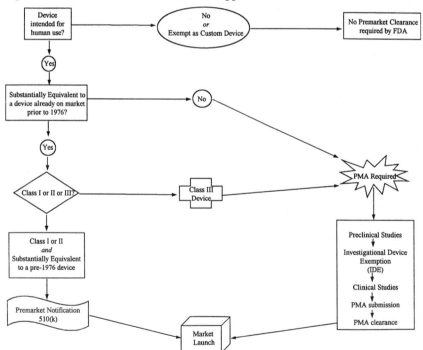

finalized until December 1984. Since that time, manufacturers and importers of medical devices must report to the FDA any incident where their product may have caused or contributed to a serious injury or may have malfunctioned. These brief descriptions of adverse events are known as MDRs (Medical Device Reports) and are frequently the subject of inquiry.

Monitoring the incidence of MDR citations to a given company, to a group of devices similar in their design and therapeutic application, or to a specific product can provide information important to legal investigators, prospective purchasers, insurers, and industry investment analysts, as well as manufacturers exploring the possibility of extending their product line. Market researchers and device developers survey MDRs to identify potential defects to avoid in designing new, competitive products and to assess perhaps unavoidable hazards and consequent product liability costs.

Reports of adverse effects associated with a well-known heart valve and with silicone breast implants pointed to the need for tighter regulatory controls. The Safe Medical Devices Act of 1990 strengthened FDA enforcement authority and expanded premarket clearance requirements. Mandatory MDR submissions now apply not only to manufacturers and importers, but also to distributors and user facilities, including hospitals, nursing homes, outpatient treatment facilities, and even individual physicians. Additional post-marketing surveillance may also be ordered by the FDA for designated devices, such as permanent implants, necessitating protocols for systematic study of safety and efficacy data after commercialization. The Act also authorizes civil penalties against manufacturers in the form of fines for violations of FDC provisions. Preproduction design validation has been added to GMP requirements and premarket approval inspections stepped up. Alleged violations have delayed clearance for more than 25% of PMAs in recent years.

Another important change affects the 510k process. Manufacturers must now obtain a "substantial equivalence" order from the FDA before beginning distribution, which means that more information is now required in premarket notifications than ever before. A thorough survey of the literature and of manufacturer data available on the predicate device showing its safety and efficacy must be certified and summarized, along with submission of information demonstrating comparability in design, technological characteristics, and intended use. The initial effect of the new regulatory requirements was a slowdown in 510k authorizations and, in many cases, a shift to full PMA preparation and submission for many more products. However, through a program of systematic reclassification, the FDA has also exempted many low-risk medical devices from premarket review. By February 1996, more than 550 categories of products, representing nearly three-fourths of all Class I devices and one-third of all those classified, could be marketed without prior agency clearance. Unimpeded commercialization is authorized for items such as examination lights, patient scales, pacemaker chargers, and dental floss.

Medical Device Amendments enacted in 1992 gave the FDA enforcement authority for both mandatory and discretionary post-market surveillance studies. The types of adverse events that must be reported (MDRs) were spelled out, for the first time, in these amendments, which also codified a new, broader statutory definition of serious injury. Subsequent regulations authorized under the 1992 legislation specify more than twenty types of devices subject to mandatory post-approval tracking, including vascular graft and tracheal prostheses, pacemakers, implantable defibrillators and infusion pumps, breathing frequency monitors, and silicone-filled prostheses. The objective of newly mandated tracking rules is to protect consumers by enabling manufacturers to locate users, should a product problem be discovered.

What does all this mean to the information seeker and provider? More questions arise when more people are affected by the law. Many queries about devices will, in fact, focus on information needed for regulatory compliance or require access to data readily available only in FDA documents. Knowledge of the marketing authorization process and of specialized terminology used to refer to important factors in that process should prompt you to ask appropriate questions in order to clarify what information is needed and to solicit background on the rationale behind a request that may influence the format and content of your response. If an inquiry involves locating device approvals, familiarity with government regulations is important in resource selection, since the legal classification of a device (I, II, or III, 510k or PMA) influences the type and amount of information available and the terminology needed to retrieve it.

Another type of question to anticipate relates to device authorizations in the European Community. Under the EC Medical Devices Directive of 1995 (effective June 1998), companies must obtain a CE mark to indicate their product's compliance with safety requirements outlined in Union law and consequent clearance to market throughout the EC. Non-CE-marked devices in the supply chain before the effective date can, however, be sold until June 30, 2001. As with EC drug law, official registration does not necessarily equate to unimpeded trade until reimbursement authorities in targeted markets accept a given product. Some countries have imposed further requirements for additional quality assurance imprimaturs beyond the CE mark. The result has been frustration on the part of manufacturers and confusion on the part of practitioners. At minimum, you may be asked to confirm CE mark and International Standards Organization (ISO) status for a given device. Such questions can be answered by consulting the *Medical Device Register* (13.8, 15.24) or by calling the manufacturer.

The Mutual Recognition Agreement (MRA) effective in December 1998 also promises to be a topic of inquiry. MRA is intended to facilitate transatlantic trade by reducing costs to governments of implementing separate regulatory requirements. The agreement will enable participating countries to rely on one another's enforcement procedures regarding good manufacturing practices for medical devices. The first step in accomplishing this goal is mutual acceptance of various government groups as Conformity Assessment Bodies or CABs, enabling them to serve as third party reviewers for licensing applications by companies who wish to market devices in designated jurisdictions. Some of the existing European notified bodies under EC drug and device law will be selected by the FDA as CABs for EC companies seeking 510k clearance in the United States. In parallel, U.S.-based CABs will stand in for EC reviewers to expedite U.S. companies' obtaining CE marks for their products and meeting ISO standards. The first three years under MRA have been referred to as a confidence building period, during which regulators will exchange information on premarket notifications, reports of inspections and adverse events, and evaluations of quality systems controls.

4.44 *The 510(k) Register.* 2 v. Rockville, MD: Diogenes, 1986–. Annual.

Produced by the publishers of the online database *Diogenes* (16.1), *The 510(k) Register* offers a complete listing of the more than 79,000 premarket notifications cleared by the FDA since May 1976. Entries are indexed by generic product name (e.g., catheter adapter) and by the FDA-assigned 510k number, both cross-referenced to a third, company name index. Listings under each company name are arranged by K numbers and include product name and therapeutic class, FDA determination date, and substantial equivalence decision. Company names have been standardized and edited to facilitate access. Two appendices offer assistance in locating categories of products: through a permuted keyword index to FDA codes, and by listing codes under pertinent FDA Advisory Panel or Committee names (e.g., immunology, hematology, orthopedic panels, etc.). Individual monthly updates issued between each annual, cumulative edition of *The 510(k) Register* are available at the FDA Web site and through the *Diogenes* database.

The most up-to-date and complete source of PMA device approvals is a newsletter known as *The Gray Sheet*, where notices are usually indexed within one week of FDA announcement.

4.45 *Medical Devices, Diagnostics, and Instrumentation Reports: The Gray Sheet.* Chevy Chase, MD: F-D-C Reports, 1975–. Weekly.

In addition to coverage of all original and supplemental PMAs authorized by the FDA, *The Gray Sheet* is legendary for its timely and thorough reporting of other device industry news, including commentary on regulatory developments, other relevant FDA activities such as Advisory Panel meetings, company sales performance and personnel changes, and device recalls. This newsletter is also available online as part of the *F-D-C Reports* database (15.10).

4.46 *Diogenes FDA Medical Devices on Cd-ROM.* Rockville, MD: Diogenes, 1993–. Quarterly.

A subset of the *Diogenes* (16.1) online database, *FDA Medical Devices on Cd-ROM* lists all 510k notifications and PMA approvals. It also includes the full text of Medical Device Reports (MDRs). Annual subscriptions offer quarterly updates consisting of a single, cumulative replacement compact disc accessible through SilverPlatter software.

All publicly available regulatory source material related to medical devices is accessible online. Refer to Chapter Sixteen for a discussion of key databases, which include: *Diogenes*, *F-D-C Reports*, *Health Devices Alerts*, the *Federal Register*, and the *FDA Home Page* on the Internet. These online sources extend the scope of document coverage to include not only 510ks, PMAs, MDRs, and device recalls, but also FDA Guidelines, Warning Letters, Establishment Inspection Reports, background documents related to recalls, and Summaries of Safety & Efficacy (SS&E, comparable to the Summary Basis of Approval or SBA issued for new drugs).

4.47 *Shepherd's System for Medical Device Incident Investigation & Reporting.* Brea, CA: Quest Publishing, 1992–.

Shepherd's System™ is designed to guide medical centers, manufacturers, importers, and distributors through incident investigation, analysis, and FDA-mandated reporting requirements, with an objective of minimizing liability exposure and preventing future incidents. Updated periodically as needed, the looseleaf binder includes the full text of government reporting and tracking regulations, along with detailed discussion of responsibilities for training, recordkeeping, and developing organizational policy and procedures.

4.48 Matsutani Y, ed. *Medical Device Regulations in Japan.* Tokyo: Yakuji Nippon, 1993.

Compiled to answer typical questions regarding relevant regulations in Japan, this book explains the application process for device approval, good clinical practice for trials, testing methods for electrical medical devices, safety requirements, and import licensing procedures. Manufacturers and traders interested in tapping into the lucrative Japanese market for devices are likely to benefit from these English-language guidelines prepared by the director of the medical device division of the Ministry of Health and Welfare.

Keeping Up-to-Date on Regulatory Developments

New sources for monitoring regulatory developments of importance to the pharmaceutical industry are created every year, and many titles also disappear within a few months after their introduction. Those that survive share some important characteristics in common: timeliness (frequency of publication as well as up-to-date reporting), evaluative analysis of events by qualified experts, and good writing that can transform often difficult-to-understand government documents or lengthy Congressional testimony into interesting narrative summaries meaningful to their readers' contextual areas of responsibility. Newsletters that merely cite the availability of FDA documents or tabulate recent agency actions are not good investments, since anyone can produce similar compilations from publicly available online databases today. On the other hand, publications from F-D-C Reports exemplify the best in value-added reporting of healthcare regulatory and business news.

4.49 *Prescription Pharmaceuticals and Biotechnology: The Pink Sheet*. Chevy Chase, MD: F-D-C Reports, 1939–. Weekly.

Prescription Pharmaceuticals and Biotechnology: The Pink Sheet has already been mentioned as the original source of information on new drug and biologic approvals and trademarks now segregated under the separate title *Pharmaceutical Approvals Monthly* (4.19). *The Pink Sheet* has also spawned at least two other specialty newsletters (4.52–4.53) in the course of its long and successful publication history, during which it has undergone three title changes (*Ethical and OTC Pharmaceuticals* until 1982, *Prescription and OTC Pharmaceuticals* until 1993). It is highly respected for thorough reporting on regulatory affairs, sales data, significant R&D advances, and virtually all news affecting the ethical drug industry in the United States, making it a core resource for competitive intelligence. *The Pink Sheet* is also an excellent source for notices of product recalls and well-written summaries of trade association activities.

Since its introduction online in 1989, most information professionals will find it easier or more cost-effective to consult in machine-readable format, where the problem of less-than-fully-informative titles listed in the table of contents of each twenty-page hardcopy issue is overcome by full-text keyword accessibility. (Refer to Chapters Fifteen and Sixteen for a discussion of the *F-D-C Reports* database.)

4.50 *FDA Week*. Washington, DC: Inside Washington Publishers, 1995–. Weekly.

4.51 *U.S. Regulatory Reporter*. Waltham, MA: Parexel, 1984–. Monthly.

Inside Washington's *FDA Week* is narrower in scope than *The Pink Sheet*, confining itself to disseminating news of current and forthcoming agency activities. The *U.S. Regulatory Reporter* also focuses solely on FDA activities and, unlike the F-D-C publication, does not analyze commercial implications. Extensive reporting and commentary on significant Congressional events found in *The Pink Sheet* is also omitted in this Parexel publication. The *Reporter*'s pullout sections, literally newsletters-within-newsletters, are entitled "Biologics and Biotech Regulatory Report" and "Regulatory Review." The Review supplement supplies executive summaries of rulings, proposals, approvals, announcements, and other FDA actions. Benchmarking studies of FDA divisional performance are a specialty of the *U.S. Regulatory Reporter*, which also regularly features in-depth interviews with agency drug reviewers and policy-makers. Its monthly, rather than weekly, update schedule reflects an emphasis on retrospective analysis.

4.52 *Nonprescription Pharmaceuticals and Nutritionals: The Tan Sheet.* Chevy Chase, MD: F-D-C Reports, 1993–. Weekly.

4.53 *Toiletries, Fragrances, and Skin Care: The Rose Sheet.* Chevy Chase, MD: F-D-C Reports, 1980–. Weekly.

Both *The Tan Sheet* and *The Rose Sheet* are part of the full-text *F-D-C Reports* database online (15.10). Each was originally a spin-off of *The Pink Sheet* (4.49), necessitated by the volume of government and trade activity to be reported in each of their respective markets and the seemingly insatiable demands of regulatory and market research personnel in industry for up-to-date specialty news reporting. Coverage of *Nonprescription Pharmaceuticals and Nutritionals* includes FDA and Federal Trade Commission (FTC) activities, enforcement actions (warning letters, recalls), relevant Congressional hearings, and a broad spectrum of business and financial news: e.g., Rx to OTC switches, litigation regarding advertising claims, product testing results, company stock performance, sales and earnings reports, and regular listings of trademarks. *Toiletries, Fragrances, and Skin Care* has a comparable scope, adding in news of new product launches (omitted in *The Tan Sheet* because OTC introductions are included, instead, in *Pharmaceutical Approvals Monthly*, 4.21).

4.54 *Quality Control Reports: The Gold Sheet.* Chevy Chase, MD: F-D-C Reports, 1967–. Monthly.

It should be evident from discussion earlier in this chapter that the Food and Drug Administration's preference for informal communication of manufacturing and related quality control standards means that enforcement documents such as Warning Letters and Establishment Inspection Reports require close monitoring. This task is the function and forte of *Quality Control Reports: The Gold Sheet.* Not only does this newsletter alert readers to the availability and content of these FDA documents, but it also identifies trends and evaluates their potential effects on production and profitability. This valuable resource is also available on CD-ROM. Good complements to *The Gold Sheet* for current awareness by quality control professionals are two newsletters from Washington Business Information, *Drug GMP Report* and *The GMP Letter* (devices), accessible online in the *Diogenes* database (16.1)

4.55 *Health News Daily.* Chevy Chase, MD: F-D-C Reports, 1989–. Daily.

Published each business day, *Health News Daily* is, in many ways, a precursor of other F-D-C newsletters, highlighting Congressional and FDA activities that will often be reported upon again, perhaps in fuller format, in *The Pink Sheet* (4.49), *The Gray Sheet* (4.45), etc. In executive briefing style, major events are summarized in each six- to seven-page issue. Although the emphasis is on legislative and regulatory developments, selected late-breaking business news items are also covered, such as mergers and acquisitions or management personnel changes. Brief notes on litigation and jurisprudence are often included, along with a calendar of forthcoming meetings of professional societies and government advisory bodies scheduled in "Washington This Week." *Health News Daily* is available in both paper and fax subscriptions, as well in full-text format for *ad hoc* access online (15.11).

4.56 *Health Policy and Biomedical Research: The Blue Sheet.* Chevy Chase, MD: F-D-C Reports, 1957–. Weekly.

The Blue Sheet focuses on government health policy coverage related to clinical and basic biomedical research, public health professions education and supply, funding, and ethics. Weekly issues typically include announcements of industry/academia collaborations (e.g., clinical trials, outcomes research), reports of hearings on Capitol Hill, requests for proposals (RFPs) and grants awards, and discussion of public health trends. The latter often contains valuable epidemiologic statistics. Regularly-issued supplements compile detailed listings of RFPs, grants, and contracts awarded by the U.S. National Institutes of Health. NIH research grants are organized by broad subject categories, such as aging, alcohol abuse, child health, and diabetes (there is no separate category for drug-related investigations). Each entry identifies the grant recipient (academic or corporate institution/organization) and location, chief investigator name, topic to be studied, and amount awarded. Selective coverage is also given in the Supplement section to the availability of health-related government-owned inventions available for licensing. *The Blue Sheet* is a particularly good source for early news of clinical trials and of clinical practice guidelines. This publication is among the family of full-text newsletters also available in the *F-D-C Reports* (15.10) database online. Complementary online resources with a similar subject orientation include the *Washington Drug Letter* in *Diogenes* (16.1) and *Health Legislation & Regulation* in the *IAC Newsletter Database* (15.15).

4.57 *Weekly Pharmacy Reports: The Green Sheet.* Chevy Chase, MD: F-D-C Reports, 1951–. Weekly.

Rounding out the long list of F-D-C current awareness sources is *Weekly Pharmacy Reports: The Green Sheet.* Each four-page issue highlights federal and state government legislation and regulation related to the profession, as well as activities of national and state pharmacy associations, reimbursement and drug pricing issues, and new drug introductions. This type of subject coverage is not replicated anywhere else, but complementary resources with a trade (community or retail setting) slant include the magazines *Drug Topics* and *American Druggist*.

4.58 *ERA News.* Richmond, Surrey, England: European Pharma Law Centre, 1991–. Monthly.

4.59 *The Regulatory Affairs Journal.* Camberley, Surrey, England: Regulatory Affairs Journals Ltd, 1992–. Monthly.

The European Pharma Law Centre (EPLC) provides its subscribers with a monthly newsletter dedicated to reporting on the regulatory situation in the various EC countries and differences between them. Coverage also includes the outcome of legal suits at the national level and in the European Court of Justice, the structure and organization of national healthcare systems, as well as individual governments' policies regarding pricing and reimbursement, control of clinical trials, intellectual property protection, advertising, competition and company law, the environment, and occupational health and safety. Articles are aimed at senior managers who are not necessarily legally trained, but who are interested in the development of the pharmaceutical industry in Europe. Hardcopy publication began in 1991, and the full text of *ERA News* (formerly entitled *EPLC Update*) was added to the *PHIND* (15.9) database online in 1996, with retrospective coverage dating from March 1994.

The Regulatory Affairs Journal (RAJ) is broader in scope, with contributions from news correspondents located in forty-five countries constituting nineteen key markets. In addition to reporting on changes in global pharmaceutical regulations, *RAJ* provides expert commentary and guidance on their significance and practical implementation in each of its seventy-page issues. A six-year full-text archive of this journal is also searchable on CD-ROM, where it is updated quarterly. Owned by PJB Publications (suppliers of *Scrip* and *Clinica*), the publisher also issues a *RAJ-Devices* journal.

Summary: Implications for the Information Provider

What emerges from this chapter's review is the extraordinarily close relationship between regulatory developments and business outcomes. Most publications designed to keep readers up-to-date on government activities affecting the drug, device, and related industries also analyze their commercial implications, for reasons that should, at this point, be fairly obvious. Additional candidate titles for tracking business-related regulatory, legislative, and judicial news online are identified in Chapter Fifteen. Figure 4.6 is a selective survey of pertinent sites on the Internet. In-depth discussion of the *FDA Home Page* is reserved for Chapter Sixteen, where it is examined in the context of other regulatory databases.

Gaining familiarity with regulatory milestones and recent issues, as well as the specialized terminology used, is essential to effective drug information provision. Disclosure and availability of requested information is linked with the drug and device development process, which, if well understood, can assist in resource selection and access methodologies employed, including appropriate nomenclature. The next chapter delves further into the topic of resource selection, examining types of literature available and major factors to consider when evaluating the bibliography.

Figure 4.6   Legal and Regulatory Specialty Sites on the Internet

- *Biotech Law Web Server*
  ⇨ http://www2.ari.net/foley
  Maintained by the law firm of Foley & Lardner (Jacksonville, Florida), this site is a pathfinder to others of potential interest, providing informative annotations about their scope and content. It also features news items and numerous full-text commentaries and analyses related to patent law. For example, an IP Resource Center provides free access to articles from the *Biotechnology Law Report* about recent legislative fine-tuning of patent terms, about searching for prior art on the Internet, and about the impact of electronic publication on patent rights. Other menu options include a patent primer (U.S.), a European intellectual property (IP) law page, and a Therapeutics page.

- *European Medicines Evaluation Agency (EMEA)*
  ⇨ http://www.eudra.org
  The EMEA Web site offers the full text of all European Public Assessment Reports (EPARs), as well as agency guidelines and standard operating procedures, a calendar of forthcoming meetings, and a directory of personnel.

- *FDA Home Page*
  ⇨ http://www.pjbpubs.co.uk/eplc/eplc.html.
  See Chapter Sixteen, Regulatory Resources Online, for a detailed discussion.

- *Food and Drug Law Institute*
  ⇨ http://www.fdli.org
  The catalog of publications at this site includes detailed descriptions, tables of contents, and sample pages for preview. Back issues of *FDLI Update*, a bimonthly newsletter, can be downloaded in PDF format (1997 +). After a moratorium of six months, tables of contents and article abstracts of archived issues of the *Food and Drug Law Journal* are also available free of charge from 1993 forward. This site's Academic section includes a hot-linked list of law schools offering food and drug law courses, as well. Under Services, the well-annotated directory of related Internet resources goes beyond the standard inventory of government URLs to include associations, legal document centers, and other pathfinders.

- *HIMA (Health Industry Manufacturers Association)*
  ⇨ http://www.himanet.com
  HIMA's Industry Topics icon leads to many press releases, commentary, and position papers regarding FDA actions. This site also provides detailed descriptions of major publications, such as the *1997 Global Medical Technology Update* and the *HIMA Emerging Market Report*. Other features include a dictionary of medical technology acronyms and an unannotated, but thorough, Links section.

- *National Association of Boards of Pharmacy*
  ⇨ http://www.nabp.net
  Under a "Who We Are" option, you'll find a complete directory of boards of pharmacy responsible for official licensure of pharmacists. The list includes all states, U.S. protectorates, Canada, Australia, and New Zealand. A *PPAD™* icon leads to the *Pharmacist and Pharmacy Achievement and Discipline Database*, where a search for named individuals or establishments can find a history of disciplinary action, if any (probation, suspension or revocation of license, etc.).

- *Pharmaceutical Online Regulatory and Legislative Issues Index*
  ⇨ http://news.pharmaceuticalonline.com/regulatory-articles
  Look here for timely reporting of key court decisions and important FDA actions, as well as new drug approvals. *Pharmaceutical Online*'s Web Resource Center shows ratings by users of hotlinked sites.

- *Pharmacy Times Callout Column*
  ⇨ http://www.pharmacytimes/callout.html
  The *Callout* column in this monthly retail magazine focuses on cases studies in pharmacy practice law.

- *RAinfo*
  ⇨ http://www.medmarket.com/tenants/rainfo/rainfo.htm
  Don Kafader's legendary subject hub is designed to provide a comprehensive set of links to regulatory-related Internet sites worldwide focusing on drugs and devices. Information is organized into four categories: U.S., Rest of World, ICH (harmonization), and MOUs (Memoranda of Understanding) between the FDA and other countries. In addition to an FDA matrix, U.S. links include the House, Senate, Judiciary, states, OSHA, DEA, DOT, DEA, FCC, and USDA. An International Sites icon leads to a fully annotated directory.

- *Regulatory Affairs Professionals Society (RAPS) Online*
  ⇨ http://www.raps.org
  RAPS' list of related links offers worldwide coverage by country. The Resource Center (online bookstore) includes government publications dealing with the regulation of biologics, drugs, and medical devices from the United States, Europe, and other countries. Forthcoming conferences, educational opportunities, and job postings round out selections.

- *U.S. Pharmacist*
  ⇨ http://www.uspharmacist.com
  This respected monthly journal now includes a regular column on pharmacy law. A search of back issues (September 1996 +) will also uncover many related feature articles of potential interest. For example, a contribution by Shepard *et al* in the July 1997 issue reviews U.S. versus Mexican drug regulation.

References

1. Shah DN, Goldstein S. New drug applications. In: Swarbrick J, Boylan JC, eds. *Encyclopedia of pharmaceutical technology*. v.10. New York: Marcel Dekker,1994:223–260.

2. Edwards C. Nonprescription drugs. In: Swarbrick J, Boylan JC, eds. *Encyclopedia of pharmaceutical technology*. v.10. New York: Marcel Dekker,1994:283–301.

3. *Generic drug industry handbook*. New York: Lehman Brothers, 1994:5.

4. Panel considers impact of 1984 law on drug development and availability. *BNA Patent, Trademark & Copyright Law Daily* 1996 Mar 6: *BNA Daily News* database record accession no. 00847469.

5. Asbury CH. Orphan drugs. In: Swarbrick J, Boylan JC, eds. *Encyclopedia of pharmaceutical technology*. v.11. New York: Marcel Dekker,1995:161–184.

6. Haffner ME. Orphan drug development update. *Drug Inf J* 1996;30:29–34.

7. USA to adopt fast-track for cancer drugs. *Marketletter* 1996 Apr 8: *IAC PROMT* record no. 06105723.

8. Chowhan ZT. Pharmacopeial harmonization: A progress report. *Drug Inf J* 1996;30:451–459.

9. *Office of Drug Evaluation: Statistical report.* Washington, DC: Food and Drug Administration, 1978–. Annual.

10. *Third annual performance report to Congress, FY95: Prescription Drug User Fee Act of 1992.* Washington, DC: Food and Drug Administration, 1995.

11. Beales JH. Marketing information and pharmaceuticals: New uses for old drugs. In: *Competitive strategies in the pharmaceutical industry.* Washington, DC: American Enterprise Institute, 1996.

12. DiMasi JA, Brown JS, Lasagna L. An analysis of regulatory review times of supplemental indications for already-approved drugs: 1989–1994. *Drug Inf J* 1996;30:315–337.

13. McMann GL. Liability aspects of drugs and devices. In: Swarbrick J, Boylan JC, eds. *Encyclopedia of pharmaceutical technology.* v.8. New York: Marcel Dekker,1993:403–416.

14. Peck JC, Rabin KH, eds. *Regulating change.* Washington, DC: Food and Drug Law Institute, 1989:8.

15. DeMarco C. *Pharmacy and the law.* 2nd ed. Germantown, MD: Aspen Systems, 1984:1.

16. Fink JL, Simonsmeier LM. Laws governing pharmacy. In: Gennaro AR, ed. *Remington's pharmaceutical sciences.* 19th ed. Easton, PA: Mack Publishing, 1995:1892–1912.

17. Feinberg JL. Complying with OSHA's hazard communication standard. *Consult Pharm* 1991 May;6(5):444–448.

18. Hazard communication standard. *29CFR* 1910.1200, Appendix C.

19. Panel considers impact of 1984 law. *BNA Daily News* database record accession no. 00847469.

20. Szycher M. Medical devices. In: Swarbrick J, Boylan JC, eds. *Encyclopedia of pharmaceutical technology.* v.9. New York: Marcel Dekker,1994:263–285.

Additional Sources of Information

Anderson BJ. May pharmacists fill prescription of physician licensed in another state? *JAMA* 1974;227:215.

Angorn RA. Foreign prescriptions: Legal or illegal? *Leg Asp Pharm Pract* 1982 Nov/Dec;5:1–2.

Angorn RA. When is a pharmacist a manufacturer? *Leg Asp Pharm Pract* 1985 Jan/Feb;8:1–3.

Basara LR. Pharmacists, patient education, and OBRA '90: results of a national survey. *APhA Annual Meeting* 1994 Mar;141:97.

Basara LR, Montagne M. *Searching for magic bullets:orphan drugs, consumer activism, and pharmaceutical development.* Binghamton, NY: Pharmaceutical Products Press, 1994.

Bass IS, Young AL. *The Dietary Supplement Health and Education Act: a legislative history and analysis.* Washington, DC: The Food and Drug Law Institute, 1995.

Bogumill MT. Pharmacists' responsibility under the Poison Prevention Packaging Act. *Am J Hosp Pharm* 1992;49:1392,1394.

Brushwood DB. The duty to counsel: Reviewing a decade of litigation. *Drug Intell Clin Pharm* 991;25:195–203.

Brushwood DB. Grounds for revocation or suspension of a pharmacist's license. *Am Pharm* 1982;NS22:574.

Brushwood DB. Liability for unauthorized prescription refills. *US Pharmacist* 1988;13:29–32.

Brushwood DB. An overview of pharmacist malpractice litigation. In: *Pharmacy law annual.* Vienna, VA: American Society for Pharmacy Law, 1988:3–47.

Brushwood DB. Patient injury and attempted link with pharmacist's negligence. *Am J Hosp Pharm* 1993;50:2382–2385.

Brushwood DB. The pharmacist's drug information responsibility after McKee v. American Home Products. *Food Drug Law J* 1993;48:377.

Brushwood DB, Abood RR. Third class of drugs. *US Pharmacist* 1985;10:34,36–39,88.

Campbell NA. Legal implications for the community pharmacist distributing nonprescription drug products. *Contemp Pharm Pract* 1981;4:216–219.

Collins ML, ed. *CANDA 1995: an international regulatory and strategy report.* Waltham, MA: Parexel, 1994.

Compilation of food and drug laws. 2 v. Washington, DC: The Food and Drug Law Institute, 1996.

Coons SJ, Fink JL. The pharmacist, the law and self-testing products. *Am Pharm* 1989;NS29:705.

Currie WJC. *New drug approval in Japan.* Waltham, MA: Parexel, 1998.

Currie WJC, Logren M. *New drug approval in the European Union: The EMEA.* Waltham, MA: Parexel, 1998.

Currie WJC, Logren M. *A practical guide to the EMEA.* Waltham, MA: Parexel, 1996.

De Suso MJG. *New drug approval in Spain.* Waltham, MA: Parexel, 1997.

Donohue TF, Sprouse CR. *Drug formularies and the pharmaceutical industry.* Waltham, MA: Parexel, 1995.

Drugs available under treatment IND. *FDA Drug Bull* 1988 Aug;18:14–15.

Dunne JF. The role of the World Health Organization. In: Pickering WR, ed. *Information sources in pharmaceuticals.* London: Bowker-Saur, 1990:307–336.

Enright SM. Perceived liability [with managed care]. *Am J Hosp Pharm* 1992;49:418–420.

Erickson SH, et al. Use of drugs for unlabeled indications. *JAMA* 1980, 243:1543–1546.

Evens RP, Flynn J, Mapes D. Preventing the pitfalls in planning phase IV clinical trials: a biotechnology experience. *Drug Inf J* 1996;30:583–591.

Evers PT. *New drug approval in the United Kingdom.* Waltham, MA: Parexel, 1995.

FDA interim index to evaluations for prescription drugs as published in the Federal Register. Volume X. Rockville, MD: Food and Drug Administration, Bureau of Drugs, 1982.

FDA interim index to evaluations published in the Federal Register for NAS-NRC reviewed prescription drugs. Volume IX. Cumulative up to Jan 1, 1980. Rockville, MD: Food and Drug Administration, Bureau of Drugs, 1980.

Ferreira I. *New drug approval in Brazil*. Waltham, MA: Parexel, 1995.

Fincham JE, Wertheimer AI. *Pharmacy and the U.S. health care system*. Binghamton, NY: Pharmaceutical Products Press, 1991.

Fink JL. Child-resistant closures: liability concerns. *US Pharmacist* 1988;13:42–45.

Fink JL. Dispensing FDA-approved drugs for non-approved uses. *US Pharmacist* 1977;2:24,26.

Fink JL. Legal issues related to telephoned prescriptions. *Leg Asp Pharm Pract* 1987 Winter;10:10–12.

Fink JL. Review of studies of malpractice claims based on prescribing. *Leg Asp Pharm Pract* 1987 Sep/Oct;10:9–11.

Fink JL. Subpoenas and discovery of pharmacy records. *Am Pharm* 1987;NS27:879–882.

Fleming TR. Surrogate endpoints in clinical trials. *Drug Inf J* 1996;30:545–551.

Foster TS. Drug product selection—part 4: selecting therapeutically equivalent products: special cases. *Am Pharm* 1991;NS31:825–830.

Gardner JS. Post-marketing drug surveillance. *US Pharmacist* 1988;13:40–47.

Greenberg RB. Medical device amendments of 1976. *Am J Hosp Pharm* 1976;33:1308–1311.

Greenberg RB. The Prescription Drug Marketing Act of 1987. *Am J Hosp Pharm* 1988;45:2118–2126.

Hammel RW. The legal status of prescription orders originating in another state. *Am J Pharm* 1978;150:185–190.

Hare D, Foster TS. The Orange Book: the Food and Drug Administration's advice on therapeutic equivalence. *Am Pharm* 1990;NS30:403–405.

Harrison J. Legal and regulatory constraints upon pharmaceutical business. In: Pickering WR, ed. *Information sources in pharmaceuticals*. London: Bowker-Saur, 1990:197–241.

Haunholter JA. Negligence and the pharmacist: a consideration of some of the aspects. Part I-III. *Can Pharm J* 1978;13:12–16,57–61,100–104.

Hayes TH. Non-approved uses of FDA-approved drugs. *JAMA* 1970;211:1750.

Hinze C, Sickmuller B. *New drug approval in Germany*. Waltham, MA: Parexel, 1995.

Kahan JS. *Medical devices: obtaining FDA market clearance*. Waltham, MA: Parexel, 1995.

Kaluzny EL. Legal liability for failure to dispense or refill a prescription. *US Pharmacist* 1978;3:24,26,28,96.

Kessler DA. Regulation of investigational drugs. *N Engl J Med* 1989, 320:281–288.

Kessler DA, et al. Federal regulation of medical devices. *N Engl J Med* 1987, 317:357–366.

Konor CA. FDA enforcement of the Prescription Drug Marketing Act. *US Pharmacist* 1991;16:37–38,40,42.

Lee SC. *New drug approval in South Korea*. Waltham, MA: Parexel, 1995.

Liang FZ, Greenberg RB, Hogan GF. Legal issues associated with formulary product selection when there are two or more recognized drug therapies. *Am J Hosp Pharm* 1988;45:2372–2375.

Liu RH, Goldberger BA, eds. *Handbook of workplace drug testing*. Washington, DC: American Association for Clinical Chemistry, 1995.

Mandl FL, Greenberg RB. Legal implications of preparing and dispensing drugs under conditions not in a product's official labeling. *Am J Pharm* 1976;33:814–816.

Mathieu MP, Cadden S. *New drug approval in North America: the U.S. and Canada*. Waltham, MA: Parexel, 1998.

McMahon E. *New drug approval in Canada*. Waltham, MA: Parexel, 1995.

Medical device submissions handbook. 6 v. Washington, DC: Health Industry Manufacturers Association, 1995.

Meyer MC. Drug product selection—part 2: Scientific basis of bioavailability and bioequivalence testing. *Am Pharm* 1991;NS31:587–592.

Molzon JA. What kinds of patient counseling are required? *Am Pharm* 1992;NS32:234–241.

Myers MJ. Treatment IND's. *US Pharmacist* 1988;13:32,37–38,82.

Myers MJ, Fink JL. Legal considerations in establishing third and fourth classes of drug products. *FDC Law J* 1976;31:4–10.

Newquist DL. *Products Liability Reporter*. Chicago: Commerce Clearing House, 1963–, biweekly.

Nightingale SL, Morrison JC. Generic drugs and the prescribing physician. *JAMA* 1987;258:1200–1204.

Parker RE, Martinez DR, Covington TR. Drug product selection—part 1: History and legal overview. *Am Pharm* 1991;NS31:524–540.

Parker RE, Martinez DR, Covington TR. Drug product selection—part 3: The Orange Book. *Am Pharm* 1991;NS31:655–664.

Parkinson C, Lumley CE. What can be learned from experience gained using the old European concertation procedure? *Drug Inf J* 1996;30:441–450.

Podell LB. Legal implications of preparing and dispensing approved drugs for unlabeled indications. *Am J Hosp Pharm* 1983;40:111–113.

Pumpian PA. Schedule V controlled substances. *US Pharmacist* 1976;1:8–9.

Sanborn MD, Godwin HC, Pessetto JJ. FDA drug classification system. *Am J Hosp Pharm* 1991;48:2659–2662.

Schwartz JI, Fink JL. Legal issues associated with pharmacokinetic software. *Am J Hosp Pharm* 1989;46:120–124.

Scott C, Ivers-Read G. *New drug approval in France*. Waltham, MA: Parexel, 1996.

Sherman M, Strauss S. How drugs are moved from Rx to OTC status. *US Pharmacist* 1988;13:69–76,78,80.

Sherman M, Strauss S. Regulation of medical devices. *US Pharmacist* 1983;8:10,12,14,16.

Simonsmeier LM. Legal implications when mailing prescription drug products. *US Pharmacist* 1980;5:9–10,23.

Simonsmeier LM. Legal significance of drug interactions. *Contemp Pharm Pract* 1981;4:211–215.

Sonnenreich MR, Mener JM. State substitution laws—a lawyer's view. *US Pharmacist* 1977;2:18–22.

Sonnenreich MR, Shaw DF. State substitution laws: update on pharmacist liability. *US Pharmacist* 1978;3:24,26–29,86.

Spilker B. Phases of clinical trials and phases in drug development. *Drug News & Perspectives* 1996 Dec;9(10):601–606.

Stewart JE. Mailing controlled substances. *Leg Asp Pharm Pract* 1983 Jul/Aug;6:2–3.

Strauss S, Sherman M. Orphan drugs. *US Pharmacist* 1987;12:46–56.

Strauss S, Sherman M. Regulations pertaining to expiration dating of drug products. *US Pharmacist* 1985 Apr;10:40–42,44,46–47,70.

Strom BL. Generic drug substitution revisited. *N Engl J Med* 1987 Jun;316:1456–1462.

Susina SV. When drugs are used for unapproved indications. *Leg Asp Pharm Pract* 1980;2:2–3.

Swafford WB, White BD, Hamner ME. Pharmacy malpractice: a review of indices of care. *US Pharmacist* 1980;5:8–10.

Tabusso G, Peviani N. *New drug approval in Italy.* Waltham, MA: Parexel, 1995.

Uchida K. Orphan drugs in Japan. *Drug Inf J* 1996;30:171–175.

Use of approved drugs for unlabeled indications. *FDA Drug Bull* April 1982;12:4–5.

Valentino JG. Legal implications of USP dispensing information. *US Pharmacist* 1978;3:24–32,76.

White BD, Hamner ME. Out-of-state prescriptions: A dilemma for the pharmacist. *US Pharmacist* 1979;4:10–13,15,68.

Williams KG. Pharmacist's duty to warn of drug interactions. *Am J Hosp Pharm* 1992;49:2787–2789.

Witmer DR, Liang FZ. Reporting of adverse drug reactions and physician liability. *Am J Hosp Pharm* 1992;49:538,544.

Young FE, et al. FDA's new procedures for use of investigational drugs in treatment. *JAMA* 1988;259:2267–2270.

5

Evaluating Drug Information Sources and Developing a Search Protocol

Competent literature research, like clinical investigation, should have a protocol. The protocol is, essentially, a detailed plan of action to achieve a goal, and the goal in this context is finding answers to drug information questions. The first step in developing a search protocol is defining the question or problem.

Figure 5.1 lists types of questions typically encountered. Use it to identify the general categories into which most of your requests, current or anticipated, fall. Printed resources annotated in this *Guide* are organized into comparable general categories to assist in resource selection. Learning to analyze and classify an information request is a practical first step in developing a systematic plan for consulting the succession of resources likely to be needed. For example, a physician might ask for information about use of drug Z in the treatment of condition Y. First, determine what type of name drug Z is (drawing on your experience and the discussion in Chapter Two). Next, use identification sources to check for alternate names under which drug Z might be indexed in the literature. Notes on sources in Chapter Three should help in selecting the best reference(s), based on the type of name you've been given as a starting point. Then, consult therapeutics information sources (Chapter Six). Unless you already know that use of drug Z in condition Y is an approved indication, choose sources that include details on both approved and off-label uses. Dosage information will probably be needed, as well as determining availability (manufacturer), so select compendia that include both types of data.

This example illustrates how careful question analysis and classification will help in formulating an efficient search protocol. It also shows how knowledge of resource scope, access points, and documentation will be put to good use on a day-to-day basis in selection decisions. Just as the quality of a clinical study is affected by criteria for inclusion/exclusion of patients to test the effects of treat-

107

Figure 5.1   Types of Drug Information Questions

Identification and Nomenclature
    domestic drug identification
    foreign (non-U.S.) drug identification
    physical identification from description/observation of dosage form
    investigational drugs

Therapeutics
    indications
    off-label uses
    dosage
    pharmacology and metabolism
    contraindications
    natural medicine—pharmacognosy, homeopathy
    patient medication counseling

Side Effects
    adverse reactions
    drug-drug interactions
    food-drug interactions
    drug-laboratory test interference
    poisoning/toxicity
    potential teratogenicity, carcinogenicity
    incompatibilities (parenterals)
    drug use and lactation

Marketing and Business Data
    product availability
    industry statistics
    company statistics
    pharmacoeconomics
    country statistics
    product licensing
    line extensions
    historical data, history of drugs, pharmacy

Regulatory Affairs
    approvals
    recalls
    regulations
    product patent numbers, expirations, extensions
    generic substitution
    controlled substances

ment, standards applied to resource selection should be appropriate to match information needs. In addition, a search plan, like a clinical protocol, should be critically assessed for adequate sample size and representation, in this case not of the patient population, but of the bibliographic options in a given subject category.

Structure and Organization of the Literature: Scaling the Pyramid

One way of visualizing bibliographic demography is a pyramid, as shown in Figure 5.2. There are three basic types of publications populating the scientific literature landscape. The largest group is primary sources, which include patent applications, conference papers, journal articles, case reports, correspondence, technical reports, and theses. They are characteristically narrow in scope, focusing on communicating details about a single subject. The volume of primary literature in the health sciences is enormous. Attempting to answer questions by drawing on reprint files built by systematic scanning of a set of journals, however carefully selected, is information malpractice. The sample size is simply too small to represent the total population of information available. As Oxman[1] points out in the first installment of a valuable *JAMA* series of users' guides to the medical literature (see Additional Sources at the end of this chapter), "the amount of time required to maintain an up-to-date file of clinical articles is formidable. . . . New methods for retrieving current medical literature are rendering personal filing systems nonessential, if not obsolete."

An adequate survey of the primary literature requires use of one of the other two types of publications depicted in the pyramid. Secondary literature selects, rearranges into meaningful categories, and summarizes primary sources: i.e., it indexes and abstracts the literature. Bibliographies and review articles are forms

Figure 5.2 Structure of the Scientific Literature

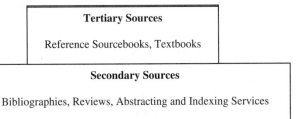

of secondary literature in microcosm. Online bibliographic databases such as *MEDLINE* (14.1), *EMBASE* (14.4), *BIOSIS Previews* (14.6), and *SciSearch* (14.7) represent secondary literature at the macro level.

Unfortunately, rapid developments in the application of computer technology to the literature search process have led to overreliance on secondary sources. Menu-driven and graphical user interfaces (GUIs) to databases on compact disc have lowered the barriers to their frequent use previously imposed by command language and costs associated with online connect time. To a certain extent, the recent vogue for evidence-based medicine (EBM), with its emphasis on critical analysis of clinical data to establish standards of care or practice guidelines, also seems to have engendered distrust or dismissal of tertiary sources. Intent on exercising their evaluation skills, proponents tend to rush headlong for the primary literature, often through fairly cursory searches of secondary sources such as *MEDLINE*. This observation is not intended as EBM bashing, but rather as a precautionary statement to medical and pharmacy educators and students. Evidence is likely to be incomplete when inadequate attention is given to the preliminary route that must be carefully charted to arrive at a definitive clinical pathway.

The expression "blinded by science" might be justifiably applied to both technology driven and curricula-induced secondary source dependency. In handling the majority of drug information questions arising in medical practice settings, the goal is rapid problem resolution. Bibliographic databases are not necessarily the best means of achieving that goal. Lists of references retrieved must be painstakingly quality-filtered to identify items likely to contain answers, which must then be tracked down and read to isolate facts needed. Individual entries in indexing sources, even when accompanied by author abstracts, are often poor indicators of actual content in articles cited.

Successful search protocols usually scale the information pyramid to the topmost tier. Consulting a good reference work first can save time, especially when citations to the primary literature are provided to back up information presented. The function of tertiary sources is to compile, evaluate, and distill information from a broad range of primary sources, thus mediating the search process on behalf of their users. For example, the majority of human toxicity and poisoning data is easily accessible in tertiary sources. Unless a substance is new or the route of exposure novel, general reference works will have gathered and assessed data available in primary sources on the toxicity of specific compounds.

When, then, is use of secondary sources really needed? When a more extensive bibliography is requested, when a topic is so new that it is unlikely to be covered in standard reference sources, or when you suspect that newly published data will augment information presented in an older tertiary source, consulting abstracting and indexing services is sound information practice.

Source Evaluation Checklist

Regardless of which tier in the information pyramid is selected as the most appropriate means of obtaining an answer, there remains the problem of choosing the best sources from the multiplicity of publications available. The checklist in Figure 5.3 identifies important factors to be weighed when evaluating scope, content, and access points.

Many items listed are interrelated. For example, if a source covers only single-entity drugs, it cannot offer thorough indexing for over-the-counter (nonprescription) medications, many of which contain combinations of active ingredients. By the same token, if generic names are preferred access points, indexing of OTC products will require extensive brand name cross referencing. Lab code/investi-

Figure 5.3   Checklist for Evaluating Drug Compendia and Basic Reference Sources

Scope
- [ ] U.S. drugs
- [ ] foreign drugs
- [ ] other chemicals
     excipients, cosmetics, household products
- [ ] other: biologics, diagnostics, botanicals,
     homeopathics, nutritionals, devices,
     radiopharmaceuticals, etc.
- [ ] veterinary drugs
- [ ] approved products
- [ ] drugs under investigation
- [ ] discontinued drugs
- [ ] single entities
- [ ] combination products
- [ ] prescription drugs
- [ ] over-the-counter products
- [ ] multisource drug products (generic drugs)
- [ ] approved indications
- [ ] off-label uses

Indexing/access points
- [ ] nonproprietary names
     USAN, INN, BAN
- [ ] brand names
- [ ] laboratory codes
- [ ] chemical names
- [ ] CAS registry numbers
- [ ] therapeutic classes
- [ ] pharmacological action
- [ ] diseases/symptoms/conditions
- [ ] manufacturers

Content
- [ ] molecular or empirical formula
- [ ] structural formula
- [ ] physical and chemical properties
- [ ] proprietary preparations
- [ ] manufacturer address/telephone
- [ ] Rx versus OTC status
- [ ] price/cost
- [ ] indications
- [ ] dosage
- [ ] details re off-label uses

Content (continued)
- [ ] pharmacology
- [ ] adverse effects/toxicology
- [ ] interactions
- [ ] comparative/evaluated data
- [ ] abstracts, literature extracts
- [ ] bibliographic references
- [ ] patent information
- [ ] extras: controlled substances,
     sugar/alcohol content, bio-
     equivalency, orphan drugs

timeliness
- [ ] frequency of updates
- [ ] up-to-date documentation

- [ ] **Authority/credibility**

gational drug number indexing usually indicates that a source is not limited to approved, on-the-market products only.

Checking off certain items on the list will lead to other questions. If combination products are indexed, do brand name entries indicate quantities or percentages of active ingredients? If indications and dosage are given, is information about investigational or off-label, as well as officially approved, uses included? If a source identifies manufacturers or distributors of substances, does it also contain a directory of all companies or organizations referenced, with addresses and telephone numbers?

If generic names are preferred in indexing, what nomenclature standard is cited (USAN, INN, BAN)? If chemical names are indexed, are these names permuted for access by name fragments? If the source groups or classifies drugs by therapeutic or pharmacological action, what reference standard is used (*AHFS*, *MeSH*, etc.)?

Documentation and Credibility

Other factors which deserve consideration when evaluating reference sources are documentation and credibility. Are bibliographic citations included in a source, and is the bibliography up-to-date? Are primary or secondary (or even tertiary) sources listed? Are citations complete and easy to use? Some reference tools make follow-up unnecessarily laborious due to obscure, unexplained abbreviations and nonstandard citation format. How is the bibliography presented? A general, unnumbered list at the end of a chapter is less useful for ready-reference purposes than a text which documents supportive citations with superscripts or bracketed numbers throughout. Have citations been evaluated? Some sources grade clinical studies, for example, by degree of importance or significance.

How trustworthy is the author's judgment likely to be? Educational attainments, previous and current employment experience, and past publication record are indicators. The fact that an author is associated with a well-known educational institution, medical center, or pharmaceutical company, or that the publication is sponsored by a professional society, may affect your evaluation of source credibility. Some publishers' imprints also serve as imprimaturs of quality.

How frequently are new editions planned? In drug information, timeliness is important. Looseleaf services have a potential for more comprehensive coverage than infrequently issued bound monographs. Yet, although evidence of timely updating is important, a bibliography that cites older references is not necessarily out-of-date. For example, resources that list significant adverse reactions or interactions may cite older references. Once an undesirable side effect has been reported, few further incidents may appear in the literature, because practitioners will avoid inducing the known adverse effect, and journal editors eschew restating the obvious in space dedicated to case reports.

Thus, a bibliography on possible interactions or adverse effects associated with established drugs may not list many recent references and still be credible. Similarly, human toxicity or poisoning literature may be quite dated and still contain valid information. In fact, much of the primary documentation of plant poisonings is found in older sources. Observed effects are the same, whether exposure occurred thirty years ago or six months previously, although diagnosis and treatment methodology will differ with the passage of time.

Guides to the Literature

Studying literature written about literature can be useful preparation for drug information provision and evaluation of resources. This book is but one example of guides to pharmaceutical resources available today. Annotated bibliographies are another popular publishing format.

5.1 Wood EH, Martin L, eds. *A Guide to Drug Information and Literature: An Annotated Bibliography*. Los Angeles: Norris Medical Library, University of S. California, 1991.

5.2 Andrews T. *Guide to the Literature of Pharmacy and Pharmaceutical Sciences*. Littleton, CO: Libraries Unlimited, 1986.

Originally compiled as a teaching aid for pharmacy students, Wood and Martin's *Guide* has been expanded to assist readers with responsibility for collection development. It includes sections on guides to the literature, indexing and abstracting services, computer databases, textbooks, general drug information sources, evaluative and comparative resources, therapeutics, adverse reactions/drug interactions/toxicology, laws and regulations, news, and the pharmaceutical industry. Standardized, structured annotations describe each reference's scope, arrangement, content, and use, but do not provide commentary on relative utility (other than that inherent in the selection of resources to feature).

Andrews' annotated bibliography is much more extensive and evaluative. The *Guide to the Literature of Pharmacy and Pharmaceutical Sciences* is divided into three sections: 1) reference works, with chapters dedicated to format classes such as dictionaries and encyclopedias, directories and catalogs, handbooks and manuals; 2) source material by subject area, where chapters address historical works, pharmacy practice, drug abuse, and similar topics; and 3) other (databases, journals, etc.). It includes separate author/title and subject indexes for easy access to descriptions of specific publications.

5.3 Fishman DL. Drug Information Sources. In: Roper FW, Boorkman JA, eds. *Introduction to Reference Sources in the Health Sciences*. 3rd ed. Metuchen, NJ: Medical Library Association and The Scarecrow Press, 1994: 143–171.

Fishman's chapter on drug information sources is an excellent introduction to the literature and to factors that affect accessibility, such as nomenclature diversity and regulatory status. Annotations are presented in the context of practical discussion of potential applications for the forty core references that are singled out for comment. Separate sections highlight guides to the literature, sources for drug identification, comprehensive treatises and textbooks, commercial sources of drug information, professional sources, official compendia, adverse effects/ toxicology/poisoning ready-reference aids, drug interactions, foreign drugs, publications appropriate for patients and the public, and secondary services (primarily computerized databases). *Introduction to Reference Sources in the Health Sciences* is obligatory reading for information professionals, but can also contribute valuable background for nonlibrarians. In addition to Fishman's outstanding contribution, chapters on indexing and abstracting services, electronic bibliographic databases, handbooks and manuals, and medical and health statistics will provide useful overviews relevant to any frequent user of the medical literature.

5.4 Pickering WR, ed. *Information Sources in Pharmaceuticals*. London: Bowker-Saur, 1990.

Despite its title, *Information Sources in Pharmaceuticals* offers little practical guidance on core collection evaluation or day-to-day applications. Its twenty chapters are, rather, essays on literature and information generation and needs in given subject areas, such as biologicals and biotechnology, toxicology, or drug metabolism, viewed primarily from a United Kingdom perspective. End-of-chapter bibliographies vary greatly in quality, but generally suggest scant attempt on the part of contributors to survey available information sources, especially newer titles. Tables embedded in discussion are used as a vehicle to identify relevant bibliography, but titles alone often appear, unsupported by full bibliographic details. For example, tables of equipment and reagent directories and of biotechnology company directories list only a publisher or author/editor for each source.

But, like the curate's egg, this book is good in parts. A chapter on information needs in technical development and production areas of industry includes brief annotations for major works such as *Beilstein* and the *Dictionary of Organic Compounds*. Tables here list journals useful for biotechnology, those relevant to product formulation, etc., with brief notes on the scope of each. The chapter on intellectual property is a good introduction to the topic, discussing how and why patent and trademark information is important to the pharmaceutical industry, as well as its drawbacks. The portion of the book devoted to marketing and business information is enhanced with informative, annotated charts of resources, but suffers from a distressing absence of copy editing that permitted repeated references to an important database by a misspelled title (*PROMPT*, instead of *PROMT*) and offers no background bibliography.

Discussion of "Post-Marketing Experience with Drug Products" offers insight into the challenges of managing data on marketed medications, including screening of published literature, analysis of spontaneous adverse events reports, and epidemiologic techniques to evaluate and report on both. Harrison's chapter on "Legal and Regulatory Constraints upon Pharmaceutical Business," already cited among Additional Sources in this *Guide*, fills in background on drug regulations and official government sources in the United Kingdom. Dunne's contribution on "The Role of the World Health Organization," also previously cited, complements Harrison with a more global view of the structure and control of national drug markets, harmonization of regulatory requirements, information exchange efforts, and other international collaboration.

Barry's chapter on "Publicly Available Information on Marketed Drugs" is a broad overview of electronic and printed media, with brief notes on sources mentioned. What is particularly refreshing is this author's open declaration of opinion on increasingly popular sources, such as *MEDLINE* on CD-ROM: "The search software rarely matches the online version in quality and sophistication, and the documentation is often clumsy and confusing. . . ."[2] Given Barry's degree of experience and success in the field (head of a literature section at Burroughs Wellcome), her perspective on trends carries weight.

The final portion of *Information Sources in Pharmaceuticals* consists of chapters devoted to information needs and availability in various countries or regions, including Australia, South America, Central Africa, and the People's Republic of China. Authors representing the U.S. scenario wrestled with the broadly stated scope of this section, in the end offering little practical advice on resource selection or use. Contributors representing Japan actually list more, and better, English-language ready-reference compendia than do the U.S. contributors to this section.

5.5 Brizuela BS, Hesp JA. Drug Information. In: Gennaro AR, ed. *Remington's Pharmaceutical Sciences*. 19th ed. Easton, PA: Mack Publishing, 1995: 42–51.

In an effort to delineate the structure of the literature as it relates to information retrieval, Brizuela and Hesp group references by publication format, rather than subject area or potential application. Such an arrangement detracts from the value of their introduction. For example, dictionaries such as *Webster's* and Bowman's *Dictionary of Pharmacology* (5.21) are presented cheek by jowl with the *USP Dictionary* (3.1) and *Marler* (3.13). Under ready-reference sources, publications as diverse as the *Handbook of Clinical Drug Data* (6.19), *Hayes Druggist Directory* (13.22), *Merck Index* (3.5), and the *World Pharmaceuticals Directory* (13.2) make strange bedfellows indeed. Secondary source coverage is cursory, identifying only five pharmaceutical and four toxicological databases or database collections (e.g., Micromedex *CCIS* and *TOXNET*). In a textbook intended for healthcare professionals and students preparing for pharmacy practice, a stronger dose of information science would not be incompatible with other sciences, which are covered far more thoroughly.

5.6 Strickland HB, Jepson MH, Reid BJ. *Keyguide to Information Sources in Pharmacy*. London: Mansell Publishing, 1989.

In the *Keyguide to Information Sources in Pharmacy*, the authors attempt to produce a book "which we would like to have had when we all started our professional careers." Aimed at librarians and information workers, Part I discusses the history and scope of the subject specialty literature and educational requirements for the practice of pharmacy. Part II divides bibliographic annotations into brief sections featuring directories, dictionaries, encyclopedias, textbooks, and the like. The list of pharmacopeias, drug indexes, and other reference compendia covered is quite short, accompanied by scope notes that are neither evaluative nor comparative. The *Keyguide* also lists both English and non-English-language journals by country.

5.7 Millares M, ed. *Applied Drug Information: Strategies for Information Management*. Vancouver, WA: Applied Therapeutics, 1998.

Applied Drug Information: Strategies for Information Management would be an excellent choice for a textbook to be used in drug information courses at pharmacy schools or colleges. Millares is a PharmD supervisor at Kaiser Permanente's drug information center and an adjunct faculty member at the University of Southern California. Experience as a preceptor to students and residents is evident in the organization of this practical workbook for information problem solving. Each chapter contains case studies that walk readers through the process of defining and classifying queries, then retrieving, analyzing, and disseminating answers. Participating authors' credentials and written contributions demonstrate hands-on familiarity with topics addressed. These include not only literature research methodologies, but also skill-building introductions to clinical literature evaluation, concepts of pharmacoeconomics, current issues in formulary management, clinical practice guideline development, and data analysis for healthcare systems.

The first four chapters provide an overview of basic information resources and their effective use. The opening contribution by James and Millares is an outstanding introduction to the process of responding to drug information inquiries. A checklist of background information to obtain for each typical category of question is especially useful. Even more valuable are the brief, but pithy, narrative tours of the literature provided in discussions of case study questions. Comparative and evaluative commentary on a few key ready-reference sources is found here, rather than in the annotated bibliography relegated to the back of the book.

Yes, the list of recommended resources in *Applied Drug Information* is widely separated from illustrations of putting the collection to work. Billed as a comprehensive catalog, the bibliography is a sound, but definitely selective, basis for collection building. Organized by subject, citations to each of the 107 titles included are accompanied by a brief description and pricing information. Thirty-two sources bear an asterisk to indicate the authors' recommendation for core status. The list of hardcopy abstracting and indexing services is distressingly brief, including only seven titles, two of which are separate *Excerpta Medica* sections and one of which is the *Readers Guide to Periodical Literature*(!). Selections under CD-ROM and other computer databases are even more limited.

Fortunately, the chapter on medical and pharmaceutical databases, at the front of the book, fills in the conspicuous blanks left by consulting this portion of the appendix. Ritchey, the medical librarian author, introduces twenty online databases and, in eight case studies, illustrates practical distinctions among them. In a separate chapter on *MEDLINE*, White introduces computer search basics, such as Boolean logic and the concept of controlled vocabulary. Examples here are confined to MEDLARS command mode, which may discourage novice end users more likely to prefer friendlier search interfaces. However, White's coverage of *MEDLINE* fundamentals is a good overview of an admittedly difficult topic.

A chapter on the Internet as a drug information tool tackles another daunting task with panache. It contains particularly good examples of when the World Wide Web will be useful, including inquiries centering on natural products, current news, travel medicine, treatment guidelines, consumer-oriented product information, recent FDA decisions, and epidemiology. The author also reports on a study of 2,478 questions received at a large drug information center over a three-month period. Only 10% of problems posed clearly called for Internet usage, but 75% of these carefully pre-qualified questions were answered successfully on the Web. These data give an accurate picture of the relative value of the Internet in classic drug information center work. Case studies also show the limited, but vital, role of this research tool. A huge collection of bookmarks is assembled in Appendix 2 of *Applied Drug Information*, but annotations have, unfortunately, been omitted.

Aside from the limited scope of its list of hardcopy and machine-readable secondary sources in the appendix and the placement of bibliographic annotations far away from pertinent discussion, this textbook has few flaws. Perhaps because of the high standard set, errors, when detected, tend to grate. One database name is, for example, repeatedly misspelled: *IAC PROMPT* [sic], instead of *PROMT.* More important, the chapter dedicated to current issues in formulary management contains a few misleading statements. The contributing author mentions use of *The Pink Sheet* to forecast and track drugs through the approval process. Not once, but twice, the text states that *The Pink Sheet* is "not indexed" and cites this as a barrier to effective use. While it is true that this newsletter does not provide a self-contained index, it is certainly indexed extensively online.

Nor will consulting the index of *Applied Drug Information* help this author locate discussion of *Pink Sheet* indexing included 200 pages earlier, in Ritchie's chapter on major databases. Titles are not permuted for easy access, so there is no entry under P. (The user would have to look under FDC, instead.) A thirteen-page index in a 600-page book immediately raises alarm signals. Closer examination does nothing to dispel fears that many of the practical tips embedded in the text will be lost to readers with less than prodigious memories. There are, for example, no entries for key topics such as brand names, natural products, consumers, drug approvals, or off-label indications—all of which are, indeed, singled out for discussion earlier in the volume. Finally, the publisher was extremely parsimonious in the printing and binding of this book. The inner margin is almost nonexistent, requiring readers to semi-mutilate their copies in order to view the beginning and end words on each line.

Lest this fault finding leave an unfavorable impression of Millares's textbook, it's worth repeating that *Applied Drug Information: Strategies for Information Management* is an excellent choice to support courses in pharmacy schools and, to a lesser degree, begin core collection development.

5.8   Ascione FJ, Manifold CC, Parenti MA. *Principles of Drug Information and Scientific Literature Evaluation*. Hamilton, IL: Drug Intelligence Publications, 1994.

5.9   Watanabe AS, Conner CS. *Principles of Drug Information Services*. Hamilton, IL: Drug Intelligence Publications, 1978.

A 1993 survey of drug information courses in U.S. pharmacy curricula revealed that only 26.8% of respondents reported use of a required textbook.[3] The fact is, very few texts on the topic have been published, beyond locally produced manuals. Watanabe and Conner were among the first to delineate the discipline as a separate specialty requiring the development of extra skills. Ascione, Manifold, and Parenti have contributed a sound successor to Watanabe and Connor's excellent textbook. Both publications are designed for use as learning/teaching tools in pharmacy education.

The more recent work reflects the current emphasis on critical analysis of available information regarding possible treatments, with the bulk of its coverage devoted to drug literature evaluation. Separate sections also address topics related to developing and operating a drug information center, such as funding and quality assurance. Discussion devoted to the process of answering questions offers guidance on basic skills and highlights the systematic approach, but this is not a source to turn to for a substantive examination of the secondary or tertiary bibliography and techniques needed to access it. The main emphasis of *Principles of Drug Information and Scientific Literature Evaluation* is on primary sources, with a useful checklist for assessment of clinical drug trials. Appendices list U.S., Canadian, and European drug information centers and reproduce forms for reporting adverse effects to the FDA. Information about electronic bulletin boards is also included.

Although bibliographic references in Watanabe and Conner's textbook are now dated, other materials included are timeless in their practical approach to the everyday challenges of drug information work. *Principles of Drug Information Services* contains numerous examples of problem solving and competency-based practicum exercises that could serve as models for updated versions to be incorporated into a course syllabus.

5.10 Sewell W. *Guide to Drug Information*. Hamilton, IL: Drug Intelligence Publications, 1976.

Another model others could strive to emulate is Sewell's classic *Guide to Drug Information*. Its charts and tables can still be helpful today in identifying key comparison points among major resources, provided that citations are updated by users and publications introduced since its 1976 imprint are taken into consideration. According to Fishman (5.3), a new edition is in the planning stages.

5.11 Sewell W et al. *Basic Booklist and Core Journals for Pharmaceutical Education*. 6th ed. Bethesda, MD: American Association of Colleges of Pharmacy, 1998.

Less well known, but nonetheless useful, is the *Basic Booklist*. First published in 1963, previous editions were also issued in 1969, 1983, 1986, and 1996. It is the product of the Libraries/Educational Resources Section of the American Association of Colleges of Pharmacy, whose members survey pharmacy educators and librarians nationwide to obtain suggestions for this lengthy bibliography. Citations are arranged by subject area, with category labels based on a review of curricula at representative schools. This characteristic leads to frequent replication of entries, but a unified title index is also included in the 1998 edition. The list identifies more than 900 books and has added core journal titles to its coverage in recent years. Although no annotations are supplied with source citations, the *Booklist*'s breadth and peer-reviewed roots make it a useful adjunct to other tools for collection development. The entire text is available for downloading in PDF format, free of charge, from AACP's Web site. It can be found under the References (rather than Publications) section at http://www.aacp.org.

5.12 *Doody's Health Sciences Book Review Journal*. Oak Park, IL: Doody Publishing, 1993–. Bimonthly.

Book reviews published in monthly issues of *Unlisted Drugs* (3.8) have already been mentioned as a valuable aid in ongoing collection development. *Doody's Health Sciences Book Review Journal* is no substitute. Coverage of pharmacy and pharmaceutical titles is meager, at best, especially when compared to much more timely and thorough monitoring of new publications in other subject areas found in this otherwise admirable source. Reviewers too often tend to invoke the *PDR* for comparison to the few drug ready-reference books covered, raising doubts on the part of this reader, at least, about the validity of assessments made within such a limited conceptual context.

5.13 Wexler P, ed. *Information Resources in Toxicology*. 2nd ed. New York: Elsevier, 1988.

Because pharmaceutical literature draws on resources from other subject disciplines, guides to bibliography in toxicology, chemistry, and the biological sciences can also provide helpful background information. Among the best is Wexler, who aptly describes his work as "a sourcebook, a kind of 'Whole Toxicology Catalog,' " in contrast to what a library cataloger might call an "annotated bibliography and directory." By whatever name, *Information Resources in Toxicology* is definitely a book worth acquiring and studying. Part I, dedicated to U.S. publications, begins with a fascinating history of toxicology information systems, then proceeds to an extensive annotated bibliography of books, journals, newsletters, popular works, computerized information sources, and audiovisuals. Wexler also provides background on government toxicology regulations and lists organizations, educational programs, mutagenicity testing laboratories, and poison control centers.

Part II is devoted to international sources, presented in comparable country-by-country (sixteen in all) compilations of books, organizations, educational programs, and research labs. Wexler's and contributing authors' annotations for individual publications are brief and descriptive, rather than evaluative. Guidance on resource selection is offered only in the form of asterisked citations, which represent the editor's recommendations. Strategically placed literary quotations related to poisons, drawn from writers as diverse as Shakespeare, Keats, and Lewis Carroll, enliven this massive, but well-organized, guide to the literature. No further embellishment is needed to make *Information Resources in Toxicology* an interesting and valuable contribution to the study of medical bibliography.

5.14 Wiggins G. *Chemical Information Sources*. New York: McGraw-Hill, 1991.
5.15 Maizell RE. *How to Find Chemical Information*. 3rd ed. New York: Wiley-Interscience, 1998.
5.16 Bottle RT, Rowland JFB, eds. *Information Sources in Chemistry*. 4th ed. London: Bowker-Saur, 1993.

Wiggins' *Chemical Information Sources* is intended as a textbook to support formal classroom instruction for undergraduates. With strong emphasis on online sources, it includes many practical tips from an author well versed in this subject area. Maizell's *How To* guide takes a classic approach, offering a thorough introduction to chemistry's many handbooks and hardcopy indexes. Online systems and databases, the Internet, and CD-ROMs are covered, but the emphasis in *How to Find Chemical Information* is, as the title implies, on developing good techniques and skills in data searching, regardless of the medium.

Like another Bowker-Saur publication reviewed earlier in this chapter (5.4), *Information Sources in Chemistry* suffers, somewhat, from the uneven treatment accorded different aspects of the topic by contributing authors. One chapter is, however, dedicated to the pharmaceutical industry, where the information needs of various departments, including process development, analytical development, formulation, and production personnel are outlined.

5.17 Davis EB, Schmidt D. *Using the Biological Literature: A Practical Guide.* 2nd ed. New York: Marcel Dekker, 1995.

5.18 Powell RH. *Handbooks and Tables in Science and Technology.* 3rd ed. Phoenix, AZ: Oryx Press, 1994.

Davis and Schmidt furnish more than 1,935 literature citations, many with brief annotations, in *Using the Biological Literature.* Arranged by subject categories, contents address broad topical areas of the bibliography, including biochemistry and biophysics, molecular and cell biology, genetics, microbiology, immunology, anatomy, and physiology (among others). Discussion identifies key periodical titles for each subject and, when focusing on secondary sources, describes indexing policies and searching strategies.

Powell's *Handbooks and Tables in Science and Technology* includes, in its annotated listing of more than 3,500 sources, relevant items in the fields of medicine, biology, and chemistry. As its title implies, the focus of this guide is on reference publications, including government documents, that tabulate and compile numeric data. Entries are arranged alphabetically by title, but indexes by subject and author/editor are provided.

5.19 *Encyclopedia of Health Information Sources.* 2nd ed. Detroit: Gale Research, 1993.

The *Encyclopedia of Health Information Sources* attempts to provide a collection development tool with narrow, topical headings used to organize the bibliography of 6,715 items. The listing of books, journals, newsletters, and even online databases is an extremely eclectic mixture, including primary, secondary, and tertiary sources. The result can sometimes be an unpalatable stew, from the information professional's point of view. Consider, for example, resources listed under the general heading Drugs, where Directories include *AHFS Drug Information* (6.5), *The Red Book* (3.15), *Drugs Available Abroad* (10.29, another Gale publication), and *Edmund's Prescription Drug Prices. The Merck Index* (3.5) and *USP Dictionary* (3.1) are listed as "Encyclopedias," and the *American Drug Index* (3.6) is identified as a handbook, in company with the *PDR* (6.10) and *USP DI* (6.5). Under Drug Interactions, every one of the standard reference publications (7.8–7.12) is ignored in favor of just one resource, *AHFS* again.

Subject terms used to organize this bibliography imply that the intended audience is a nonprofessional one. Consumer-oriented, popular terminology is, however, supplemented with cross references from more technical/scientific terms (e.g., apnea—see sleep disorders). Regardless of the target audience, its serious omissions and undoubted oddities in organization make the *Encyclopedia of*

Health Information Sources a poor guide to basic bibliography on drugs for consumers, librarians, and medical professionals alike.

Although some of the better guides to the literature cited in this chapter do
address online databases, in-depth coverage of this important category of pharmaceutical information resources is available in bibliographies accompanying
Chapters Fourteen to Sixteen. However, one form of publication that should, perhaps, be mentioned here is what might be called Internet "pathfinder" sources.

Internet Pathfinders

The lack of organization and maze-like attributes of the Internet are already legendary. Despite the increasing sophistication of search engines being introduced
as front ends to help users locate relevant material, retrieval software is still ap-
pallingly primitive when compared to fee-based online services available since
the 1970s. Unless a topic can be encapsulated in one or two unambiguous and
highly specific terms, approaching the Internet by way of system-wide search
engines is often a waste of time. What's often needed, instead, is a front end that
mediates the exploration process by introducing a subject-oriented structure to
organize resources into logical units. This type of Web page is often referred to
as a subject hub.

The primary purpose of a subject hub is to provide a road map to other sources
on the information superhighway. It does so by compiling and classifying references to topically related sites and constructing hypertext ("hot") links as a direct
route to accessing them. These pathfinders fulfill the dual functions of an index
and a guide to the literature through the quality-filtering inherent in their selection of resources and identification of sites whose titles alone might not indicate
their potential relevance. The best pathfinders result from systematic examination
of sources by compilers whose background and experience closely match that of
their intended audience. Hence, indexing sites created by, and intended for, members of the general public (such as *Yahoo!*) are usually inadequate starting points
for pharmaceutical users.

HEALTHWEB: Pharmacy & Pharmacology (Purdue University)
 ⇨ http://thorplus.lin.purdue.edu/hw

HEALTHWEB: Pharmacy & Pharmacology exemplifies the benefits of subject
expertise matched to a clearly defined audience. Reference sources assembled
under Pharmacy Practice focus on the information needs of clinical and public
service pharmacists. Drug information sites predominate, supplemented with toxicity resources and quality-filtered herbal and consumer-oriented links. Brief annotations add to the utility of this excellent subject hub produced by Bill Running
and Vicki Killion at Purdue's Pharmacy, Nursing and Health Sciences Library.

Useful Pharmacy Links (Dalhousie University, Canada)
 ➪ http://is.dal.ca/~pharmwww/links
Drug Information Resources for Pharmacists
 ➪ http://www.dal.ca/~pharmwww/druginfo

Lengthier than Purdue's list of subject sites, *Useful Pharmacy Links* is subdivided into categories devoted to "all-round" pharmacy resources, specialized Web pages (e.g., Antimicrobial Use Guidelines, Cholesterol Information Collection), patient information and support groups, pharmacy schools, education resources (learning modules, software, etc.), mailing lists, organizations, drug manufacturers, online publications (e-journals), and monographs. Entries are briefly annotated, and some evaluative commentary is interjected.

Dalhousie's Web site also includes a separate pathfinder by MacCara *et al.* entitled *Drug Information Resources: A Guide for Pharmacists.* It is basically a guide to the hardcopy literature, complemented with hotlinks to Internet URLs. The lengthy list of reference sources is divided into twenty-three categories that reflect areas of frequently asked questions. The title of each book is linked to a full bibliographic citation, which is, in turn, usually linked to a pertinent Web site, such as the publisher's. This bibliography includes a selection of useful journal articles, as well.

World Wide Web Virtual Library: Pharmacy (University of Oklahoma)
 ➪ http://www.pharmacy.org

In the *World Wide Web Virtual Library: Pharmacy*, David Bourne, Associate Professor of Pharmacy at the University of Oklahoma, has assembled an impressive index to Internet sites, conceptually unified by their emphasis on clinical education and practice. Hotlinked entries are organized under the categories: schools, associations, journals, jobs, databases, community pharmacy pages, conferences, hospital pages, pharmaceutical companies, and miscellaneous. The latter includes software suppliers, hardcopy publishers, consulting firms, and other service vendors. In addition to Web pages, a selection of Gopher, Telnet, and other dial-up sources are annotated, as well as listservs and newsgroups. In general, however, scope notes are omitted from this pathfinder, which leaves to the user the laborious task of separating the luxury models from the lemons in the large catalog provided.

PharmWeb (University of Manchester, UK)
 ➪ http://www.pharmweb.net

The product of a self-confessed computer hobbyist, *PharmWeb* has grown to become one of the most used subject hubs since its initial launch in December 1994 by Dr. Antony D'Emanuele of the University of Manchester (UK). With a stated purpose of serving both the patient and the health professional, home page menu choices closely match categories offered in Bourne's *Virtual Library:*

Pharmacy, with the addition of consumer information and a Eurocentric slant. The *PharmWeb* Yellow Pages is a cross-disciplinary and global gateway to many supplementary hubs, including alternative medicine, biotechnology, chemistry, pharmacognosy, and veterinary medicine sites. The emphasis is, however, on companies and commercial enterprises. The list of drug information sources is very short and omits many relevant items.

What makes a visit to *PharmWeb* particularly worthwhile is a section entitled "Pharmacy and the Internet." It includes the full text of D'Emanuele's monthly column in the *International Pharmacy Journal* (January 1995–February 1997), plus a selection of well written articles from other publications. *PharmWeb* has also been enhanced with a specialized search engine, PharmSearch, for accessing the Internet.

The Virtual Pharmacy Center—Martindale's Health Science Guide
   ➪ http://www-sci.lib.uci.edu/~martindale/Pharmacy.html

Size is the main drawback to the *Virtual Pharmacy Center* in Jim Martindale's *Health Science Guide* series. Accessing this list during normal workday, prime-time hours can be extremely time-consuming, making the opening screen's embellishments of weather reports and general news less than welcome. The reward at the end of the wait is a huge subject hub with a scope encompassing pharmacology, toxicology, and professional pharmacy practice. Among Internet sources identified are medical dictionaries and glossaries, chromosome maps and genome databases, course and tutorial sites (including online calculators and case studies), patents, physicians/hospitals worldwide, and images/animation sites.

Many entries are hierarchically arranged, so that users can proceed directly to pertinent portions of home page menus. For example, Martindale offers, within the CDC collection of biosafety documents, separate direct links to guidelines for shipment of dried blood spot specimens, importation permits for etiologic agents, and packaging and shipping of biomedical material. Notes on source content also assist in site selection, but annotations tend to quote directly from linked sites' opening statements—often an inaccurate gauge of worth or lack thereof.

HSLS Pharmacy, Pharmacology & Therapeutics (University of Pittsburgh)
   ➪ http://www.hsls.pitt.edu/intres/health/pharm.html

Compiled by Charles Wessel, a member of the University of Pittsburgh health science library staff, this pathfinder is one of many from the same author. Each is characterized with logical organization and informative annotations. This contribution is relatively modest in scope, but does, nonetheless, help uncover some unique sources not identified in other hubs discussed here.

PharmInfoNet PharmLinks
   ➪ http://pharminfo.com/phrmlink.html

Also comparatively narrow in the range of its coverage, Mediconsult's *PharmInfoNet* is arguably one of the better subject hubs currently available. Its

PharmLinks index to other resources is thoroughly annotated, very well organized, and, unlike several other commercially sponsored source lists, has no difficulty in distinguishing between popular and professional information. Sections address biotechnology, drug information, drug R&D, general medical resources, general pharmaceutical sites, U.S. government URLs, relevant associations, pharmaceutical companies, and U.S. pharmacy schools and education. In addition, several other options make the *PharmInfoNet* home page more than a jumping-off place. Its drug database and publications section will be singled out for discussion in Chapter Six.

Pharmacy Internet Guide (University of Sydney, Australia)
➪ http://www.library.usyd.edu.au/Guides/Pharmacy/index.html

Produced by the University of Sydney Library staff, the *Pharmacy Internet Guide* is intended to cover subject areas central to the interests of Pharmacy Department faculty and Pharmacy Library users. Accordingly, selections include pharmaceutics, pharmaceutical chemistry, and pharmacy practice resources, as well as sites with substantive information relevant to pharmacokinetics and biotechnology. Worldwide directories of colleges of pharmacy head the list of categories used to organize the *Guide*, followed by pharmaceutical organizations, associations, and companies. Entries in subsequent categories are what make this pathfinder a valuable addition to academically oriented subject hubs. The selection of pharmacy and herbal/medicinal plant sites shows discrimination, and brief descriptions of source content will undoubtedly assist users in further prescreening before follow-up.

Pharmacy Web Australia (The Pharmacy Guild of Australia)
➪ http://www.pharmacyweb.com.au

Operated from Tasmania by Mark Dunn, under commercial sponsorship, *Pharmacy Web Australia* reflects these retail roots in its greater emphasis on providing directories to community pharmacies/pharmacist sites and country-specific government and drug information resources. It promotes participation in discussion groups for either community or consultant pharmacists and includes a networking directory and a category dedicated to other mailing lists and newsgroups. With "aims to be a comprehensive Australian pharmacy Internet resource," this hub could be a complement, but not a competitor, to the University of Sydney's *Guide* (see previous entry).

Medical Matrix
➪ http://www.medmatrix.org/

Under the "Rx Assist" button, *Medical Matrix* compiles a ranked, peer reviewed, and annotated list of drug ready reference sources on the Internet. Although one might disagree with rankings and starred ratings, the collection is a small, but good, starting point. In a separate Pharmacotherapeutics section, more than 100 additional selections are assembled in categories for searches, news, fulltext/multimedia, abstracts, textbooks, major sites/link pages, practice guidelines/FAQs, cases, patient education, directories, educational materials, classifieds, and forums. Many titles found here could equally well have been classified in Rx Assist. Another potential pitfall to beware of is double entries for the same source within the same category, but with different titles (and rankings). For example, during one visit, "Top 200 Prescriptions" and "Drug Monograph Search at RxList" both appeared, although these are, essentially, references to the same site. A second drawback in *Medical Matrix* is that no clear distinction is made in many annotations between consumer sources and professional materials.

Selected Internet Resources for Pharmacists (University of Nebraska)
  ➪ http://www.unmc.edu/library/pharm/netpharm.html

Theresa Arndt, librarian at the University of Nebraska Medical Center, adds considerable value to this brief list of *Selected Internet Resources for Pharmacists* by providing links to criteria for evaluating Web-based information, as well as to externally-produced recommendations on how to cite electronic media. In addition, informative annotations for other sites enhance this attractively presented subject hub. Categories covered are: general sources and directories (other subject directories), government sites of interest to pharmacists, patient information, professional associations, pertinent commercial home pages (including pharmaceutical companies), standards of practice/medication safety resources, and pharmaceutical care.

IDIN's Links (Iowa Drug Information Network)
  ➪ http://idin.idis.uiowa.edu/idinlink.htm

University of Iowa resources head *IDIN's Links* from compiler Kevin Moores, followed by categories for medical/pharmacy information sites, journals and newsletters, clinical practice guidelines, evidence-based medicine resources, professional associations, companies, U.S. government titles, and patient education sites. Equivalent to six pages in hardcopy format, this URLography omits any indicators of content beyond titles.

Sara's Pharmacy Page
  ➪ http://www.geocities.com/NapaValley/7458/pharmacy.htm

As its title indicates, *Sara's Pharmacy Page* is the product of an individual. The author, Sara Hancock, is a PharmD employed at a hospital pharmacy in St. Louis. There are several excellent subject hubs on the Internet maintained as personal projects by practicing pharmacists on behalf of the profession. This particular example stands out because it provides sound guidelines for novices new to the Web. Opening sections discuss the benefits and limitations of Internet drug information for pharmacists, basics of server technology, advice on navigating to useful sites, and recommendations for assessing content of medical information found. The remainder of *Sara's Pharmacy Page* is a quality-filtered collection of hotlinks to health news sources, general pharmacy sites, seachable drug information databases, relevant online journals, and, in separate lists, consumer-oriented and healthcare provider-oriented drug resources. Pointers to other directories and search engines round out this pathfinder.

MedWeb Pharmacy and Pharmacology (Emory University)
⇨ http://WWW.MedWeb.Emory.Edu/MedWeb/default.htm

Maintained by the Emory University Health Science Center Library (Atlanta, Georgia), *MedWeb* bibliographies of Internet sites are somewhat difficult to navigate, due to a plethora of poorly defined subject categories. Vocabulary used intermingles "condition" terms (e.g., allergies, arthritis) with fields of specialization (anesthesiology, biochemistry), and publication types (advice columns, catalogs, tutorials). Would subject hubs, for example, be classified under Guides, Lists of Internet Resources, or Sites? With 123 subdivisions currently listed under Pharmacology, efficient use of *MedWeb* is nearly impossible. Pertinent links are scattered, perhaps inevitably, under multiple headings.

Oddities in category application on the part of the site's organizers are repeatedly encountered. For example, the *U.S. Pharmacopeia*, the *Australian Prescription Products Guide*, the *Nurses Drug Reference Center*, and a South African database of package inserts are the sole (and strangely mixed) selections under the term Pharmacopoeias. Under Pharmacy and Pharmacology (which is, to confuse matters further, used as both a main heading and subcategory label), nearly 600 hotlinks are a mishmash of company, association, and other sites, including individual book table of contents. Annotations are cryptic, often absent, and give little indication that any attempt has been made to prescreen sites. Nonetheless, the size and diversity of this collection make it worth visiting. *MedWeb* is undergoing reorganization as of January 1999, so watch for future improvements. Because the URL for the pharmacy and pharmacology hub seems to change frequently, only the home page address is included here as a base for further exploration.

Karolinska Institute Drug Therapy (Sweden)
⇨ http://www.mic.ki.se/Diseases/e2.html

Poor organization also characterizes the Karolinska Institute subject hub. Sites gathered under Drug Therapy (beginning on the second screen at this URL) are listed in random order. Apart from noting the sponsor or author of each resource, hotlinks are unembellished by this pathfinder's editors. However, the selection is huge and includes many sources not easily found elsewhere.

Edmund's Home Page
⇨ http://www.li.net/~edhayes/ed.html

Ed Hayes is a hospital pharmacist at SUNY-Stony Brook with a long-standing history as an Internet guide. His *Home Page* is a more eclectic pathfinder than those of many of his peers. Sources in pharmacy, dentistry, nursing, chiropractic, general medicine, the biosciences, and nutrition are singled out in separate sections, as are poison control centers, medical newsgroups and the Press, general reference aids, and pharmaceutical companies with indigent patient programs. A new section presents, in tabular format, information on drugs that interfere with laboratory tests. Aside from a few editorial comments ("Super Site—Don't Miss This One"), indexes for each discipline are presented without scope notes. However, *Edmund's Home Page* selection in pharmacy is informative and interesting, if too abbreviated.

Hardin Meta Directory of Pharmacy & Pharmacology
⇨ http://www.lib.uiow.edu/hardin/md/pharm.html

Hardin's various meta directories are frequently cited as a good place to start if you'd like to compare subject hubs on your own. With a goal of identifying "the best sites that list the sites," Hardin divides the directory into large, medium, and small pathfinder pages. Within each category, sources are generally ranked by connection rate, i.e., at least 80% of URLs compiled at a given hub will successfully link users with resources. In other words, less than 20% broken links found by line-checking software and random manual testing earns a pathfinder the "Clean Bill of Health Award." The resulting list is decidedly lean and mean. Aside from noting the author or institution responsible for each link, Hardin's entries lack descriptions. Only twenty-five hubs are currently identified in the *Meta Directory of Pharmacy and Pharmacology*. Reviews of several are deliberately omitted from this chapter because their scope is comparatively limited or their selection lacks discrimination.

The Mining Company: Pharmacology
⇨ http://pharmacology.miningco.com

The Mining Company's designated human guide for its pharmacology collection is Mary Ann Elchisak, an Associate Professor of Pharmacology at Purdue University. This site has earned a number one rating, in terms of size and connect rate, by Hardin. More significant, from a subject viewpoint, are two bonuses found here in the form of brief introductions to locating and interpreting specific types of information on the Internet: *Clinical Trials, Understanding Them and Finding Them* (June 1998) and *How to Do Specific Drug Searches* (March 1998). Both are consumer-oriented, as is the bulk of other content identified here. Categories include A–Z drug name searches and another source locator organized by therapeutic class (analgesics to urogenital). The contents of directories labeled General-Consumers and General-Professionals are nearly identical, which detracts somewhat from the utility of this hub as a launch pad for healthcare professionals.

However, other features have made this a popular site. For example, new drug approvals in the United States are accessible via both alphabetical and chronological lists, currently dating back to January 1998. Hotlinks for each product lead to informative press releases from manufacturers. U.S. pharmacy school home pages are indexed state by state. Source lists assembled in other categories devoted to drug safety and regulation are relatively modest in scope, but do offer brief annotations. Beyond dilution due to an attempt to serve two essentially incompatible target audiences, the chief drawback to *The Mining Company: Pharmacology* hub is its linking technology. The producer masks URLs from users. The address shown for any site visited is always simply The Mining Company, making it impossible to establish personal bookmarks for direct access in the future.

Yahoo! Health: Pharmacy

⇨ http://www.yahoo.com/Health/Pharmacy/

Consumer orientation accounts for *Yahoo!*'s apples and oranges (lions and lemons?) approach to science, typially mixing hobbyist home pages side-by-side with rigorously peer-reviewed resources. However, as a commercial enterprise dependent on the Internet audience, *Yahoo!* must be checked periodically for new sources that might otherwise be missed. Its Pharmacy section divides links for drugs and medications under "Types" and "Specific drugs & medications." Clicking on "Types" leads to a menu of seventeen classes of products, mixing pharmacological action (beta blockers), therapeutic effect (asthma), and dosage form (lozenges) terminology. Links for psychedelics and stimulants far outnumber all other drug types.

In the separate directory of more than 400 "Specific drugs & medications," *Yahoo!* has constructed a similar hodgepodge of products. Psilocybe mushrooms are cheek-by-jowl with major brand names, and numerous hot links for methamphetamines and marijuana are presented in dubious company with diaper rash ointments. In general, *Yahoo!* users must have the skill (and patience) to winnow out serious science from substance abuse sites in this subject hub's regrettable medley defined as Pharmacy.

This comment should prompt reexamination of the role of subject hubs in day-to-day problem solving. Their size often renders them impractical for use in quick-reference queries. Like guides to the hardcopy literature, Internet pathfinders are useful in preparation for drug information provision and identifying locations where answers can be found in the future. Allocating time to explore and evaluate linked sites in advance is the best way to ensure effective application of Internet resources. Experienced users create bookmarks as they go along, essentially constructing their own customized sub-Nets to match anticipated needs. Better pathfinders permit users to register for automatic e-mail updates informing them of additions or alterations. In this way, systematic (and tedious) revisits to slow-loading subject hubs can be avoided. This is also the rationale behind provision of full addresses for each site described in this book, rather than referring readers back to pathfinders highlighted here. A cumulative directory of these and sites evaluated in other chapters is included at the end of Appendix B.

Keeping up-to-date on newly introduced Internet sources or changes in existing home pages will be a constant challenge. Many of the newsletters designed to assist users in this task are too general in scope and tend to focus on medicine, instead of the multidisciplinary needs of pharmacy practitioners or pharmaceutical industry knowledge workers.

PharmaPages—Internet Issues in the Pharmaceutical Industry
➪ http://www.pjbpubs.co.uk/ppages/index2.html

PJB publications comes to the rescue with its *PharmaPages*, a free online newsletter devoted to covering the latest developments on the Internet of potential interest to the industry. Each month, it reviews new sites and business applications/implications. Forthcoming Internet conferences relevant to pharmaceuticals are listed in a worldwide Diary section, and reviews of recent meetings help readers stay in touch with emerging issues. Another regular feature is a summary of important information picked up on *sci.med.pharmacy* and *sci.med.telemedicine* newsgroups. A concluding directory of URLs in each issue streamlines current awareness. Another helpful user aid is a glossary of Web-speak and related technology terms reprinted with each issue.

Pharmacy Times—Pharmacists on the Net
➪ http://www.pharmacytimes.com/net.html
U.S. Pharmacist—Cyberpharmacist
➪ http://www.uspharmacist.com

Other good sources of Internet news are monthly columns in the trade press. Contributed by Ann Letner, *Pharmacists on the Net* appears at the *Pharmacy Times* Web site. *U.S. Pharmacist* also launched a *Cyberpharmacist* column in January 1997 and is archiving back issues for free viewing.

Guides to the Terminology of Pharmacy and Related Disciplines

The glossary in this volume attempts to define specialized terminology associated with the discipline of drug information, but cannot hope to encompass all vocabulary likely to be needed by users preparing to embark on a career in this specialty or striving to enhance their effectiveness as literature research mediators. Putney and Roper[4] have compiled a very good core list of terminology sources in medicine, including general dictionaries; etymology sourcebooks; reference aids to identification of syndromes, eponyms, and quotations; foreign language translation tools; terminology textbooks; medical word finders; inverted (concept) dictionaries; and guides to the acronyms and abbreviations with which the literature is rife. However, additional titles annotated below will complement coverage of-

Figure 5.4   Best Bets among Internet Pathfinders

- *HEALTHWEB: Pharmacy & Pharmacology (Purdue University)*
    ⇨ http://thorplus.lin.purdue.edu/hw
- *Useful Pharmacy Links (Dalhousie University, Canada)*
    ⇨ http://is.dal.ca/~pharmwww/links
- *World Wide Web Virtual Library: Pharmacy (University of Oklahoma)*
    ⇨ http://www.pharmacy.org
- *PharmWeb (University of Manchester, UK)*
    ⇨ http://www.pharmweb.net
- *The Virtual Pharmacy Center—Martindale's Health Science Guide*
    ⇨ http://www-sci.lib.uci.edu/~martindale/Pharmacy.html
- *HSLS Pharmacy, Pharmacology & Therapeutics (University of Pittsburgh)*
    ⇨ http://www.hsls.pitt.edu/intres/health/pharm.html
- *PharmInfoNet PharmLinks*
    ⇨ http://pharminfo.com/phrmlink.html
- *Pharmacy Internet Guide (University of Sydney, Australia)*
    ⇨ http://www.library.usyd.edu.au/Guides/Pharmacy/index.html
- *Medical Matrix*
    ⇨ http://www.medmatrix.org/

---

fered in general medical terminology publications. (See also Chapter Ten for multilingual guides.)

5.20 Laurence DR, Carpenter JR. *A Dictionary of Pharmacology and Clinical Drug Evaluation.* London: UCL Press, 1994.

Laurence and Carpenter's dictionary is meant to reflect common usage and explain terms employed by pharmacologists beyond the strictly technical vocabulary of the discipline. Examples of vernacular expressions defined include "abuse liability," "carrier," "additive responses," and "salami publication." Always erudite, at times pedantic, and often humorous, entries entice users to browse, as well as turn to this book for more conventional quick look-ups. For example, the definition of soma cites an intoxicating plant used in Hindu ritual and also refers to Huxley's use of the term, in *Brave New World*, to describe an imaginary social drug that could be taken to provide holidays from reality without adverse effects. Under routes of administration, wry wit leavens the long list of keywords: "Virtually every route that ingenuity can devise and technology can allow has been used, e.g., ... The terms are generally self-evident and a comprehensive list would be wearisome." Characteristically puckish, the humor, at times, verges on the supercilious, exemplified in two extra definitions included in the entry for statistician. "Unjustly: a tedious fellow. . . . Less unjustly: a person who can draw a mathematically precise line from an unwarranted assumption to a foregone conclusion." Aside from its occasional preciosity, *A Dictionary of Pharmacology and Clinical Drug Evaluation* is a good (albeit lively) guide to specialized terminology.

5.21 Bowman WC, Bowman A, Bowman A. *Dictionary of Pharmacology*. Oxford: Blackwell Scientific Publications, 1986.
5.22 Fincher JH, et al. *Dictionary of Pharmacy*. Columbia, SC: University of S. Carolina, 1986.

The Bowman family's *Dictionary of Pharmacology* is another source readable in and of itself, rather than as a mere adjunct to reference work. Its compact format and clear, concise style enhance its utility. The broad cross section of vocabulary selected for inclusion is a strength; e.g., acaricide, Acceleranstoff, Ames test, autoindicator tissues, and zero-order kinetics.

Recognizing that pharmacy is an applied field encompassing physical, chemical, biological, social, behavioral, economic, and administrative sciences, Fincher and colleagues also set out to provide more than a scaled-down medical dictionary. Terms and expressions defined embrace dosage form technology, medicinal chemistry, pharmacology, and pharmacognosy. Additional sections supply weights and measures equivalents (apothecary, avoirdupois, metric, and Imperial British systems), translate common abbreviations and acronyms, and interpret Latin abbreviations sometimes used in medication orders. For example, "a c" is explained as "medication order meaning before meals or food after the Latin *ante cibos* or *ante cibum*." Some vocabulary associated with drug abuse (e.g., yellow jackets) is also covered in the *Dictionary of Pharmacy*.

5.23 Pashos CL, Klein EG, Wanke LA, eds. *ISPOR LEXICON*. Princeton, NJ: International Society for Pharmacoeconomics and Outcomes Research, 1998.

The *ISPOR LEXICON*™ defines key terms used in the literature of pharmacoeconomics and outcomes research. It is intended as a reference tool both for practitioners in the field as well as users of their publications. Published by a nonprofit organization formed in 1995 to promote scientific investigations into pharmacoeconomics and assessments of health outcomes, the *LEXICON* can be ordered directly from the Society, as described on their Web page at http://www.ispor.org/publications/lexicon/index.html.

5.24 *EuroBABEL*. Richmond, Surrey, England: European Pharma Law Centre, 1998.

An apt title sums up the dilemma many people face in trying to cope with the growing list of acronyms and abbreviations associated with European Union regulatory developments. *EuroBABEL* defines those used in the pharmaceutical, agricultural, veterinary, and medical healthcare sectors. The text of each acronym is given in the original language from which it was derived, with further English-language explanations added, when needed. More than 5,000 entries illustrate the impetus behind this EPLC publication.

5.25 Lewis RA. *Lewis' Dictionary of Toxicology.* Boca Raton, FL: CRC Press, 1998.

Lewis' Dictionary of Toxicology is based on terms found in more than 600 core journals, 15,000 reprints of scientific papers, and other reference sources. The resulting 1,700-page selection embraces a wide variety of related fields, including biochemical, clinical, comparative, developmental, forensic, immunological, nutritional, neurological, pharmacological, and veterinary toxicology vocabulary. Regulatory terminology and official abbreviations are also covered. Each entry categorizes definitions and usage by field, with extensive cross references for synonyms and related entries.

5.26 Hodgson E, Mailman RB, Chambers JE. *Dictionary of Toxicology.* 2nd ed. New York: Van Nostrand Reinhold, 1998.

The *Dictionary of Toxicology* includes entries for general chemicals (e.g., aniline), classes of drugs (anesthetics, anticholinesterases), popular terms (angel dust), theories (Cornfield and Ryzin model = low-dose extrapolation), and explanations of various kinetic equations used in toxicology. In common with other dictionaries listed in this section, this guide to terminology could be useful to the information intermediary in fleshing out the often sparse language of search requests from specialists, offering assistance in understanding concepts and in predicting alternative terms likely to be used in the literature and indexing.

5.27 Walker JM, Cox M. *Biotechnology: A Dictionary of Terms.* 2nd ed. Washington, DC: American Chemical Society, 1995.

Acknowledging at the outset that biotechnology means different things to different people, Walker and Cox outline in their dictionary's preface the spectrum of related disciplines involved in the commercialization of biological processes and systems in manufacturing, service industries, and management of the environment that constitute biotechnology applications today. Microbiologists, biochemists, pharmacologists, chemical engineers, and other scientists must typically collaborate in the development of practical biotechnologies and, to do so, will need to understand one another's subject specialty jargon.

Biotechnology: A Dictionary of Terms incorporates terminology from diverse disciplines to meet this need. Changes in the field since the first edition was published by ACS in 1988 are reflected in expansion of definitions to include new applications of processes previously defined, as well as introduction of many additional entries to encompass new technology such as polymerase chain reaction, gene therapy, growth factors as therapeutic agents, and the like. A welcome enhancement is a clear key to pronunciation of each term, a feature often omitted in specialized glossaries of this type.

Figure 5.5   Free Glossaries on the Internet

- *Glossary of Terms and Symbols Used in Pharmacology*
   ⇨ http://www.bumc.bu.edu/www/busm/pharmacology/Programmed/
Framedglossary.html
   Edward W. Pelikan, MD, is the author of this glossary originating from Boston University's Department Of Pharmacology and Experimental Therapeutics. It is browsable by alphabetic letter and full of hotlinked cross references between separate entries.

- *BioTech Life Sciences Dictionary*
   ⇨ http://biotech.chem.indiana.edu/pages/dictionary.htm
   Developed by Indiana University staff members and contributors, this illustrated dictionary includes more than 8,300 terms used in a variety of life science disciplines, including biochemistry, biotechnology, botany, cell biology, genetics, ecology, limnology, pharmacology, toxicology, and medicine. Both main entry keywords and character strings found in definitions can be searched via the form at the URL given above.

- *BioTech Chemical Acronyms Database*
   ⇨ http://129.79.137.107/cfdocs/libchem/titleu.cfm
   A product of Indiana University's Chemistry Library, this database is designed for specific acronym/abbreviation look-ups.

- *PharmInfoNet Glossary*
   ⇨ http://pharminfo.com/glos_ab.html
   PharmInfoNet's Glossary, browsable by alphabetic letter, is the most general in scope of Internet guides listed here. It defines many basic anatomical and medical terms, as well as drug nomenclature, and often (but not always) includes a key to pronunciation. Illustrations accompany selected entries, and others incorporate hotlinked cross references to related information included on other pages of the *PharmInfoNet* Web site.

- *Medical Technology-Related Acronyms*
   ⇨ http://www.himanet.com/resource/acronyms.htm
   The Health Industry Manufacturers Association provides this key to acronyms used in the medical device/technology industry.

- *Dictionary of Epidemiology*
   ⇨ http://www.kings.ca.ac.uk/~js229/glossary.html
   Edited by Jonathan Swinton, this dictionary focuses on defining terms from the perspective of ecological epidemiology and reflects U.K. usage. It is published by the University of Cambridge and can be browsed by alphabetic letter.

- *PharmaPages Glossary*
   ⇨ http://www.pjbpubs.co.uk/ppages/index2.html
   Each issue of *PharmaPages*, a PJB newsletter dedicated to Internet issues in the pharmaceutical industry, includes a glossary of the highly specialized vocabulary and numerous abbreviations/acronyms used in publications about the Web and related topics.

5.28 Steinberg ML, Cosloy SD. *Dictionary of Biotechnology and Genetic Engineering.* New York: Facts on File, 1994.

Steinberg and Cosloy also aim at serving the nomenclature needs of a wide-ranging audience, extending their reach to include "high school and college students, lawyers, physicians, scientists, teachers, librarians, or others" attempting to keep abreast of advances reported in the media. Their *Dictionary of Biotechnology and Genetic Engineering* includes both basic and technical terminology, defining terms in a way that readers with only an elementary knowledge of biology and biochemistry will be able to follow.

References

1. Oxman AD, Sackett DL, Guyatt GH. Users' guides to the medical literature I. How to get started. *JAMA* 1993 Nov;270(17):2094.

2. Barry C. Publicly-available information on marketed drugs. In: Pickering WR, ed. *Information sources in pharmaceuticals.* London: Bowker-Saur,1990:275.

3. Mullin BA et al. Comparison of drug information course curricula in schools and colleges of pharmacy. *Am J Pharm Educ* 1995;59:55–59.

4. Putney T, Roper FW. Terminology. In: Roper FW, Boorkman JA, eds. *Introduction to reference sources in the health sciences.* 3rd ed. Metuchen, NJ: Medical Library Association and the Scarecrow Press, 1994:121–134.

Additional Sources of Information

A proposal for structured reporting of randomized controlled trials. *JAMA* 1994 Dec 28;272:1926–1931.

Alla B, Livesay B. *How to use Biological Abstracts, Chemical Abstracts, and Index Chemicus.* Aldershot, England: Gower, 1994.

Amerson AB. Clinical drug literature. In: Gennaro AR, ed. *Remington's pharmaceutical sciences.* 19th ed. Easton, PA: Mack Publishing, 1995, 1837–1841.

Bauer F. Internet resources for chemistry. *Coll & Res Lib News* 1996 Dec at http://www.ala.org/acrl/resdec.html.

Brandon AN, Hill DR. Selected list of books and journals for the small medical library. *Bull Med Libr Assoc* 1997 Apr;85:111–135. Updated biennially.

Collier H, ed. *Recent advances in chemical information.* Cambridge: Royal Society of Chemistry, 1992.

Coombs J. *Dictionary of Biotechnology.* 2nd ed. New York: Stockton Press, 1992.

Courtois MP, Goslen AH. Internet resources in biology. *Coll & Res Lib News* 1996 Jul at http://www.ala.org/acrl/resjul96.html.

Frisse ME, Florance V. A library for internists IX: Recommendations from the American College of Physicians. *Ann Intern Med* 1997 May 15;126(1):836–846. Updated triennially.

Guyatt GH, Sackett DL, Cook DJ. Users' guides to the medical literature II. How to use an article about therapy or prevention. A. Are the results of the study valid? *JAMA* 1993 Dec;270(21):2598–2601.

Guyatt GH, Sackett DL, Cook DJ. Users' guides to the medical literature II. How to use an article about therapy or prevention. B. What were the results and will they help me in caring for my patients? *JAMA* 1994 Jan;271(1):59–63.

Guyatt GH, Sackett DL, Sinclair JC, Hayward R, et al. Users' guides to the medical literature IX. A method for grading health care recommendations. *JAMA* 1995 Dec;274(22):1800–1804.

Hart JL, Hart GE. Biotechnology resources [on the Internet]. *Coll & Res Lib News* 1997 Dec at http://www.ala.org/acrl/resdec97.html.

Hayward RS, Wilson MC, Tunis SR, Bass EB, Guyatt G. Users' guides to the medical literature VIII. How to use clinical practice guidelines. A. Are the recommendations valid? *JAMA* 1995 Aug;274(7):570–574.

Health care on the Internet. Binghamton, NY: Haworth Press, v. 1–, 1997–.

Jaeschke R, Guyatt G, Sackett DL. Users' guides to the medical literature III. How to use an article about a diagnostic test. A. Are the results of the study valid? *JAMA* 1994 Feb;271(5):389–391.

Jaeschke R, Guyatt GH, Sackett DL. Users' guides to the medical literature III. How to use an article about a diagnostic test. B. What are the results and will they help me in caring for my patients? *JAMA* 1994 Mar;271(9):703–707.

Laupacis A, Wells G, Richardson WS, Tugwell P. Users' guides to the medical literature V. How to use an article about prognosis. *JAMA* 1994 Jul;272(3):234–237.

Levine M, Walter S, Lee H, Haines T, et al. Users' guides to the medical literature IV. How to use an article about harm. *JAMA* 1994 May;271(20):1615–1619.

Naylor CD, Guyatt GH. Users' guides to the medical literature X. How to use an article reporting variations in the outcomes of health services. *JAMA* 1996 Feb;275(7):554–558

Nowels D. Whose data are these, anyway? *Arch Fam Med* 1995 Nov;4(11):935–936.

Oxman AD. Checklists for review articles. *Brit Med J* 1994 Sep 10;309:648–650.

Oxman AD, Cook DJ, Guyatt GH. Guidelines for reading literature reviews. *Can Med Assoc J* 1988;138:697–703.

Oxman AD, Cook DJ, Guyatt GH. Users' guides to the medical literature VI. How to use an overview. *JAMA* 1994 Nov;272(17):1367–1371.

Richardson WS, Detsky AS. Users' guides to the medical literature VII. How to use a clinical decision analysis. A. Are the results of the study valid? *JAMA* 1995 Apr;273(16):1292–1295.

Richardson WS, Detsky AS. Users' guides to the medical literature VII. How to use a clinical decision analysis. B. What are the results and will they help me in caring for my patients? *JAMA* 1995 May;273(20):1610–1613.

Snyder DE, ed. *The Interpharm international dictionary of biotechnology and pharmaceutical manufacturing*. 2nd ed. Buffalo Grove, IL: Interpharm, 1992.

Strickland-Hodge B. *How to use Index Medicus, Psychological Abstracts, and Excerpta Medica*. Aldershot, England: Gower, 1994.

Van Camp AJ. Finding health science books and book reviews online. *Online* 1993 May;17:120–123.

Wolman Y. *Chemical information, a practical guide to utilization.* 2nd ed. New York: John Wiley & Sons, 1988.

Wyatt HV, ed. *Information Sources in the life sciences.* 4th ed. London: Bowker-Saur, 1994.

6

Pharmacology and Therapeutics Reference Sources

Consulting reference sources listed in this chapter can save hours of research in the secondary literature. These compendia assemble information on therapeutic use of drugs, precautions, and pharmacology. Some sources base their content on thorough retrospective surveys of the literature, followed by independent expert analysis and evaluation of available bibliography to create summaries of known uses. Others are derived from manufacturer-supplied and FDA-approved professional package insert/labeling information, limiting their scope to officially sanctioned indications only. Types of drug names used in indexing also differ, assessment of which will influence whether consultation of nomenclature sources discussed in Chapter Three is a necessary preliminary step to effective use. The checklist in Figure 5.3 will assist in evaluating each source's potential utility. Discussion here focuses on distinctive features of a selection of compendia and highlights differences in scope among major resources only.

An International Compendium

Any core collection of drug information sources should have at least one ready-reference guide to international drug prescribing and use. Current medical practice transcends geopolitical boundaries, in that it recognizes therapeutic regimens beyond those approved by local government authorities. As we enter the twenty-first century, information service must support global exploration of the literature to examine all possible treatment options. A good place to start is *Martindale*.

6.1 Reynolds, JEF, ed. *Martindale: The Extra Pharmacopoeia*. 31st ed. London: The Pharmaceutical Press, 1996.

Martindale is named for its original editor, William Martindale, a London pharmacist and former president of the Pharmaceutical Society of Great Britain. Since 1883, each new edition of *The Extra Pharmacopoeia* has been eagerly awaited by drug information providers. Larger libraries will want to retain older editions, as well, for the valuable historical perspective they can provide, always reinforced with references to the primary literature of the day.

Compiled since 1933 by the staff of the Pharmaceutical Society, *Martindale* is international and ecumenical in scope. It covers both human and veterinary prescription and nonprescription drugs, single-entity and combination products, drugs still under investigation, as well as those on the market, and some discontinued medicinals still of interest. Its scope includes listings for both active and inactive pharmaceutical ingredients, including coloring, flavoring, and sweetening agents; preservatives; surfactants; solvents; stabilizing and suspending agents; and emulsifying or emollient bases used in the preparation of medications. Information on otherwise elusive products, such as contrast media, nutritional supplements, and vitamins, is also provided.

The overall arrangement is by therapeutic class; Part 1 of the volume organizes material into fifty-four chapters reflecting clinical or pharmaceutical applications. Each section begins with a general introduction to the featured category of drugs, with discussion on choice of therapeutic agent. Monographs for individual compounds follow, each compiling extensive nomenclature data, including generic names (identifying BAN, USAN, INN status), laboratory codes, chemical names, CAS registry number, and molecular formula/weight. References to compendial status, when applicable, cite one or more of seventeen official pharmacopeias. Physical and chemical properties, solubility, and storage data complete the first portion of each *Martindale* monograph. More extensive chemical and analytical data, included in earlier editions, has been removed, reflecting the strong clinical orientation of this "extra" pharmacopeia.

The main portion of each drug monograph is devoted to abstracts of the literature regarding the compound's uses (including off-label indications), absorption and fate, adverse effects, interactions, and toxicity. Documentation is extensive: 26,300 + bibliographic citations back up the 11,000 + reviews and abstracts. Each of the more than 4,500 monographs for generic entities in Part 1 ends with a list of proprietary names, with British brand names heading the entries. Part 2 adds 800 monographs on substances not easily accommodated in the therapeutic category arrangement of Part 1. Compounds featured here include some drugs no longer used clinically, nondrug substances of potential interest in pharmacy and medicine, and selected toxic substances (e.g., pesticides, insecticides) whose effects may require drug therapy. Part 3 is a new section first introduced in the 30th edition of *Martindale* and is devoted to providing details on 62,500 single- and multi-ingredient proprietary preparations from any of seventeen countries. Proprietary name entries identify manufacturer, active ingredients, and summarize indications, but do not attempt coverage of all dosage forms or list quantities of each ingredient in preparations covered. These omissions mean that further follow up is needed to identify equivalents of products featured in this portion of *Martindale*.

The massive (more than 300-page) index is a monument to editorial quality, which has ensured that every brand, generic, and chemical name, investigational drug number, therapeutic or pharmacological category, and disease or condition mentioned in preceding monographs is an access point, adding up to more than 131,500 index entries. Cross references cite both page and column number, but users will find that locating relevant entries in the densely printed monograph sections of the volume can still be difficult. *Martindale* also includes an extremely useful international directory of manufacturers and distributors, giving full mailing addresses for 4,800 companies, clinics, and other organizations cited in drug entries.

Few reference books have become the subject of popular fiction, but *The Extra Pharmacopeia* has earned this distinction. It is mentioned as being part of the scene-of-crime kit of the policeman protagonist, Detective Chief Inspector George Masters, in no fewer than four novels[1-4] written by British author Douglas Clark. Masters quotes *Martindale* as the source for such diverse facts as 1) how to extract a toxin from convallaria (lily of the valley), 2) what effects topical administration of the veterinary analgesic etorphine hydrochloride might have in humans, 3) whether the solubility and toxicity of cyanide would be sufficient to cause death when a treated rope is held momentarily in a weekend sailor's teeth, and 4) which of several emetics could be successfully disguised, with fatal effect, in a thimbleful of liqueur.[5] These examples illustrate the breadth and depth of this compendium's scope, and the first points to one of its particular strengths: coverage of "natural" drugs, toxins, and herbal remedies. This feature accounts for its popularity not only among writers of mystery fiction, but also among drug information professionals asked to locate references to medical uses and toxic properties of plant and animal extracts, which are reemerging as self-medications much favored by the patient population.

Marketed as an online database since 1987 and also available on CD-ROM, *Martindale* in machine-readable format offers users annual updates and the ability to locate groups of compounds based on factors other than those singled out for organization and indexing in the hardcopy volume. The Pharmaceutical Society has developed a hierarchical thesaurus of more than 9,600 descriptors for use as index terms in the database, but not provided in its printed counterpart. Nonetheless, acquisition of *Martindale* in print is a wise investment. It should be noted that, despite its title, this publication has no official government standing or legal status; it is not a book of standards users might equate with the "pharmacopeia" designation. Yet, many would agree that it sets a standard other drug information sources would do well to emulate. Indeed, *Martindale: The Extra Pharmacopoeia* has earned the status of a *vade mecum*, without which no pharmaceutical collection is complete.

Core Collection for Access to U.S. Pharmacotherapeutic Information

Anyone who attempts to single out, from the long list of ready-reference publications available today, sources that can be regarded as essential must approach the task with some trepidation. However, feedback from users of the previous edition of this *Guide* indicated that more advice on collection development would be welcome. Participants in drug information courses for which the *Guide* has served as a textbook have repeated this request. Therefore, while acknowledging that an appropriate core collection is a matter of opinion and very much dependent on user community information needs and expectations, this section identifies resources that can be considered best bets. Selection is based on factors discussed in Chapter Five, reinforced by hands-on experience with these references and ongoing interaction with users requesting assistance in answering drug information questions. Annotations will, hopefully, provide enough information to support assessments of whether a recommended title is really the best choice to match your needs.

6.2 *Drug Facts and Comparisons*. St. Louis: Facts and Comparisons, 1947–. Monthly.

Drug Facts and Comparisons® is an up-to-date compendium of objective information about most drugs on the market today in the United States: more than 16,000 Rx and 6,000 OTC products. Tabbed section dividers assist in access to the therapeutic class arrangement, but a comprehensive drug name index (USAN and brand) is also provided. Monographs for generic entities within each therapeutic class focus on prescribing information, offering sections on actions, indications, contraindications, warnings and precautions, drug interactions (including lab test interferences), adverse effects, patient information, overdosage, and administration/recommended dosage data.

Tables follow each set of monographs, grouping marketed products by dosage and strength. These tables aid quick comparisons among available therapeutic options, noting cost, Rx versus OTC status, package sizes and dosage forms, quantities of each active ingredient in combination products, and distributors. Controlled substance schedules are also noted for applicable products, and sugar-free preparations are consistently identified. The cost index used in tables is based on minimum daily dose at wholesale price without discounts, calculated anew for each table of comparable products, to serve as an indicator of relative, rather than actual, cost.

Several features set *Drug Facts and Comparisons* apart from many other commercial compendia. 1) Adverse effects information includes incidence data, when available. Instead of the usual undifferentiated litany of ills associated with most drugs, ranging from diarrhea to death, incidence data assist in evaluating the likelihood and severity of side effects. Tables inserted in monographs compile facts for quick comparisons of side effects. 2) Discussion of indications covers off-label or investigational uses, sometimes (but not always) with dosage. 3) Additional tables are often included to compare pharmacokinetic data for drugs in a given therapeutic category. 4) Product summary charts concluding each section save time in locating equivalents or comparable products and, in general, streamline drug selection decisions by gathering together influential facts, such as relative cost, sugar-free preparations, etc. 5) Information is timely. Monthly updates to the looseleaf service include a "Keeping Up" news section that frequently features newly-approved drugs or those nearing commercialization, along with announcements of new strengths, new dosage forms, or new indications that will be incorporated into the main monograph section in future revisions. A recent issue of Keeping Up offered a table summarizing data on AIDS drugs in development, including R&D status (e.g., Phase II). 6) Once largely limited to pharmaceuticals sold in the retail, community pharmacy marketplace, *Drug Facts and Comparisons* has expanded its scope to encompass many hospital products. For example, a section on biologics covers immune serums, antitoxins and antivenins, vaccines, allergenic products, and *in vivo* diagnostics (tuberculin tests, skin test antigens). Biologics available only from the Centers for Disease Control (CDC) are included, as are NCI investigational agents available outside specialty protocols. Listings for *in vitro* and *in vivo* diagnostic aids cover home test kits, as well as those intended for professional office use (e.g., pregnancy tests, occult blood screens).

Beyond drug directory listings, *Drug Facts and Comparisons* adds reference material on controlled substance regulations, FDA risk categories for drug use in pregnant women, management of acute overdosage and severe hypersensitivity reactions, normal laboratory values, and a key to standard abbreviations. It also includes a complete table of orphan drugs. The Manufacturers/Distributors Index is actually a directory (no page or product cross references) with addresses and telephone numbers. A dosage form/packaging format trademark glossary is unique. It identifies brand names for items such as unit-dose packs (e.g., Accu-Pak, Ciba Geigy) or sustained-release preparations (Dura-Tab, Chronotab, etc.).

The drawbacks? No bibliographic references accompany monographs. Consultation of cumulative indexes, issued quarterly, must be followed up by a check of subsequent monthly indexes. Brand names identified in the separate trademark glossary are not also listed in the general drug name/class indexes. Finally, the looseleaf binder is a monster, requiring two hands and a table to use.

The awkwardness of the binder leads some prospective purchasers to opt for the annual, hardbound edition of *Drug Facts and Comparisons*, thereby sacrificing the important advantage of timely updates. Ideally, both looseleaf and hardbound versions of *Facts* should be acquired: the annual volume to establish an archival record of marketed products, the looseleaf subscription to provide the most up-to-date prescribing information. This resource has also recently been issued on CD-ROM, updated quarterly.

6.3 *Mosby's GenRx*. St. Louis: Mosby: Denniston Publishing, 1990–. Annual, with quarterly supplements.

Formerly titled *Physicians' GenRx*, this annual compendium includes entries for all FDA-approved prescription drugs (1,700 in the 1998 edition), including (but not limited to) generic products. Monographs, arranged alphabetically by USAN, are officially authorized professional package inserts, but have been augmented with references to unapproved uses. These off-label uses cannot, by law, be integrated into FDA-approved labeling, so the compromise reached in this source is to list them at the top of monographs, flagged with asterisks, and to include off-label uses as part of indexing. No dosage or precautions data are supplied for unofficial indications. Other additions to monographs include systematic identification of 1) DESI review drugs rated as "unproved efficacy"; 2) orphan drugs; 3) top-sellers in the United States, e.g., top 20, top 100; 4) scheduled drugs, i.e., II, III, IV, V; 5) FDA risk category in pregnancy; 6) date approved, from April 1982 forward; 7) patent expiration dates, from December 1986 through December 2004; 8) FDA's NDA code, e.g., 1P, 4S; 9) NDC; 10) *Orange Book* (4.42) therapeutic equivalency rating; and 11) drugs with worldwide sales in U.S. dollars of more than $100 million, $500 million, or $1 billion.

Mosby's GenRx monographs also designate federal procurement eligibility (i.e., covered by Medicaid rebate) and other formulary coverage, naming major managed care organizations on whose reimbursable lists the featured drugs are included. Entries identify federal maximum allowable costs (MAC) and Health Care Financing Administration (HCFA) reimbursement codes. Pricing information (comparable to *Red Book* data, 3.15) and cost of therapy information are included, as well. The latter cost factor is explained as a benchmark based on assumptions from labeling administration instructions. Sometimes, a drug's cost of therapy is also compared to cost of hospitalization.

In addition to a directory of certified poison control centers in the United States and Canada, a company directory is also included. Manufacturer data have been enhanced in *Mosby's GenRx*, beyond the expected name-and-address listing. A Supplier Profiles section includes, when available, product sales volume, total number of employees, revenues and net income for the past five years, and executive personnel names for more than 850 public and private companies. To assist in visual identification of 1,260 solid dosage forms, a photograph section and index to tablet/capsule imprints replicated from The Medicine Chart section of *USP DI* (6.5) was added in 1995 and continued in later editions. Other recent enhancements include comparative drug charts, a directory of AIDS drug assistance programs, a list of withdrawn drugs, and a list of sound alike/look alike drugs.

Finally, one integrated index offers access, by nonproprietary and brand names, manufacturers, pharmacological action, therapeutic use, and disease state, to information regarding the 30,000 drug products included in the scope of this

2,500-page volume. Keyword index entries bring together useful lists of the top-selling 100, 200, 300, and 400 medications in the United States. The index also provides all U.S. brand names ever used for drugs listed in *Mosby's GenRx*, including those no longer available. A recent enhancement has been foreign brand names used in any of 137 countries (10,000 names in 1998). However, this addition does not mean that *Mosby's GenRx* covers foreign drugs. Users should bear in mind that its scope, though admirable, is confined to marketed U.S. Rx drugs only.

Updates to the annual hardcopy volume currently consist of quarterly supplements. *Mosby's GenRx* is also available in a variety of machine-readable formats, including CD-ROM and Internet/Intranet implementations, with networking and site licensing an option (see http://www.mosby.com).

6.4 *AHFS Drug Information.* Washington, DC: American Society of Health-System Pharmacists, 1989–. Annual, with quarterly supplements.

Professional society publications in the field of drug information have the advantage of sound scholarship, reinforced by rigorous peer review, and a reputation for authoritative evaluation associated with the imprimatur of the sponsoring organization. The American Society of Health-System Pharmacists (ASHP, formerly the American Society of Hospital Pharmacists) is a prolific and highly respected publisher in this subject specialty. Their imprint has long been regarded as a guarantee of quality.

AHFS Drug Information is no exception. Formerly published under the title *American Hospital Formulary Service* (1959 +), this compendium is more selective in scope than other resources described thus far in this section. It focuses on better known (rather than all) products in use in the United States, with the objective of providing unbiased and evaluated monographs to assist healthcare professionals in rational drug therapy. Arranged by therapeutic categories, each group of monographs in preceded by a general overview of the drug class and factors to consider in prescribing decisions. Entries for individual substances include alternate nonproprietary name(s), structural formula, and thoroughly researched discussion of pharmacology, including absorption, distribution, metabolism, and excretion. Both investigational (off-label) and approved uses are discussed, with full details regarding dosage and precautions. A list of U.S. proprietary preparations and their manufacturers concludes each monograph.

Drug classes covered include many for which comparable authoritative and evaluative discussion is not readily available, such as radiopharmaceuticals, parenterals, and selected biologics/vaccines. The primary emphasis is on prescription drugs, but some OTC agents, such as nutritional supplements and vitamins, are included in the scope of *AHFS*. The research and evaluation process imposes some constraints on rapid addition of monographs for new drugs, but supplements to annual volumes are issued periodically throughout the year.

AHFS Drug Information is also available online as part of the *Drug Informa-*

tion Fulltext database (14.18), where users will find that supportive bibliography for each monograph, omitted in the hardcopy volume, is available for immediate display. CD-ROM editions, generally updated less frequently, are offered by several vendors. MedAxon combines *AHFS Drug Information* with First DataBank's *National Drug Data File* (*NDDF*) on compact disc. *Stat!-Ref* supplements *AHFS* with *Mosby's GenRx* and the *Merck Manual of Diagnosis and Therapy* on a single CD-ROM, updated semiannually.

One measure of the quality of this publication is that many hospitals adopted it as their standard for therapy and product selection in the days when institutional formularies were more prevalent. The *AHFS* classification scheme developed for the arrangement of drugs by therapeutic/pharmacological category is also used in other drug information sources, and many practitioners advocate its use in organizing personal reprint or drug information center files.

6.5 *USP DI: United States Pharmacopeia Dispensing Information. Volume 1: Drug Information for the Health Care Professional.* Rockville, MD: United States Pharmacopeial Convention, 1982–. Annual, with monthly updates.

With coverage of approximately 11,000 generic and brand name products, volume 1 of *USP DI®* is narrower in scope than *Drug Facts and Comparisons* (6.2) and *Mosby's GenRx* (6.3). Like *AHFS Drug Information*, *USP DI*'s peer review accounts, in part, for its greater selectivity. Each monograph in *Drug Information for the Health Care Professional* is subjected to an approval process representing the consensus of thirty-five expert advisory panels and involving the contributions of more than 700 volunteers drawn from the fields of medicine, pharmacy, dentistry, and nursing. Scientific, professional, consumer, and trade organizations provide input, as does the federal government. The result is a thoroughly investigated collection of authoritative monographs cited in federal, and some state, statutes as a basis for development of formularies and drug utilization review under Medicaid. It is this quasi-official status and its well-written, structured, and attractively presented reference material that earns this volume a place in the core collection. (Note: A Spanish-language version of *USP DI Volume 1*, entitled *Información de Medicamentos para el Profesional Sanitario*, is also being published by the Ministerio de Sanidad y Consume de España.)

Each generic substance entry is organized in an outline format, with category headings covering indications, dosage, drug interactions and precautions, side/ adverse effects, pharmacology/pharmacokinetics, patient consultation, and available dosage forms. Reference material on indications addresses both labeled and unlabeled (if judged to be medically accepted) uses. Two separate indexes offer access by drug names (USAN and both U.S. and Canadian brand names) and indications.

Appendices compile information about new products and uses, orphan drugs, biologics, and issues related to total parenteral nutrition (such as TPN product stability, precipitates, compatibility, compounding, and container requirements). Also appended are a directory of poison control centers in the United States and a listing of the U.S. Veterans' Administration system for classifying drugs. A chapter devoted to Drug Utilization Review describes the DUR process, providing a framework for criteria development, useful definitions, background bibliography, and selected case studies.

Annual subscribers automatically receive monthly updates containing tables of additional products and indications, offering brief interim entries until full monographs can be developed. *USP DI Update* issues also provide information on newly accepted unlabeled indications, which are not FDA-approved, but which the USP advisory panels consider to be part of currently accepted medical practice. Another valuable extra in updates is a cumulative six-month list of human and veterinary drug recalls announced by the FDA, as well as recalls of selected medical devices used in ambulatory care medical settings. Monthly issues also announce new USAN designations.

In December 1994, the American Medical Association and the U.S. Pharmacopeial Convention announced plans to combine *Drug Evaluations* and *USP DI* into a joint database, to provide a national source of consistent information for use by physicians, pharmacists, and other practitioners. *AMA Drug Evaluations*, published from 1971 through 1995, was well known for its critical assessment of therapeutic options, backed up by thorough surveys of available scientific data. The result of the AMA/USP agreement has been integration of this comparative therapeutic information into *USP DI*. AMA-derived monographs, organized by disease conditions or symptoms, provide an overview of alternative drug therapies.

Still another strategic alliance was announced in September, 1998. The *USP DI* database and licensing of its trademark has been sold to Thomson Healthcare. Thomson's subsidiary publishers already include Medical Economics (*Physicians Desk Reference*) and Micromedex (*DRUGDEX, POISINDEX*, etc.). Under the new agreement, the U.S. Pharmaceopeial Convention will retain oversight of *USP DI* content through ongoing work with its expert advisory panels. Micromedex will assume product development, marketing, and distribution responsibilities. What effect this collaboration will have on future publication is unknown, but the 19th edition of *USP DI* is scheduled for release in January 1999.

Meanwhile, numerous online and Internet versions of this important publication continue to be introduced. Implementations extract drug monographs from the hardcopy resource and make them accessible through a variety of user interfaces. InteliHealth, HealthAnswers, and HELIX Web sites each added *USP DI Volume I* in 1998 (see http://www.usp.org/did). Dialog launched its online version in 1996, with the content structured in an entirely different way than the printed counterpart. It concatenates separate entries for nonproprietary names into approximately 800 master monographs covering drug classes. For example, information on cimetidine, famotidine, nizatidine, and ranitidine is coalesced into a single master entry on Histamine H2-Receptor Antagonists (Systemic). Refer to Chapter Fourteen for further details about this *USP DI* database (14.19).

6.6 Covington TR, ed. *Handbook of Nonprescription Drugs.* 11th ed. Washington, DC: American Pharmaceutical Association, 1998.

6.7 Knodel LC, ed. *Nonprescription Products: Formulations and Features.* Washington, DC: American Pharmaceutical Association, 1998–. Annual.

OTC products (also known as "patent medicines") are the poor stepchildren of pharmaceutical information services. Nonprescription medications tend to be either ignored or very selectively covered in publications prepared for health science professionals, perhaps because caregivers have, traditionally, been less actively involved in the self-medication decisions of their patients. The FDA's designation of OTC versus prescription status is based, in part, on whether adequate directions for safe and effective use, without medical supervision, can be written for the average layperson. This distinction generally limits drugs approved for OTC use to those indicated for treatment of relatively minor and self-limiting conditions that either do not require assessment by a physician for diagnosis or do not require treatment that should be monitored by a medical doctor. Nevertheless, proponents of holistic medicine and family practitioners may be called upon for advice in treating such ailments, as will community pharmacists, especially those practicing in independent, rather than chain store, settings. Information services to support their needs will benefit greatly from inclusion of a professionally oriented, noncommercial OTC drug reference compendium in their core collection.

Because pharmacists are, in fact, the only health professionals who receive formal, university-level training in nonprescription pharmacotherapy, it is not surprising that by far the best guide to OTC drug use is prepared under the auspices of the American Pharmaceutical Association. First published in 1967, new editions of the APhA *Handbook of Nonprescription Drugs* have steadily grown in size and quality with each revision, issued every two to four years. The 11th edition includes well-written introductory material on the self-care movement and patient assessment and consultation. The thirty-three chapters that follow are each dedicated to providing thorough background on, and unbiased evaluation of, nonprescription products in a given therapeutic category.

Intended to increase professional competence and expand patient services, each chapter's discussion begins with assessment criteria ("Questions to ask the patient . . ."), and proceeds to review the epidemiology, etiology, anatomy, and physiology of the condition. Factors to be considered in product selection are itemized and weighed dispassionately from both a scientific and psychosocial perspective. For example, a chapter on diabetes care includes discussion of nondrug care (exercise, diet, recommendations for travel), covering behavioral issues and patient education. Similarly, a chapter on OTC contraceptives also covers noninvasive or nondrug methods, including rhythm, fertility awareness, and condoms. Numerous charts, figures, drawings, and other illustrative materials greatly enhance the information content of the *Handbook of Nonprescription Drugs*.

APhA began separate publication of supplementary *Product Updates* in 1995, in order to facilitate annual revision of product listings without re-issuing the main narrative volume. *Nonprescription Products: Formulations and Features* is the new name for the companion volume. It covers more than 3,500 brand name OTCs, organizing information into tables designed to assist in comparisons of ingredients present in each formulation and their respective quantities.

Frequently requested information is systematically identified in *Formulations and Features* tables, which flag sugar-free, gluten-free, and aspirin-free products, as well as those where cholesterol, caffeine, dyes, fluoride, fragrance, lactose, preservatives, purine, sodium, or sulfite are absent. Products containing phenylalanine are also identified. (Note: cost information is omitted.) Listed brand name preparations represent a sample of better-known products available in each of the eighty-two functional categories covered, rather than a comprehensive catalog. A general index offers unified access by both brand and generic drug names. Appendices include a directory of information sources for both pharmacists and patients, listing associations (professional and self-help), publishers, and drug companies. Two new tables added in the 1998–99 update bring together miscellaneous diagnostic test kits and, in a separate listing, various dietary supplements.

Several classes of products and conditions not covered elsewhere in the professional reference literature are accorded authoritative assessment in the *Handbook of Nonprescription Drugs*. Its scope and overall quality are unparalleled, making this volume and its *Formulations and Features* annual update valuable additions to the core drug information collection. Counterparts for Canadian products would be good investments for libraries near the border: the *Compendium of Nonprescription Products* (10.21) and *Nonprescription Drug References for Health Professionals* (9.45), both published by the Canadian Pharmaceutical Association. The Royal Pharmaceutical Society's *Non-Prescription Medicines* (10.23) handbook provides comparable assistance to U.K. information providers.

Alternative Selections and Additional Bibliography

Several ready-reference publications could serve as acceptable alternatives to core collection titles discussed above, or qualify as strong add-on candidates when a larger selection of resources is desired. Other compendia featured in this section of the *Guide* will, perhaps, fill in gaps in the problem-solving capabilities of collections already established.

6.8 *PDR Generics*. Montvale, NJ: Medical Economics, 1995–. Annual.

Debuting in 1995 from the publishers of the *PDR* (6.10), *PDR Generics*™ differs from its partial namesake in that it includes information on virtually all prescription drugs currently on the market, rather than a selection of products, and
it compiles information on both approved and off-label uses. This behemoth
(3,500-page) volume includes *Red Book* (3.15) cost data (average unit prices and
average prices for standard package sizes), *Orange Book* (4.42) bioequivalence
rating, and controlled substance schedule as part of product entries. Prescribing
information in individual drug monographs represents a synthesis of FDA-
approved labeling (standard package insert) and of peer-reviewed data on unapproved uses, derived from *DRUGDEX®* (6.14). Unlike *DRUGDEX*, *PDR Generics* does not supply bibliographic references in support of this portion of its
monographs, but does reproduce summaries of study results and differentiates
among adverse drug reactions by citing incidence data. A bonus is that structural
formulas accompany entries for single-entity products.

PDR Generics offers a separate listing of FDA pregnancy category drugs, and
appendices which include directories of drug information centers and poison information centers, as well as a summary of new molecular entities approved in
the previous year. This summary identifies NDA numbers for each NME, date of
NDA filing, date of first action by the FDA, number of months to the first action,
date of approval, and number of months to approval. Appendix material also features brief descriptions of FDA drug classification (i.e., P, S, E, AA, V). A section
devoted to Additional Alternatives at the back of the volume lists brand and generic alternatives beyond those identified in the How Supplied segment of drug
monographs in the main product information portion of *PDR Generics*.

The product identification guide in this new Medical Economics compendium
lists more than 6,000 imprint codes. Color photographs of 1,500 products, organized by generic name, augment the imprint code aid to visual identification of
solid dosage forms. *PDR Generics* perpetuates the indexing arrangement of the
Physicians' Desk Reference. Drug brand and generic name indexing is separated
from product category (therapeutic/pharmacological) access, and a third index is
devoted to indications (2,300 in all). Given its much broader scope (40,000 single
and multisource drug products), *PDR Generics'* manufacturers directory (including both address and telephone numbers) is, however, far more extensive than the
PDR's.

A point-by-point comparison of features annotated here will show that *PDR
Generics* is a competitor to *Mosby's GenRx*, but differs in its arrangement of indexes, method of presenting off-label indications information, number of extra
facts systematically added to monographs (e.g., fewer trade-related flags, such as
top-seller indicators, formulary identifiers, patent expiration dates), and manufacturer directory data compilation. Some of these differences may disappear in future editions of both resources, but, for the moment, must be taken into account
when deciding whether this is a complement to, or substitute for, *Mosby's GenRx*.

6.9 *Physicians' Desk Reference for Nonprescription Drugs.* Montvale, NJ: Medical Economics, 1979–. Annual.

Overlap between the *Physicians' Desk Reference for Nonprescription Drugs*® and APhA's *Handbook of Nonprescription Drugs* (6.6) is far less obvious. The *PDR* compendium is a collection of manufacturers' product information, totally unlike the *Handbook*'s comparative and evaluative approach designed to assist in patient counseling and product selection. The two sources also differ in the number and types of OTC preparations represented. The Medical Economics publication contains detailed information on 700 products marketed by eighty-six manufacturers. Its first section indexes participating companies, listing their OTC products and address and telephone numbers for emergency contacts. Section 2 is a product brand name index, Section 3 a product category index by indication (e.g., acne, allergy relief), and Section 4 an index to active ingredients, accessible by generic name.

This member of the growing family of *PDR* publications provides the popular identification guide, with full color actual-size photographs, arranged alphabetically by manufacturer, of more than 1,000 products. Helpful appendices include an FDA telephone directory and a name/address/phone listing of state boards of pharmacy and drug information centers. The product information (monograph) portion of the volume is, however, still limited to package insert data for a relatively small selection of drugs, whose suppliers pay for their listings in this volume. Entire categories of OTC products covered in the *Handbook of Nonprescription of Drugs* are omitted here. APhA's *Handbook* includes, for example, otic preparations to treat ear conditions beyond the scope of "OTC PDR" listings, and personal care products, such as depilatories, not found in the Medical Economics publication's listing. Also absent is structure and content to assist in product comparisons and unbiased evaluations.

Nonetheless, the *Physicians' Desk Reference for Nonprescription Drugs* can be regarded as a useful complementary resource. Particularly noteworthy is its inclusion of products from major homeopathic companies, such as Boiron and Standard Homeopathic, and from purveyors of other hard-to-find drug categories, such as nutritional supplements (including shark cartilage) and natural vitamins. This coverage of otherwise elusive, but often requested, information makes this compendium a strong candidate for inclusion in collections that must support service to the general public.

6.10 *Physicians' Desk Reference.* Montvale, NJ: Medical Economics, 1947–. Annual.

It may seem surprising that the *Physicians' Desk Reference* (*PDR*) was not listed earlier in this *Guide* as part of the recommended core collection. For many years, mass distribution free-of-charge to physicians ensured that the *PDR* exerted a strong influence on prescribing patterns, while, at the same time, performing the much-needed service of broadly disseminating labeling/package insert information to the practitioners for whom it was prepared. Giveaways also guaranteed the *PDR*'s visibility in physicians' office reference collections, lending it value in the eyes of patients. By the time Medical Economics began marketing the *PDR* in bookstores serving the general public, an audience of increasingly health-conscious consumers was ready and waiting. If they stock no other drug information source, public libraries nearly always reserve a place on their shelves for the *PDR*, in direct response to user requests. Why, then, is it not listed here among best bets?

First of all, it's important to recognize that the *Physicians' Desk Reference* is a highly selective listing of therapeutic options available on the U.S. market today (4,000 prescription drugs from 250 manufacturers). Product representation is limited, due to fees assessed by the publisher for inclusion in *PDR* listings. Even among companies who choose to participate and are included in the *PDR*'s manufacturer directory, users will find drugs listed that are not featured later in the volume in the detailed product information section. Economics play a major role in *PDR* coverage, essentially equating it with a paid advertising and marketing vehicle.

Once this fact is recognized, there's a tendency among users to suspect commercial bias in the product information provided in the *Physicians' Desk Reference*. This belief is unfounded or, charitably viewed, considerably overstates the case. The *PDR* simply reproduces FDA-approved prescription drug labeling. There is no latitude in government regulations regarding therapeutic claims made or adverse effects identified. Label content has been (somewhat wryly) described as "representing the least common denominator of disagreement between attorneys from the drug company and those from the Food and Drug Administration."[6] Claims cannot exceed indications for which proof of safety and efficacy have been proven, and documented adverse effects cannot be omitted. Although the format and layout of information (e.g., boxed highlighting, bold or italic typeface), chosen by companies but still prescreened by the FDA, may influence readers to notice some data elements more than others, the content is not, strictly speaking, advertising. The bias accusation can only be accurately applied to the presence or absence of listings for marketed products, based on payment for inclusion.

The *PDR*'s limitation to package inserts can, however, safely be cited as a second reason for also-ran rather than must-have status here. Package inserts vary greatly in quality from company to company. For example, adverse effects information can simply be relayed as a catalog of conditions, ranging in severity from a temporary rash or gastrointestinal disturbance to anaphylactic shock, and varying in likelihood from common occurrences to extremely rare incidents. Some drug sponsors include incidence data, when available, in their labeling. Further desirable enhancements seen more often today than in past inserts are bibliographic references, statistical tables and charts, a chemical structure, and a list of educational materials. Many companies also labor long and hard to produce well-written inserts, which adds considerably to their value in communicating pharmacology and therapeutics information. But what no amount of effort can change is that official labeling must omit discussion of unapproved uses, however prevalent and accepted they are in current medical practice. Sources that extend their content beyond package insert data must, therefore, be given higher precedence than the *Physicians' Desk Reference* when efficient problem solving, and collection development to support it, is the goal.

The arrangement of the *PDR* has also added to its detractors. There are three wholly separate indexes: a manufacturer index/directory, a brand/generic name index, and a product category index. The latter favors therapeutic over pharmacological terminology, although it is a mixture of both. The product category section ends with a useful list of unit-dose systems covered in the volume. Another helpful feature is a visual product identification guide, which includes 2,000 color photographs. Less helpful is the organization of this section, which is by manufacturer, rather than by imprint code or other distinguishing characteristics, such as color, that are obvious starting points in this difficult type of identification. A separate section in the *PDR* is devoted to diagnostic products in common use. Appendices list poison control centers, discontinued products, FDA telephone numbers, and keys to controlled substance categories (i.e., schedules) and FDA use-in-pregnancy ratings. The agency's Adverse Event Report form is also included in the *PDR*. Two supplements per year, issued in May and September, are available for separate purchase. The entire PDR library (6.9, 6.10, 6.12, and 7.13) is also available in CD-ROM format, with an option to add on *The Merck Manual* and *Stedman's Medical Dictionary* to the subscriber disc.

Despite its limited coverage, in terms of number of products listed and indications discussed, the *Physicians' Desk Reference* remains the most widely recognized U.S. drug compendium. For this reason, it may be prudent to include it in collections. Dissenters have argued that the only way to wean practitioners from too-heavy reliance on this source is to eliminate it from their shelves and substitute reference tools broader in scope, less overtly commercial in origin, and more evaluative in their presentation of material necessary to support scientific product selection. This radical approach to "user education" may be necessary in reference collections serving the public. (Refer to Chapter Nine for further discussion of drug information for the consumer or patient.)

6.11 *ImmunoFacts: Vaccines & Immunologic Drugs*. St. Louis: Facts and Comparisons, 1995–. Looseleaf, updated semiannually.

It seems appropriate that the year marking the 200th anniversary of Jenner's landmark work with cowpox and smallpox (credited with awakening the medical establishment to the advantages of vaccination) was also the release date of a new reference compendium dedicated to compilation of data regarding this increasingly important category of drug therapy. *ImmunoFacts* assembles, in nearly 100 detailed monographs, information needed by professionals who prescribe, dispense, or administer vaccines. Each entry describes approved indications, unlabeled uses, limitations, contraindications, adverse reactions (including statistics on frequency and severity), potential drug interactions, and pharmacological/dosing characteristics (route and site, booster recommendations, onset, duration, protective level). Both pediatric and adult dosages are routinely specified, along with summaries of pertinent clinical studies (alas, without references to primary sources) and facts regarding use in elderly, pregnant, or lactating patients. The Pharmaceutical Characteristics section of monographs lists dose forms, packaging, solvent, adjuvant, preservative, allergen, and excipient data, as well as physical appearance, storage/stability guidelines, and shelf life.

A particularly exciting bonus in *ImmunoFacts* monographs is a lengthy section devoted to disease epidemiology, where domestic and international incidence statistics are compiled, accompanied by discussion of susceptible pools (data on populations at risk), target for 2000 (U.S. goals set in *Healthy People 2000*), transmission media/means, incubation, and communicability. The concluding portion of monographs outlines historical milestones in disease prevention and the specified vaccine's development, date of first U.S. licensing, national policy on use, and pharmacoeconomics considerations, ending with citations to one or two recent review articles.

Monographs cover all vaccines, toxoids, globulins, immunologic mediators and modulators, hypersensitivity agents, and related nonimmunologics in use in the United States. Descriptions of selected investigational and international drugs are also included. Dozens of charts facilitate comparisons of brand name preparations and quick identification/assessment of drug interactions, summarizing effects, management, significance, validity, and frequency of the latter. One semiannual update to the looseleaf volume and two issues of an informative newsletter are offered as part of annual subscriptions to *ImmunoFacts*.

Booster Shots, the semiannual companion newsletter, highlights recent developments in immunology, citing references to emerging off-label uses, cost-effectiveness studies, epidemiological studies, and progress in immunization programs, along with new drug approvals, new indications added (supplemental NDAs), an update on trademarks, changes in FDA or U.S. Department of Agriculture practices or policies, company news, relevant Internet sites, and related professional association guidelines (e.g., the American Veterinary Medical Association's revised recommendations for vaccinating horses).

6.12 *Physicians' Desk Reference for Ophthalmology*. Montvale, NJ: Medical Economics, 1972–. Annual.

6.13 *Ophthalmic Drug Facts*. St. Louis: Facts and Comparisons. Annual.

The *Physicians' Desk Reference for Ophthalmology* departs from the expected *PDR* norm by organizing information into therapeutic (indications) categories and including numerous tables and charts to assist in product comparisons and selection. Coverage encompasses not only drugs, but also selected medical devices, such as suture materials, lenses, and diagnostic tests. Separate indexes offer access by manufacturer name, brand name, product category, and active ingredients (USAN). Indexes also help users locate instrumentation and equipment and patient education materials. Additional reference materials provided in this helpful volume are a listing of vision standards for various occupations and a color vision screening chart. Another unusual feature is that, although the *PDR for Ophthalmology* is intended for a health professional audience, it also includes advice for patients.

Ophthalmic Drug Facts replicates many of the features that have made *Drug Facts and Comparisons* (6.2), from the same publisher, an indispensable reference source: similar drugs are compared side-by-side in detailed, evaluative monographs, and sections devoted to individual therapeutic categories typically include useful charts and tables to assist in product selection and assessment. Mydriatics and cycloplegics, antiallergics, antibiotics, glaucoma agents, surgical and nonsurgical adjuncts, anti-inflammatory and anti-infective agents, and systemic drugs are among categories featured. Extras include a special section on contact lens care, a chapter on orphan and investigational drugs, an excellent glossary, and a manufacturer directory.

6.14 *DRUGDEX*. Denver: Micromedex, 1978–. Annual.

DRUGDEX® is part of an automated (CD-ROM or Intranet) collection of databases, known as CCIS (Computerized Clinical Information System, marketed by Micromedex), but is also available for separate purchase. It consists of two subfiles: Drug Evaluation Monographs and Drug Consults. Monographs resemble those found in *Drug Information Fulltext* (14.18), the online counterpart of *AHFS Drug Information* (6.4). Each reviews a single generic entity's known uses (both FDA-approved and off-label), dosage, precautions, pharmacokinetics, interactions, and adverse reactions, and is accompanied by relevant bibliographic references. Accessible by generic names, brand names, or indications, Drug Evaluation Monographs have been prepared for both approved drugs and a selection of investigational agents, prescription and OTC preparations, and U.S. as well as non-U.S. medications (although coverage of the latter is relatively limited). Current scope statistics cite 1,800 products. The Drug Consults portion of the *DRUGDEX* system is its most unusual feature. "Consults" anticipate inquiries on current drug-related topics and provide ready-made responses, backed up by brief bibliographies and cross-referenced to pertinent Drug Evaluation Monographs.

When using *DRUGDEX*, it's important to check dates at the end of Monographs or Consults, to verify when they were written and last updated. Consults, in particular, tend to have a relatively short shelf life and should be supplemented with a search for recent references obtained from more up-to-date online sources (e.g., *MEDLINE*, *EMBASE*, and other databases discussed in Chapter Fourteen). Fishman[7] also warns that, because CCIS is designed for *ad hoc* use without reliance on training or printed documentation, search protocols are highly structured and limited to on-screen menu choices. This characteristic can sometimes lead to missed data, due to inappropriate or inadequate user entries/responses (e.g., failure to follow up cross references under a generic name).

6.15 Rakel RE. *Conn's Current Therapy*. Philadelphia: W.B. Saunders, 1949–. Annual.

With its focus on problems encountered in primary care, *Conn's Current Therapy* emulates the now deceased *AMA Drug Evaluations*. Tables identify preferred drugs and 1,000 best therapies for more than 300 medical conditions. Off-label indications, footnoted as lacking official approval, are cited, as are some non-U.S. drugs and investigational agents. Product selection recommendations must be followed up by consultation of other sources, as *Conn's Current Therapy* limits its discussion to generic entities. The index omits brand names, instead offering access by USANs and disease/condition terms. A new feature added to Appendices in the 1995 edition (and continued thereafter) is a list of drugs approved by the FDA during the previous year. Another recent enhancement is a list of the 200 drugs most frequently prescribed in the United States, including brand names, manufacturers, and relative cost indicators ($–$$$$).

6.16 *Therapeutic Choices*. 2nd ed. Ottawa: Canadian Pharmaceutical Association, 1998.

Therapeutic Choices is narrower in scope, focusing on management of about 100 common medical conditions. Both pharmacologic and non-drug treatment options are discussed, based on the clinical experience of more than 100 contributing Canadian physicians and pharmacists. Chapters are organized into sections devoted to psychiatric, neurologic, eye, cardiovascular, respiratory, gastrointestinal, musculoskeletal, skin, endocrine, blood, and fluid or electrolyte disorders. Other topics singled out for separate discussion are infectious diseases, drugs in pregnancy and lactation, antineoplastics, vitamins and minerals, and symptom control. Chronic fatigue syndrome and HIV infection are examples of new material added in the second edition of *Therapeutic Choices*, which also adds pharmacoeconomic considerations to its appendices. Dosage adjustment in renal impairment, abbreviations for microorganisms, and a glossary of other abbreviations are the subject of other appendices.

6.17 *The Medical Letter on Drugs and Therapeutics*. New Rochelle, NY: The Medical Letter, 1959–. Biweekly.

It's unusual for a brief newsletter to achieve recognition as a valuable reference source worth archiving, but *The Medical Letter* is often accorded this distinction. Each biweekly issue features one or two topics, evaluating published data and delivering the informed opinion of *The Medical Letter* clinical consultants. For example, a recent issue focused on drugs of choice for cancer chemotherapy and included in its discussion off-label (unapproved, but accepted) indications. *The Medical Letter* also frequently summarizes drug selection data in tabular format, facilitating quick comparisons of recommended agents on factors such as adverse effects, costs, etc. An annual index offers brand and generic name access, as well as cross references from drug class terms and subject descriptors. *STAT!-Ref*, from Teton Data Systems, supplies *The Medical Letter* (v. 30 forward) as part of its CD-ROM collection.

6.18 Ringer DL. *Physicians' Guide to Nutriceuticals*. Omaha, NE: Nutritional Data Resources, 1998–. Annual.

According to its Web site, Nutritional Data Resources is a company founded in 1995 with the express purpose of publishing the nutraceutical industry's first third-party product-specific compendium. The result is the *Physicians' Guide to Nutriceuticals* (*PGN*), a 286-page publication with coverage of more than 200 dietary supplements and herbal remedies on the market in the United States. Entries in its main Product Information section include descriptions, ingredients, intended uses, warnings, interactions data, summaries of selected clinical studies, and information on how each product is supplied and where it can be purchased. This section is organized alphabetically by company, but a separate product name index provides access by brand names. A Universal Index enables look-ups by generic terminology (e.g., plant names) and specific health conditions (arthritis, cholesterol). An opening company index functions as a directory, providing mailing and e-mail addresses, telephone numbers (voice and fax), and Web site URLs, when available.

A Quick Reference Guide in the *PGN* lists vitamins, minerals, and herbs cross referenced to U.S. RDA, when applicable, and to claimed biological functions or health benefits (conditions, symptoms). The volume also includes a glossary of 400 terms and a section devoted to Studies and References. Organized by product, bibliographic data indicate that a broad spectrum of sources have been used to support functional claims. The mixed quality of references cited show that follow-up searches and evaluation of the literature would be desirable, to establish credibility and authority. Unfortunately, users of the *Physicians' Guide to Nutriceuticals* will not be restricted to healthcare professionals equipped by education or inclination to investigate further. For example, customer comments available at a noted electronic bookstore site on the Internet show that consumers have contributed the bulk of reviews. On the other hand, the publishers of *PGN* plan to limit free access to quarterly updates online to licensed practitioners only (see http://www.mitec.n4/~manager/index.html).

Several clinical reference sources identified in Chapter Twelve's discussion of pharmacognosy would be alternatives worth examining for collections intended to support practitioners (see 12.9–12.18). *The Honest Herbal* (9.19) or the *American Pharmaceutical Association's Practical Guide to Natural Medicines* (9.20) would be supplementary titles for consumers.

Handbooks

Drug information handbooks are compact quick-reference guides that anticipate common problems in drug therapy and provide concise answers. Given their fast facts orientation, handbooks can be valuable additions to core library collections, if judiciously selected.

6.19 Anderson PO, Knoben JE, eds. *Handbook of Clinical Drug Data.* 8th ed. Stamford, CT: Appleton & Lange, 1997.

Anderson and Knoben's *Handbook of Clinical Drug Data* has, by its eighth edition in 1997, achieved the stature of a classic reference source in pocket-sized, albeit 900-page, format. A multitude of tables add to its utility, including compilation of normal laboratory values and of extensive pharmacokinetic parameter data, plasma levels, and quick-reference material on adverse drug reactions. This handbook features reviews of more than 700 drugs, including many new antivirals, cardiovascular and cancer chemotherapy agents, and products produced by biotechnology, backed up by references to more than 3,300 bibliographic citations. Drug monographs are arranged by therapeutic class. A detailed subject index assists readers in quick access to drug data.

6.20 Lacy C, Armstrong LL, Ingrim N, Lance LL, eds. *Drug Information Handbook.* 6th ed. Hudson, OH: Lexi-Comp, 1998.

Produced in partnership with the American Pharmaceutical Association, Lexi-Comp's *Drug Information Handbook* provides concise prescribing information in monographs arranged alphabetically by generic name. Helpful cross references from brand names to USAN are included in the main body of the text, rather than embedded in a back-of-the-book index. This handbook's index focuses, instead, on providing access to individual drug entries by therapeutic categories. In most ready-reference manuals of this type, the appendices are the chief feature that will add to their value, since information compiled in monographs (which omit bibliographic references) is readily available elsewhere. Appendices in this volume include drug dosage measurement aids (body surface area, etc.), a key to abbreviations and measurements, normal laboratory values, vaccine/immunization guidelines, a controlled substance list, and an index to Canadian and Mexican brand names. Numerous tables will assist in answering commonly asked questions, such as which medications discolor feces or urine, what dosage forms should not be crushed, and queries related to drug compatibility in parenteral nutrition. Another particularly useful feature, all too often overlooked in other ready-reference publications, is the pronunciation key provided for each of the generic names listed in monographs covering more than 1,000 medications.

6.21 Fischer DS, et al, eds. *The Cancer Chemotherapy Handbook.* 2nd ed. Norwalk, CT: Appleton & Lange, 1994.

6.22 Perry MC, ed. *The Chemotherapy Source Book.* 2nd ed. Baltimore: Williams & Wilkins, 1997.

6.23 Skeel RT, Lachant N, eds. *Handbook of Cancer Chemotherapy.* 4th ed. Philadelphia: Little, Brown, 1995.

All three of the source books listed here focus on medications used in oncology practice. Drug monographs in *The Cancer Chemotherapy Handbook* refer to nonstandard experimental therapies and dosing schemes, when relevant. Entries also provide information on antitumor activity and mechanisms of action, dosage, preparation, stability, adverse effects and potential interactions, and special precautions. Nursing considerations in cancer chemotherapy are singled out in a separate section of the Appleton & Lange *Handbook.*

Perry organizes chemotherapeutic techniques by cancer type and by drug. *The Chemotherapy Source Book* begins with an overview of issues in drug development, resistance, and clinical trial design and interpretation. Drug administration and handling, as well as management of toxicity, are addressed in separate sections. In the *Handbook of Cancer Chemotherapy,* Skeel and Lachant summarize treatment regimens of choice for specific cancers. Also included are sections on supportive care, with coverage of adjuvants for nausea and vomiting, infections, pain, and psychological problems.

6.24 Coustan DR, Mochizuki TK. *Handbook for Prescribing Medications During Pregnancy.* 3rd ed. Philadelphia: Lippincott-Raven, 1998.

The *Handbook for Prescribing Medications During Pregnancy* is intended as a desktop reference aid, with drug profiles for nearly 200 medications in common use in the United States, including entries for both prescription and OTC products. Arranged alphabetically by generic name, monographs provide dosage information for both approved and off-label indications, each concluding with a brief list of references as recommended reading. Three appendices expand coverage by adding profiles for vitamins and minerals, antineoplastic agents, and industrial chemicals. Another appendix focuses on immunization of the obstetric patient. The *Handbook* includes a drug classification index, employing both therapeutic and pharmacological terms as access points, and a separate drug name index, listing both generic and brand names. (For expanded coverage of this specialized area of therapeutics, see also *Drugs in Pregnancy and Lactation,* 7.19.)

6.25 Bennett WM, Aronoff GR, Golper TA, Morrison G, et al. *Drug Prescribing in Renal Failure: Dosing Guidelines for Adults.* 3rd ed. Philadelphia: American College of Physicians, 1994.

6.26 Schrier RW, Gambertoglio JG. *Handbook of Drug Therapy in Liver and Kidney Disease.* Boston: Little, Brown, 1991.

The tabular organization that is a hallmark of pharmacotherapeutic handbooks is used to convey needed facts for ready reference in the American College of

Physicians' *Drug Prescribing in Renal Failure: Dosing Guidelines*. Drug entries in tables are listed alphabetically by generic name (no brand names are cited or indexed) under subdivisions based on similarity of structure and pharmacological action. For example, the section of tables devoted to antihypertensive and cardiovascular agents provides separate listings for adrenergic and serotoninergic modulators, ACE inhibitors, beta blockers, and vasodilators. An identical classified arrangement is used in this handbook's concluding bibliography, to assist in quick location of primary source articles. The volume also supplies, in an introductory section, a review of basic biochemical and physiological effects of drugs in patients with renal disease.

Drug dosing in both renal and hepatic failure is the topic of Schrier and Gambertoglio's text. Here, drugs are organized by treatment category. Charts highlight information on dosage adjustments and dialysis of drugs. The *Handbook of Drug Therapy in Liver and Kidney Disease* also discusses drug-induced hepatic and renal, as well as electrolyte, disorders.

6.27 Benitz WE, Tatro DS. *The Pediatric Drug Handbook*. 3rd ed. Philadelphia: Mosby, 1995.

6.28 Barone MA, ed. *The Harriet Lane Handbook*. 14th ed. St. Louis: Mosby Year Book, 1996.

The *Pediatric Drug Handbook* is a concise compilation of information on drugs commonly used in pediatric practice, grouped by organ system or disease condition. Each generic name entry lists commercially available preparations and provides dosage and administration data, including recommended routes, dilutions, and regimens, accompanied by bibliographic references. Tables in this handbook offer assistance in drug selection by summarizing important information for quick comparisons. The drug generic/brand name index helps users distinguish between main monograph references and citations to tables through the use of different typefaces.

Originally created to serve as a manual for pediatric house officers at the Harriet Lane Service of the Children's Medical and Surgical Center at Johns Hopkins Hospital, *The Harriet Lane Handbook* has, fortunately, been made available to a much wider audience since its debut in 1950. Its formulary section is particularly useful, beginning with a brand name index cross referenced to generic name entries in a subsequent table. The latter shows available forms and strengths, dose and route, and includes notes regarding contraindications and important side effects. Bibliographic references for this section include *The Pediatric Drug Handbook* (6.27), *Drug Facts and Comparisons* (6.2), *AHFS Drug Information* (6.4), the *PDR* (6.10), *Handbook of Clinical Drug Data* (6.19), the *Pediatric Dosage Handbook* (6.27), and the *Handbook on Extemporaneous Formulations* (6.39). Another section on special drug topics contains a table of maternal drugs contraindicated in breast feeding.

6.29 Graef JW, ed. *Manual of Pediatric Therapeutics.* 6th ed. Philadelphia: Lippincott-Raven, 1997.

6.30 Pagliaro LA, Pagliaro AM. *Problems in Pediatric Drug Therapy.* 3rd ed. Hamilton, IL: Drug Intelligence Publications, 1995.

The *Manual of Pediatric Therapeutics* is a collaborative effort of staff at Boston's Children's Hospital. The approach here is, for the most part, centered around treatment options for specific conditions, organized into chapters on renal, cardiac, endocrine system, infectious, allergic, hematologic, neurologic, and behavioral disorders, as well as prepubertal and adolescent gynecology, and metabolic diseases. Separate sections also address well child care, acute care and poisoning, management of the normal and of the sick newborn, and fluids and electrolytes. Following general principles at the beginning of each chapter is discussion, in outline format, of disease management. A formulary concludes the volume.

Problems in Pediatric Drug Therapy is much more medication oriented. Problems addressed include drug administration by various routes, potential teratogenesis resulting from drug exposure during pregnancy, excretion in human breast milk (presented in tabular format), treatment of common pediatric poisonings (salicylates, caustic poisons, hydrocarbons, acetaminophen, iron), and abusable psychotropic drug use among children and adolescents. A series of tables compile useful adverse reaction data, such as categories of drugs for which sudden termination of therapy may result in adverse effects, those implicated in neonatal jaundice, diseases and clinical conditions that can be caused by commonly used pediatric medications, and a lengthy cross reference chart listing drugs and their associated reactions. That monographs in a chapter devoted to pediatric drug interactions are contributed by Hansten (see 7.8) is an assurance of the quality of this publication.

6.31 Takemoto CK, Hodding JH, Kraus DM, eds. *Pediatric Dosage Handbook.* 5th ed. Hudson, OH: Lexi-Comp, 1998.

6.32 Young TE, Mangum OB. *Neofax: A Manual of Drugs Used in Neonatal Care.* 11th ed. Bethesda, MD: American Society of Health-System Pharmacists, 1998.

Recommended dose information found in the current literature provides the basis for data presented in 615 medication monographs in the *Pediatric Dosage Handbook*. Similar in organization to Lexi-Comp's *Drug Information Handbook* (6.20), this ready-reference guide includes neonatal dosing, drug administration issues, and extemporaneous preparations in its coverage. Structured entries, arranged alphabetically by generic (USAN) name, supply a guide to pronunciation, common brand names and other synonyms, therapeutic class, approved uses, applicable controlled substance restrictions, information on pregnancy risk factors (FDA categories), contraindications, warnings, precautions, adverse reactions/

interactions, stability, mechanism of action, pharmacodynamics, pharmacokinetics, usual dosage, reference levels for therapeutic and toxic serum concentrations, laboratory test (assay) interferences, and patient-oriented, as well as nursing, information. Available dosage forms and strengths conclude each monograph, followed by bibliographic references, with an emphasis on dosage literature. An appendix compiles quick-reference tables, guidelines, and conversion information. This volume's index focuses on drug brand and synonym name access, rather than the therapeutic categories found in the *Drug Information Handbook.*

Neofax assembles information on antibiotics, biologicals, nutritionals, and many other classes of drugs used in neonatal care. This spiral-bound handbook from ASHP summarizes quick-reference data likely to be needed, including indications, administration and dosage, monitoring, basic pharmacology, adverse effects, and compatibility.

6.33 Theesen KA. *The Handbook of Psychiatric Drug Therapy for Children and Adolescents.* Binghamton, NY: Pharmaceutical Products Press, 1995.

6.34 Maxmen JS, Ward NG. *Psychotropic Drugs: Fast Facts.* 2nd ed. New York: W.W. Norton, 1995.

Information on psychotropic agents is organized into six chapters in *The Handbook of Psychiatric Drug Therapy for Children and Adolescents*: CNS stimulants, antidepressants, antipsychotics, lithium, benzodiazepines, and other agents. Indications, pharmacology, efficacy, pharmacokinetics, dosage, adverse effects, drug interactions, and monitoring guidelines systematically provided for each agent discussed are backed up by end-of-chapter references. Available brands and prices are also cited. Monitoring guidelines are detailed, giving baseline assessments and practical instructions for parents, as well as prescribers. Index entries include drug and company names side-by-side with indications terminology, ensuring that this easy-to-read text is equally easy to use when surveying therapeutic options.

Written by MDs and intended for health science professionals, *Psychotropic Drugs: Fast Facts* exemplifies the better features of handbook publications. Although largely a derivative compilation of data that can be found elsewhere, *Fast Facts* distills needed information into numerous tables summarizing, for example, pharmacology and side effects data. Separate sections address drug classes in a standardized, predictable format. Product selection tables list generic name, brand(s), cost (dollars/dose), manufacturer, available dosage form(s), strength(s), and physical description for each medication, along with incidence data (percentage of patients affected) for side effects. Two appendices provide cross references from generic to brand names and therapeutic class and from brand to generic names and drug class. This spiral-bound volume also brings together information on prescribing in pregnancy and lactation, on possible psychotropic drug effects on laboratory tests, and on interactions. Each drug monograph includes a section labeled Nurses' Data, intended to inform staff about observing patients on medication. Additional notes remind medical staff of what patients and their families need to know about prescribed psychotropic medications, such as administration in relation to meals, how to deal with forgetting a dose, and how to cope with immediate side effects. Unfortunately, bibliographic references do not accompany each chapter, but are, instead, included in one integrated alphabetic list at the back of the book.

6.35 Semla TP, Beizer JL, Higbee MD, eds. *Geriatric Dosage Handbook.* 4th ed. Hudson, OH: Lexi-Comp, 1998.

6.36 Ahronheim JC. *Handbook of Prescribing Medications for Geriatric Patients.* Boston: Little, Brown, 1992.

Information on more than 740 medications in the *Geriatric Dosage Handbook* is presented in thirty-three-point, structured monographs comparable to other Lexi-Comp/APhA handbooks discussed in this section (6.20, 6.31). Special considerations when prescribing or using medication in older adults are the primary focus, including changes in pharmacokinetics or pharmacodynamics, monitoring parameters, exact dosing guidelines, nursing implications, and brief patient information instructions. References to sources used to verify information accompany each generic name entry. The *Handbook*'s overall dictionary arrangement is punctuated with cross references from brand names and other synonyms. Its index offers access to drugs by their therapeutic classification. Appended reference materials duplicate many found in other volumes in this series (e.g., tablets that should not be crushed or altered, drugs known to discolor feces or urine), augmented in this handbook with a compilation of federal OBRA regulations regarding recommended maximum doses of hypnotics, antipsychotics, anxiolytics, and antidepressants. Numerous charts will assist prescribers in comparing factors such as potency, half life, onset of action, and side effects for medications featured earlier in separate monographs.

Following a brief introduction to drug use in the elderly, Ahronheim's *Handbook of Prescribing Medications for Geriatric Patients* presents information in thirty-three short chapters dedicated to categories of drugs, citing a selection of brand name preparations, along with generic names discussed (both of which are accessible through the index). Coverage includes both approved and off-label, but accepted, uses. The author recommends supplementation of recommended readings listed at the end of each chapter with consultation of other "standard reference material, such as the *Physicians' Desk Reference.*"

6.37 Phelps SJ, Hak EB. *Guidelines for Administration of Intravenous Medications to Pediatric Patients.* 5th ed. Bethesda, MD: American Society of Health-System Pharmacists, 1996.

ASHP's *Guidelines for Administration of Intravenous Medications to Pediatric Patients* includes monographs for 146 drugs, arranged alphabetically by USAN. Entries compile information on brand names, dosage, and concentration.

Each of the more than 1,700 references in the extensive bibliography, which concludes this handy spiral-bound volume, is numbered for easy location from superscripts provided in the text of monographs. A back-of-the-book index offers access by both brand and generic names.

6.38 Nahata MC, Hipple TF. *Pediatric Drug Formulations*. 3rd ed. Cincinnati, OH: Harvey Whitney Books, 1997.
6.39 Committee on Extemporaneous Formulations, Special Interest Group on Pediatric Pharmacy Practice. *Handbook on Extemporaneous Formulations*. Bethesda, MD: American Society of Hospital Pharmacists, 1987.
6.40 McCrea J, et al. *Extemporaneous Oral Liquid Dosage Preparations*. Toronto: Canadian Society of Hospital Pharmacists, 1988.

As Nahata and Hipple point out, only about one-fourth of drugs marketed today are actually approved by the FDA with specific indications for use in children. Yet many more are, in fact, prescribed for pediatric patients. This fact means that pharmacists are frequently faced with the responsibility for extemporaneous formulations, because no suitable dosage forms may be available for this special population. *Pediatric Drug Formulations* addresses this critical area of pharmacy practice, critical due to the careful measurements required, the possibility of intoxication if errors occur, and challenges presented by stability issues when dosage forms are altered. This excellent handbook provides instructions for preparation, storage, and labeling of more than sixty oral, rectal, and intravenous (IV) formulations with documented stability data.

Other works with the same mission are ASHP's *Handbook on Extemporaneous Formulations* and the Canadian Society of Hospital Pharmacists' *Extemporaneous Oral Liquid Dosage Preparations*. Both, however, are more limited in scope, with coverage of oral suspensions and liquids only. ASHP's handbook provides information for fifty-one formulations, CSHP's for 139 formulations. The latter classifies entries by the availability of published stability data. Figure 6.1 identifies Web sites with additional formulation facts available free of charge.

6.41 Reynolds L, Closson RG. *Extemporaneous Ophthalmic Preparations*. Vancouver, WA: Applied Therapeutics, 1993.
6.42 Trissel LA. *Trissel's Stability of Compounded Medications*. Washington, DC: American Pharmaceutical Association, 1996.

Methods for preparing fifty-four formulations are provided in *Extemporaneous Ophthalmic Preparations*. Reynolds and Closson suggest strengths and appropriate vehicles, discussing stability issues and special precautions. In *Stability of Compounded Medications*, Trissel offers another overview of general stability considerations. Other sections address properties (pH, solubility, etc.), compatibility with other products, and commercial availability. As might be expected

Figure 6.1   Free Sources of Compounding Information on the Internet

- *Compounding Formulas from the Recent Journal Literature*
  ⇨ http://www.dal.ca/~pharmwww/compound

  Kilby Rogers and Elizabeth Foy at Dalhousie University (Canada) have compiled a collection of full-text references published from 1997 forward in the *International Journal of Pharmaceutical Compounding, American Druggist, Pharmacy Times*, and *U.S. Pharmacist*. The list is organized by main ingredient name and, in some cases, by indication or dosage form. They hope to update the bibliography on a quarterly basis.

- *Compounding Hotline*
  ⇨ http://members.aol.com/pharmtimes/com.html

  The retail journal *Pharmacy Times* hosts a regular compounding hotline column well worth monitoring. Martin Erickson of Paddock Laboratories is the author of responses to reader questions, all of which are retrospectively archived at the URL shown above.

- *Contemporary Compounding*
  ⇨ http://users.aol.com/mefrancom/contcmpd.html

  Martin Francom, a pharmacist in Washington state, maintains a menu of tips and hints, as well as formulas for an assortment of specific capsules, nasal sprays, and gels at the Web site entitled *Contemporary Compounding*. Archives from an ongoing compounding hotline and a compounders' discussion forum can also be viewed. General techniques for the extemporaneous preparation of various dosage forms have been compiled here, drawn from the writings of Loyd Allen, Professor and Head of the Pharmaceutics and Medicinal Chemistry Department at the University of Oklahoma College of Pharmacy.

- *Secundum Artem Index*
  ⇨ http://www.paddocklabs.com/SECUNDUM/secarndx.html

  Paddock Laboratories provides another impressive collection of Allen's work in the online newsletter *Secundem Artem*. Lengthier monographs at this Internet site often review the physiology and function of a given type of preparation as useful background to preparation methods. Ultimate administration and supportive counseling are also discussed. In a recent contribution devoted to veterinary compounding, Allen surveys important regulatory issues and guidelines, the marketplace for individualized medications for animals, and sample formulations.

---

from an editor of the classic *Handbook on Injectable Drugs*, this volume reviews and summarizes the published literature on the topic of compounded formulations.

6.43 Allen LV. *The Art, Science, and Technology of Pharmaceutical Compounding*. Washington, DC: American Pharmaceutical Association, 1998.

The *Art, Science, and Technology of Pharmaceutical Compounding* is a practical guide for pharmacists who must prepare extemporaneous formulations needed in care of terminally ill, pediatric, or geriatric patients. Published by the

APhA, it includes discussion of legal and regulatory issues, facility and equipment requirements, and safety considerations. Allen provides step-by-step instructions for preparing all dosage forms and gives sample formulations for each. Compounding veterinary medications is among topics addressed.

Another special topic that a core drug information collection should be prepared to handle is immunization, with special reference to international travel. Although the U.S. Centers for Disease Control (CDC) and the World Health Organization (WHO) of the United Nations both publish, periodically, vaccination requirements and health recommendations for travelers, the American College of Physicians has also contributed an outstanding handbook on the subject.

6.44 *Guide for Adult Immunization*. 3rd ed. Philadelphia: American College of Physicians, 1994.

This brief *Guide* includes sections on immunizations for healthy adults, for special populations (pregnant women, nursing home residents, selected occupational and "lifestyle" groups, such as veterinarians, IV drug users/abusers), and for accidental or unavoidable exposures (e.g., animal, snake, or spider bites). Discussion highlights clinical issues regarding specific vaccines. Appendices include a table of immunobiologics and schedules for adults and a list of products, with dates licensed, manufacturers, and telephone numbers. Another appendix provides an extremely valuable index to *Morbidity and Mortality Weekly Report (MMWR)* citations for follow-up on specific recommendations for immunizations. Content of other appendices includes a chart compiling state immunization requirements in the United States, a list of state and territorial health departments, and pointers to other sources of vaccine information, such as government agencies and a few hardcopy reference sources. Bibliographic references for facts cited throughout the *Guide for Adult Immunization* are included at the end of the volume. This handbook is well organized, attractively presented, and eminently readable.

6.45 Centers for Disease Control. *Health Information for International Travel*. Atlanta, GA: CDC, 1989–. Annual.

Intended for use by public health departments, physicians, travel agencies, international airlines, shipping companies, and others who must advise global travelers, the CDC's annual compendium (known as "The Yellow Book") presents vaccination and certificate requirements in a country-by-country listing. A separate section organizes recommendations for vaccination and prophylaxis by disease, itemizing thirty-two communicable conditions, from AIDS to yellow fever. Another section shows the geographic distribution of potential health hazards to travelers. General Hints cover a necessarily diverse set of topics, such as WHO guidelines for blood transfusion, swimming precautions, warnings regarding contaminated goatskin handicrafts, and measures to protect against mosquitoes and other arthropod vectors, motion sickness, travelers' diarrhea, or risks of infected food and drink.

Information is also provided on the importation of human remains, the importation or reentry of pets (dogs, cats, nonhuman primates, turtles), and emerging infectious diseases. *Health Information for International Travel* concludes with useful definitions of terms and both a subject index and an index by country. It should be noted that, given the nature of rapid disease transmission in the increasingly well-traveled world today, information in publications such as the two annotated here should be updated through voice or fax information service offered by the CDC or consultation of their World Wide Web page on the Internet. The full text of *The Yellow Book* can be downloaded in PDF format or viewed in HTML at http://www.cdc.gov/travel. Other reference material at this URL is a *Summary of Health Information for International Travel*, known in some circles as "The Blue Sheet" (not to be confused with the F-D-C newsletter).

6.46 Isada CM, Kasten BL, Goldman MP, Gray LD, Aberg JA. *Infectious Diseases Handbook, including Antimicrobial Therapy and Laboratory Diagnosis*, 2nd ed. Hudson, OH: Lexi-Comp, 1996.

6.47 Conte JE. *Manual of Antibiotics and Infectious Diseases*. 8th ed. Baltimore: Williams & Wilkins, 1995.

The *Infectious Diseases Handbook* is one of a series of publications produced in partnership with the American Pharmaceutical Association (see also 6.20, 6.31, 6.35). In separate sections, it covers common diseases and recommendations for their empiric treatment, common microorganisms, testing procedures necessary for diagnosis, and anti-infective agents available in the United States. Extensive cross referencing between sections encourages efficient use. For example, the entry for a specific organism will refer to an approved laboratory test for its accurate detection and to appropriate antimicrobial drugs for treatment. Monographs on individual agents each include a pronunciation key, brand names, notation of whether a generic form is available, organisms for which it is the drug of choice or an alternative, FDA pregnancy risk rating, contraindications, adverse reactions and percentage of incidence, toxicology, drug interactions, mechanism of action, pharmacokinetics, usual dosage, monitoring parameters, patient information, and dosage forms/strengths.

References to Selected Readings also accompany each monograph. Pertinent U.S. Department of Health and Human Services clinical practice guidelines are assembled in an appendix. Judging from the bibliography of sources cited in its introduction, it is evident that most information in the *Infectious Diseases Handbook* is derivative of other publications annotated earlier in this chapter. Titles cited include *Drug Facts and Comparisons* (6.2), *AHFS Drug Information* (6.4), *USP DI* (6.5), the *Handbook of Nonprescription Drugs* (6.6), *Physicians' Desk Reference* (6.10), *Drug Interactions Facts* (7.10), and the "*Handbook of Objectionable* [sic] *Drugs*" (7.31).

Similarly, Conte's *Manual of Antibiotics and Infectious Diseases* performs the valuable service that most handbooks provide of incorporating "a variety of source materials ordinarily found in many different locations." Information compiled is divided into eleven sections. The first section is devoted to entries for individual antibiotics, including availability (companies, brand names), use, adult and pediatric dosage, adverse reactions, and interactions. Section 2, Empiric Antibiotic Therapy, organizes information into tables (subdivided by organ systems and organisms), recommends drugs of choice and alternatives, and includes dosage. Data on therapy of established infection in Section 3 are also presented in tables by infecting organism. Sections on prophylactic antibiotics and AIDS and HIV infections are followed by "Antibiotic Susceptibilities," featuring a chart summary of organisms commonly encountered in human infectious diseases and their susceptibility to antimicrobial agents. The opposite side of the coin, bacterial resistance, is then depicted in both graphical and tabular summaries of epidemiology and resistance patterns of organisms. Guidelines for the clinical use of immunobiologic agents distributed by the CDC are supplied in Section 8. Concluding portions of the *Manual* focus on parasitic diseases, tuberculosis, and sexually transmitted diseases, respectively. One drawback detected in its otherwise admirable organization is that brand names cited in the body of the text are not listed in the index.

6.48 *Handbook of Antimicrobial Therapy*. New Rochelle, NY: The Medical Letter, 1994.

6.49 Peter G, ed. *Report of the Committee on Infectious Disease*. 24th ed. Elk Grove, IL: American Academy of Pediatrics, 1997.

6.50 Yoshikawa TT, Norman DC, eds. *Antimicrobial Therapy in the Elderly Patient*. New York: Marcel Dekker, 1994.

The *Handbook of Antimicrobial Therapy* reprints recommendations previously published in *The Medical Letter* (6.17). Given this respected provenance, it is used by many physicians to identify drugs of choice and dosing schedules for the treatment of bacterial and parasitic diseases. The American Academy of Pediatrics publishes its own recommendations in a periodic report sometimes called "The Red Book." Both active and passive immunization are discussed. Summaries for each of more than 200 diseases cover etiology, epidemiology, clinical manifestations, diagnostic tests, treatment, and control in children.

Noting that infections are among the top ten causes of death in the geriatric population, the editors of *Antimicrobial Therapy in the Elderly Patient* concisely describe contributory factors, such as comorbidity, organ failure, systemic disease, malnutrition, and senescence of components of the human immune system. The majority of this book's chapters address use of major classes of antibiotics, with particular attention to the pharmacodynamics of individual medicinal agents in aged patients, who are likely to be more susceptible to side effects and especially vulnerable to drug interactions in "settings of geriatric polypharmacy."

Additional sections examine the use of antibiotics in nonhospital venues, such as community outpatient facilities, in-home patient care, and nursing homes. Numbered references interpolated throughout discussion will encourage follow-up consultation of the excellent bibliographies that conclude each chapter. This feature, along with its overall layout and length, places *Antimicrobial Therapy in the Elderly Patient* beyond the handbook or ready-reference manual class of publications, signaling transition here into another important source of pharmacotherapeutic information, textbooks.

Encyclopedic Works and Textbooks

In contrast to ready-reference handbooks, good pharmacology and therapeutics textbooks invariably provide extensive discussion, supported by lengthy bibliographies. By going beyond the product-by-product approach seen in many publications annotated thus far in this chapter, textbooks will perform the valuable service of summarizing background material likely to be requested from time to time by students and others seeking an authoritative introduction to, or review of, selected categories of drugs and related topics. By acquiring one or more of the following encyclopedic works, drug information providers can save hours of redundant research in secondary publications.

6.51 Hardman JG, Gilman AG, Limbird LE, eds. *Goodman and Gilman's The Pharmacological Basis of Therapeutics*. 9th ed. New York: McGraw-Hill, 1996.

No reputable guide to pharmaceutical reference sources would be complete without citing *Goodman and Gilman*, long considered the preeminent U.S. textbook on pharmacology and therapeutics. First published in 1941, its emphasis remains on therapeutic advances made possible by newly marketed drugs, with selective coverage of agents still under investigation. Accordingly, the ninth edition features new chapters on serotonin receptor agonists and antagonists, treatment of migraine, and ocular pharmacology. Chapters now begin with a synopsis and end in a prospectus, pointing in the latter to conceptual advances or therapeutic options still new, but included with the intent of helping readers search the biomedical literature for updated information before publication of the tenth edition. The appendix of pharmacokinetic data includes 335 agents, with ninety-one new entries. Bibliography cited by contributing authors gives preference to review articles, literature on new drugs, and original contributions in controversial fields.

Chapter Three in *Goodman and Gilman* includes a brief discussion of sources of drug information. After acknowledging that the *PDR* (6.10) is most often used, Nies and Spielberg single out *USP DI* (6.5), *Drug Facts and Comparisons* (6.2), and *The Medical Letter* (6.17) as worthy of special consideration. Two sources cited by Nies in the previous edition are, curiously, no longer mentioned: *AHFS Drug Information* (6.4) and *Clin-Alert* (7.6). The list of journals judged to be objective and "not supported by drug manufacturers" remains a short one. Titles recommended by Nies and Spielberg on this basis include *Clinical Pharmacology and Therapeutics, Drugs, New England Journal of Medicine, Annals of Internal Medicine, JAMA, Archives of Internal Medicine, British Medical Journal, Lancet,* and *Postgraduate Medicine.*

6.52 Gennaro AR, ed. *Remington's Pharmaceutical Sciences.* 19th ed. 2 v. Easton, PA: Mack Publishing, 1995.

Several chapters from *Remington's* have already been cited in this *Guide*, which should provide an indication of its undisputed stature in the world of pharmacy. Although a large portion of this mammoth (now two-volume) textbook is devoted to monographs for individual drugs, its chief value in day-to-day pharmaceutical information service lies in its coverage of topics such as pharmaceutics, pharmaceutical chemistry, testing and analysis, and preparations and their manufacture. Here, users will find authoritative discussion of concepts such as bioavailability, sterilization, stability, packaging materials, quality assurance, and quality control. *Remington's* also provides an orientation to the practice of pharmacy, with chapters on its historical evolution, ethics, and other useful introductory overview material. New additions to coverage in the nineteenth edition include community pharmacy economics and management, pharmacoeconomics, and alternative health care.

Particularly noteworthy is Tischio's chapter on pharmacogenetics, which offers a valuable table compiling information on pharmacogenetic conditions, identifying mode of inheritance (e.g., autosomal dominant or recessive), frequency of occurrence in the general population, and drugs producing an abnormal response. Der Marderosian's chapter on biotechnology and drugs reviews basic biological milestones that helped paved the way for modern developments and cites specific applications in pharmacognosy. The same contributor, supported by coauthor Kratz, compiles a useful primer on another hot topic, alternative health care, tracing the rise (or resurgence) of consumer interest in complementary therapies and providing brief descriptions of options as diverse as acupuncture, aromatherapy, Ayurvedic medicine, iridology, and reflexology. Tables summarize reasons for the current popularity of alternatives to conventional therapies, as well as reasons for criticism. Another table compiles examples of foods with purported medical properties.

Chapter 80, Pharmaceutical Necessities, by Reilly, can help answer many challenging questions that arise when extemporaneous formulations are required. The author provides information on agents of little or no therapeutic value, but with undoubted utility in compounding and manufacturing. For basic information on often elusive categories of substances, such as antioxidants, preservatives, coloring and flavoring agents, emulsifiers, suspending agents, ointment bases, and diluting agents, *Remington's* is the first stop.

Monographs for conventional therapeutic and medicinal agents are arranged in broad pharmacological/therapeutic classes. Each entry includes USAN, chemical name, a structural formula, empirical formula, CAS RN, common U.S. brand names, manufacturers, molecular weight, references to patents or other literature on method of preparation, physical description, solubility data, uses, dose, and dosage forms. Indexing is exhaustive, as users of *Remington's* since the first edition in 1886 have come to expect of this encyclopedic reference source. Nearly every chapter is accompanied by extensive references to precedents, as well as suggested readings. Along with the subject matter being addressed, some contributing authors also discuss information sources and supply helpful glossaries of terms (e.g., biotechnology, alternative healthcare vocabulary).

6.53 Mutschler E, Derendorf H. *Drug Actions: Basic Principles and Therapeutic Aspects*. Stuttgart: Medpharm, 1995.

The first English-language edition of a popular German textbook, *Drug Actions* is in many ways a European counterpart of *Goodman and Gilman* (6.51). Part A deals with general pharmacology, covering principles of pharmacokinetics, pharmacodynamics, pharmacogenetics, side effects, interactions, chronopharmacology (biorhythm of drug effects), drug development, and clinical trials. Part B addresses pharmacology in specific classes of drugs, such as hypnotics and muscle relaxants, with emphasis on drug structure/activity relationships. An overview of anatomy, physiology, and pathology precedes each drug class, focusing on organ systems affected. Part C covers toxicology, general emergency management of poisoning, and specific poisons, including biotoxins and zootoxins (e.g., mushrooms, snakes). An appendix lists INNs of drugs discussed in the text, identifying brand names in the United States, Great Britain, and Sweden. Entries for brand names in the back-of-the-book index refer users to this appendix chart, after which it is necessary to return to the index for page references, which are only fully compiled under the preferred generic name. Aside from this slight flaw in indexing, information in *Drug Actions* is very attractively presented, with numerous figures and tables enhanced with color graphics.

6.54 Munson PL, ed. *Principles of Pharmacology: Basic Concepts & Clinical Applications*. New York: Chapman & Hall, 1995.

Munson's *Principles of Pharmacology* is the brainchild of an *ad hoc* committee of distinguished pharmacologists originally convened in Geneva by the founding director of the WHO Collaborating Center for Research and Training in Neurosciences. According to the introduction, it was conceived as a "concise reference book"—but the reality is that this is one of the largest tomes readers are ever likely to encounter on contemporary library shelves. This description extends beyond the physical (1,789 pages, 3.5 inches thick) to the metaphorical: a huge scope compared to many other textbooks. For example, this volume includes a major section on the pharmacology of nutrients and nutritional diseases, with ten chapters on topics such as fat-soluble vitamins, macrominerals, enteral and parenteral feeding, starvation, undernutrition, and trauma. Discussion of dermatopharmacology is similarly thorough, encompassing fourteen chapters on pertinent classes of drugs (e.g., retinoids, antihistamines, antimicrobials, topical antiacne products), including "adjuvant treatments and other medicaments in the 'gray' area between medicine and toiletries."

The toxicology section singles out occupational and environmental hazards for special consideration, along with chapters on pesticides, mycotoxins, chemical carcinogenesis and mutagenesis, reproductive toxicity and teratology, risk assessment, and systemic antidotes. Pharmacology in special patient populations examines not only pediatrics and geriatrics, but also AIDS, Alzheimer's, and critical care. Other extras include coverage of natural medicinal products and a section devoted to government regulation of drugs in the United States, the European Community, and Japan. Despite an awe-inspiring total of 121 chapters (some quite brief), *Principles of Pharmacology* is well organized and well written. Contributors from seventeen countries each supply extensive lists of references to support discussion, cited by superscripts within the text. Their bibliographies include research reports, reviews, monographs, and symposia.

6.55 Rowland M, Tozer TN. *Clinical Pharmacokinetics: Concepts and Applications*. 3rd ed. Philadelphia: Lea & Febiger, 1995.

6.56 Ritschel WA, ed. *Handbook of Basic Pharmacokinetics*. 5th ed. Washington, DC: American Pharmaceutical Association, 1998.

Much more modest in scope than *Goodman and Gilman* (6.51), *Drug Actions* (6.53), or *Principles of Pharmacology* (6.54), Rowland and Tozer's *Clinical Pharmacokinetics* is, nonetheless, a good candidate for a textbook likely to complement basic drug information collections in hospitals. Its focus is on providing background material for effective monitoring and interpretation of plasma concentrations and their use as a guide to drug therapy. Coverage includes absorption and disposition kinetics, therapeutic regimens, physiologic concepts and kinetics, individualization (e.g., variability in response due to genetics, age, weight, disease, or interacting drugs), and discussion of dose and time dependencies, as well as dialysis. Designed for use as a programmed learning text, each chapter begins with educational objectives and ends with study problems to test achievement, with answers provided at the end of the book. Examples used consistently feature currently prescribed drugs.

Despite its title, Ritschel's *Handbook of Basic Pharmacokinetics* is closer to a textbook than a handbook in its approach to conveying information to its users, although it does present much of its data in tabular format. An appendix compiles pharmacokinetic parameters of important drugs, covering more than 300 medications.

6.57 Katzung BG, ed. *Basic and Clinical Pharmacology*. 7th ed. Stamford, CT: Appleton & Lange, 1997.

Intended as a textbook for medical, pharmacy, and other health science students, *Basic and Clinical Pharmacology* includes "special features to make it useful to house officers and practicing clinicians," starting with a moderately sized, paperbound format. Sections devoted to broad drug groups (e.g., autonomic, cardiovascular-renal) concentrate on the choice and use of medications in patients and on monitoring their effects. At the end of each chapter is a list of preparations available in the United States (released through 1996), including brand and generic names, along with dosage forms. Other chapter topics include toxicology, perinatal and pediatric pharmacology, geriatric pharmacology, dermatology, the therapeutic and toxic potential of OTC drugs, and rational prescribing/prescription writing.

Appendix 1 is a table of vaccines, immune globulins, and other biologic products, organized by pathogen or disease target. Data supplied in each entry identify type of agent (live virus, polysaccharide, or killed bacteria), route of administration, dosage and administration schedule for primary immunization, and duration of effect. The second appendix tabulates important drug interactions, drawn from sources such as Horn and Hansten (7.8) and *Drug Interaction Facts* (7.10). Enhanced by numerous charts and other illustrative graphics, highlighted in color, this textbook, in its back-of-the-book index, also systematically lists generic and brand names from earlier tables of preparations. One drawback perhaps worth noting is that bibliographies concluding each chapter in *Basic and Clinical Pharmacology* are not numbered or directly coordinated with the preceding text. This style of documentation, though common, offers less incentive to student readers to use and peruse the undifferentiated lists of references presented in alphabetical order.

6.58 Brody TM, Larner J, Minneman KP, eds. *Human Pharmacology: Molecular to Clinical*. 3rd ed. St. Louis: Mosby, 1998.

The introduction in *Human Pharmacology: Molecular to Clinical* repeats the aims and claims of Katzung's (6.57) textbook: content organization for students that matches the framework of standard professional curricula, a focus on drug classes, use of tables to summarize factual data, and an intent to provide residents and practicing physicians with easy access to clinical information related to drug use. Chapter-by-chapter discussion of broad drug classes is consistently presented under the headings: therapeutic overview, mechanisms of action, pharmacokinetics, relation of mechanisms of action to clinical response, side effects, clinical problems, and toxicity. Departures in content, compared to Katzung, are first apparent in two extra features: inclusion of representative questions for student self-assessment and, in many chapters, a concluding section devoted to New Directions, which points to future drug developments and anticipated uses. More significant are chapters on gene therapy and novel drugs produced by recombinant biotechnology, as well as a section on nutritional aspects of pharmacology (not separately covered by Katzung). More liberal use of color is another plus, offset by the negatives of shorter bibliographies and less information on marketed preparations.

6.59 Herfindal ET, Gourley DR, Hart LL, eds. *Textbook of Clinical Pharmacy and Therapeutics: Drug and Disease Management.* 6th ed. Baltimore: Williams & Wilkins, 1996.

6.60 Hart LL, Gourley DR, Herfindal ET, eds. *Workbook for Clinical Pharmacy and Therapeutics.* 6th ed. Baltimore: Williams & Wilkins, 1996.

Because of its companion *Workbook* presenting nearly 200 cases to reinforce background material covered in the main volume, the *Textbook of Clinical Pharmacy and Therapeutics* provides an excellent foundation on which to build knowledge and analytical skills necessary to function effectively in a clinical environment. The opening section includes discussion of pharmacokinetics, adverse drug reactions and interactions, lab tests, patient education and disease monitoring, and biotechnology. Other sections address specific disease classes or body systems, as well as immunizations, drugs in pregnancy and lactation, and transplantation. New chapters in the sixth edition focus on patient counseling, gynecologic cancer, and racial and ethnic differences in response to drugs. Cases in the accompanying *Workbook* are organized in sections paralleling the textbook and are intended to help users develop therapeutic decision-making skills.

6.61 Machlin LJ, ed. *Handbook of Vitamins.* 2nd ed. New York: Marcel Dekker, 1991.

A particularly elusive category of therapeutic substances, in terms of drug ready-reference service, is vitamins. It is, then, refreshing to find a good textbook dedicated to their pharmacology. Chapters by various contributors to the *Handbook of Vitamins* review the chemistry, analytical and assay procedures, metabolism, biochemical function, signs of deficiency, and nutritional requirements of vitamins A, B-6, B-12, D, E, K, C, thiamin, riboflavin, nicotinic acid, biotin, pantothenic acid, folic acid, choline, and carnitine. Factors that influence each vitamin's status are also discussed, including drugs and other organic compounds. Discussion covers the efficacy of pharmacological doses, as well as hypervitaminosis. Supported by a bibliography of 3,200 references to the primary literature, the *Handbook of Vitamins* will save time in answering many quick-reference questions. The concluding chapter adds to its potential value by providing background on substances originally described in the scientific literature as vitamins, but later found to be identical to other essential nutrients or mixtures of others. Substances covered include vitamins M, B11, T, G, and F, as well as the "pseudovitamins" B17 (laetrile, amygdalin), B15 (pangamic acid), B13 (orotic acid), and H3 (Gerovital).

Therapeutic Drug Compendia for Nurses

Any and all of the core collection resources featured earlier in this chapter are appropriate for use by physicians, pharmacists, and other health science professionals, including nurses. However, some individuals responsible for collection development advocate purchase of additional drug compendia specifically compiled for nurses, and several publishers have shown themselves more than willing to capitalize on this acquisition policy. The resulting publications are largely derivative of more comprehensive sources annotated above, presenting subsets of available drug data with an emphasis on nursing implications. The following references represent only a small sample of drug compendia compiled for nurses. Consult Brandon and Hill's list published biennially in *Nursing Outlook*,[8] "Books of the Year" in the January issue of the *American Journal of Nursing*,[9] and the bibliography at the end of this chapter for additional hardcopy sources.

6.62 *Nurses Drug Facts*. St. Louis: Facts and Comparisons, 1995–. Annual.

The outcome of a collaboration between the American Nurses Association and a respected publisher already mentioned several times in this chapter, *Nurses Drug Facts* is a particularly attractive example of publications of this type. Vividly enhanced with color highlighting and eye-catching icons, monographs convey key pharmacological and nursing considerations in a succinct, clearly written format designed for rapid assimilation by care-givers. This book's alphabetic listing by generic name represents a more practical arrangement than the therapeutic category approach found in many other sources. Labeled, unlabeled (not officially approved), and orphan drug uses are all identified (when applicable) in the indications portion of each monograph. The interactions section in each entry lists suspected agents alphabetically. Side effects are organized by body system and include "most life-threatening" and "most-common" adverse reactions. Nursing Considerations consistently highlight administration and storage guidelines, assessment/intervention recommendations, signs and symptoms of overdose, and advice on patient/family education.

This volume's appendices include FDA pregnancy categories, normal laboratory values, a list of drug names that look alike and sound alike, oral dosage forms that should not be crushed or chewed, and directions for management of acute overdosage and acute hypersensitivity. Nonproprietary product name monographs represent coverage of a total of 4,500 branded U.S. products, encompassing a selection of investigational drugs and AIDS drugs still under development. A visual identification section, arranged by color of solid dosage forms, depicts more than 900 medications. *Nurses Drug Facts* also features tables of combination drugs and an orphan drug table. It is sold as part of a two-volume set, appropriately accompanied by *Patient Drug Facts* (9.40). Accordingly, specific page cross-references to the latter are incorporated into the patient/family education segment of each *Nurses Drug Facts* monograph.

A *Nurses Drug Information* CD-ROM issued annually by the same publisher incorporates direct click-on links to patient monographs in English and Spanish. The user interface enables searching by trade or generic name, indication, or other keywords. Like Facts & Comparisons' CD-ROM version of the *American*

Drug Index, Nurses Drug Facts on disc offers audio pronunciations of nonproprietary names—a definite bonus.

6.63 Loebl S, Spratto GR, Woods AL. *The Nurse's Drug Handbook.* 7th ed.
      Albany, NY: Delmar, 1994.

The *Nurse's Drug Handbook* organizes information on more than 1,000 drugs
into tables arranged by therapeutic class. Brief narrative annotations highlight
important instructions and nursing implications. An introductory section provides an overview of pharmacology basics, including side effects and drug interactions. Other chapters discuss the nursing process and considerations in drug
therapy, with special attention to administration by different routes and drug response in special populations (geriatric, pediatric, pregnancy). Counseling patients in order to promote compliance is stressed. The *Handbook* also includes a
glossary, bibliography, and index by generic and brand names. Appendices compile commonly used laboratory test values, food-drug interaction data, a controlled substance list, a directory of poison control centers, FDA pregnancy categories, and information on computing areas of burns.

6.64 Skidmore-Roth L. *Mosby's 1996 Nursing Drug Reference.* St. Louis:
      Mosby, 1995–. Annual.

Mosby's Nursing Drug Reference is more ambitious in its scope, presenting
drug data in standard monograph format. Entries, arranged alphabetically by generic name, each include a pronunciation key, brand names, pharmacological/
therapeutic class, and a summary of information on action, side effects, contraindications, dosage and routes, available forms, and treatment of overdose. Reference to controlled substance schedule is made, when applicable, and laboratory
test interferences are also noted. An icon is used to indicate which drugs should
not be crushed before administration. Appendices list abbreviations and formulas
for drug calculation, as well as FDA pregnancy categories and a controlled substance chart. Focusing on the most common prescription and OTC drugs, *Mosby's Nursing Drug Reference* offers access to them via an index of 1,300 generic
and 4,500 brand names. Drug updates, consisting of abbreviated monographs for
newly approved products, are released on a quarterly basis (free of charge) at
http://www1.mosby.com/Mosby/nursing_drug_updates.

6.65 Shannon MT, Wilson BA, Stang CL. *Govoni & Hayes Drugs and Nursing
      Implications.* 8th ed. Norwalk, CT: Appleton & Lange, 1995.

Govoni & Hayes Drugs and Nursing Implications also offers a monograph approach and easy-to-use alphabetic arrangement by generic name. Each entry lists
brand names and discusses actions and uses, absorption and fate, adverse reac-
tions/interactions, including diagnostic test interferences, contraindications and
precautions, dosage, routes of administration, and nursing implications. Appendices include schedules of controlled substances, the list of FDA pregnancy catego-

ries, a glossary, a key to abbreviations, and a bibliography. The index to this volume is not confined to generic and brand names, but also includes pharmacological and therapeutic terms as access points to drug monographs.

6.66 Spratto GR, Woods AL. *PDR Nurse's Handbook*. New York: Delmar, 1995–. Annual.

The 1999 *PDR Nurse's Handbook* represents a collaboration between Medical Economics and Delmar Publishing (6.63), both now owned by Thomson International. The new edition opts for a simple A–Z arrangement by generic name. Coverage is still limited to the most commonly used drugs dispensed in hospitals and at retail. However, both on- and off-label indications are cited. In addition to the by-now-standard monograph sections devoted to contraindications, adverse reactions, interactions, dosage/administration instructions, and dosage forms available, individual entries add nursing considerations such as assessment (step-by-step guidelines for ensuring patient tolerance to prescribed dosage), interventions (procedures for identifying and handling side effects), evaluation (how to assess drug efficacy), and patient communication. Also included are more than 200 color photographs to assist in visual identification of selected products. A CD-ROM version of the *PDR Nurse's Handbook* is also available, and a companion database with free monthly updates has been launched on the Web (see next section).

Drug Handbooks on the Internet

Good (and gratis) ready-reference professional pharmacotherapeutics sources are few and far between on the Internet. Although generally more limited in scope compared to many hardcopy publications described in this chapter, Web compendia could, however, be useful complements where and when access to printed materials is not available. Figure 6.2 identifies best bets. Consumer-oriented drug information databases are discussed in Chapter Nine.

RxList
  ⇨ http://www.rxlist.com

RxList provides professionally oriented drug information on more than 4,000 U.S. products in approximately 300 monographs and is searchable by both brand and generic names in one integrated index. A new Keyword search capability enables access to the full text of all database entries by symptom terminology, side effects, interactions, etc. Best of all, *RxList* monographs are derived from *Mosby's GenRx* (available elsewhere for a fee).

A separate section, labeled RxList-ID, facilitates searching by dosage form imprint codes. This excellent Web site also offers Top 200 lists for 1997, 1996, and 1995, each ranked by prescription volume in the United States (per *American*

Druggist data) and cross referencing top brands to company names and nonproprietary designations. The latter are hotlinked to full drug monographs. In contrast, drug class or category searches simply lead to lists of common indications and side effects. *RxList* is maintained by Neil Sandow, now manager of automated technologies for a pharmaceutical distributor. He was previously employed as a hospital pharmacy director in the San Francisco Bay area.

InteliHealth—U.S. Pharmacopeia Dispensing Information
   ⇨ http://ipn.intelihealth.com/ipn

Unlike the University of Washington's *Federated Drug Reference* site (see next entry), *InteliHealth* is decidedly commercial in look and feel, replete with frames and distracting advertisements. However, it does provide access to several key reference sources in its Professional Network, including *Taber's Cyclopedic Medical Dictionary*, complete with illustrations, and Volume I of *U.S. Pharmacopeia Dispensing Information—Drug Information for the Health Science Professional*. The interface enables searches by either brand or generic name. Correct spellings of either type of nomenclature can also be located by browsing an integrated alphabetic index. The pitfall in this method of accessing the database is that the index provides no cross references from brand to generic names, or from generic names to *USP DI* monograph titles that cover them, but that bear "class" titles. For example, no index entry appears for captopril or enalapril, because these drugs are covered in the ACE inhibitor monograph. However, using the *InteliHealth* search form, relevant *USP DI* monographs will be located.

Users will also find three other USP databases available at this site: 1) *USP DI Volume II: Advice to the Patient*, 2) Patient Education Leaflets, and 3) Medicine Charts (photos of dosage forms). Search capabilities offered to consumers are more "forgiving" than the interface constructed for Volume I. Either brand or generic names can be submitted to the search engine, and separate alphabetical indexes of each type of name are also offered for browsing.

Federated Drug Reference—U.S.Pharmacopeia Dispensing Information
   ⇨ http://kirk.hslib.washington.edu/fdr

FDR is an experimental service for drug reference under development by a collaborative team at the University of Washington. It currently includes the full *USP DI Volume I—Drug Information for the Health Science Professional*, the University's own formulary, Washington State's Basic Health Care Plan Formulary, and links to selected external sources (e.g., Micromedex, *MEDLINE*, and the FDA). Accessible by either brand or generic drug name, the database offers the option to display individually labeled sections of otherwise lengthy *USP DI* monographs.

RxMed
   ⇨ http://www.rxmed.com/index.html

Dubbed The Website for Family Physicians, this Canadian resource includes "drug monographs for all medications" drawn from an undisclosed source. Its opening menu under Prescribing Information permits browsing of an alphabetic list mixing brand and generic names for quick selection. A separate index to U.S. drug information also includes both brand and generic names as hotlinks. The source of U.S. prescribing data appears to be *Mosby's GenRx*, although this connection is unacknowledged by Web authors. *RxMed* offers the option to print out patient instruction sheets, but these are not particularly attractive examples of this genre on the Web.

PDR Nurse's Handbook
⇨ http://www.nursespdr.com/members/database/content.html

Delmar, publisher of the *Nurse's Drug Handbook* (6.63) and new collaborators with Medical Economics on the *PDR Nurse's Handbook* (6.66), is currently offering an online counterpart free of charge. However, full nursing considerations included in the hardcopy are not in the gratis online version. Nonetheless, the entries supplied convey all basic professional package insert information in an easy-to-use and beautifully formatted package. They also provide Client/Family Teaching Tips, such as timing of administration in relation to meals.

Drug brand or nonproprietary name searches in the *PDR Nurse's Handbook* produce a ranked list of results where the main monograph appears first, followed by a link to the relevant drug class entry, and additional links to other monographs that cite the drug, usually as an interacting agent. Queries using drug category keywords, such as beta blockers, produce a list of individual agents in the category, each accompanied by notes on action/kinetics, uses, contraindications, special precautions, overdose management, and potential interactions. Another search option is clicking on a generic name in an A–Z drug listing.

The *PDR Nurse's Handbook* Web site is also retaining monographs recently removed from the current hardcopy edition to make room for coverage of new drugs. Archived entries are listed alphabetically in a separate brand and generic name index. The bonus is that these monographs incorporate the full text of nursing considerations omitted in entries found in the other portion of the database. Delmar is using the Web to post monthly drug updates between hardcopy editions. Coverage includes newly approved medicines, new uses, new combinations, and safety alerts regarding side effects and interactions.

Medscape Drug Search from First DataBank
⇨ http://www.medscape.com/misc/formdrugs.html

The source behind *Medscape Drug Search* is the *National Drug Data File* (*NDDF*) from First DataBank, with coverage of an impressive 200,000 drug products. The interface facilitates searching by brand or generic name, as well as disease or condition terms. Another welcome enhancement is that monographs cite both approved and off-label indications. Patient education versions of each professional insert can also be printed. Clicking on hotlinks embedded in the text for Indications keywords produces a list of other drugs used in treatment, those to avoid in patients with certain conditions, and drugs implicated in etiology of the named disease, when applicable.

NDDF entries also cite potential drug-drug, drug-food, or drug-lab test interactions. Links to interaction monographs yield ratings of significance level, a description of mechanism of action and clinical effects, plus discussion of predisposing factors, patient management, and bibliographic references. The easiest way to locate these separate monographs for specific interactions is via hypertext links found in *NDDF* medication entries, rather than trying to use the awkward and confusing Interactions Search module currently offered on *Medscape*. Another unhelpful portion of the interface is advising visitors to use the built-in medical dictionary at this site, if they're unsure how to spell a drug or disease name. For diseases, this recommendation is fairly sensible; for drugs, it's downright silly, as few generic or brand names appear in *Merriam-Webster's Desktop Dictionary* (the source used).

Clinical Pharmacology Online
⇨ http://www.cponline.gsm.com/

Gold Standard Multimedia's *Clinical Pharmacology Online*, after more than a year of gratis availability, has switched to paid subscription access. However, excerpts from full monographs are still provided free of charge, with coverage limited to the most common and classic medications in clinical practice. These are searchable by brand or generic name. Alternatively, segments of the alphabetic index to brand or nonproprietary names can be browsed to locate available entries. Abbreviated records begin with a structural formula and a color photograph of the finished dosage form, continue with a description that provides an intro-

---

Figure 6.2   Best Bets among Free Drug Ready-Reference Sources on the Internet—For Healthcare Professionals

- *RxList*
  ⇨ http://www.rxlist.com

- *InteliHealth—U.S. Pharmacopeia Dispensing Information Volume I*
  ⇨ http://ipn.intelihealth.com/ipn

- *RxMed*
  ⇨ http://www.rxmed.com/index.html

- *PDR Nurse's Handbook*
  ⇨ http://www.nursespdr.com/members/database/content.html

- *Medscape Drug Search from First DataBank*
  ⇨ http://www.medscape.com/misc/formdrugs.html

---

ductory overview, and conclude with sections devoted to mechanism of action and pharmacokinetics. Numbered links to supportive bibliographic references are a nice extra.

Complete monographs, now available to paid subscribers only, include dosage for both approved and off-label indications, contraindications, interactions, adverse reactions, and absolute and relative cost data. Information on more than 500 frequently prescribed drugs is drawn from a subset of this publisher's *Clinical Pharmacology CD-ROM*. Summaries of pharmacology are derived from standard reference texts such as *USP DI*, *AHFS*, *Drug Facts and Comparisons*, and the *PDR*.

Drug INFONET℠
⇨ http://www.druginfonet.com/

This relatively small database is a collection of 127 professional package inserts supplied by manufacturers and approved by the FDA. It can be searched by brand or generic name, ailment keywords, company names, or other concept terms. Scrolling through the browsable brand name index is also an option, where each entry includes generic name, dosage form, and manufacturer.

Infomed Drug Guide
⇨ http://www.infomed.org/100drugs/

Based on the book *100 wichtige Medikamente* published by Infomed-Verlags AG in Switzerland and Germany, information at this Web site has been translated into English and made accessible via a browsable index to nonproprietary names. The result is an attractively formatted professional ready-reference tool compiling lengthy monographs supported by bibliographic references and tables summarizing pharmacokinetics and dosage data. An unusual feature is commentary by *Infomed* editors on the relative utility of each drug featured, accompanied by ratings on its Lifetime Value, Symptomatic Value, and Safety.

South African Electronic Package Inserts
⇨ http://home.intekom.com/pharm

As its name implies, this resource limits its scope to manufacturer-provided and government approved package inserts for medications licensed for marketing in South Africa. With coverage of both over-the-counter and prescription drugs, it is a large and diverse collection. Especially noteworthy are numerous inserts supplied for herbal preparations, accessible by any of the common plant names listed as active ingredients. There are, in fact, three ways to locate product information at the site: an alphabetical list of nonproprietary names, a comparable directory of brand names, or pharmacological/therapeutic class terms as given by manufacturers. Malahyde Information Systems, the database provider, warns that the latter can be an unreliable method, due to unpredictable variations in terminology used. They also warn that not all medicines marketed in South Africa are, as yet, represented in *Electronic Package Inserts*.

DrugBase
⇨ http://www.drugbase.co.za/

DrugBase is identical in its stated coverage of manufacturer-provided package inserts for medicinals registered in South Africa. Like the *Electronic Package Inserts* (*EPI*) file annotated above, it, too, incorporates both OTC and Rx product information. But the collection compiled here seems to be smaller and does not include the many herbal products seen in *EPI*. On the other hand, the interface is more sophisticated, accepting brand or generic names, company names, and disease or condition keywords as directly searchable queries. Package inserts have also been thoroughly indexed and systematically structured into sections offered for individual display (e.g., composition, pharmacological classification, indications, dosage).

PharmInfoNet DrugDB
⇨ http://pharminfo.com/drugdb

DrugDB is a database created by VirSci Corporation as an index to further information found at other locations on the *PharmInfoNet* (Pharmaceutical Information Network) site. Separate, browsable A–Z indexes of generic or brand names permit quick scans for pertinent entries. Very brief *DrugDB* monographs identify only brand name, manufacturer, therapeutic class, and indication. However, many listings are supplemented with hotlinks to *Medical Sciences Bulletin®* reviews or other original publications found at this URL, such as mechanism of action tables.

Internet Mental Health
⇨ http://www.mentalhealth.com

In addition to providing professional reviews of diagnosis, treatment, and related research findings for fifty common mental disorders, *Internet Mental Health* compiles official Canadian package insert information for sixty-seven of the most commonly used psychiatric drugs. Medications covered are indexed by both brand and nonproprietary names in a browsable alphabetic list. Monographs are supplemented with summaries of research results found in literature published from 1991 through 1995, with full bibliographic references supplied. Another source of drug data at *Internet Mental Health* is a large collection of articles and booklets gathered in a separately labeled Magazine section. Once in this section, click on Medications to view options. This site is the product of Philip W. Long, MD, a psychiatrist based in Vancouver, British Columbia.

ECPHIN (European Community Pharmaceutical Information Network)
⇨ http://ecphin.etomep.net

The *European Community Pharmaceutical Information Network* is a database of all registered medicinal products in Europe. It can be searched by ECPHIN number, CAS registry number of active ingredient, brand name, generic name, company, pharmaceutical form classification, and/or anatomic/therapeutic category (ATC). Indexes of dosage forms and ATC coding can be viewed as picklists to assist in narrowing down a query. Results show all medicinal product (trade) names, associated authorization holders (companies), country where approved, and ECPHIN number. Package size, pricing, date of marketing clearance, storage guidelines, and shelf-life are also compiled.

References

1. Clark D. *Sick to death.* New York: Harper & Row, 1983:148.
2. Clark D. *Plain sailing.* London: Victor Gollancz, 1987:119–120.
3. Clark D. *Vicious circle.* New York: Harper & Row, 1985:211.
4. Clark D. *Heberden's seat.* New York: Harper & Row, 1984:162.
5. Snow B. Martindale online: drug information in a detective's toolkit. *Database* 1988 Jun;11:90–98.
6. Hollister LE. AMA Drug Evaluations subscription (book review). *JAMA* 1991 Jul 17;266:424.
7. Fishman DL. Computerized clinical information system: CCIS from Micromedex. *Database* 1992 Apr;15:58–63.
8. Hill DR. BrandonHill selected list of nursing books and journals. *Nurs Outlook* 1998 Jan-Feb;46(1):7–16.
9. Books of the year. The most valuable texts of 1997 as chosen by AJN's panel of judges. *Am J Nurs* 1998 Jan;98:69–70.

Additional Sources of Information

Allen LV. *Contemporary compounding compendium.* 3 v. New York: Jobson Publishing, 1993–1996.
Allwood M, Stanley A, Wright P, eds. *The cytotoxics handbook.* 3rd ed. Washington, DC: American Pharmaceutical Association, 1997.
Arndt KA. *Manual of dermatological therapeutics.* 5th ed. Boston, MA: Little, Brown, 1995.
Belanger D, Bedard M, Morris ME. *Intravenous drug therapy manual.* Ottawa: Ottawa General Hospital, 1997.
Bernstein JG. *Handbook of drug therapy in psychiatry.* 3rd ed. St. Louis: Mosby, 1995.
Bezchlibnyk-Butler KZ. *Clinical handbook of psychotropic drugs.* 8th ed. Toronto: Hogrefe & Huber, 1998.
Bressler R, Katz MD, eds. *Geriatric pharmacology.* New York: McGraw-Hill, 1993.
Bloom HG, Shlom EA. *Drug prescribing in the elderly.* Baltimore: Williams & Wilkins, 1993.

Bruel HP. *Clinical pharmacology in the elderly.* New York: Springer Verlag, 1996.

Chernow B. *The pharmacologic approach to the critically-ill patient.* 3rd ed. Baltimore: Williams & Wilkins, 1994.

Collett DM, Aulton ME, eds. *Pharmaceutical practice.* New York: Churchill Livingstone, 1996.

Connors KA, Amidon GL, Stella VI. *Chemical stability of pharmaceuticals.* New York: John Wiley, 1986.

Craig CR, Stitzel RE, eds. *Modern pharmacology: with clinical applications.* 5th ed. Philadelphia: Lippincott-Raven, 1997.

Datta S. *Obstetric and anesthesia handbook.* 2nd ed. St. Louis: Mosby, 1995.

Delafuente JC, Stewart RB, eds. *Therapeutics in the elderly.* Cincinnati, OH: Harvey Whitney Books, 1995.

Dental practitioners' formulary 1992–94. London: The Pharmaceutical Press, 1992.

DiPiro JT et al., eds. *Pharmacotherapy: A pathophysiologic approach.* 3rd ed. New York: Elsevier Science Publishing, 1997.

Freeman-Clark JB, Queener SF, Karb VB. *Pharmacological basis of nursing practice.* 4th ed. St. Louis: Mosby, 1993.

Fuentes RJ, Rosenberg JM, Davis A, eds. *Allen & Hanbury's athletic drug reference.* Durham, NC: Glaxo Wellcome, 1995.

Gage P, Pickett FA. *Mosby's dental drug reference.* St. Louis: Mosby-Year Book, 1998. Annual.

Gahart BL, Nazareno AR. *Intravenous medications.* St. Louis: Mosby, 1998. Annual.

Gleicher N, ed. *Principles and practices of medical therapy in pregnancy.* 2nd ed. New York: Appleton & Lange, 1992.

Greene RJ, Harris ND. *Pathology and therapeutics for pharmacists: A basis for clinical practice.* London: The Pharmaceutical Press, 1993.

International medical guide for ships, including the ship's medicine chest. 2nd ed. Geneva: World Health Organization, 1988.

International travel and health: vaccination requirements and health advice. Geneva: World Health Organization, 1994.

Janicak PG, Davis JM, Preskom SH, Ayd FJ. *Principles and practice of psychopharmacology.* 2nd ed. Baltimore: Williams & Wilkins, 1997.

Kayne SB. *Homeopathic pharmacy.* Philadelphia: Churchill Livingstone, 1997.

Keltner NL, Folks DG. *Psychotropic drugs.* 2nd ed. St. Louis: Mosby, 1997.

King RE. *Dispensing of medication.* 9th ed. Easton, PA: Mack Publishing, 1984.

Ledward RS, Cruikshank SA. *Drug treatment in gynecology.* 2nd ed. St. Louis: Mosby, 1995.

Mammen GJ, ed. *Clinical Pharmacokinetics drug data handbook.* 3rd ed. Auckland, NZ: Adis International, 1998.

Mandell GL, Douglas G, Bennett JE. *Principles and practice of infectious diseases: Handbook of antimicrobial therapy.* New York: Churchill Livingstone, 1992.

Mason P. *Handbook of dietary supplements: vitamins and other health supplements.* Cambridge, MA: Blackwell Science, 1995.

Mathewson-Kuhn M. *Pharmacotherapeutics: a nursing process approach.* 3rd ed. Philadelphia: Davis, 1994.

McCue JD, Tessier EG, Gaziano P, Lamhut P. *Geriatric drug handbook for long-term care.* Baltimore: Williams & Wilkins, 1993.

McHenry LM, Salerno E. *Mosby's pharmacology in nursing.* 19th ed. St. Louis: Mosby, 1995.

Needle R, Sizer T. *The CIVAS handbook, the centralized intravenous services reference.* London: The Pharmaceutical Press, 1998.

Omoigui S, ed. *The anesthesia drugs handbook.* 2nd ed. St. Louis: Mosby, 1995.

Omoigui S, ed. *The pain drugs handbook.* St. Louis: Mosby, 1995.

Onofrey BE, Skorin L, Holdeman NR. *Ocular therapeutics handbook.* Baltimore: Williams & Wilkins, 1997.

Pies RW. *Handbook of essential psychopharmacology.* Washington, DC: American Psychiatric Press, 1998.

Plotkin SA, Mortimer EA, eds. *Vaccines.* 2nd ed. Philadelphia: W. B. Saunders, 1994.

Rayburn WF. Chronic medical disorders during pregancy: Guidelines for prescribing drugs. *J Reprod Med* 1997;42(1):1–24.

Reiss BS, Evans ME. *Pharmacological aspects of nursing care.* 5th ed. Albany, NY: Delmar, 1996.

Requa-Clark B, Holroyd SV, eds. *Applied pharmacology for the dental hygienist.* 3rd ed. St. Louis: Mosby, 1995.

Rubin P, ed. *Prescribing in pregnancy.* 2nd ed. London: BMJ Publishing Group, 1995.

Speight TM, Holford NHG. *Avery's drug treatment.* Auckland, NZ: Adis International, 1997.

Spratto GR, Woods AL. *Delmar's NDR: Nurse's drug reference.* Albany, NY: Delmar, 1997. Annual.

Stahl SM. *Essential psychopharmacology: Neuroscientific basis and clinical applications.* Cambridge, NY: Cambridge University Press, 1996.

Stoklosa MJ, Ansel HC. *Pharmaceutical calculations.* 10th ed. Philadelphia: Lea & Febiger, 1995.

Sutton JD. *IV drug guide for nurses.* Norwalk, CT: Appleton & Lange, 1993.

Turkowski BB, Lance BR, Janosik JE, eds. *Drug information handbook for nursing.* Hudson, OH: Lexi-Comp, 1998.

The use of essential drugs. Model list of essential drugs. 8th list. Geneva: World Health Organization, 1995.

Vitamin supplements. *Med Lett Drugs Ther* 1998 Jul 31;40(1032):75–77.

Walton JG, Thompson JW, Seymour RA. *Textbook of dental pharmacology & therapeutics.* 2nd ed. New York: Oxford University Press, 1994.

White J, Garrison MW. *Basic clinical pharmacokinetics handbook.* Vancouver, WA: Applied Therapeutics, 1994.

WHO drug information. Geneva: World Health Organization, 1987–. Quarterly.

WHO model prescribing information: Drugs used in anesthesia. Geneva: World Health Organization, 1989.

WHO model prescribing information: drugs used in mycobacterial diseases. Geneva: World Health Organization, 1991.

WHO model prescribing information: drugs used in parasitic diseases. 2nd ed. Geneva: World Health Organization, 1995.

WHO model prescribing information: drugs used in sexually transmitted diseases and HIV infection. Geneva: World Health Organization, 1995.

Wills S. *Drugs of abuse.* London: The Pharmaceutical Press, 1997.

Winter ME. *Basic clinical pharmacokinetics*. 3rd ed. Vancouver, WA: Applied Therapeutics, 1994.

Wynn RL, Meiller TF, Crossley HL. *Drug information handbook for dentistry*. Hudson, OH: Lexi-Comp, 1996–. Annual.

Young LY, Koda-Kimble MA, eds. *Applied therapeutics: The clinical use of drugs*. 6th ed. Vancouver, WA: Applied Therapeutics, 1995.

Young LY, ed. *Physical assessment: A guide to evaluating drug therapy*. Vancouver, WA: Applied Therapeutics, 1994.

Zaloga GP. *The critical care drug handbook*. 2nd ed. St. Louis: Mosby, 1996.

Zambito S. *Manual of dental therapeutics*. St. Louis: Mosby, 1991.

Zimmerman TJ, Kooner KS, Sharir M, Fechter RD. *Textbook of ocular pharmacology*. Baltimore: Williams & Wilkins, 1997.

Practicum 2

This practicum exercise will help you evaluate your ready-reference source selection skills and review information presented in Chapters Four through Six. Questions posed can be answered without actual reference to hardcopy sources. Suggested answers are included in Appendix E.

Directions: Assume that you have available for your use all of the sources cited in previous chapters. Unless otherwise indicated, your response to each question should consist of:

    a. a list of sources to be consulted, with order of priority indicated, and

    b. a brief explanation of the rationale behind your selection of resources and sequence of consultation.

1. Is Vitamin D ever used for topical treatment of leg ulcers? Is so, what is the recommended dosage and concentration?
2. Does Brand X toothpaste contain any alcohol?
3. In the state of Connecticut, can syringes or injection needles be sold outside a pharmacy?
4. What is MO-911? Find the first reference to this name.
5. A community pharmacist needs to identify a U.S. source for wild cherry bark extract.
6. Is tolnaftate sodium soluble in alcohol?
7. Is paregoric a controlled substance? If so, on what schedule does it appear?
8. Has mistletoe ever been used therapeutically? Find supportive references, if possible.
9. When was Brand Y reformulated?
10. What sugar-free laxatives are available? Which is the least expensive?
11. Can a pharmacist legally fill a foreign prescription order, if it turns out to be for a product that is sold over-the-counter in the United States?
12. What are some bases for hydrophilic ointments?
13. Has OTC antacid Z been associated with photosensitivity reactions?

14. A group of researchers need to know if their animal testing facilities are suitable for conducting preclinical investigations under contract to a pharmaceutical manufacturer preparing for an IND.
15. Where might a consumer find comparative information on diaper rash products?
16. Where can I find pronunciations of drug names?
17. A pharmacist needs to know if a scheduled drug can be sent via the U.S. postal service for intrastate delivery to the patient for whom it was prescribed.
18. A hospital pharmacist has been asked to investigate the possibility of preparing an oral preparation intended for adults in an alternative form for administration to a child, either orally or intravenously.
19. A law firm needs to find out what companies marketed Drug B in tablet form in 1980. What were the approved indications and dosage?

Side Effects: Sources of Adverse Drug Reactions and Interactions Information

It's sometimes easy to forget that the basis of efficacious drug therapy is induction of a side effect. Early remedies were often discovered by observing beneficial effects following exposure to certain plants. Several modern medicines can trace their origin to unexpected incidents occurring during the course of therapy and later transformed to advantageous outcomes through adjustments in dosage or route of exposure. Side effects are inherent to the concept of administration of exogenous agents to induce changes in body response. Harnessing the powerful effects of chemical substances to good use is the objective of pharmaceutical research, where finding an acceptable balance between benefit and risk is, at times, a scientific tightrope walk, given wide variations in patient response. Genetic factors, age, gender, body weight, and overall physical fitness can each be influential in determining the dividing line between efficacy and potential harm.

Virtually all drugs have been associated with untoward side effects in humans. Commonly observed conditions are also often experienced by people not undergoing drug therapy, such as nausea, headache, nasal congestion, or skin rash. Thus, establishing a definite cause-effect link between medication use and adverse experiences can be difficult. Despite careful preapproval testing, many adverse effects are not detected until a drug is introduced into commerce. As Nies and Spielberg[1] have pointed out, the scope of clinical trials required prior to launch is necessarily limited, due to time, cost, and ethical constraints. Adverse events uncovered after a drug's clearance for marketing are delayed risks or those likely to occur in fewer than one out of 1,000 administrations, both requiring long-term use in a larger and more diverse population to manifest themselves.

The FDA recognized the importance of post-launch surveillance when it created an official mechanism for voluntary adverse drug reaction (ADR) reporting by healthcare professionals, first established in 1960. Although Phase IV studies can uncover previously unsuspected effects, spontaneous reporting also plays a vital role in monitoring marketed drugs. As Rossi *et al.*[2] have observed, none of the Phase IV trials designed for cimetidine, cyclobenzapine, or prazosin detected unknown ADRs, but the voluntary reporting network did. Regrettably, experience has shown that only "a small proportion of drug-related events occurring in clinical practice" are actually relayed through this system, with the U.S. reporting rate averaging 25% of that seen in Denmark, 40% of that in Canada, and 50% of U.K. figures.[3] Griffin's 1986 review of ADR reporting systems in fifteen countries placed the United States as ninth in a ranking of frequency of voluntary submissions per million of population and fifteenth in the number of ADR reports per physician.[4] Furthermore, a survey published in 1988[5] found that only 57% of physician respondents were aware of the FDA's voluntary ADR submission system, despite the fact that official forms had been reprinted in the AMA's *Drug Evaluations* since 1983, in the *PDR* since 1987, and disseminated by direct mail by the FDA to licensed practitioners at least once a year.

Clearly, accurate data on the overall incidence of drug adverse reactions are not available. Studies of hospital admissions have, nonetheless, provided consistent indicators of their magnitude. Those most frequently cited date from the 1970s.[6-8] In 1971, Melmon estimated that 18–30% of all hospitalized patients experience an unintended drug effect and that the duration of their hospitalization was nearly doubled as a consequence. "In addition, three to five % of all admissions to hospitals are primarily for a drug reaction, and 30% of these patients have a second reaction during their stay."[9] Talley[10] underscored the extent of the problem in an oft-quoted 1974 *JAMA* report, estimating that approximately one million patients are hospitalized and 140,000 deaths occur each year in the United States as a direct result of medication use.

Data from more recent studies show that the frequency of drug-related iatrogenic admissions and inpatient ADR incidents has remained stable in subsequent years. Analyzing ADR rates reported in articles published from 1966 through 1989, Einarson[11] concluded that drug-induced hospitalizations account for 5% of all admissions. Complications from drug therapy were the most common adverse event in hospitalized patients, constituting 19% of such events, in the Harvard Medical Practice Study, published in 1991.[12] Morbidity and mortality associated with medication use and misuse (both physician-induced and patient noncompliance) has been estimated to cost $76.6 billion in the ambulatory setting in the United States, the largest component in this cost-of-illness model being drug-related hospitalizations.[13] Despite this staggering price tag, it is unlikely that the general public would measure the impact of adverse drug effects solely in terms of dollars.

Investigations into causes are equally disturbing. Out of the 5.4% admissions attributable to iatrogenic disease in Lakshmanan's findings published in 1986, the author concluded that 48% "were avoidable."[14] The Harvard Medical Practice Study found that 45% of serious or life-threatening ADRs were preventable.[15]

Results reported by Bates[16] in 1995 showed that 6.5% of adult nonobstetrical patients admitted suffered an adverse drug reaction, 28% of which were due to errors. (Note: Error is not equivalent to medical negligence in tort law.) Leape's analysis of these data reveal that lack of knowledge of drugs and how they should be used was the most common cause, accounting for 35% of preventable and potential ADRs.[17] Examples include incorrect doses, forms, frequencies, routes, and errors in choice of drug.

Such statistics are a clarion call to action for information providers, as well as primary care-givers. Although some adverse effects are inevitable, many can be prevented, or their severity reduced, by better-informed prescribing and therapeutic monitoring. Pharmacotherapeutic reference sources reviewed in the previous chapter address this information need by including discussion of contraindications, precautions, and known side effects. However, book collections supporting healthcare practitioners should also include publications specifically designed to facilitate retrieval of adverse reaction data. Such resources are the focus of this chapter.

Adverse Reactions Information Sources

The best known source of side effects data is commonly referred to by the name of its first editor, Meyler, who was associated with its compilation from publication of the first edition in English in 1952 through the seventh edition in 1972.

7.1 Dukes MNG, ed. *Meyler's Side Effects of Drugs*. 13th ed. Amsterdam: Elsevier, 1996.

7.2 Aronen JK, Van Boxtel CJ, eds. *Side Effects of Drugs Annual*. Amsterdam: Elsevier, 1977–.

Individual chapters in *Meyler's Side Effects of Drugs* deal with pharmacologically related drugs, rather than those with similar adverse effects. Each is introduced with a monograph on the drug class, then is supplemented by specific data on individual agents in the class "insofar as their adverse effects deviate from the general pattern." Structured entries provide a predictable format that assists in quick location of information on general and toxic reactions, hypersensitivity, tumor-inducing effects, risk situations (contraindications), interactions, and interference with diagnostic routines. Rapid access is further assisted by separate indexes to both side effects and drug names (generic names, usually INN, preferred).

Meyler's coverage includes a chapter devoted to drugs used in "non-orthodox" medicine, with side effects and interactions data on many plants used therapeutically, substances of animal origin, minerals, vitamins, special diets, and nutritional therapies. Another noteworthy chapter on "miscellaneous drugs and materials" covers surgical and dental materials and appliances, dietary preparations and sweeteners, as well as side effects of dyes and colorants.

Each edition of *Meyler's* reports new observations since the last compilation and summarizes, but does not entirely replicate, important data from previous volumes. This means that it's wise to retain older editions. Since 1977, annual updates have been published to bridge the gap between main editions, which are issued every three to four years. Monographs in annual volumes often feature special reviews that revise previous conclusions, when new data discredit older findings. Cumulative access to *Meyler's* (dating from the 9th edition through the end of 1995) is available online in Elsevier's *SEDBASE*, where drug name indexing is augmented with cross references from Marler's *Pharmacological and Chemical Synonyms* (3.13) and bibliographic references are enhanced with abstracts drawn from *EMBASE* (14.4). In hardcopy format, *Meyler's* uses a coded scheme for citing supportive bibliography. References embedded in the text are accompanied by one of four different designations representing editorial evaluations of the depth of coverage and clinical evidence presented in cited sources. Such indicators are intended to assist users in assessments of clinical risk. Aptly subtitled "An Encyclopedia of Adverse Reactions and Interactions," *Meyler's* has no rival in its broad-ranging scope and authoritative survey of the literature, making it a recommended core collection acquisition.

7.3 Benichou C, ed. *Adverse Drug Reactions: A Practical Guide to Diagnosis and Management*. New York: John Wiley, 1994.
7.4 Davies DM, ed. *Textbook of Adverse Drug Reactions*. 4th ed. New York: Oxford University Press, 1991.

As its title implies, the intended audience for *Adverse Drug Reactions: A Practical Guide to Diagnosis and Management* is the primary care-giver, who, when confronted with various clinical manifestations, must answer the question: Could it be drug-related? Benichou's text outlines how to direct etiologic investigations and establish a positive diagnosis, exploring nondrug-related causes and how they can be ruled out, as well as delineating which chronological and clinical criteria might suggest a medication-induced reaction. Discussion generally focuses on classes of drugs, rather than specific products, and is presented in an easy-to-read two-column format, with essential information on the left and comments or complementary explanations on the right. Liver test abnormalities, unusual hematologic values, cutaneous reactions, acute renal failure, and psychiatric disorders are each accorded a separate chapter.

Part II of the *Practical Guide* deals with regulatory and technical issues, such as international reporting requirements for ADRs (presented in quick-reference tables), pharmacovigilance in the European Community, harmonization efforts among nations in communicating safety information for marketed drugs, and World Health Organization ADR terminology. Detailed examination is given to the important topic of imputability of unexpected or toxic reactions and weighing the evidence of intrinsic factors (e.g., chronological implicators) against extrinsic data. Discussion of the latter focuses on "scoring" of bibliographic data and introduces a new method for causality assessment: RUCAM (Roussel Uclaf Causality Assessment Method). It is only in this section of the book that the reader becomes aware of the fact that its contents have been translated from the original French edition. For example, "semiology" (i.e., symptomatology), defined as "the clinical or paraclinical picture which may or may not be evocative of the role of the drug," must be weighed against "the existence of validated risk factors" in the complex RUCAM system. Aside from occasional language difficulties, the *Practical Guide* is a noteworthy contribution to the adverse reaction reference shelf.

Davies' *Textbook of Adverse Drug Reactions* is another good source for background on general principles and possible mechanisms for interactions and adverse effects. Organized by body systems/effects, this book is also geared to the clinician, with its disease-oriented rather than drug-oriented approach. Discussion includes treatment and management of effects. One useful appendix lists adverse reactions associated with excipients. Refer to *Adverse Reactions to Drug Formulation Agents* (7.18) and Additional Sources at the end of this chapter for other publications addressing the effects of nontherapeutic ingredients.

7.5 *Reactions*. Auckland, New Zealand: ADIS Press, 1979–. Biweekly.
7.6 *Clin-Alert*. Medford, NJ: Clin-Alert, 1962–. Semimonthly.

Reactions™ is the best source for current awareness of drug side effects and interactions. An annual subscription to this extremely timely and informative newsletter in hardcopy format includes two quarterly, one six-month, and an annual cumulative index. The full text of *Reactions* is also available online, updated daily (14.26). Each issue begins with Views and Reviews, consisting of well written essays analyzing observed trends. For example, one issue offered a review of ADR impacts in the previous year, outlining the results of increased scrutiny by regulatory agencies worldwide and summarizing resulting withdrawals of approved indications and major labeling/data sheet changes. The Reactions Update portion of each issue cites references drawn from a survey of 2,000 international medical journals and features original, detailed abstracts for each source cited. Entries are arranged alphabetically by generic drug name. ADIS editors add value by flagging first reports and those documenting serious adverse effects. In the *Reactions Annual* sent as a free supplement to each year's subscription, reports published during the previous twelve months that offered new or significant data are summarized in full, while briefer references are included for others.

Clin-Alert is also an excellent current awareness source, although considerably more modest in scope (and price) than *Reactions*. Each issue offers ten to fourteen in-depth abstracts of significant case reports published in the recent primary literature.

7.7 Miller RR, Greenblatt DJ, eds. *Drug Effects in Hospitalized Patients: Experiences of the Boston Collaborative Drug Surveillance Program 1966–1975*. New York: Kreiger, 1976.

Part of the continuing problem of a high incidence of adverse effects is the lack of well publicized, large scale, and long-term surveillance necessary to increase awareness of potential reactions. Systematic study of adverse effects did not begin until the mid-1960s. The Boston Collaborative Drug Surveillance Program dates from this era and remains one of the most valuable and frequently-cited sources of epidemiological data. Miller and Greenblatt's compilation is useful for its documentation of less common side effects, information about which may not be reported elsewhere. Results of 20,000 hospital admissions and 200,000 drug orders are tabulated.

Reference Sources for Drug Interactions

Combination or concurrent drug therapy often takes advantage of one drug's modification of the effects of another. A second drug may be prescribed to enhance the effectiveness of another or to reduce its adverse effects. Thus, many drug-drug interactions are intentional or beneficial. However, an increasingly mobile and cost-conscious consumer/patient population can lead to unplanned and undesirable interactions. Individuals may be consulting several different physicians and alternative healthcare providers, obtaining medication from a variety of sources, and using both prescription and nonprescription remedies without fully disclosing their concurrent use to prescribers. When diet and other environmental factors are added to the mixture, the result may be a confusing clinical condition difficult to attribute to any single agent.

Tracking down data on possible interactions can be equally challenging. Several sources cited in the previous section include information on interactions, as well as adverse effects associated with single drug agents. However, no core drug collection is complete without one or more of the following specialty publications.

7.8 Horn JR, Hansten PD, eds. *Hansten and Horn's Drug Interactions Analysis and Management*. Vancouver, WA: Applied Therapeutics, 1997–. Updated quarterly.

Hansten is a name long associated with drug interactions publication, beginning with a small paperbound compendium published in 1971. By its 5th edition in 1985, Hansten's *Drug Interactions* had been translated into Japanese, German, Spanish, and Portuguese. The current looseleaf successor is equally highly regarded, though somewhat more awkward to use. The basic arrangement is by interacting drug class, scattering references to some drugs' potential interactions throughout the volume. For example, cimetidine interactions are discussed under antacids, anticoagulants, antidepressants, barbiturates, benzodiazepines, beta blockers, etc. Only use of the generic name index brings all references to potential interactions together. Many brand names are also included as cross references in the index. A further drawback is that, unlike the revised/replacement pages issued for most looseleaf services, material provided in quarterly *Drug Interactions Newsletter* updates is not designed for interleaving with the bulk of reference material. Updates and supplements in separate issues renders consultation of the index doubly important, or relevant material could easily be missed.

Horn and Hansten have written extensively about pitfalls in evaluation of drug interaction literature. Perils include inappropriate extrapolation of data from normal subjects to the patient population or from one member of a drug class to all members in the class, inadequate assessment of the significance of case reports, failure to account for sequence of administration or to consider the effect of dose or that of the indication for which a drug is prescribed. (Some interactions occur when a drug is used for one purpose, but not when it is employed for another indication.) That both editors have devoted considerable attention to literature evaluation and risk assessment is evident in the quality of drug class monographs included in *Drug Interactions Analysis and Management*.

7.9 Zucchero FJ, Hogan MJ, eds. *Evaluations of Drug Interactions*. St. Louis: Professional Drug Systems, 1990–. Bimonthly.

Zucchero and Hogan's *Evaluation of Drug Interactions* is also an outstanding reference resource, but suffers somewhat from its packaging in a very fat looseleaf binder that requires two hands to hold open. Aside from this physical barrier, the arrangement is sometimes rated as more user-friendly by nonpharmacist users. Organized into eighteen broad drug category sections, monographs are arranged alphabetically by generic names of interacting drugs (unfortunately, brand name cross references are omitted). Each entry includes discussion of related drugs, the mechanism of interaction, recommendations for management, and bibliographic references. A useful feature of this volume, which is produced under the auspices of the APhA, is summation of interaction data into tables, where coding also indicates the clinical significance of each effect reported. First DataBank also markets a machine-readable version of *Evaluations of Drug Interactions* (see http://www.firstdatabank.com/drug/edi.html).

7.10 *Drug Interaction Facts*. St. Louis: Facts & Comparisons, 1983–. Updated quarterly.

Drug Interaction Facts is perhaps the simplest to use of the three looseleaf sources, due to its single integrated index of interacting agents, listing both generic and major brand names. Significant and substantiated drug interactions are indicated by boldface type in the index. Monographs, arranged by drug classification, are concise summaries of effects, providing data on the importance, severity, and rapidity of the interaction, mechanism of action, and recommended management. Bibliographic references are also included. In addition to publication in hardcopy format, *Drug Interaction Facts* is available from Micromedex on CD-ROM or magnetic tape. The advantage of computer-assisted access through the *DRUG-REAX*™ system is that as many as fifteen drugs can be checked simultaneously in all permutations and combinations to locate possible interactions.

7.11   Stockley IH. *Drug Interactions*. 4th ed. London: The Pharmaceutical Press, 1996.

Stockley's *Drug Interactions* provides individual drug-drug or drug-food synopses organized into twenty-three chapters grouped by therapeutic or pharmacological class of the major agent affected (e.g., anticoagulant drug interactions, immunosuppressants). Such an arrangement means, once again, that the quality of the index is critical. Fortunately, all interacting pairs of agents are accessible by both USAN and BAN. Chapters on drug classes also compile brief tables cross-referencing brand and generic names, but back-of-the-book indexing omits proprietary designations, except for combination products. Each of the more than 2,000 drug monograph entries begins with a one- or two-sentence abstract, followed by a summary of available clinical evidence, mechanism of the interaction, discussion of its importance and management, and bibliographic references.

7.12   *DRUG-REAX*. Denver: Micromedex, 1996–. Annual.

The *DRUG-REAX*® system, marketed in machine-readable form for networking, has the advantage of enabling users to check for possible interactions by entering more than one suspected agent as a starting point. Cross-matching capabilities extend, in fact, up to 128 concurrent search factors. Drug-drug, drug-food, drug-disease, drug-ethanol, and drug-lab assay interactions are all covered, along with their clinical significance. *DRUG-REAX* also includes information on excipients implicated in interactions or hypersensitivity reactions. Results of searches are drug-specific, rather than class-oriented, to assist users in accurate interpretation of data.

7.13   *The PDR Companion Guide*. Montvale, NJ: Medical Economics, 1998–. Annual.

The PDR Companion Guide (formerly *PDR Guide to Drug Interactions, Side Effects, Indications*, 1993–) is simply a separately published index to the current year's edition of the *Physicians' Desk Reference* (6.10), the *PDR for Nonprescription Drugs* (6.9), and the *PDR for Ophthalmology* (6.12). It cannot be used independently of its parent volumes to retrieve summaries of interaction or adverse effect data. Indexing, though thorough, is limited by the comparatively selective coverage of products that characterizes the *PDR* set of publications and by the uneven quality of their package inserts (see discussion in Chapter Six). The introduction acknowledges that product labeling varies in scope of interactions reported, and that cross-sensitivity reactions and effects of laboratory test results are not included. *The PDR Companion Guide* does offer a food interactions index with relevant entries by dietary item (e.g., chocolate, anchovies). Its Side Effects index also provides access to 3,600 reactions cited in the *PDR* and its sister volumes. Other sections include a Generic Availability Table, an Off-Label Treatment Guide, a Daily Cost of Therapy Guide, and an International Drug Guide naming U.S. equivalents for approximately 14,000 foreign medications.

Specialized Adverse Effects Publications

More specialized resources can be useful acquisitions for drug information collections where depth, as well as breadth, is important. Many are designed to address hot or hard-to-find topics, such as drugs and human lactation, drug-nutrient interactions, iatrogenic conditions affecting the eye, and adverse reactions to drug formulation agents (excipients) and cosmetics. In addition, Figure 7.1 identifies two bonuses found on the Internet related to the subject focus of this chapter.

7.14 Grant WM. *Toxicology of the Eye.* 4th ed. Springfield, IL: Charles C. Thomas, 1993.
7.15 Fraunfelder FT. *Drug-Induced Ocular Side Effects and Drug Interactions.* 4th ed. Philadelphia: Lea & Febiger, 1995.

Grant's *Toxicology of the Eye* has become a reference textbook classic, providing information on the adverse effects of more than 16,000 drugs, chemicals, metals, minerals, plants, and other biotoxins on the eye. Discussion includes systemic side effects resulting from eye medications. Fraunfelder's work, citing only human ocular side effects, is less research-oriented and more practice-oriented than Grant. *Drug-Induced Ocular Side Effects and Drug Interactions* incorporates data from the National Registry of Drug-Induced Ocular Side Effects, collected over a twelve-year period. Arranged by therapeutic categories (e.g., analgesics, anesthesia), entries list side effects in probable order of importance, based on their recorded incidence.

References are included for each drug's side effects, with an emphasis on compiling the best and most current bibliography, as evaluated by the author. The drug name index includes both generic and proprietary nomenclature, providing access by all recognized generic designations (not just United States), as well as by domestic and foreign brand names (for each of which, country of origin, not manufacturer, is cited). The volume also includes an index to side effects, but no separate index to interactions. A new feature in this edition of Fraunfelder's work is a section on drug-related systemic side effects from medications used primarily by ophthalmologists.

7.16 Ciraulo DA, Shader RI, Greenblatt DJ, Creelman WC, eds. *Drug Interactions in Psychiatry.* 2nd ed. Baltimore: Williams & Wilkins, 1995.

Drug Interactions in Psychiatry is arranged by drug class, with a back-of-the-book index to generic names of interacting drugs. Brand name cross-references are, unfortunately, omitted. Each drug class section concludes with a bibliography of references to the primary literature.

7.17 De Groot AC, Wyland JW, Nater JP. *Unwanted Effects of Cosmetics and Drugs Used in Dermatology.* 3rd ed. Amsterdam: Elsevier, 1994.

Unwanted Effects of Cosmetics and Drugs Used in Dermatology presents information on side effects in a standardized format with subheadings for each organ system affected. One chapter features a thirty-page tabulation of cosmetic ingredients and synonyms. Drugs covered include dermal implants, chemical face peels, and agents used in cryotherapy and laser therapy. This edition expands its coverage of systemic drugs to include new products in the dermatologist's armamentarium, such as retinoids, itraconazole, terbinafine, and cyclosporin A. Standard patch test concentrations and vehicles are cited throughout this comprehensive work, which is copiously referenced and well indexed for easy use.

7.18 Weiner M, Bernstein IL. *Adverse Reactions to Drug Formulation Agents.* New York: Marcel Dekker, 1989.

Nontherapeutic components in drug formulations are sometimes implicated in clinical side effects. *Adverse Reactions to Drug Formulation Agents* compiles

---

Figure 7.1 Two Specialized Adverse Effects Publications on the Internet

---

- *Cutaneous Drug Reaction Database*
  ⇨ gopher://gopher.Dartmouth.EDU:70/00/Research/BioSci/CDRD/README.

  The Internet harbors a hidden gem, the *Cutaneous Drug Reaction Database*, at a gopher site maintained by the Dartmouth-Hitchcock Medical Center in Lebanon, New Hampshire. Author Jerome Z. Litt, M.D., has gathered together, for reference purposes, information on drug reactions that have skin manifestations. Offered free of charge and updated annually, the collection organizes entries by drug generic names. Data include brand name (also searchable), pharmacological category, half-life, and a list of skin, hair, nail, and related effects, each accompanied by a bibliographic reference to a primary source. The search mechanism accepts keyword queries, or the database can be scanned quickly for a pertinent nonproprietary name.

- *MotherRisk*
  ⇨ http://www.motherrisk.org/publi/a_n.htm

  Toronto's Hospital for Sick Children offers an excellent bibliography on the topic of drugs and lactation at its *MotherRisk* Web site.

---

data on allergic and nonallergic effects associated with individual pharmaceutical excipients, including color additives, coatings, and flavors. This book also contains a helpful section on reactions to materials used in medical devices. An appendix reprints the FDA's 1988 list of inactive ingredients, coordinating 3,400 substances with route of administration and CAS registry number.

Drugs and Lactation

Drug excretion in human milk is one of the most common subjects of adverse reaction queries. Several journal articles provide extensive bibliographies on this topic. A file containing reprints of such articles is useful to have on hand in anticipation of frequent inquiries. Refer to Additional Sources of Information at the end of this chapter for a bibliography of reviews (see also Figure 7.1).

7.19 Briggs GG, Freeman RK, Yaffe SJ, comps. *Drugs in Pregnancy and Lactation*. 5th ed. Baltimore: Williams & Wilkins, 1998.

Drugs in Pregnancy and Lactation summarizes findings from clinical trials and case reports, drawing heavily from information compiled on 50,000 mothers in the Boston Collaborative Perinatal Project (Heinonen, 8.29). These data are augmented by outcome statistics gathered from a larger surveillance study of 229,000 pregnancies, conducted from 1985 through 1992 and involving 250 drugs. This reference guide is arranged alphabetically by USAN, with more than 800 monographs presenting basic information in six parts: 1) nomenclature, 2) pharmacological class, 3) risk factor, a system categorizing chemical entities by potential for harm, defined at the beginning of the book, 4) fetal risk summary, 5) breast feeding summary, and 6) bibliographic references. The index includes cross references from brand names, including those used outside the United States. Quarterly updates are available by subscription.

7.20 Bennett PN, ed. *Drugs and Human Lactation*. 2nd ed. Amsterdam: Elsevier, 1996.

Bennett also offers an extensive review of the literature in *Drugs and Human Lactation*, subtitled "A comprehensive guide to the content and consequences of drugs, micronutrients, radiopharmaceuticals, and environmental and occupational chemicals in human milk." Findings of a three-year study by a WHO Working Group are used as the basis of recommendations on the safety of drugs cited. Opening chapters focus on the effects of drugs on milk secretion and composition and determinants of drug transfer into human milk, as well as disposition in the nursing child. Monographs on 234 drugs are followed by sections devoted to vitamins, minerals, and essential trace elements, radiopharmaceuticals, and other chemicals. This Elsevier publication also compiles a lengthy bibliography of relevant clinical trials and case reports.

7.21 Kauffman RE, et al. "Transfer of Drugs and Other Chemicals into Human
      Milk." *Pediatrics* 1994;93:137–150.
7.22 Taddio A, Ito S. "Drug Use During Lactation." In: Koren G, ed. *Mater-
      nal-Fetal Toxicology: A Clinician's Guide.* 2nd ed. New York: Marcel
      Dekker, 1994: 133–219.

In "Transfer of Drugs and Other Chemicals in Human Milk," the American
Academy of Pediatrics Committee on Drugs identifies agents excreted and describes their possible effects on the infant or on lactation, citing 312 bibliographic
references. This summary updates and revises a list published in the same journal
in 1989. Taddio and Ito, in reviewing the safety of commonly-used medications
in lactating ambulatory patients, summarize findings in the literature to date and
compile an extensive list of primary information sources (331 references). Their
chapter in *Maternal-Fetal Toxicology* includes a forty-five-page table of data obtained from clinical trials and other studies, listing 125 drugs in a therapeutic
class arrangement.

7.23 Hale T. *Medications and Mother's Milk.* 4th ed. Amarillo, TX: Pharmsoft
      Medical Publishing, 1997. Annual.

Hale provides a brief quick-reference handbook in *Medications and Mother's
Milk.* Drugs are listed alphabetically by brand and generic name in this annual
publication. Data compiled include drug elimination half-lives and milk/plasma
ratios. Hale also relays American Academy of Pediatrics recommendations.

Food-Drug Interactions

Another hot topic to anticipate is food-drug interactions. "Drug-nutrient interactions can be defined as events that result from chemical, physical, physiological
or pathophysiological relationships between nutrients and drugs. These events are
important when they diminish the intended response to a therapeutic drug; when
the nutritional status of an individual is impaired; or when it causes an acute or
chronic drug toxicity."[18] Although Hansten (7.8), *Meyler's* (7.1), and other general side effects sources index drug-food interactions, Roe and Basu offer more
in-depth background on the topic.

7.24 Roe DA. *Diet and Drug Interactions.* New York: Van Nostrand Reinhold,
      1989.
7.25 Basu TK. *Drug-Nutrient Interactions.* New York: Croom Helm, 1988.
7.26 Roe DA. *Handbook on Drug and Nutrient Interactions.* 5th ed. Chicago:
      American Dietetic Association, 1994.

In *Diet and Drug Interactions,* Roe provides information on mechanisms responsible for food interference with drug absorption and metabolism. This well-
referenced textbook discusses compatibility reactions, the effects of drugs on nu-

tritional status, and the influence of patient nutritional status on drug disposition. Basu's *Drug-Nutrient Interactions* includes brief tables, but is not designed as a quick-reference aid. Separate sections are devoted to drugs affecting food intake, absorption, carbohydrate metabolism, lipid metabolism, protein and amino acid metabolism, drug-vitamin interactions, mineral interactions, and possible adverse effects resulting from the pharmacological use of vitamins. Portions of this discussion address only classes of drugs, rather than individual agents. Basu also covers nutrition and experimental carcinogenesis and has compiled an extensive bibliography for further follow up. Roe's *Handbook,* published by the American Dietetic Association, offers a ready-reference, drug-by-drug approach.

7.27   Bodwell CS, Erdman JW, eds. *Nutrient Interactions.* New York: Marcel Dekker, 1988.

7.28   Garrison RH, Somer E. *The Nutrition Desk Reference: NDR.* 3rd ed. New Canaan, CT: Keats Publications, 1995.

Nutrient Interactions publishes the proceedings of a symposium sponsored by the Institute of Food Technologists and the International Union of Food Science and Technology. Editors Bodwell and Erdman arrange their material into sections devoted to energy-nutrient interactions, amino acid interactions, mineral interactions, nutrient-food additive and nutrient-drug interactions, and vitamin-vitamin interactions. For ready-reference purposes, *The Nutrition Desk Reference* may appeal more to health science professionals. Garrison and Somer provide an introduction to vitamin and mineral supplements, diet and disease relationships, and discuss important drug-nutrient interactions. (Refer to Additional Sources for further background bibliography.)

Drug-Laboratory Test Interactions

Laboratory test modifications associated with drug therapy fall into two major categories: 1) chemical interference due to test-reagent interactions adversely affecting analytical results, and 2) physiological/biological alterations, where drug effects on the patient alter test outcome, leading to false negatives or false positives.[19] Test methodology employed is important background information for efficient data retrieval in this subject area. As Evans[20] has pointed out, significant changes in methodology for clinical laboratory tests rapidly outdate information sources for drug-lab test interferences. Thus, searching major medical databases online will augment and update coverage of the literature available in hardcopy format.

7.29   Young DS, ed. *Effects of Drugs on Clinical Laboratory Tests.* 4th ed. Washington, DC: American Association of Clinical Chemistry, 1995.

Effects of Drugs on Clinical Laboratory Tests is a popular compilation of (and index to) references to the published literature on both chemical and physiological alterations in lab test results. It includes material on both frequently used tests and those infrequently performed in the United States, but still used elsewhere. The directory is organized into five sections. The first is a cross-reference index to laboratory test names, the second an index to drug brand and generic names, as well as selected drug classes, such as anticonvulsants. The third and fourth sections organize interaction entries by preferred test names or by selected drug names, respectively. Each entry includes a drug name, the body fluid or analyte measured, and information on whether the effect is a physiological or pharmacological (*in vivo*) effect, or an analytical interaction affecting the measurement procedure (*in vitro* effect). A brief description of the mechanism of the effect follows, and each entry concludes with a reference number. The fifth section lists more than 3,000 bibliographic references by number, documenting the nearly 40,000 drug-lab test interactions cited.

7.30 Salway JG, ed. *Drug-Test Interactions Handbook*. New York: Raven Press, 1990.

The arrangement of the *Drug-Test Interaction Handbook* attempts to address the complexity of this specialized area of drug information. Salway's *Handbook* divides interaction references into three parts centering on the type of specimen used, presenting information in color-coded sections which address, respectively, blood specimens (pink pages), urine specimens (yellow), and other clearance studies (blue). Within each part, tests covered are presented in classified groups. Two "matrices" introduce each part and serve as quick-reference indexes to subsequent listings. The first lists interactions by test type, the second by drug. Individual interaction entries summarize data on method of analysis used, dose, duration, and subject population, and cite primary literature sources (3,969 in all). Modifications of test results are classified into categories distinguishing between increases or decreases in biological effects and increases or decreases due to analytical interference. Two appendices provide integrated alphabetical lists of drugs covered in previous sections, and of tests cited.

Parenteral Incompatibilities

Although the phrase "therapeutic incompatibility" is sometimes used to describe situations where the response to one or more drugs in a patient is of a different nature than that intended by the prescriber, the term incompatibility is more commonly employed in the pharmaceutical literature to describe a distinct type of interaction. Incompatibility usually refers to physical or chemical interactions between two or more substances outside the body, before administration. The term customarily implies studies of parenteral solutions, but it may also appear in publications discussing the stability of other dosage forms.

"Parenteral" is defined as any route of administration other than the oral-gastrointestinal (enteral) tract, but general usage of the term excludes topical administration. Intravenous (IV), intramuscular (IM), and subcutaneous (SC) are examples of parenteral routes. The term is derived from the Greek *para enteron*, which can be roughly translated as "beside the intestine." A synonym for parenteral is injectable.

To avoid multiple injection sites in hospitalized patients, parenteral drugs are frequently administered in solutions combining more than one medication. Therapeutic agents are, for example, typically added to large volume nutrient or electrolyte solutions known as IV additives. Incompatibility questions arise in this admixture context. Physical incompatibility often leads to visible, recognizable changes in injectables, such as formation of a precipitate, haziness, or altered color. Solubility, storage conditions permitting dehydration or salting out, and temperature changes may all affect physical incompatibility. Chemical incompatibilities may be more difficult to detect. Changes associated with oxidation-reduction, acid-base, or hydrolysis problems often exhibit no outward signs in admixtures affected. Yet either type of incompatibility (physical or chemical) can lead to lack of uniformity in dosage and to reduction in bioavailability of active ingredients in parenterals.

Information on incompatibility is often found in stability studies. Stability describes the capability of a product (a combination of formulation, dosage form, and container) to maintain predetermined physical, chemical, and therapeutic qualities or specifications over time. Stability studies are initiated to determine shelf life, consequent expiration dating, and recommended storage conditions for a product. Retention of potency and efficacy are key issues to investigators.

Thus, incompatibility data may be needed not only for given admixtures, but also for specified storage conditions: light, temperature, containers, and closures. Packaging and drug delivery system components can undergo physical and chemical changes, leading to migration of their ingredients to the medications they contain. Permeation or "breathing" in containers or closures may occur, and moisture penetration or loss is not uncommon. Clearly, the topic of incompatibility is "much broader and more involved than one drug interacting with another drug."[21]

Despite the fact that many factors may contribute to parenteral incompatibilities, one hardcopy reference source has compiled data on most physical or chemical interactions of this type.

7.31 Trissel LA. *Handbook on Injectable Drugs.* 10th ed. Bethesda, MD: American Society of Health-System Pharmacists, 1998.

No professional drug information collection should be without Trissel's *Handbook on Injectable Drugs*, which covers 303 products, listed alphabetically by generic name, and compiles more than 2,000 references to relevant bibliography. Each monograph provides information on products available (brands, manufacturers, forms, sizes, strengths), dosage, administration, stability (storage requirements, temperature and light effects, pH), compatibility (both drugs and excipient interactions), and preparation. Cross references to *AHFS Drug Information* (6.4) therapeutic classification numbers assist in follow-up for additional information, such as pharmacology. Well-organized tables facilitate quick-reference use of the *Handbook*, listing products and solutions with which each featured drug is compatible, grouped by infusion solutions, intravenous solutions, syringes, and y-sites.

A separate section, first introduced in the 1992 edition, is devoted to parenteral drugs available outside the United States (names cited are primarily those in use in the United Kingdom). Additional sections focus on a selection of investigational drugs and on parenteral nutrition solution formulas. The index includes entries for all drug names cited: brand, generic, and code designations. Supplements issued between biennial editions supply new entries into the compatibility tables and add new drug monographs. A subset of Trissel's data is published in a *Pocket Guide to Injectable Drugs*, which contains 127 monographs. Updates to the full hardcopy edition are also available to online and CD-ROM users in the *Drug Information FullText* database (14.18), which provides integrated full-text access to both the *Handbook on Injectable Drugs* and *AHFS Drug Information*.

7.32 Turco SJ. *Sterile Dosage Forms, Their Preparations and Clinical Implications*. 4th ed. Baltimore: Williams & Wilkins, 1994.

7.33 Leff RD, Roberts RJ. *Practical Aspects of Intravenous Drug Administration*. 2nd ed. Bethesda, MD: American Society of Hospital Pharmacists, 1992.

7.34 Lindley CM, Deloatch KH. *Infusion Technology Manual: A Self-Instructional Approach*. Bethesda, MD: American Society of Hospital Pharmacists, 1993.

Turco's *Sterile Dosage Forms* is generally considered the most authoritative textbook to support education and reference work regarding parenteral preparations. *Practical Aspects of Intravenous Drug Administration* is a brief (54-page) guide to IV drug delivery systems, with emphasis on their implications for the nurse, pharmacist, and physician, and discussion of special clinical problems and their management. *The Infusion Technology Manual*, intended for pharmacy and nursing students, addresses basic concepts in fluid dynamics and standards for parenteral drug therapy. Chapters begin with learning objectives and end with self-assessment questions, with answers provided at the back of the *Manual*, which also includes a list of infusion control device manufacturers and a bibliography. This self-instructional training tool can be purchased as a package accompanied by a 48-minute videotape.

References

1. Nies AS, Spielberg SP. Principles of therapeutics. In: Hardman JG, Gilman AG, Limbird LE, eds. *Goodman and Gilman's The pharmacological basis of therapeutics*. 9th ed. New York: McGraw-Hill, 1995:57.

2. Rossi AC, Knapp BE, Anello C, O'Neill RT et al. Discovery of adverse drug reactions. A comparison of selected phase IV studies with spontaneous reporting methods. *JAMA* 1983;249(16):2226–2228.

3. Edlavitch SA. Adverse drug event reporting; Improving the low U.S. reporting rates. *Arch Intern Med* 1988 Jul;148:1499–1503.

4. Griffin JP. Survey of the spontaneous adverse drug reaction reporting schemes in fifteen countries. *Br J Clin Pharmacol* 1986;22(Supp 1):83S–100S.

5. Rogers AS, Israel E, Smith CR, et al. Physician knowledge, attitudes, and behavior related to reporting adverse drug events. *Arch Intern Med* 1988 Jul;148:1596–1600.

6. Miller RR. Hospital admissions due to adverse drug reactions: A report from the Boston Collaborative Drug Surveillance Program. *Arch Intern Med* 1974;134:219–223.

7. Caranasos GJ, Stewart RB, Cluff LE. Drug-induced illness leading to hospitalization. *JAMA* 1974;228:713–717.

8. Porter J, Jick H. Drug-related deaths among medical inpatients. *JAMA* 1977;237:879–881.

9. Melmon KL. Preventable drug reactions—causes and cures. *N Engl J Med* 1971 Jun;284(24):1361–1368.

10. Talley RB. Drug-induced illness. *JAMA* 1974;229:1043.

11. Einarson TR. Drug-related hospital admissions. *Ann Pharmacother* 1993 Jul–Aug;27:832–840.

12. Leape LL, Brennan TA, Laird N, et al. The nature of adverse events in hospitalized patients: Results of the Harvard Medical Practice Study II. *New Engl J Med* 1991;324;377–384.

13. Johnson JA, Bootman JL. Drug-related morbidity and mortality: a cost-of-illness model. *Arch Intern Med* 1995;155:1949–1956.

14. Lakshmanan MC, Hershey CO, Breslau D. Hospital admissions caused by iatrogenic disease. *Arch Intern Med* 1986 Oct;146:1931–1934.

15. Leape LL, 377–378.

16. Bates DW, Cullen D, Laird N, et al. Incidence of adverse drug reactions and potential adverse drug events: implications for prevention. *JAMA* 1995;274:29–34.

17. Leape LL, Bates DW, Cullen DJ, et al. Systems analysis of adverse drug events. *JAMA* 1995 Jul 5;274:35–43.

18. Basu TK. *Drug-nutrient interactions*. New York: Croom Helm, 1988:vii–viii.

19. Hopkins LE. Introduction to clinical laboratory test interactions. *Hosp Pharmacy* 1971 Aug;6:30–32.

20. Evans GO. Changes in methodology and their potential effects on data banks for drug effects on clinical laboratory tests. *Ann Clin Biochem* 1985 Jul;22:397–401.

21. Tousignaut DR. Parenteral incompatibilities. In: *Proceedings of the 12th annual DIALOG users conference—Update '85.* v. 1. Palo Alto, CA: Dialog Information Services, 1985:126.

Additional Sources of Information

Alcohol- and drug-related visits to hospital emergency departments: 1992 National Hospital Ambulatory Medical Care Survey. Vital and Health Statistics Series: Advance Data Reports, no. 251. Hyattsville, MD: NCHS, 1994.

Atkin PA, Shenfield GM. Medication-related adverse reactions and the elderly: a literature review. *Adv Drug React Toxicol Rev* 1995;14(3):175–191.

Bates DW, O'Neil AC, Boyle D, et al. Potential identifiability and preventability of adverse events using information systems. *J Am Med Inform Assoc* 1994;1:404–411.

Baum C, Faich GA, Anello C, et al. Differences in manufacturer reporting of adverse drug reactions to the FDA in 1984. *Drug Inf J* 1987;21:257–266.

Born GV et al. *Drug-induced hepatotoxicity. Handbook of experimental pharmacology* v. 121. New York: Springer-Verlag, 1996.

Breathnach SM, Hinter H. *Adverse drug reactions and the skin.* Cambridge, MA: Blackwell, 1992.

Caird FI, Scott PJW. *Drug-induced diseases in the elderly; A critical survey of the literature.* New York: Elsevier, 1986.

Classen DC, Pestotnik SL, Evans RS, Burke JP. Computerized surveillance of adverse drug events in hospital patients. *JAMA* 1991 Nov;266(20):2847–2851.

D'Arcy PF. Adverse reactions and interactions with herbal medicines. Part 1. *Adv Drug Reac Toxicol Rev* 1991;10:189–208; Part 2. 1993;12:147–162.

De Smet P, ed. *Adverse effects of herbal drugs.* 3 v. New York: Springer-Verlag, 1992–1996.

De Smet P. Adverse effects of herbal remedies. *Adv Drug Reac Bull* 1997 Apr;183:695–698.

Descote J, ed. *Drug-induced immune diseases.* Amsterdam: Elsevier, 1990.

Farrell GC. *Drug induced liver disease.* New York: Churchill Livingstone, 1994.

Friedman RB, Young DS. *Effects of disease on clinical laboratory tests.* 3rd ed. Washington, DC: American Association for Clinical Chemistry, 1997.

Florence AT, Salole EG, eds. *Formulation factors in adverse reactions.* London: Butterworth, 1990.

Griffin JP, Weber JCP. Voluntary systems of adverse reaction reporting: part 2. *Adv Drug React Acute Poison Rev* 1986;1:23–55.

Guslandi M, Braga PC, eds. *Drug-induced injury to the digestive system.* New York: Springer Verlag, 1993.

Korstanje MJ. Drug-induced mouth disorders. *Clin Exp Dermatol* 1995 Jan;20(1):10–18.

Lang AE, Weiner WJ, eds. *Drug-induced movement disorders.* Mt. Kisco, NY: Futura Publications, 1992.

Miller JJ, ed. *CRC handbook of ototoxicity.* Elkins Park, PA: Franklin Book, 1985.

Roujeau JC, Stern RS. Severe adverse cutaneous reactions to drugs. *New Engl J Med* 1994 Nov;331(19):1272–1285.

Snow B. SEDBASE online for drug side effects and interactions. *Database* 1989 Feb;12:85–94.

Stricker BH, ed. *Drug-induced hepatic injury.* 2nd ed. New York: Elsevier, 1992.

Swanson M, Cook R. *Drugs, chemicals and blood dyscrasias.* Hamilton, IL: Drug Intelligence Publications, 1977.

Van Camp AJ. SEDBASE–A Caduceus update. *Database* 1992 Dec;15(6):94–96.

Worthington EL, Lunin LF, Heath M, eds. *Index-handbook of ototoxic agents, 1966–1971.* Ann Arbor, MI: UMI Books on Demand, 1973.

Young DS. *Effects of preanalytical variables on clinical laboratory tests.* 2nd ed. Washington, DC: American Association for Clinical Chemistry, 1997.

Drugs and Lactation

Anderson PO. Drug use during breast feeding. *Clin Pharm* 1991 Aug;10:594–624. [578 refs]

Atkinson HC, Begg EJ. Prediction of drug distribution into human milk from physico-chemical characteristics. *Clin Pharmacokinet* 1990;18:151–167. [102 refs]

Atkinson HC, Begg EJ, Darlow BA. Drugs in human milk. Clinical pharmacokinetic considerations. *Clin Pharmacokinet* 1988;14:217–240. [255 refs]

Bailey B, Ito S. Breast-feeding and maternal drug use. *Ped Clin N Amer* 1997 Feb;44(1):41–54.

Berglund F, Flodh H, Lundborg P, Prame B, Sannerstedt R. Drug use during pregnancy and breast feeding. *Acta Obstet Gynecol Scand* 1984;63 Supp 126;1–55. [207 refs]

Brooks PM, Needs CJ. Antirheumatic drugs in pregnancy and lactation. *Baillieres Clin Rheumatol*1990;4:157–171. [111 refs]

Buist A, Norman TR, Dennerstein L. Breastfeeding and the use of psychotropic medication: a review. *J Affect Disord* 1990;19:197–206. [55 refs]

Friedman JM, Polifka JE. *The effect of drugs on the fetus and nursing infant: A handbook for health care professionals.* Baltimore: Johns Hopkins Press, 1996.

Goldberg HL. Psychotropic drugs in pregnancy and lactation. *Int J Psychiatr Med* 1994;24:129–147. [88 refs]

Kacew S. Adverse effects of drugs and chemicals in breast milk on the nursing infant. *J Clin Pharmacol* 1993 Mar;33:213–221. [81 refs]

Lee JJ, Rubin AP. Breast feeding and anesthesia. *Anesthesia* 1993;48:616–625. [109 refs]

Murray L, Seger D. Drug therapy during pregnancy and lactation. *Emerg Med Clin North Am* 1994 Feb;12(1):129–149. [68 refs]

Nation RL, Hotham N. Drugs and breast feeding. *Med J Aust* 1987;146;308–313. [82 refs]

Nice FJ. Breast feeding and medications: update. Part 2. *Pharm Times* 1989 Jan;55:92–99,101–103. [135 refs]

Parke AL. Antimalarial drugs, pregnancy and lactation. *Lupus* 1993 Feb;2:PS21–S23. [23 refs]

Pons G, Rey E, Matheson I. Excretion of psychoactive drugs into breast milk. Pharmacokinetic principles and recommendations. *Clin Pharmacokinet* 1994;27:270–289. [132 refs]

Smith IJ, Wilson JT. Infant effects of drugs excreted into breast milk. *Pediatr Res Commun* 1989;3:93–113.

Spigset O. Anesthetic agents and excretion in breast milk. *Acta Anaesth Scand* 1994;38:94–103. [70 refs]

Stockton DL, Paller AS. Drug administration to the pregnant or lactating woman: a reference guide for dermatologists. *J Am Acad Dermatol* 1990;23:87–103. [139 refs]

Thomas J. Factors controlling drugs in human milk. *Aust J Pharm* 1992 May;73:329–332,345–347. [162 refs]

Food-Drug Interactions

Bates ER, Florit GP. Medication administration and its relationship to meals. *Pharm Times* 1996;62(3):55–58,64–68.

Drug-nutrient interactions. *Can Pharm J* 1994;127:86–96.

Guay DRP. Drug-nutrient interactions. *Can Pharm J* 1985;118:336–339. [34 refs]

Ioannides C, Lewis DVP, eds. *Drugs, diet and disease.* New York: Ellis Horwood, 1995.

Mason P. Diet and drug interactions. *Pharm J* 1995 Jul 15;255:94–97.

Neuvonen PJ, Kivisto KT. Food-drug interactions: a review. *Med J Aust* 1989;150:36–40. [79 refs]

Pepin SM. Databases of potential drug-enteral nutrition product interactions. *Am J Hosp Pharm* 1994;51:1965.

Poirier TI, Giudici RA. Evaluation of drug-feed/nutrient interactions microcomputer software programs. *Hosp Pharm* 1991 Jun;26:533–535,538–540.

Pronsky ZP. *Food-medication interactions.* Pottsdown, PA: Medical Surveillance, 1997.

8

Side Effects: Sources of Poisoning and Toxicology Information

The distinction between side effects defined as "adverse reactions" and those termed "poisoning" is related to dosage. Adverse reactions can occur in normal usage, when a drug is correctly administered in accepted dosage range for therapeutic, diagnostic, or prophylactic purposes. Poisoning refers to harmful side effects of drugs resulting from dosages beyond recommended levels of safe use. Toxicology, the experimental study of these effects, involves testing to determine the margin of safety in drug dosage or acceptable limits of exposure to other environmental agents. From an historical perspective, toxicology is an outgrowth of pharmacology and is still linked with the latter in formal instruction programs. However, toxicology information resources discussed in this chapter are not restricted to coverage of pharmaceutical adverse effects. Drug information providers should anticipate queries about the poisoning potential of many nonmedicinal chemicals, such as biotoxins and household or industrial products.

Quick-Reference Sources for Poisoning Therapy

Handbooks intended for emergency use provide quick access by commonly used drug or chemical names, describe signs and symptoms of poisoning to assist in diagnosis, and summarize treatment recommendations in a concise format.

8.1 Olson KR, ed. *Poisoning & Drug Overdose*. 2nd ed. Norwalk, CT: Appleton & Lange, 1994.

8.2 Leikin JB, Paloucek FP, eds. *Poisoning & Toxicology Handbook*. 2nd ed. Hudson, OH: Lexi-Comp, 1996.

8.3 Viccellio P, ed. *Handbook of Medical Toxicology*. Boston: Little, Brown, 1993.

Poisoning & Drug Overdose, a collaborative effort of the faculty and staff of the San Francisco Bay Area Regional Poison Control Center, is an excellent example of this type of publication. Its small size reinforces its objective of providing a practical ready-reference manual dedicated to the management of poisoning, with information presented in four sections. The first section focuses on emergency treatment, guiding the reader from initial response to physical diagnosis, laboratory tests, and methods of decontamination. Section Two is devoted to 150 drugs and other poisons most commonly encountered in emergency admissions, discussing pathophysiology, toxic dose, clinical presentation, and specific treatment. Section Three, Therapeutic Drugs and Antidotes, describes use and side effects of sixty widely used products. Section 4 presents data in tabular format on 500 industrial chemicals, including health hazard summaries, CAS registry numbers, ACGIH threshold limit values, National Fire Protection Association hazardous class codes, and physical descriptions for each chemical. Generic drug names, chemical names, and numerous brand names are integrated into the detailed subject term index concluding *Poisoning & Drug Overdose*.

Leikin and Paloucek's *Poisoning & Toxicology Handbook* was also developed by clinicians currently practicing in nationally recognized poison control centers. Five cross-referenced sections address, respectively, medicinals, nonmedicinals, biologicals, the laboratory, and antidotes. The medicinals section compiles toxicodynamics/kinetics, drug interactions, and laboratory reference range data for individual drugs, including some products recently approved by the FDA. The scope of the nonmedicinals section encompasses alcohols, herbicides, inhalation toxins, fungicides, and rodenticides, citing CAS registry numbers and DOT identification numbers. Plants, venoms, mushrooms, and food-borne toxins are all included in the biologicals section. The laboratory portion of this handbook identifies key diagnostic tests to aid in determining effects, as well as analytical toxicology methods, such as tissue testing for drugs. An appendix assembles clinical data on a variety of topics: drug-induced seizures, porphyrinogenic drugs, vital signs, drug-induced arrhythmias, and pregnancy risk implications.

Viccellio's *Handbook of Medical Toxicology*, by devoting its first two sections to general aspects of the topic, would appear to be less emergency-oriented. Opening chapters address, for example, epidemiology and prevention, pharmacokinetics, principles of toxin elimination, and special considerations in pregnancy. Remaining sections cover specific toxic entities, presented in classified groups: industrial and household chemicals (aldehydes, hydrocarbons, metals), medical/ therapeutic toxins (e.g., salicylates, vitamins, ergotamines), psychiatric drugs, drugs of abuse, environmental toxins (carbon monoxide, food-borne substances, botulism, foreign bodies), as well as animal and plant toxins. Supportive references (numbered in previous discussion) and selected readings conclude the volume. The appendix also presents material on differential diagnosis of poisonings—eminently appropriate in a handbook whose dedication page bears the

Hippocrates quote: "Life is short, the art long, experience treacherous, judgment difficult."

8.4 Dreisbach RH, Robertson WO. *Handbook of Poisoning: Prevention, Diagnosis and Treatment.* 12th ed. Los Altos, CA: Appleton & Lange, 1987.

8.5 Arena JM, Drew RH, eds. *Poisoning: Toxicology, Symptoms, Treatments.* 5th ed. Springfield, IL: Charles C. Thomas, 1986.

8.6 Plunkett ER. *Handbook of Industrial Toxicology.* 3rd ed. New York: Chemical Publishing, 1987.

8.7 Sittig M. *Handbook of Toxic and Hazardous Chemicals and Carcinogens.* 3rd ed. 2 v. Park Ridge, NJ: Noyes Data, 1991.

Dreisbach and Robertson's *Handbook of Poisoning* is divided into sections on agricultural poisons, industrial hazards, household hazards, medicinal poisons, and animal and plant hazards. A detailed index enables user to locate individual substance entries quickly. This handbook also includes a summary of emergency first aid that can be carried out by laypeople. It is more concise and better referenced than Arena and Drew's huge *Poisoning* compendium, which focuses on symptoms, with less emphasis on rapid access to treatment information.

Plunkett's *Handbook of Industrial Toxicology*, as its name implies, provides emergency response data for suspected nontherapeutic substance poisonings. Each monograph includes a physical description of the chemical, identifies settings where occupational exposure is likely to occur (e.g., textile finishing, laboratory research), and offers a concise summary of route of entry, mode of action, signs and symptoms, diagnostic tests (often none), and treatment. Entries also give a threshold limit value (TLV), toxicity rating, and briefly describe preventive measures. One or two bibliographic references accompany each monograph, each of which is accessible by common names and synonyms listed in this compact volume's index.

Sittig's *Handbook of Toxic and Hazardous Chemicals and Carcinogens*, like Plunkett's work, arranges entries in dictionary format and provides first-aid information. References accompanying each of the 1,300 monographs also cite applicable government regulations. Each entry, presented in a concisely structured outline format, supplies synonyms, permissible exposure limits in air and permissible concentrations in water, information on medical surveillance, determination in air and water, personal protection measures, and suggested disposal methods. Sittig has also compiled an index to 178 carcinogens in the *Handbook*.

Although their older publication dates may cause some practitioners to question their utility, all four of the quick-reference guides discussed above are considered classics and are repeatedly cited in more recently issued poisoning management sources. Two other revered icons in the world of clinical toxicology are Gosselin's *Clinical Toxicology of Commercial Products* and *Sax's Dangerous Properties of Industrial Materials*.

8.8 Gosselin RE, Smith RP, Hodge HC. *Clinical Toxicology of Commercial Products: Acute Poisoning.* 5th ed. Baltimore, MD: Williams & Wilkins, 1984.
8.9 Lewis RJ. *Sax's Dangerous Properties of Industrial Materials.* 9th ed. 3 v. New York: John Wiley & Sons, 1996.

Clinical Toxicology of Commercial Products, by virtue of its sheer bulk, is less handy to use than a brief handbook in an emergency situation, but remains, nonetheless, a useful reference tool to retain in book collections on poisoning. Section I provides first aid and general emergency treatment information, intended for rapid response, which can later be followed up with supportive treatment described in Section IV. Section III is a Therapeutics Index, outlining recommended measures for handling exposures to general classes of ingredients. If a brand name is known for the agent suspected to have caused the emergency, Section V's Trade Name Index offers access to an impressive range of household and workplace product information, identifying ingredients in various brands of cleansers, car care preparations, floor finishes, and many over-the-counter medications and personal care products (e.g., deodorants, moisturizers, hair sprays, shampoos).

When a brand name is unknown, but an application or use can be deduced from the setting where a poisoning occurred (e.g., garage, kitchen), information provided in Section VI, General Formulations, will assist in subsequent treatment. Typical ingredients and toxicity ratings for products such as shoe polishes, laundry detergents, windshield de-icers, and varnish removers can be identified using this section. Section II, the Ingredient Index, rates individual ingredients by degree of toxicity using a six-point scale defined in the introduction, where probable lethal oral doses in humans are also given. Section VII is a directory of manufacturer names and addresses for emergency contact, when more information is needed. Inside both the front and back covers is a much-needed graphic guide showing how to use this manual. Although formulations for many of the brand name products cited may have changed by now, it's important to bear in mind that toxicity ratings for named ingredients remain the same.

Sax's Dangerous Properties of Industrial Materials provides quick hazard analysis and handling information for more than 20,000 chemicals used in industry. Analysis includes toxicity data, as well as radiation and fire hazards, identifying probable routes of exposure (e.g., inhalation) and countermeasures (adequate ventilation) for each substance. Recommendations for storage, safe handling, and shipping are also included.

8.10 *POISINDEX.* Denver, CO: Micromedex, 1974–. Quarterly.
8.11 *TOMES Plus.* Denver, CO: Micromedex. Quarterly.

Ideally, every emergency room or hospital pharmacy and every academic medical library would have access to the world's premier poison information resource, *POISINDEX®*. Available in CD-ROM or magnetic tape format, this database brings together information from each of the publications listed above, and many more, including citations to the primary literature. Its initial development was the result of a collaboration between the Rocky Mountain Poison Control Center and the University of Colorado Health Sciences Center. Today, entries are reviewed by an editorial board of subject experts from any of twenty countries, ensuring that treatment protocols are internationally recognized and that products covered are representative of the worldwide marketplace.

POISINDEX identifies both active and inactive ingredients in more than 750,000 commercial preparations, including pharmaceuticals, as well as biological toxins, such as plants, fungi, and snake venoms. Access is facilitated by thorough indexing of synonyms, including brand, generic, chemical, botanical, "street," and other names. Each substance entry is linked with one or more of approximately 800 poisoning management documents, which cover clinical effects, range of toxicity, and treatment protocols. Easy-to-use menus assist in rapid transitions from product identification to therapeutic data. Protocols summarize emergency first-aid and long-term treatment, pharmacology and kinetics, and suggested laboratory tests. Pertinent references to the primary literature are cited, along with citations to standard textbooks and respected compendia, such as *Sax's Dangerous Properties of Industrial Materials* (8.9) and *Clinical Toxicology of Commercial Products* (8.8).

Micromedex's *TOMES Plus®* (Toxicology, Occupational Medicine, and Environmental Series) database complements *POISINDEX* by providing detailed information for managing hazardous chemicals in the workplace. In addition to emergency patient treatment protocols, *TOMES* compiles data needed for compliance with government regulations and for correct response to accidental chemical release into the environment. It includes, for example, extensive fire-fighting data, such as whether chemicals or water are required to extinguish or control fires where the target substance is present, and what types of protective clothing and other measures are recommended. The intended audience for such information extends beyond clinicians to industrial hygienists and others responsible for corporate chemical safety programs. Numeric and regulatory data typically supplied reflect this broader orientation, including TLVs promulgated by the American Conference of Governmental Industrial Hygienists (ACGIH), PELs (Permissible Exposure Limits) set by the U.S. Occupational Safety and Health Administration (OSHA), and U.S. Department of Transportation (DOT) shipping standards.

Both *TOMES Plus* and *POISINDEX* are part of the CCIS® (Computerized Clinical Information System) databank, which includes more than twenty databases available to users in customized combinations or as separate subscriptions. *DRUGDEX* (6.15) and *IDENTIDEX* (10.1) are other resources accessible through the same master software, if desired. Although *POISINDEX* and *TOMES Plus* contain little information that is not available elsewhere, their strength lies in synthesis and standardized search software. Entries bring together needed data from a broad spectrum of resources, evaluating, interpreting, and summarizing results of literature research that would otherwise take much more time to retrieve and analyze. As Fishman has observed, "Micromedex likes to advertise its database as a 44-foot textbook, but a more accurate simile would be to a small personal reference library."[1] In fact, the library equivalent to *POISINDEX* and *TOMES Plus* is beyond the scope of most personal, and even hospital, reference collections. Subscriptions are, in consequence, expensive ($15,000), but included in the price is access not only to an outstanding compilation of factual information, but also to evaluation of data by toxicologists and its integration into concise, authoritative monographs.

Textbooks in Clinical Toxicology

Textbooks provide background material and instruction in the principles of a subject of study, but are not designed for quick reference. Nonetheless, textbooks are often inc luded in drug information collections for the extensive data they provide on chronic poisoning and prognosis.

8.12 Klaassen CD, ed. *Casarett and Doull's Toxicology: The Basic Science of Poisons*. 5th ed. New York: McGraw-Hill, 1995.

Casarett and Doull's Toxicology is arguably the best known textbook in the field. Its material is organized into seven units. Unit 1 introduces the general principles of toxicology, including risk assessment, and provides an overview of the history and scope of the discipline. Unit 2 is devoted to the disposition of toxicants, discussing absorption, distribution, excretion, and toxicokinetics. It also includes a section on standard animal toxicity tests, e.g., acute lethality, skin and eye irritations, sensitization, subacute, subchronic, chronic, developmental/reproductive, and mutagenicity tests. Tables summarize typical cost data (in U.S. dollars) of such descriptive toxicity tests and flag those required for U.S. drug registration submissions, as well as those considered prerequisites in meeting minimum worldwide registration requirements. Unit 3 covers nonorgan-directed toxicity, including chemical carcinogenesis and genetic/developmental toxicology. Unit 4's discussion of target organ toxicity devotes separate chapters to the immune system, blood, liver, kidney, respiratory system, the eye, etc.

Unit 5 covers specific toxic agents, subdividing discussion into broad classes of substances, such as pesticides, metals, solvents and vapors, radiation and radioactive materials, plants, and animal toxins. Unit 6 addresses the topic of environmental toxicology (air, water, and terrestrial), and Unit 7 is dedicated to applications of toxicology, such as food, analytic/forensic, clinical, occupational, and regulatory uses. Unit 7 is likely to be the most useful section of *Casarett and Doull* for information professionals using this book to prepare for better reference service. The fifth edition, marking the twentieth anniversary of this legendary text, includes a new appendix compiling recommended limits for exposure to chemicals, with 1994–95 recommendations on TLVs from ACGIH and 1989 PELs from OSHA, drinking water recommendations from the 1994 National Primary Drinking Water standards, and Health Advisories from the EPA. Readers are advised to supplement these data with consultation of primary sources cited, since the appendix does not attempt to replicate all information provided in them.

8.13 Ellenhorn MJ, ed. *Ellenhorn's Medical Toxicology: Diagnosis and Treatment of Human Poisoning.* 2nd ed. Baltimore: Williams & Wilkins, 1997.

Ellenhorn's Medical Toxicology is another contender for gold standard status among clinicians and practitioners. Five major areas of coverage include principles of poisoning management, drugs, home, chemicals, and natural toxins. Each of seventy-four chapters follows a uniform format highlighting factors such as pharmacokinetics, pathophysiology, clinical presentation, laboratory findings, and treatment, all supported with bibliographic references (more than 8,000 in all). New chapters in this second edition extend its scope to include several additional classes of drugs (AIDS, antivirals, gastrointestinals), arts and crafts supplies, veterinary products poisoning, and blood transfusions. Appendices provide manufacturers' telephone numbers, OSHA recommendations, and a glossary of terminology.

8.14 Goldfrank LR, ed. *Goldfrank's Toxicologic Emergencies.* 6th ed. Stamford, CT: Appleton & Lange, 1998.

Goldfrank's Toxicologic Emergencies is another well respected textbook of clinical toxicology. In addition to in-depth discussions of specific antidotes or antagonists at the end of each chapter, it includes a management section with chapters on principles of nontoxic ingestions and techniques to prevent absorption and enhance elimination. Principles of care for special populations are another enhancement, covering perinatal, pediatric, geriatric, and AIDS patients.

Case Study chapters remain the heart of this text, emphasizing practical patient management immediately after case descriptions. Written by and for attending emergency physicians in New York City, *Goldfrank's* problem-solving approach ensures its applicability in other locales. Coverage includes specific information on various types of prescription and nonprescription medications, alcohols, drugs of abuse, food poisoning, botanicals, farm toxicology, heavy metals, household toxins, marine envenomation, pesticides, and occupational/environmental toxins. Furthermore, multiple choice questions in the workbook portion of this 1,500-page volume will help prepare readers for board certification or recertification.

8.15 Haddad LM et al., eds. *Clinical Management of Poisoning and Drug Overdose.* 3rd ed. Philadelphia: W.B. Saunders, 1998.

8.16 Gossel TA, Bricker JD. *Principles of Clinical Toxicology*. 3rd ed. New
      York: Raven Press, 1994.

Clinical Management of Poisoning and Drug Overdose will also provide a
thorough introduction to the field, again in the form of a massive textbook. Coverage includes developmental, neonatal, and geriatric toxicology and an expanded section on environmental toxicity. Gossel and Bricker devote eight chapters to drug toxicity and a comparable number to other chemicals and
environmental toxins. Their third edition of *Principles of Clinical Toxicology* includes information on new antidotes (e.g., flumazenil for benzodiazepine derivatives) and recommends changes in treatment for managing some types of toxic
ingestions. Replete with figures, tables, and references, chapters also feature case
studies and pose questions to enhance use of the text in medical and pharmacy
educational programs. Appendices include tables of vital signs, normal clinical
laboratory test values, and list therapeutic, toxic, and lethal blood concentrations
for various agents.

Sourcebooks in Analytical Toxicology

Analytical procedures play an important role in poisoning diagnosis and treatment. Reference collections supporting laboratory investigators involved in rapid
screening for suspected toxins, drug abuse testing, therapeutic drug monitoring,
or research into pharmacokinetics will need sourcebooks for methods of drug
analysis.

8.17 Moffatt AC, ed. *Clarke's Isolation and Identification of Drugs*. 2nd ed.
      London: The Pharmaceutical Press, 1996.
8.18 Clarke EG, ed. *Isolation and Identification of Drugs*. London: The Phar-
      maceutical Press, v.1, 1969, v. 2, 1975.

Clarke's Isolation and Identification of Drugs sets the standard for sourcebooks of this type. It includes rapid screening techniques for the hospital bio-
chemist, more precise methods likely to be needed by forensic scientists whose
findings must withstand courtroom examination, and simple analytical techniques appropriate for chemists engaged in fieldwork. The section on rapid
screening gives quick methods for identifying drugs responsible for 90% of poisoning incidents and offers guidelines in cases of emergency, both when there is
strong presumptive evidence of the identity of the drug, and when there is no clue
to its identity.

Part 1 in the second edition includes eighteen chapters on specific analytical
techniques and allied subjects, such as drug abuse in sports. Part 2 compiles analytical and toxicological data for 1,300 drugs and related substances, in monograph form. Entries are arranged by BAN, USAN, or INN and include synonyms,

such as selected proprietary names and CAS registry numbers. With the exception of CAS RNs, alternative nomenclature is included in the index to monographs. Part 3 supplies sixty-six indexes of analytical data, tabulated in numerical order, for chromatography, spectrophotometry, and mass spectrometry. Indexes of molecular weight and melting point round out this section. Part 4 is an appendix of reagents and proprietary test materials referred to in Parts 1 and 2. A concluding forty-eight-page index with nearly 12,500 entries ensures ready accessibility to the contents of the preceding 1,200 pages.

One important fact to bear in mind is that monographs for many substances covered in the first edition of *Clarke's* are not replicated in the second, so it's a good idea to retain the original two-volume set, issued separately in 1969 and 1975. When it was first published, this outstanding reference source was suitably dubbed "An Extra Pharmacopoeia Companion Volume." It remains an unrivaled compilation of data essential for detecting, identifying, and quantifying the presence of most drugs in pharmaceutical formulations, body fluids, or postmortem material. The section devoted to drug disposition in the body discusses absorption, distribution, excretion, major metabolites, therapeutic and toxic concentrations, and gives values for pharmacokinetic parameters such as half-life. Abstracts from clinical studies are also included in *Clarke's* drug monographs.

8.19 Baselt RC, Cravey RH. *Disposition of Toxic Drugs and Chemicals in Man*. 4th ed. Foster City, CA: Chemical Toxicology Institute, 1995.

Baselt and Cravey's *Disposition of Toxic Drugs and Chemicals in Man* complements *Clarke's* coverage with information on pesticides and industrial chemicals frequently responsible for poisoning incidents, as well as drugs. Arranged alphabetically by generic name, each entry shows the structure of the featured compound, summarizes its occurrence (where it is on the market, if at all) and uses, and provides blood concentration data, information on metabolism and excretion, type of toxicity, and analysis. Cases and incidents are cited in narrative discussion. Bibliographic references accompany each monograph, and an index offers some cross references from common brand names and alternate generic names.

8.20 Flanagan RJ, Braithwaite RA, Brown SS, Widdop B, de Wolff FA. *Basic Analytical Toxicology*. Geneva: World Health Organization, 1995.

Reflecting World Health Organization objectives, *Basic Analytical Toxicology* is intended to assist laboratory staff in hospitals lacking the support of specialized analytical toxicology services. It covers a range of simple tests known to produce rapid and reliable results for the management of poisoning emergencies. Qualitative tests for poisons include a three-part series appropriate in cases where the identity of the toxin is unknown. These tests can be used to detect poisons either in biological samples or in powders or tablets found near the patient. Step-by-step instructions describe methods of testing for 113 specific poisons or groups of toxins, ranging from pesticides to pharmaceuticals, plant toxins to industrial chemicals. All techniques and procedures have previously been performed by laboratory technicians in developing countries, in order to ensure accurate results using relatively unsophisticated equipment, without access to expensive reagents or a continuous supply of electricity. Entries for individual toxins also provide information on clinical signs of poisoning and recommended treatment.

8.21 Adamovics JA, ed. *Analysis of Addictive and Misused Drugs.* New York: Marcel Dekker, 1995.

8.22 Wilson J. *Abused Drugs II: A Laboratory Pocket Guide.* Washington, DC: American Association for Clinical Chemistry, 1994.

Analysis of Addictive and Misused Drugs highlights the latest technologies used in testing, including immunochemical analysis, biosensors, thin-layer gas chromatography, high performance liquid chromatographic methods, capillary electrophoresis, and robotics. The appendix supplies an alphabetic listing of more than 400 controlled substances, providing a sample matrix, suggested handling procedures, and mode of detection for each. Chapters contributed by experts in the field include discussion of sports drug testing programs and approaches to solving forensic problems in developing countries with limited resources. Enhanced by numerous tables, figures, and equations, this book is a practical guide that can also support scholarly research, compiling more than 1,700 bibliographic references to the primary literature.

Abused Drugs II, necessarily more limited in scope as a "Pocket Guide," nonetheless compiles toxicological data frequently needed, including solubility, structure, progressive symptomology, methods of administration, duration of effect, mode of treatment, principle metabolites, half life, volume of distribution, clearance, percentage excreted unchanged in urine, associated toxic blood levels, suggested methods of analysis, and DEA schedule for each drug listed. Information on individual substances is organized into ten drug classes: stimulants, opiates, barbiturates, hallucinogens, sedatives/hypnotics, benzodiazepines, antipsychotics/antidepressants, solvents, analgesics, and anabolic steroids.

Teratogenicity Information Sources

Congenital anomalies rank sixth among causes of death in the United States.[2] Current estimates are that 3% of all newborns exhibit some form of birth defect, and that 10% of such defects are caused by *in utero* exposure to a teratogenic agent.[3] More than 2,500 publications per year address this complex area of toxicology.[4] Ready access to the literature on reproductively active chemicals can play an important role in prevention of birth defects.

Before administering drugs during pregnancy, practitioners must assess the possibility of teratogenesis. Dosage and the stage of development of the fetus are important factors in this assessment. Often, the only information available on potential effects will be derived from animal studies. Jelovsek, Mattison, and Chen[5] offer a useful analysis of the relationship between animal tests and identification of human teratogens. Variations in species susceptibility can make extrapolation difficult. Kimmel and Gaylor[6] offer insight into how acceptable exposure levels are determined.

Understanding of influential factors in teratogenesis has been acquired relatively slowly. Of the few known human teratogens (including nineteen drugs), most were definitely linked to congenital anomalies only in the wake of the thalidomide tragedy (post-1961). The legacy of thalidomide is, perhaps, partly responsible for unnecessarily alarming articles in popular magazines, which are often a source of misinformation to patients. Gunderson-Warner and others[7] surveyed fifteen such publications and found that out of fifty-six articles about pregnancy exposures, thirty-one (55%) were misleading or inaccurate.

Confusion sometimes arises from the fact that the bulk of evidence on human teratogenic effects is derived from isolated case reports by physicians. Sources based on systematic surveys of professional publications and subsequent assessment of such reports for validity are needed. Data from animal studies are easier to find, but *ad hoc* forays into the literature through secondary sources (abstracting and indexing services) can easily miss critically important research. Acquiring one or more of the reference sources annotated in this section is essential, if information (as well as medical) malpractice is to be avoided.

8.23 Shepard TH. *Catalog of Teratogenic Agents*. 8th ed. Baltimore: Johns Hopkins University Press, 1995.

Most literature research on potential toxicity of specific substances to the fetus should begin with Shepard's *Catalog of Teratogenic Agents*, which compiles data on 2,200 agents, including chemicals, drugs, and physical factors, such as viruses, hyperthyroidism, cigarette smoking, spray adhesives, and biotin deficiency. The importance of Shepard's *Catalog* is, perhaps, underscored by the fact that it is included in Micromedex's *REPRORISK® System*, a collection of machine-readable databases available in CD-ROM and magnetic tape format for licensed multiuser access through local area networks or mainframe computer systems.

Because negative data can be as important as positive indicators of teratogenicity, *Catalog* coverage encompasses a considerable number of nonteratogenic agents. Therefore, it's important to remember that the presence of an agent in the *Catalog* does not necessarily indicate that it is a potential teratogen. Shepard has attempted to cite all agents that have been studied for teratogenicity in animals or humans. The volume's introduction supplies a short list of proven, as well as possible and "unlikely" teratogenic agents in human beings. Also included is a chart with comparative time periods of embryonic and fetal development in humans and in experimental animals. This annotated, compact graphic will assist users in the difficult process of extrapolation from animal data to evaluate risk in humans. Approximately 1,200 agents have been identified by Shepard as producing congenital anomalies in experimental animals, but only forty are known to cause defects in humans.

Simplified chemical names, following *Merck Index* standards, are the primary access points in alphabetically arranged entries, but cross references are also provided from other names, including proprietary designations. A slightly daunting convention for alphabetizing name entries can lead to some confusion: single, preceding letters, numbers, or Greek symbols are disregarded, so that 1-beta-D-arabinofuranosyl-5-fluorocytosine is listed in the A portion of the *Catalog*. Each monograph begins with a summary of published data or issues, followed by bibliographic references, and includes a CAS registry number, when relevant. Back-of-book index entries refer to Shepard *Catalog* numbers, rather than page numbers. The author index is not limited to first authors, but, instead, offers access to all author names in cited references. The subject index is intended to augment alternative substance name access by offering drug classification terms as extra cross references. For example, ACE inhibitors is an extra pointer to the *Catalog* entry for captopril (but not also for enalopril).

8.24 Schardein JL. *Chemically Induced Birth Defects*. 2nd ed. New York: Marcel Dekker, 1993.

Shardein's *Chemically Induced Birth Defects* complements Shepard's compendium by organizing data into tables and listing current reproductive and teratology testing requirements for chemicals in the United States. Material is organized into eighteen chapters, which group drugs by therapeutic use, and eleven additional chapters devoted to other classes of chemicals, such as pesticides, metals, and food additives. Each drug chapter begins with an introductory overview of the therapeutic class, citing pregnancy categories assigned by the FDA (see Figure 8.1) and data on prescription prevalence and sales, to reinforce the importance of the information presented. Individual pharmacological categories of

Figure 8.1   FDA Pregnancy Categories Used in Package Inserts for Rx Drugs

Low risk	Category A	Possibility of fetal harm is remote.
↑ ↑	Category B	Results of animal reproduction studies not confirmed in controlled studies on women— no positive evidence of fetal risk in humans.
↑ ↑	Category C	Studies in women and animals not available, or studies in animals show fetal adverse effects, but no controlled studies on women are available. Drugs in this category should be administered only if potential benefit justifies risk.
↓ ↓ ↓	Category D	No positive evidence of human fetal risk, but caution advised; benefits for pregnant women may outweigh risk, if other safer drugs cannot be used in cases of life-threatening or serious disease.
High risk	Category X	Evidence of fetal risk based on human experience. Drug is contraindicated in women who are, or may become, pregnant.

drugs are then discussed, with a review of published animal and human studies and a table correlating named drugs with animal species teratogenicity data and bibliographic references. All drug names cited in individual tables throughout the book are listed in one integrated index at its conclusion, and all references cited in abbreviated form in tables are given in full form at the end of each chapter. Teratogenic reactions tabulated in various laboratory animal species are rated by the author as teratogenic (flagged with a plus + sign), equivocally teratogenic (+ −), or not teratogenic (minus − sign). Schardein estimates that out of the more than 3,300 chemicals tested, 37% have been found to be teratogenic.

8.25 Lewis RL. *Reproductively Active Chemicals, A Reference Guide.* New York: Van Nostrand Reinhold, 1991.

In *Reproductively Active Chemicals, A Reference Guide*, Lewis distinguishes between effects on the male and female reproductive systems, identifying influences on mating success, the fetus (including spontaneous abortion and transplacental carcinogenesis), and postbirth events. Each reproductive or teratogenic effect reported includes information on the dose, species exposed, exposure conditions, and the source of data. Human data are separated from animal evidence to highlight their importance; no negative study findings are cited. Coverage includes drugs, food additives, preservatives, ores, pesticides, and dyes. Some radioactive materials are also listed, but adverse events reported are chemically produced, rather than radiation-induced.

Reference Guide entries are arranged alphabetically by commonly used designation, and include CAS registry numbers, molecular formula, weight, description, and physical properties. Properties information selected for inclusion is that judged to be most useful in evaluating the potential hazard of the material and in planning for its proper storage and use (e.g., boiling point, melting point, density, vapor pressure, refractive index, flash point, autoignition temperature, lower and upper explosive limits, solubility, miscibility in water and common solvents). Two cross indexes offer access by CAS registry numbers and by synonyms, encompassing brand, generic, and chemical names, as well as drug research codes. Lewis cites more than 700 primary sources, including journals and handbooks. References employ cryptic abbreviations and a somewhat unconventional style, e.g., "ARZNAD 20, 1559, 70." Although a key to abbreviations is included at the end of the volume (ARZNAD = *Arzneimittel-Forschung* v1- , 1951–), no explanation of citation format is provided. In the sample entry, for example, the user is left to deduce that 20 is probably the volume number, 1559 a page reference, and 70 is, presumably, the year of publication.

This basic teratogenicity reference collection could be usefully expanded to include one or two textbooks and other reference aids from the selection listed below. It should also be noted that *Drugs in Pregnancy and Lactation* (7.19), discussed in the previous chapter, includes extensive data summaries regarding fetal risk.

8.26 Koren G, ed. *Maternal-Fetal Toxicology: A Clinician's Guide.* 2nd ed.
      New York: Marcel Dekker, 1994.
8.27 Folb PI, Dukes MNG. *Drug Safety in Pregnancy.* Amsterdam: Elsevier,
      1990.
8.28 Persaud TVN, Chudley AE, Skalko RG. *Basic Concepts in Teratology.*
      New York: Alan R. Liss, 1985.

Maternal-Fetal Toxicology: A Clinician's Guide is not designed for quick reference, but provides useful background on the topic in chapters contributed by various experts. One such chapter surveys drugs of choice for pregnant women, presenting recommendations in tabular format and arranging them by conditions to be treated (e.g., acne, headache, insomnia, peptic ulcer). Another chapter reviews issues involved in drug use during lactation, concluding with an extensive (44-page) table summarizing findings from clinical trials and an excellent bibliography of 331 information sources. Recognizing that millions of people in North America regularly consume medicinal plants, either as self-prescribed remedies or following the advice of naturopaths, the *Clinician's Guide* devotes a chapter to maternal-fetal toxicology of fifty plants, listing them by both common and botanical names. Another thought-provoking section addresses teratogenicity and litigation, reviewing the complex medicolegal issues involved. This book also provides a directory of teratogen information service hotlines, listing forty-five in the United States and sixteen comparable services in Canada, France, Israel, Italy, and Spain.

In well-referenced chapters devoted to categories of drugs, *Drug Safety in Pregnancy* reviews the literature pertaining to medication risks for the fetus and the pregnant woman. Bibliographic citations are coded for clinical significance, based on a critical examination and evaluative assessment of evidence presented in primary sources. Results of selected experimental studies, including animal teratology and *in vitro* findings, are discussed, when they can contribute to a better understanding of the mechanisms of fetal toxicity in the context of medication use in clinical practice. Several appendices compile drug data in tabular format, noting associations with various anomalies, including behavioral teratology. Separate indexes offer access by side effects keywords and by drug generic names.

Basic Concepts in Teratology is a textbook offering background on classification and epidemiology of developmental defects, genetic contributions to human malformations, cellular mechanisms, and the role of chemical interactions. A chapter on teratogenicity testing summarizes regulatory guidelines worldwide (as of 1985) and reviews issues such as selection of species and dosing regimens.

8.29 Heinonen OP, Slone D, Shapiro S. *Birth Defects and Drugs in Pregnancy.*
      Littleton, MA: Publishing Sciences Group, 1977.

Since much of the information available on drug and chemical hazards to human reproduction is derived from isolated case reports by physicians, any resource that compiles epidemiological data is valuable. In *Birth Defects and Drugs in Pregnancy*, Heinonen and others have reported outcomes of more than 50,000 pregnancies in drug-exposed women. Extensive tables propose risk rates based on these data. Because it was compiled from pregnancies reviewed from 1959 through 1965, this publication will not include references to newer drugs.

8.30 Barlow SM, Sullivan FM. *Reproductive Hazards of Industrial Chemicals. An Evaluation of Animal and Human Data*. London: Academic Press, 1982.

8.31 Kirsch-Volders M. *Mutagenicity, Carcinogenicity, and Teratogenicity of Industrial Pollutants*. New York: Plenum Press, 1984.

8.32 Kolb VM, ed. *Teratogens: Chemicals Which Cause Birth Defects*. 2nd ed. Amsterdam: Elsevier, 1993.

Barlow and Sullivan's *Reproductive Hazards of Industrial Chemicals* covers forty-eight industrial compounds, many in widespread use. Kirsch-Volders provides summary discussions on pollutants, dividing them into four groups: heavy metals, insecticides, monomers, and halogenated hydrocarbon solvents.

Teratogens: Chemicals Which Cause Birth Defects includes chapters on the principles and mechanisms of teratogenesis, maternal occupational exposure and spontaneous abortion, and biochemical determinants of chemical teratogenesis. A discussion of legal and ethical aspects of fetal protection policies provides an excellent summary of legal cases and of controversial issues that must be addressed in such policies. This book also includes a list of teratogenic chemicals likely to be found in undergraduate chemical laboratories. The list identifies CAS registry numbers, U.S. Department of Transportation (DOT) and *Registry of Toxic Effects* (*RTECS*) reference numbers, and brand names. Along with physical data for listed chemicals, environmental and health hazards are summarized for each substance, including TLV, biological effects in water, and biodegradability in soil. Bibliographic references to data sources are also included.

A chapter on how to obtain information on teratogenicity, contributed by staff members at Oak Ridge National Laboratory, identifies fifty-five key journal sources and recommends online search strategies. Unfortunately, databases cited represent only a sample of potentially relevant sources. Furthermore, the authors assert that ETIC and its successor DART (Figure 14.11) are "the most comprehensive of the on-line computer systems that provide access to the worldwide literature of teratology and reproductive/developmental toxicology." Although this claim is questionable, the chapter does provide a good introduction to the topic of online resources, especially for the MEDLARS-oriented user.

RTECS (8.33, 14.28) is used as the source for the list of 5,625 chemicals associated with reproductive effects that constitutes the bulk of this book (462 out of a total of 586 pages in *Teratogens: Chemicals Which Cause Birth Defects*). No information beyond chemical name and CAS RN is supplied in the list, so users would be wise to consult individual *RTECS* entries for details, to gauge the validity of these data. Another drawback to this volume is its very limited subject index. Occupying only three printed pages, subject entries appear to be author-provided keywords. Only legal and ethical issues are thoroughly indexed. The book also suffers from a similarly uneven presentation style. It is all too obviously reproduced from camera-ready copies of contributing authors' manuscripts, resulting in distractingly different typefaces and erratic reference formats, particularly that of the editor's own contribution.

Other Toxicology Reference Bibliography

Wexler's *Information Resources in Toxicology* (5.13) provides a far more extensive bibliography of potentially useful resources than is included here. However, this chapter attempts to single out major hardcopy publications found in larger drug information collections and likely to be useful in answering inquiries typically received. Relevant online and Internet databases are discussed in Chapter Fourteen.

No bibliography of toxicology reference sources would be complete without the *Registry of Toxic Effects of Chemical Substances (RTECS)*.

8.33 *Registry of Toxic Effects of Chemical Substances*. Cincinnati, OH: U.S. National Institute of Occupational Safety and Health, 1971–. Quarterly.

8.34 Sweet DV, ed. *Registry of Toxic Effects of Chemical Substances, RTECS: A Comprehensive Guide*. Upland, PA: Diane Publishing, 1993.

A publication of known toxic data mandated under OSHA regulations, *RTECS* is easier to use in machine-readable format (compact disc, magnetic tape, or online database, 14.28) than in hardcopy (paper) or microfiche alternatives formerly issued (these ceased publication in mid-1980s and 1993, respectively). Quarterly updates continue only in electronic (machine-readable) versions of this source. Sweet's *Guide* is intended to assist users of computerized versions and describes in detail the various format options.

When using *RTECS* in any form, it's important to remember that this source includes unevaluated data, requiring informed, critical assessment by qualified health science professionals of the full text of primary sources cited, before risks can be assumed. *RTECS* also typically gives lowest dose in any study cited. Negative study results are generally omitted, such as those which might have found a substance to be nonirritating.

8.35 Richardson ML, Gangolli S, eds. *DOSE: The Dictionary of Substances and Their Effects*. 7 v. Boca Raton, FL: CRC Press, 1992–1995.

Developed under the sponsorship of the Royal Society of Chemistry, *The Dictionary of Substances and Their Effects* compiles identification and toxicity data on more than 4,000 chemicals cited in official regulatory lists from the United States, Canada, the European Community, and the United Kingdom. To put this coverage in perspective, it's helpful to know that *RTECS* lists more than 140,000 compounds, the *Hazardous Substances Data Bank* (14.29) lists approximately 4,500, and *CHEMTOX* (14.30), a collection of Material Safety Data Sheets (MSDS) online, provides data on more than 10,300 substances. MDL Information System's database, MSDS-OHS (14.31), covers 56,300 chemicals, and the Canadian Centre for Occupational Safety and Health MSDS-CCOHS (14.32) collection encompasses 118,000 substances.

DOSE entries, arranged alphabetically by simplified or generic name, include alternative nomenclature, CAS RN, a structural diagram, molecular formula, and molecular weight. Physical properties data provided are melting, boiling, or flash point, specific gravity, partition coefficient, volatility, and solubility. Occurrence of the compound is briefly described (e.g., detected in river water), and information on mammalian and avian toxicity is then summarized. *DOSE* monographs also contain, when available, data on environmental fate (e.g., degradation studies, anaerobic effects, abiotic removal), ecotoxicity (effects on fish and invertebrates, bioaccumulation, nutrification inhibition), and occupational exposure (limit values, regulatory list reference numbers). Bibliographic citations conclude each monograph. Every volume includes an index of chemical names, CAS RNs, and molecular formulas, as well as a glossary of biological organisms cited. The entire seven-volume set is, unfortunately, quite expensive ($3,000). An online version of *DOSE*, updated semiannually, is also available.

8.36 Maga JA, Tu AT, eds. *Food Additive Toxicology*. New York: Marcel Dekker, 1995.

Information on food additives, although not quite as elusive as data on pharmaceutical excipients, is challenging to find. More than 2,800 compounds have, after all, been approved for use in the United States alone, and can be incorporated into 20,000 different food items. Therefore, any reputable reference publication on that class of substances used to improve color, consistency, flavor, stability, nutritional quality, or convenience in foods is welcome. *Food Additive Toxicology* compiles 1,750 literature references and includes 225 tables and other useful figures. Compounds covered include acidulants, antioxidants, curing agents, flavor potentiators, salts, modified food starches, antimicrobial agents, and "incidental" food additives, such as lead, mercury, pesticides, drug residues, packaging, and other unintentional contaminants. An index offers access by alternative names to discussion of uses and toxicity included in separate chapters in this handy volume.

8.37 *CIR Compendium*. Washington, DC: Cosmetic, Toiletry, and Fragrance Association, 1998. Annual.

Results of cosmetic ingredient reviews (CIRs) conducted since the 1970s are summarized in the *CIR Compendium*. Updated annually, this resource cumulates key data derived from more than 600 safety assessments completed by an expert panel of the international Cosmetic, Toiletry, and Fragrance Association (CTFA). Entries for each ingredient digest essential information from the Abstract, Discussion, and Conclusion sections of CIR final reports. A Quick Reference Table provides concise descriptions of the panel's findings on safe concentration levels for each ingredient, cross referenced to a complete literature citation. Both product formulators and medical practitioners can use this source to determine what substances are considered safe in dermatological applications, and at what levels. Full reports of CIR decisions regarding safety, including the basis for positive or negative assessments, have been published in the *International Journal of Toxicology*. Final reports are also part of a full-text CD-ROM database available from CTFA. The Association's Web site provides valuable background on ingredient review priorities that have evolved over the past twenty-one years. It lists each ingredient's current status and enables searching for a substance to determine its priority number (see http://www.ctfa.org).

8.38 Sheftel VO. *Handbook of Toxic Properties of Monomers and Additives.* Boca Raton, FL: CRC Press, 1995.

The scope of Sheftel's *Handbook of Toxic Properties of Monomers and Additives* includes plastics and polymeric materials used in food packaging (possible indirect food additives). Monographs on individual substances are arranged in chapters dedicated to broad classes, e.g., stabilizers, catalysts, initiators, and hardeners. Each entry provides a simplified chemical name, CAS registry number, synonyms, properties, applications, possible routes of exposure, data on acute toxicity, repeated exposure and long-term effects, reproductive toxicity, carcinogenicity, chemobiokinetics, and government regulations. The latter include applicable U.S. FDA standards and international restrictions, such as permissible migration level to food or water, provisional tolerable weekly intake, maximum permitted quantity of the residual substance in the material or article, and specific migration limits in food. Supportive bibliography is cited by numbered references throughout the handbook and reflects a thorough review of both European and American toxicology literature, augmented with a selection of Russian sources. Although monographs do not distinguish among types of names listed (a mixture of brand and generic designations), all are equally accessible in the concluding index.

8.39 *IARC Monographs on the Evaluation of Carcinogenic Risk of Chemicals to Man.* Lyon, France: International Agency for Research on Cancer, v. 1–, 1972–.

8.40 *Overall Evaluations of Carcinogenicity, An Updating of IARC Monographs Volumes 1–42.* Lyon, France: International Agency for Research on Cancer, 1987.

The *IARC Monographs*, distributed by the World Health Organization, are likely to be frequently requested, because of their cumulation of carcinogenic data on chemicals to which humans are often exposed. More than sixty volumes have been published to date. Each focuses on a group of related chemicals or other agents, such as nitroso compounds, aromatic amines, food additives, naturally occurring compounds, or solar and ultraviolet radiation. In 1987, an IARC Working Group convened in Lyon, France to reevaluate epidemiologic and experimental evidence for the carcinogenicity of 617 agents that had been previously evaluated in volumes 1–42 of the *Monographs*. Results of their work were published as Supplement 7 to the *IARC Monograph* series.

8.41 National Cancer Institute. *Survey of Compounds Which Have Been Tested for Carcinogenic Activity.* Rockvillle, MD: Technical Resources, 1941–.

8.42 National Cancer Institute. *Survey of Compounds Which Have Been Tested for Carcinogenic Activity. Cumulative Indexes.* Rockville, MD: Technical Resources, 1991.

The U.S. National Cancer Institute's *Survey* publications, sometimes cryptically referred to as PHS 149, are also extremely valuable for their compilation of references from older published literature. Presented in tabular format, these bibliographies can save much time-consuming retrospective searching of secondary sources. The 1991 volume, the latest issued at this writing, presents carcinogenesis data extracted from literature published in 1989–1990 and is 2,158 pages in length. Organized by chemical structural categories (e.g., inorganic, aliphatic, monocyclic), compounds within each class are listed alphabetically under their Chemical Abstracts Service preferred name (per the 9th Collective Index). A list of synonyms follows each CAS preferred chemical name entry, drawn from literature references cited, as well as names used in previous volumes of the PHS-149 series. Structural diagrams are also included as an aid to identification. Cumulative indexes are issued separately. The 1991 edition includes an alphabetic list of all preferred chemical names and common synonyms used in previous *Survey* volumes, cross referenced to accession numbers. This 784-page index also offers cumulative access by CAS registry numbers, listed sequentially in a separate section.

8.43 *Data from the Drug Abuse Warning Network (DAWN).* Statistical Series I. Washington, DC: Substance Abuse and Mental Health Services Administration, 1980–. Annual.

Another U.S. government source of often needed data is the annual *DAWN* (*Drug Abuse Warning Network*) report. The Substance Abuse and Mental Health Services Administration (SAMHSA) sponsors the compilation of statistics on emergency room admissions and deaths attributed to drug abuse. Data are broken down by patient age, sex, race, major metropolitan area, and drug class. Episode characteristics such as whether single- or multi-drug use is involved, drug use motivation, source and form of substance, and route of administration are also tabulated. The annual report is issued in two parts, one presenting emergency room data and a second devoted to mortality statistics submitted by medical examiners. Midyear preliminary statistics are also released, but the minimum lag time between collection and reporting is generally at least one year.

8.44 *National Household Survey on Drug Abuse.* Washington, DC: Substance Abuse and Mental Health Services Administration. Annual.

SAMHSA also publishes results of the *National Household Survey on Drug Abuse*. Each year, a representative sample of the civilian noninstitutionalized population aged twelve years and older is interviewed to determine the prevalence of illicit drug use. In 1997, 24,505 people participated in the survey, which provides estimates of the use of alcohol, marijuana, heroin, cocaine, and hallucinogens, as well as rates of tobacco cigarette smoking. Data from both this *Survey* and *DAWN* midyear, as well as annual, reports from 1993 forward are available for downloading free of charge in PDF format on the Internet. The National Clearinghouse for Alcohol and Drug Information is the source, located at http://www.health.org. Be sure to examine both the Survey and Publications sections of this site to locate all pertinent links.

A frequent query in industrial toxicology is a request for threshold limit values (TLVs). The American Conference of Governmental Industrial Hygienists (ACGIH) determines TLVs and publishes them periodically. Although ACGIH recommendations are not official, enforceable, regulatory standards until they are adopted by the Occupational Safety and Health Administration (OSHA) as PELs (permissible exposure limits), guidelines established by the ACGIH are carefully monitored in industry settings.

8.45 *Threshold Limit Values for Chemical Substances and Physical Agents and Biological Exposure Indices, 1995–1996.* Cincinnati, OH: American Conference of Governmental Industrial Hygienists, 1995. Annual.

8.46 *Documentation of the Threshold Limit Values and Biological Exposure Indices.* 6th ed. 3 v. Cincinnati, OH: American Conference of Governmental Industrial Hygienists, 1991.

8.47 LaNier M, ed. *Threshold Limit Values: Discussion and Thirty-Five Year Index with Recommendations.* Cincinnati, OH: American Conference of Governmental Industrial Hygienists, 1984.

TLVs are published each year in brief, inexpensive paperback editions. *Documentation* volumes, issued prior to 1971 under the title *Documentation of the Threshold Limit Values for Substances in Workroom Air*, are released approximately every five years. They compile background bibliography supporting ACGIH recommendations and include an index.

It's perhaps worth repeating that the *Dictionary of Toxicology* (5.26) is an excellent source of definitions for significant terms used in the discipline and explanations of key concepts. Entries also cover specific substances or groups of toxic compounds, giving their source, side effects, mechanism of action, and antidotes. Pertinent organizations, government agencies, and regulations are also covered. More than 400 diagrams and other illustrations accompany *Dictionary* entries, and a bibliography lists additional sources of information.

Biotoxins

Biotoxins include both plants (phytotoxins) and animals (zootoxins). Information resources in both areas should include good illustrations accompanied by detailed narrative descriptions, because accurate identification of the toxic source is essential for effective treatment.

8.48 Kingsbury JN. *Poisonous Plants of the United States and Canada*. 3rd ed. Englewood Cliffs, NJ: Prentice Hall, 1964.

8.49 Lampe KF, McCann MA. *The AMA Handbook of Poisonous and Injurious Plants*. Chicago: American Medical Association, 1985.

8.50 Benezra C. *Plant Contact Dermatitis*. Toronto: Marcel Dekker, 1985.

8.51 Frohne D. *A Colour Atlas of Poisonous Plants: A Handbook for Pharmacists, Doctors, Toxicologists, and Biologists*. London: Wolfe Medical, 1984.

Kingsbury's *Poisonous Plants of the United States* is the most frequently cited reference on the poisoning potential of plants, although antidotes are generally not discussed. It also makes interesting reading for other than purely pragmatic purposes. Although the photographs and line drawings are none too impressive by today's standards, Kingsbury's compilation of relevant information is practically unparalleled, covering all plants causing death or "identifiable deleterious reaction" in animals, as well as man. Algae, fungi, and ferns are included in its scope, and the background bibliography is extensive. Because of its older publication date and the fact that it has been out of print for a number of years, your library's copy of *Poisonous Plants of the United States* may need to be rescued from the circulating collection and placed where it rightly belongs, as a treasured selection on reference or reserve book shelves.

In *The AMA Handbook of Poisonous and Injurious Plants*, Lampe focuses on the management of plant poisonings, including those caused by cultivated or native plants commonly found in the United States, Canada, and the Caribbean. Section I covers those with systemic effects in humans, and Section II is devoted to plants associated with dermatitis. Mushrooms are the topic of Section III. Discussion includes notes on geographic distribution, symptoms, and treatment, backed up by references to the primary literature. Both common names and Latin binomials are provided as access points.

Benezra's *Plant Contact Dermatitis* is dedicated to treatment of the most prevalent form of adverse reaction to plants: skin effects. Discussion highlights clinical, immunological, and molecular aspects of plant-induced contact dermatitis, and includes information on patch testing. Dermatotoxic reactions to contact with tropical woods are among topics covered.

Frohne's *A Colour Atlas of Poisonous Plants* covers clinical signs and symptoms, mechanism of action, and treatment of plant exposures, in addition to supplying material to fulfill its primary purpose: identification. The *Atlas* supplements photographic aids to identification with descriptions of leaf characteristics, fruits, and other visual distinctions.

There are several free sources of botanical toxicity information on the Internet. Figure 8.2 identifies five sources, ranging from the no-abstracts, no-frills *PLAN-TOX* database to the sophisticated, interactive system developed for *Canadian Poisonous Plants*. Complementary sources focusing on plant toxicity to livestock and other domesticated animals are listed in Figure 12.1.

Although plants are associated with more poisoning cases than other biotoxins, reference publications dealing with zootoxins are often needed, particularly in coastal regions where the patient population is exposed to marine animals, and in areas where poisonous snakes and arthropods are common.

8.52 Halstead BW. *Poisonous and Venomous Marine Animals of the World.* 2nd ed. Princeton, NJ: Darwin Press, 1988.

8.53 Halstead BW. *Dangerous Aquatic Animals of the World. A Color Atlas, with Prevention, First Aid and Emergency Treatment Procedures.* Princeton, NJ: Darwin Press, 1992.

8.54 Halstead BW. *Dangerous Marine Animals That Bite, Sting, Shock, Are Non-Edible.* 3rd ed. Centreville, MD: Cornell Maritime Press, 1995.

Halstead is the best known authority on poisonous aquatic animals. *Poisonous and Venomous Marine Animals,* considered the standard reference work in this subject area, reflects recent research in its extensive bibliographies. Aids to identification include both black-and-white illustrations and a section of color plates. Individual chapters discuss various phyla or classes of hazardous marine invertebrates and vertebrates, including dinoflagellates, sponges, and corals.

Dangerous Aquatic Animals of the World extends its scope to include freshwater animals, as well as those found in marine environments, and offers a glossary with definitions of pertinent biotoxicology terms. Photographs, line drawings, and maps are supplemented with detailed descriptions of the physical environment where animals are likely to be encountered, which will help users identify specific species. Photos of patients with stings and other injuries accompany the treatment portion of this text, which was developed in collaboration with Auerbach, editor of the *Journal of Wilderness Medicine* and author of *Medicine for the Outdoors.* Another frequently cited publication by Halstead, *Dangerous Marine Animals That Bite, Sting, Shock, Are Non-Edible,* surveys pertinent references

Figure 8.2   Free Sources of Botanical Toxicity Information on the Internet

- *Botanical Dermatology Database (BoDD)*
  ⇨ http://BoDD.cf.ac.uk
  First launched in 1994, Richard Schmidt's *Botanical Dermatology Database* was, for several years, restricted to pre-authorized users only. When the ban was lifted in January 1997, searchers worldwide could benefit from this "electronic re-incarnation" of a book published in 1979 entitled *Botanical Dermatology*, by Mitchell and Rook. Separate indexes to plant names offer access by genus/species, family, or common terminology. A miscellaneous category lists algae, ant plants (myrmecophytes), bryophytes, cycads, ferns, fungi, and lichens. Clicking on a name leads to a meaty monograph summarizing known dermatological reaction data, including discussion of potential causes, references to basic chemical literature, and clinical case reports. Still under construction are dermatological indexes, which will make it easy to isolate plants that cause macro- or microtrauma mechanical injuries, as well as those associated with chemical injuries, such as allergic, airborne, or irritant contact dermatitis and photoirritants. An index to herbal remedies, listed by indication, is also promised. Still another series of access lists under development will group plants by function, such as food materials, pharmaceuticals, and fragrance/cosmetic raw materials. A phytochemical name/class index is also in the works.

- *Canadian Poisonous Plants Information System*
  ⇨ http://res.agr.ca/brd/poisonpl
  This interactive database is the work of Derek Munro, an employee of a research branch of the Canadian government dedicated to agriculture and agrifood. Coverage encompasses more than 250 plants capable of poisoning livestock, pets, or humans. After designating whether formal botanical or common names are the preferred access point, users are offered the option to search poisonous houseplants only or to limit output to records with illustrations. Another approach permits a combination of common or scientific plant name with either distribution (by province), poisonous plant parts, or toxic chemical. Records, once retrieved, provide general notes regarding poisoning by the plant, supportive references drawn from the literature, and basic nomenclature (English, French, and Latin). Record elements that follow identify toxic parts, chemicals involved, and symptoms, sequelae, and prognosis in poisoning of named types of animals, including humans. Statements in each segment are backed up by bibliography.

- *Guide to Poisonous and Toxic Plants*
  ⇨ http://chppm-www.apgea.army.mil/ento/PLANT.HTM
  The *Guide to Poisonous and Toxic Plants* was developed to support U.S. Army regulations regarding child development facilities and what should be avoided in their environs. The database organizes information into four browsable lists of house, garden, ornamental, and wild plants. Cross references from synonymous names assist in locating records. Entries for each species list common names and include a physical description, identify toxic part (e.g., leaves, fruit, stems) and detail symptoms of exposure. Treatment information is, however, omitted. This file's source bibliography includes respected authors, such as Kingsbury (8.48) and Lampe (8.49).

- *PLANTOX*
  ⇨ http://vm.cfsam.fda.gov/~djw/.
  Wagstaff's *PLANTOX* database continues the bibliography originally included in the

TOXLINE database, where a backfile of references is still maintained (see Figure 14.13). Entries are listed alphabetically by author and, as is seen in the PPBIB subfile of TOX-LINE, no abstracts are provided. This Internet site also includes a list of vascular plants reported to be toxic.

- *Poisonous Plant Databases*
  ⇨ http://www.inform.umd.edu/Medicinals/harmful.html
  Michael C. Tims of the University of Maryland maintains this subject hub, which currently lists twenty-eight sources. Entries consist of one-line hypertext links to titles, unembellished with any form of annotation.

---

back to the nineteenth century to support discussion of mechanisms of poisoning and recommended treatments.

8.55 Bucherl W, Buckley EE, Devlofeu V. *Venomous Animals and Their Venoms*. 3 v. New York: Academic Press, 1968–1971.

Bucherl, Buckley, and Devlofeu concentrate on treatment information in aid of victims of better known animals, and conclude with an intriguing chapter on animal venoms in therapy. Their work is also a good source for discussion of the chemistry of venoms and for determining the geographic distribution of cited animals. *Venomous Animals and Their Venoms* covers both vertebrates and invertebrates, with extensive material on snakes, and chapters on insects, fish, mollusks, and arthropods.

8.56 Tu AT, ed. *Food Poisoning. Handbook of Natural Toxins* v. 7. New York: Marcel Dekker, 1992.

The opening chapter in *Food Poisoning* discusses the scope of this problem from the public health point of view. Subsequent chapters address poisons of bacterial origin (e.g., staphylococcal, salmonellae, botulism) and those of plant and fungal origin (mushrooms, alkaloids, plant lectins, and mycotoxins). Part 5 deals with allergy and food intolerances, Part 6 is devoted to problems in consumption of seafood, and Parts 7 through 9 discuss, respectively, teratogenicity, antibiotic residues in food, and nitrosamines. Contributing authors cover prevalence, mechanisms of action, symptoms, diagnosis, treatment, and prevention. This book, part of an excellent series published in installments under the overall title *Handbook of Natural Toxins*, is very well-referenced (2,200 citations to the literature) and indexed. Numerous charts and tables add to its attractions.

Other volumes of the *Handbook of Natural Toxins* include *Plant and Fungal Toxins* (1983); *Insect Poisons, Allergens, and Other Invertebrate Venoms* (1984); *Marine Toxins and Venoms* (1988); *Bacterial Toxins* (1988); *Reptile Venoms and Toxins* (1991); *Toxicology of Plant and Fungal Compounds* (1991); and *Bacterial Toxins and Virulence Factors in Disease* (1995).

Occupational/Industrial Toxicology

Sax's Dangerous Properties of Industrial Materials (8.9) and handbooks by both Plunkett (8.6) and Sittig (8.7), cited earlier in this chapter, will provide a good core collection to answer most information queries related to occupational and industrial toxicology. Additional candidates for an expanded basic reference library are highlighted below.

8.57 Harbison RD, Hardy HL, eds. *Hamilton and Hardy's Industrial Toxicology*. 5th ed. St. Louis: Mosby, 1998.

8.58 Raffle PA, ed. *Hunter's Diseases of Occupations*. 8th ed. London: Oxford University Press, 1994.

Hamilton and Hardy's Industrial Toxicology features chapters on more than thirty-six metals. Biological hazards are also discussed, with an emphasis on occupational diseases and a helpful glossary of relevant terminology. *Hunter's Diseases of Occupations*, a reference classic, provides interesting background reading on the general topic of occupational toxicology, with numerous historical notes.

8.59 Rietschel RL, Dowler JF, eds. *Fisher's Contact Dermatitis*. 4th ed. Baltimore: Williams & Wilkins, 1995.

The most common occupational disease is dermatitis and *Fisher's Contact Dermatitis* is probably the best known sourcebook on the topic. It features all allergens that patients are likely to encounter, including latex and gold, as well as aquatic dermatoses. Opening chapters explain the pathogenesis of allergic contact hypersensitivity, the role of patch testing, and the effects of age, sex, and color of skin on etiology. Reactions to selected topical medications, antiseptics and disinfectants, antimicrobials, antihistamines, and corticosteroids or their vehicles are dealt with, in turn. Other chapters address dermatitis due to medications derived from plants, contact reactions to food additives and dyes, and dermatological adverse effects induced by medical devices and implants. Rietschel and Dowler also include instructions for coping with common allergens, written in language appropriate for direct dissemination to patients.

8.60 Marzulli FN, Maibach HI, eds. *Dermatotoxicology*. 5th ed. Washington, DC: Taylor & Francis, 1996.

Marzulli and Maibach's *Dermatotoxicology* is a huge compendium covering both theoretical aspects and practical test methods. Eight chapters on percutaneous absorption begin this work, followed by a chapter that describes skin metabolism of specific substances. Irritant dermatitis, chemically-induced skin hypersensitivity reactions, light-related skin effects and photoallergy, cutaneous carcinogenesis, and possible reproductive hazards in humans resulting from skin exposure to selected drugs are topics of discussion in the next sixteen chapters.

Alternatives to whole animal testing, a current hot topic, are also reviewed in this book, including *in vitro* skin and eye tests. Coverage includes methods used in industry and suggested by regulatory agencies to monitor and evaluate the safety of dermatological drugs, cosmetics, and other commercial products intended for skin contact. Drugs known to produce systemic effects following topical application are identified in the last chapter of *Dermatotoxicology*.

References

1. Fishman DL. Computerized clinical information system: CCIS from Micromedex. *Database* 1992 Apr;15:58.

2. Shardein JL. *Chemically induced birth defects*. 2nd ed. New York: Marcel Dekker, 1993:1.

3. Wassom JL, et al. How to obtain information about the teratogenic potential of chemicals. In: Kolb VM, ed. *Teratogens: chemicals which cause birth defects*. 2nd ed. Amsterdam: Elsevier, 1993:93.

4. Ibid., p. 95.

5. Jelovsek FR, Mattison DR, Chen JJ. Prediction of risk for human developmental toxicity: how important are animal studies for hazard identification? *Obstet Gynecol* 1989;74:624–636.

6. Kimmel CA, Gaylor DW. Issues in qualitative and quantitative risk analysis for developmental toxicity. *Risk Anal* 1988;8:15–20.

7. Gunderson-Warner S, Martinez LP, Martinez IP, Corey JC, et al. Critical reviews of articles regarding pregnancy exposures in popular magazines. *Teratology* 1990;42:469–472.

Additional Sources of Information

Brent RL. The law and congenital malformations. *Clin Perinatol* 1986;13:505–544.

Briggs SA. *Basic guide to pesticides: Their characteristics and hazards*. Washington, DC: Taylor & Francis, 1992.

Cockerham LG, Shane BS. *Basic environmental toxicology*. Boca Raton, FL: CRC Press, 1993.

Cronin E. *Contact dermatitis*. New York: Churchill Livingstone, 1980.

Drill VA, Lazar P, eds. *Cutaneous toxicity*. New York: Raven Press, 1984.

Edmonds LD, Layde PM, James LM, Flynt JW, et al. Congenital malformations surveillance. Two American systems. *Int J Epidemiol* 1981;10:247–252.

Foster S, Caras RA. *A field guide to venomous animals and poisonous plants*. Boston: Houghton Mifflin, 1994.

Fregert S. *Manual of contact dermatitis*. Chicago: Year Book Medical Publishers, 1981.

Friedman JM, Polifka JE. *Teratogenic effects of drugs: A resource for clinicians*. Baltimore: Johns Hopkins Press, 1994.

Gad SC, Chengalis CP, eds. *Animal models in toxicology*. New York: Marcel Dekker, 1992.

Halstead BW. *Color atlas of dangerous marine animals.* Boca Raton, FL: CRC Press, 1990.

Hayes WJ, et al. *Handbook of pesticide toxicology.* San Diego: Academic Press, 1991.

Jelovsek FR, Mattison DR, Young JF. Eliciting principles of hazard identification from experts. *Teratology* 1990;42:521–533.

Liu RH, Gadzala DE. *Handbook of drug analysis: Applications in forensic and clinical laboratories.* Washington, DC: American Chemical Society, 1997.

Maibach H, Hogan D, Dannaker CJ. *Handbook of contact dermatitis.* Boca Raton, FL: CRC Press, 1995.

Marks JG, DeLeo VA. *Contact and occupational dermatology.* 2nd ed. St. Louis: Mosby, 1997.

Matsumura F. *Toxicology of insecticides.* 2nd ed. New York: Plenum Press, 1985.

Meier J, White J, eds. *Handbook of clinical toxicology of animal venoms and poisons.* Boca Raton, FL: CRC Press, 1995.

Menendez-Botet CJ, St. Germain JM. *Hazardous waste: facts and fallacies.* Washington, DC: American Association for Clinical Chemistry, 1990.

Nisbet I, et al. *Chemical hazards to human reproduction.* Park Ridge, NJ: Noyes Data, 1983.

Olishifski JB, Harford ER, eds. *Industrial noise and hearing conservation.* Chicago: National Safety Council, 1975.

Proctor NH et al. *Chemical hazards of the workplace.* Philadelphia: Lippincott, 1988.

Rycroft RJG, Menne T, Frosch PJ, eds. *Textbook of contact dermatitis.* 2nd ed. New York: Springer-Verlag, 1994.

Smith RP. *Primer of environmental toxicology.* Baltimore: Williams & Wilkins, 1992.

Stacey NH, ed. *Occupational toxicology.* Washington, DC: Taylor & Francis, 1993.

Turner NJ, Szczawinski AF. *Common poisonous plants and mushrooms of North America.* Portland, OR: Timber Press, 1991.

Wagner SL. *Clinical toxicology of agricultural chemicals.* Park Ridge, NJ: Noyes Data, 1983.

Wang GM, Schwetz BA. An evaluation system for ranking chemicals with teratogenic potential. *Teratog Carcinog Mutagen* 1987;7:133–139.

Wassom JS. Use of selected toxicology information resources in assessing relationships between chemical structure and biological activity. *Environ Health Perspect* 1985;61:287–294.

Witorsch RJ, ed. *Reproductive toxicology.* 2nd ed. New York: Raven Press, 1995.

Worthing C, Hance R, eds. *The pesticide manual.* Cambridge, MA: Blackwell Scientific Publications, 1991.

Zakrzewski SF. *Principles of environmental toxicology.* 2nd ed. Washington, DC: American Chemical Society, 1997.

Practicum 3

This practicum exercise will help you evaluate your ready-reference source selection skills and review information presented in Chapters Seven and Eight. Questions posed can be answered without actual reference to hardcopy sources. Suggested answers are included in Appendix E.

Directions: Assume that you have available for your use all of the sources cited in previous chapters. Unless otherwise indicated, your response to each question should consist of:

   a. a list of sources to be consulted, with order of priority indicated, and
   b. a brief explanation of the rationale behind your selection of resources and sequence of consultation.

   1. A physician wants to know if a child will suffer ill effects from eating the contents of a four-ounce jar of vanishing cream.
   2. What is the LD_{50} for Drug X?
   3. Will tricyclic antidepressants, Brand ABC in particular, interact with antihistamines?
   4. Could oral amoxycillin at a dosage of two milligrams twice a day cause a false reading in a bilirubin test?
   5. Is the fruit of the weeping fig poisonous?
   6. In what percentage of patients is nausea a side effect of Drug Y?
   7. A public health nurse needs to know how long syringes prepared for administration of a given medication can be stored by a home-bound patient, if cloudiness detected in the week old preparation indicates "spoilage," and what storage conditions (temperature, light exposure) are recommended.
   8. Have collagen wound dressings been associated with congenital anomalies?
   9. What are the clinical signs of Brand X overdose, and how should it be treated?
   10. Can shoe polish (brand name unknown) cause a dermatological reaction?

9

Drug Information for the Consumer/Patient

Questions from patients about their medications are a common occurrence and one that presents special challenges to information professionals. The consequences of inappropriate answers can be therapeutic failure. Adherence to a prescribed treatment plan, usually referred to as patient "compliance," is essential to effective prevention and management of disease. Yet, as many as half of all patients issued a prescription fail to have it filled, and 30% ignore authorized refills.[1] It is estimated that nearly two million hospital admissions annually can be traced directly to noncompliance[2] and that 125,000 Americans die each year simply because they fail to take their medications as prescribed.[3]

Noncompliance can be attributed to several factors, nearly all of which center on communication and education. In an effort to ensure development and dissemination of appropriate written instructions to all Rx recipients, the FDA proposed a mandatory Medication Guide (MedGuide) program in 1995. The plan presented to Congress would have standardized data elements covered, language used, and overall format of patient package inserts (PPIs). In 1996, Congress rejected direct involvement of the government in production of mandatory PPIs for all prescription drugs, endorsing, instead, a private sector action plan. This voluntary initiative, adopted early in 1997, sets a goal of providing useful written information to at least 75% of patients issued new prescriptions by the year 2000 and 95% by 2006.[4]

Meanwhile, market forces are influencing patient behavior. It's no secret that direct-to-consumer (DTC) pharmaceutical advertising is on the rise in the United States (this practice is still banned in the European Union). Since August 1997, when the FDA relaxed constraints regarding information required about risks associated with Rx drugs advertised on television, manufacturer investment in this form of promotion has grown by leaps and bounds. The increase seen in 1997 alone was 46%, with a total of $917 million spent by the industry on DTC marketing.[5] The effect on sales of heavily promoted products is well documented. At

237

the same time, the indirect effects of DTC advertising appear to be heightened consumer awareness of medical conditions and possible treatments, with concomitant demand for readily accessible healthcare information.

While the growing phenomenon of participatory health care may ultimately lead to better compliance with prescribed medication regimens, some evidence suggests that patient empowerment could have negative effects. For example, a study conducted by Ziment Associates on behalf of *Time* magazine in 1998 revealed that one-third of 1,500 consumers surveyed believed that they could choose medications without their doctor's advice.[6] Results of this and other surveys[7] undertaken to measure the impact of DTC ads, coupled with data on the continuing prevalence of noncompliance, are compelling motivators in favor of providing consumers access to appropriate printed materials, whether or not such information is directly requested. Yet, whether your approach to patient education is proactive or reactive, whether your interest in finding good sources is personal or professional, you will encounter problems.

Thirty years ago, the advent of government-mandated patient package inserts for selected prescription products, such as oral contraceptives, brought into sharp focus barriers that can be anticipated in providing accurate and appropriate drug information to consumers. Foremost among these is difficulty in translating technical medical terminology into language easily understood by lay people. Another issue is selection of relevant data. Simply paraphrasing package inserts intended for health science professionals is not the answer, if information service, rather than mere transmission of facts, is the goal. The average consumer, when confronted with an undifferentiated list of adverse effects reported for most medications (typically ranging from diarrhea to death), is unlikely to come away better informed. Thus, promoting access to many of the drug information sources discussed thus far in this *Guide* will not satisfy consumer information needs. Yet, in introductions to library reference work, it is still not uncommon to find optimistic assertions that, although a given source is published for physicians, "it is equally clear to laypersons with patience and a medical dictionary at hand."[8]

More than a dictionary would be needed to transform the litany of ills of the flesh contained in most package inserts into practical precautions for patients prescribed the medication in question. Information in this form can have a negative effect on compliance with prescribed drug regimens. Concern about side effects is the most prevalent risk factor associated with drugs in consumers' perception.[9] What is needed is greater selectivity and evaluation of side effect data on behalf of patients, identifying not just the fact that an effect has been reported, but its likelihood, duration, severity, and importance. Sources that select and evaluate data in this manner are the focus of this chapter. Additional consumer health information available online is discussed in Chapter Fourteen.

Recommended Core Collection

It's perhaps inevitable that public library drug information collections always include the *Physicians' Desk Reference* (6.10). As publications more appropriate for patients and their families have become available, consumers should also find at least one of the following alternative sources shelved next to the *PDR*. Equally important is a thorough grasp on the part of librarians serving the general public of exactly what information is, and is not, compiled in the *PDR*, compared to other drug compendia.

First, the *PDR* does not cover all prescription drugs on the market in the United States: ". . . surprisingly, it contains gaps in information on some widely used drugs, such as ampicillin, prednisone, or propranolol, for which it simply lists the drug name, dosage, and nothing else."[10] Why? Companies must pay for copy space in this source, which means that older drugs already well known and widely prescribed are less likely to be featured than newer products requiring promotion. Second, *PDR* product information is limited to labeling and prescribing instructions prepared for health science professionals and otherwise disseminated in the form of package inserts, which are usually removed when the drug is dispensed to patients. The content of such inserts is regulated by the FDA, whose primary objective is to ensure that prescribers (physicians) receive information necessary for safe and effective use of the drug. Accordingly, only those diseases or conditions and dosage for which proof of safety and efficacy have been established, following government guidelines, are listed as indications (i.e., accepted medical applications or uses). However, patients should be aware that other uses and dosage levels may be widely recognized in the medical community and can be legally prescribed by their physician.

Another portion of *PDR* product entries that is easily misinterpreted by the layperson is the listing of side effects. It's important to remember that all drugs can be associated with adverse effects and that not all of the possible reactions listed are equally likely to occur. Sources expressly published for patients will generally supply better guidelines regarding side effects, based on expert assessment of data on their incidence, prevalence, and severity (information often absent in *PDR* entries).

9.1 *USP DI: United States Pharmacopeia Dispensing Information. Volume 2: Advice for the Patient.* Rockville, MD: U.S. Pharmacopeial Convention, 1982–. Annual, with monthly updates.

9.2 *Información de Medicamentos, Consejos al Paciente.* Madrid: Ministerio de Sanidad y Consumo de España, 1991. Update issued in 1994. Distributed in the United States by the U.S. Pharmacopeial Convention, Rockville, MD.

9.3 *The Complete Drug Reference.* Mt. Vernon, NY: Consumer Reports Books, 1998.

9.4 *The USP Guide to Medicines.* New York: Avon Books, 1998.

One such compendium is the second volume of *USP DI. Advice for the Patient* presents essential consumer-oriented drug information in concise, clearly written monographs. Emphasis is on prescription drugs, with only selective coverage of major OTC preparations. Data systematically provided in its simplified, large-type monographs include proper use and storage of medications, precautions, and identification of side effects that are significant enough to warrant reporting back to the prescribing physician. Indexed by both brand and generic names, this source also supplies a photographic section, arranged alphabetically by USAN. Color photos included in The Medicine Chart are limited to the most frequently prescribed solid oral dosage forms (capsules and tablets), preceded by a product index of both brand and generic names, as well as an index to imprint codes. *Información de Medicamentos* is a Spanish language translation of *Advice for the Patient*.

The Complete Drug Reference is the bookstore version of *USP DI Volume 2*, covering more than 10,000 prescription and OTC medications. *The USP Guide to Medicines* is a derivative publication, also including only a limited selection of monographs (2,600) from *Advice for the Patient*. With a focus on the most widely used drugs, it appears to be the successor of another USP publication entitled *About Your Medicines*, the seventh edition of which was last issued in 1993. Other installments in the new *Guide* series include *The USP Guide to Heart Medicines* and *The USP Guide to Vitamins and Minerals*, also published by Avon Books. What these guides and *The Complete Drug Reference* lack is interim monthly updates available to *USP DI* subscribers between annual editions. These updates offer introductory versions of patient education leaflets for new drugs within thirty days of product availability.

9.5 Clayman CB, ed. *The American Medical Association Guide to Prescription and Over-the-Counter Drugs.* New York: Random House, 1988.

The AMA's *Guide to Prescription and Over-the-Counter Drugs* covers fewer products than *USP DI Advice for the Patient*, but is more attractively presented. Following an opening section on understanding and using drugs, which focuses on administration and storage, a Drug Name Finder Index offers both a color identification guide (538 brand name tablets and capsules, arranged by color and size) and a listing of brand and generic names for more than 5,000 products. Next is lay language discussion of major drug groups, organized into anatomical/therapeutic/pharmacological categories, highlighting uses and mechanisms of action. Separate A–Z sections provide monographs on drugs, vitamins and minerals, abused substances, and food additives.

Drug entries are designed for quick access to practical advice on 320 medications, including an overdose danger rating, potential for dependency, information on Rx versus OTC status, and whether a product is marketed in generic form. Possible adverse effects are presented in a table, rating their frequency and likelihood, and whether or when to discuss effects with a physician. The AMA's *Guide* concludes with a glossary, index, and drug poisoning emergency advice. This publication's writing style, outstanding illustrations, and eye-catching layout make it a highly recommended choice for core collections targeting consumers.

9.6 *AARP Pharmacy Service Prescription Drug Handbook*. 2nd ed. New York: Harper Perennial, 1992.

The American Association of Retired Persons' *Prescription Drug Handbook* is another *de rigueur* selection for patient information libraries. Arranged in thirteen chapters dealing with related medical conditions (e.g., digestive disorders, respiratory problems), the *Handbook* departs from other consumer guides by deliberately omitting dosage information, explaining that this factor must be determined by the physician familiar with the patient's state of health. Each chapter concludes with a chart organizing basic drug information. Brand name access is limited to those names most commonly used, but generic names are fully indexed, with cross-references to appropriate charts; approximately 1,000 names are listed. The photo identification section is organized by color. Despite its title, the AARP *Prescription Drug Handbook* does offer coverage of selected nonprescription medications, such as aspirin, calcium supplements, and vitamins. As might be expected, its focus is on products frequently prescribed for patients over fifty years of age, with special advice for those over sixty-five.

9.7 Fried JJ, Petska S, Subak-Sharpe GJ, eds. *The American Druggist's Complete Family Guide to Prescriptions, Pills, and Drugs*. New York: Hearst, 1995.

A retail pharmacy journal published since 1871, *The American Druggist* is a logical title to be associated with drug information for consumers. The *Complete Family Guide to Prescriptions, Pills, and Drugs* opens with chapters dealing with a wide variety of medically related issues, such as how drugs work in the body, how they are tested before approval, and government controls on their use and distribution. Its introduction wisely warns patients that dietary habits, herbal remedies, homeopathic preparations, high-dose vitamins, and other OTC medications that their doctor "doesn't know about" can affect their prescribed health care. It encourages full disclosure and frank discussion with care-givers.

In chapters dedicated to categories of products such as pain-killers, antiarthritics, dietary supplements, and skin and hair preparations, tables provide detailed information on individual drugs, including dosage forms available, how they should be taken, possible side effects, precautions, and interactions. A forty-eight-page color photo section, sensibly organized by color and size, is intended to assist in identification of products most commonly prescribed. The index offers good access, by brand names, to drugs featured in preceding textual discussion and tables, but fails to flag products pictured in the photo-ID section. Nonetheless, *The American Druggist's Complete Family Guide* will be a welcome addition to public and patient education library shelves, sharing an editor with the excellent *Columbia University College of Physicians and Surgeons Complete Home Medical Guide*.

9.8 Sullivan D. *The American Pharmaceutical Association's Guide to Prescription Drugs*. Washington, DC: American Pharmaceutical Association, 1998.

9.9 Peirce A. *Parent's Guide to Childhood Medications*. Washington, DC: American Pharmaceutical Association, 1997.

The American Pharmaceutical Association's Guide to Prescription Drugs is an inexpensive and simply organized source of information on 1,000 of the most commonly prescribed medications in the United States. Arranged alphabetically by trade name and enhanced with color photographs of major brands, monographs include nonproprietary names and indicate whether or not a generic version of the product is available. Entries also cite therapeutic class, dosage forms, main uses, customary dosage, common side effects, drug interactions, allergies, and pregnancy/breast feeding precautions. This source also identifies brand names, when relevant, of other drugs within the same therapeutic category, and average price.

The *Parent's Guide to Childhood Medications* compiles essential data on more than 300 Rx and OTC drugs commonly used to treat children. Entries in this APhA publication are organized by generic name. Monographs list major brand names and dosage forms available and explain what each drug is used to treat, how and when it should be administered, how it works, and the speed with which it will take effect. Signs and symptoms of overdose are included in discussion, as are possible side effects.

9.10 Fudyma J. *What Do I Take? A Consumer's Guide to Nonprescription Drugs*. Washington, DC: American Pharmaceutical Association, 1997.

The third APhA consumer resource, *What Do I Take?*, focuses on nonprescription medications. Its arrangement is unusual, in that it organizes products by the ailments that they can be used to treat. Equally unique is provision of pharmacists' ratings of each product for effectiveness, speed of action, ease of use, minimal side effects, and duration of relief. These ratings are derived from a national survey of APhA community pharmacist members. *What Do I Take?* covers 400 OTC products used for any of seventy specific medical conditions.

9.11 *Mosby's Patient GenRx*. St. Louis: Mosby, 1999.

Mosby plans to introduce its *Patient GenRx* in 1999 in a binder designed for easy extraction and convenient photocopying of individual drug leaflets. Each leaflet will feature pictograms and bulleted information points, in an effort to enhance patient compliance. A total of 650 English-language and 450 Spanish-language monographs, each one to two pages in length, will be available in this initial edition, which will include a supplementary CD-ROM.

9.12 *Taking Your Medications Safely*. Springhouse, PA: Springhouse Corp., 1996.

With cover billing as "Hospital-tested advice from America's leading nurses," *Taking Your Medications Safely* begins with a useful section on drug self-administration, with recommendations on filling, taking, and storing prescriptions and establishing a daily schedule to encourage compliance. Illustrations show patients how to use drops and inhalers, apply ointments, and handle injections. Instructions are also included on how to check your own pulse and blood pressure, and how to check another person's. Drug monographs, organized by brand name, advise readers how to take the featured product, what side effects can occur and what can be done to relieve or prevent them, when side effects signal an emergency or require immediate medical attention, and what other drugs to avoid because of potential interactions. Entries also include appropriate warnings regarding use during pregnancy or breastfeeding, by the elderly or by athletes, as well as outlining precautions for alcohol consumption during therapy. The index to this volume reinforces its utility as a recommended core collection purchase by citing all drug names, both brand and generic, used in monographs and by supplying keyword access to drug entries by the conditions they are intended to treat. The scope of *Taking Your Medications Safely* is typical of most drug information compendia marketed directly to consumers: "common and important" Rx and OTC drugs.

9.13 Griffith HW. *Complete Guide to Prescription and Nonprescription Drugs*. 15th ed. New York: Body Press/Perigree, 1997.

For many years prior to his death in 1993, Griffith's name had been associated with high-quality patient education materials (see also 9.41). Entries in the *Complete Guide to Prescription and Nonprescription Drugs* reflect this legacy of editorial excellence, presenting information in easy-to-read chart format. Coverage includes 700 generic entries, each of which lists both U.S. and Canadian brand names representing more than 5,000 products currently on the market. Drug charts, organized by nonproprietary designations, show whether or not the medication is habit-forming, Rx or OTC, and whether it is available in a generic formulation. Notes on dosage and use describe how and when to take each drug, what it does, the time lapse to expect before the drug works, what to do if a dose is forgotten, and "don't take with" instructions. Overdose symptoms and first aid notes focus on providing similarly practical guidance.

Adverse effects listings for each medication advise what to do if they occur and draw clear distinctions between those that are life-threatening, rare, and infrequent and those that are common. The warnings and precautions section of drug charts addresses a broad spectrum of topics, such as potential effects on skin and sunlight sensitivity, prolonged administration, use in pregnancy and breastfeeding, the aged, infants and children, as well as precautions in driving, piloting, and other hazardous work. Annotations regarding interactions include alcohol, foods, tobacco, and other medications (identified by drug class, rather than individual generic names). Back-of-the-book appendices in the *Complete Guide* compile additional interactions information and a glossary. Despite its 1,100-page length, the volume is readily accessibly through an index listing generic, brand, and drug class names.

9.14 Rybacki JJ, Long JW. *The Essential Guide to Prescription Drugs, 1998.* New York: Harper Collins, 1997.

Rybacki and Long's *Essential Guide to Prescription Drugs* is comparatively limited in its scope, containing approximately 200 drug profiles for commonly prescribed medications used widely in the United States and Canada, arranged by generic name. Entries include a guide to pronunciation and information on: 1) whether a product is a controlled substance, 2) its Rx versus OTC status (some nonprescription drugs are covered), and 3) generic availability. Along with a glossary, other extras in the *Essential Guide* are a concluding collection of tables on adverse effects. Drugs that may cause photosensitivity or dysfunction/damage to the heart, lung, liver, kidney, nerves, or blood cells are the topic of separate tables. Other lists single out drugs that may adversely affect the fetus or newborn infant, behavior, vision, or sexuality.

9.15 Zimmerman DR. *Zimmerman's Complete Guide to Nonprescription Drugs.* 2nd ed. Detroit: Gale Research, 1992.

Another excellent (other than the quality of its paper) consumer drug information resource is *Zimmerman's Complete Guide to Nonprescription Drugs*, formerly titled *The Essential Guide to Nonprescription Drugs* (1988). There are three ways to approach this volume: 1) through the table of contents, where titles offer access by therapeutic class (e.g., acne medications, reducing aids); 2) a symptoms index, or 3) the main back-of-the-book index, which includes entries for symptoms, other subject keywords, and both generic and brand names. In addition, a Unit Finder in the introduction organizes titles into logical groups (baby care, body odor control, skin care). This feature is particularly helpful, because many related products are widely separated in the text under highly specific alphabetic section headings. For example, skin care items can be found under eighteen narrower headings, scattered across the alphabetic arrangement under acne, insect repellents/bite and sting treatments, styptic pencils and other astringents, sunscreens, etc.

The text in each unit of this book explains, in everyday language, many symptoms and ailments, how OTC drugs may help, and when they may not (i.e., when to consult a doctor). Following this discussion, near the end of each unit, is a table of products widely sold, compiling data on their safety and effectiveness. Zimmerman has ferreted out and reorganized results of the FDA's OTC Reviews, providing cross references to brands currently on the market and identifying those deemed safe and effective, versus those with conditional status (category 3, see Chapter 4). Encompassing more than 900 OTC preparations, this publication's scope embraces best-selling medications identified from the *Chain Drug Review* in 1992.

The range of products covered is unusually broad, from cradle cap removers to antiperspirants, hangover and overindulgence remedies to dandruff shampoos, wart paints to toothache medications. It includes many items commonly classified as toiletries, rather than nonprescription drugs. Information professionals should note that the source section at the end of Zimmerman's *Complete Guide* gathers together important references to OTC Drug Review documents: citations to panel reports, tentative final monographs, and final monographs (when available) in the *Federal Register*, plus applicable *Code of Federal Regulations* references. The author has also compiled a cumulative list of ingredients switched from Rx to OTC status as a result of FDA reviews, numbering more than 400 substances as of 1992.

9.16 Gorman JM. *The Essential Guide to Psychiatric Drugs.* 3rd ed. New York: St. Martin's Press, 1997.
9.17 Yudofsky S, Hales RE, Ferguson T. *What You Need to Know About Psychiatric Drugs.* New York: Grove Weidenfeld, 1991.
9.18 Salzman B. *The Handbook of Psychiatric Drugs, A Consumer's Guide to Safe and Effective Use.* 2nd ed. New York: Henry Holt, 1996.

Any one of these three guides to psychiatric drugs would be useful additions to a core consumer collection. Gorman's *Essential Guide to Psychiatric Drugs* is a handbook intended for potential patients and their families, written to help them understand when drug therapy may help, how long treatment should last, and what side effects can be expected. Both generic and brand names are used in the opening Drug Directory (index). Part I offers background information, with an underlying theme of "Be an informed consumer." Part II, organized by psychiatric disorder (e.g., depression, anxiety, drug abuse), is a drug ready-reference guide. Part III covers special topics, such as family, environment, genetics, weight loss and gain, sex and psychiatric drugs, and generic versus brand name product selection. Clearly written in a compassionate, but not condescending, voice, Gorman's *Essential Guide* presents often difficult-to-discuss material in a balanced and objective manner, encouraging communication between doctors and patients. This volume includes a glossary and provides a quality-filtered bibliography of suggested reading appropriate for lay people.

What You Need to Know About Psychiatric Drugs is similar in intent and scope to Gorman's *Guide* and a good complement, particularly in its section on frequently asked questions (and answers) about psychiatric drugs. Discussion is organized by disorder and suggests, when appropriate, nondrug alternatives and self-help groups, giving details on agencies for possible referrals. Individual drug monographs are attractively organized. This volume incorporates many of the better features of the AMA *Guide* (9.5), such as tables of side effects information, a glossary, and a good index to brand and generic drug names.

Salzman divides reference material in *The Handbook of Psychiatric Drugs* into six parts. The first addresses "What you need to know before taking psychiatric medications." Discussion covers distrust of psychiatrists, who is authorized to prescribe drugs of this type, and what your doctor needs to know, as well. Part Two describes how psychiatric drugs work in the body. It offers insight into the latency period, why following a drug schedule is important, and what to do about side effects. Common psychiatric disorders are the topic of Part Three, and people at particular risk are discussed in Part Four (e.g., pregnant or elderly patients, children). Part Five's coverage of drug misuse and abuse confronts misconceptions that lead to misuse and addresses dependence liability, the washout period, and signs of drug dependency. The final section (Part Six) of the *Handbook* is devoted to individual psychiatric drug profiles, followed by a glossary and index.

9.19 Tyler VE. *The Honest Herbal: A Sensible Guide to the Use of Herbs and Related Remedies*. 3rd ed. Binghamton, NY: Pharmaceutical Products Press, 1993.

Tyler, well-known coauthor of one of the classic textbooks on pharmacognosy (12.2), in recent years has devoted his considerable writing and public-speaking talents to spreading the good word about scientific investigations into natural medicines, at the same time offering equally well-informed warnings. In *The Honest Herbal*, he discusses the dangers, as well as the apparent efficacy, of popular plant-based remedies. Following brief highlights on their pros and cons and reference to pertinent laws and regulations, the bulk of the text consists of separate entries compiling information on more than 100 botanicals.

Descriptions include traditional folk uses of each herb and detailed discussion of the safety and therapeutic effectiveness of the remedy, summarized in a final value judgment by this respected authority. Selection of items covered is based on their relative public significance, as determined from literature sources and prevalence in health food stores. Thus, Chinese herbs are included, as are apricot pits (laetrile), garlic, honey, kelp, bee pollen, royal jelly, and pangamic acid ("vitamin" B15). A handy table in the final chapter of *The Honest Herbal* offers a concise at-a-glance digest of uses, validity, and safety of each herb and related remedy featured earlier in the volume. Bibliography accompanying each entry will assist users interested in more detailed study.

9.20 Peirce A. *The American Pharmaceutical Association's Practical Guide to Natural Medicines*. Washington, DC: American Pharmaceutical Association, 1998.

The American Pharmaceutical Association weighs in with a *Practical Guide to Natural Medicines* in response to its members' (and other pharmacists') need for authoritative reference material written in lay language. Peirce evaluates the effectiveness of 300 natural remedies—from acidophilus to zinc—based on scientific studies summarized in separate entries. Individual monographs describe what each product is, how it is used, and forms commercially available. Each product is then rated on a scale of one to five, where 1 indicates proven efficacy and safety and 5 warns of health hazards even within standard dose ranges.

Additional Selections

The last ten years have brought a plethora of health related publications aimed at the consumer marketplace, all of which require careful evaluation to determine their value compared to excellent sources already available, such as those annotated in the previous section. As Barry[11] has warned, many have been extravagantly oversold, although they may meet the relatively uninformed expectations of unsuspecting patients. Medical information professionals can perform a valuable service by applying their extensive training in technical literature assessment to evaluating consumer health information sources on behalf of nonsubject-specialty colleagues and their clientele.

9.21 Rees AM, ed. *Consumer Health Information Source Book*. 5th ed. Phoenix, AZ: Oryx Press, 1998.
9.22 Rees AM, ed. *Consumer Health USA*. Phoenix, AZ: v. 1–1995, v.2–1997.

Rees lends such expertise in two publications from Oryx Press. The *Consumer Health Information Source Book* will help users locate credible and appropriate books (600 are listed), magazines and newsletters (130), and pamphlets (1,400). In addition, it identifies 200 toll-free hotlines, 278 patient/family support groups, and more than forty health information clearinghouses. Rees' coverage of computer-based resources has expanded to include forty-five online and CD-ROM titles, compared to twenty-three featured in the 1994 edition of the *Source Book*. Predictably, Internet resources merit a new chapter in the fifth edition, with 139 Web sites briefly annotated. Indexed by author, title, and subject in hardcopy format, the full text of the *Source Book* is also searchable online in the *IAC Health & Wellness Database* (14.33).

Consumer Health USA, subtitled "Essential Information from the Federal Health Network," reproduces the full text of more than 150 government documents likely to help answer many information requests related to such hot topics as AIDS, chronic fatigue syndrome, diabetes, smoking, vaccines, and substance abuse. Volume 2, issued in 1997, adds another 150 documents to the collection, this time complementing government agency publications with articles from seventeen nonprofit organizations. The latest installment in the series contains new sections on stroke, musculoskeletal diseases, and connective tissue disorders.

9.23 Leber MR, Jaeger RW, Scalzo AJ. *Handbook of Over-the-Counter Drugs and Pharmacy Products*. Berkeley, CA: Celestial Arts, 1994.

Discussion of products and of issues not found in other printed consumer guides sets the *Handbook of Over-the-Counter Drugs and Pharmacy Products* apart, making it a potentially useful adjunct to the core collection of resources cited above. Examples include: bottled water; cosmetic ingredients (and the "De-laney Dilemma" in extrapolating toxicity data from animal evidence); denture cleaners (including devices); sanitary napkins and tampons; support stockings; infant feeding equipment, diapers, and wipes; do-it-yourself medical tests; heat lamps; pet products; humidifiers and vaporizers; hair dyes, brushes, dryers, and removers, including electrolysis; thermometers; and sunlamps. Following an in-troduction that encourages consumers to read labels before turning to this book, information on approximately 700 OTC ingredients is organized to match drug-store shelf arrangement (i.e., by indications). A subject index offers access by diseases, conditions, and a limited number of brand names. Generic names are primary entry points to the *Handbook*'s drug data. A brief bibliography con-cludes the volume.

9.24 *The PDR Family Guide to Prescription Drugs*. 5th ed. Montvale, NJ: Med-ical Economics, 1998.

9.25 *The PDR Family Guide to Women's Health and Prescription Drugs*. Mont-vale, NJ: Medical Economics, 1994.

9.26 *The PDR Family Guide to Nutrition and Health*. Montvale, NJ: Medical Economics, 1995.

Given the name recognition factor of the initials PDR, patients may wish to consult the Family Guide series from the same publisher. *The PDR Family Guide to Prescription Drugs*® offers drug profiles of best-selling Rx medications, ar-ranged by brand name and cross referenced from generic names. Based on infor-mation compiled in the *Physicians' Desk Reference* (6.10), profiles have been enhanced to include missed-dose instructions, storage guidelines, and a phonetic pronunciation key for brand names. The *Guide* also features twenty-three chap-ters on diagnosing and treating major health problems, such as arthritis, AIDS, high blood pressure, and heart disease.

The *PDR Family Guide to Women's Health and Prescription Drugs*™ takes a similar approach, augmenting its selected drug profiles with chapters discussing general health concerns. Contraception and fertility, premenstrual syndrome, hormone replacement therapy in menopause, osteoporosis, and sexually transmit-ted diseases are among topics addressed. A disease and disorder index supple-ments generic/brand name access to drug information. Other extras include a chart showing safety-in-pregnancy ratings of top selling drugs, a glossary of common medical terms, and a directory of self-help and women's support orga-nizations.

The newest addition to the series, *The PDR Family Guide to Nutrition and Health*™, compiles drug profiles for anticholesterol agents; diabetes, gout, and ulcer medications; diet pills; antacids; diarrhea remedies; and vitamin and min-

eral supplements. A separate section, "Nutrition, A to Z," provides brief overviews of vitamins, minerals, and trace elements, outlining minimum requirements, upper limits on megadosing, and signs and symptoms of toxicity. The
remainder of the text devotes considerable attention to weight control, special
diets, and meal planning. A fat, cholesterol, and calorie counter is included, along
with a guide to reading the new food labels, directories of nutritional groups and
poison control centers, and a glossary of nutrition keywords. All three of these
PDR Family Guides also supply the ever popular drug identification color photograph sections.

9.27 Burger A. *Understanding Medications: What the Label Doesn't Tell You*.
Washington, DC: American Chemical Society, 1995.

The American Chemical Society would seem to be an unlikely source of medical information intended for consumers/patients, but Burger's long association
with ACS as editor/founder (1959–1971) of the *Journal of Medicinal Chemistry*
accounts for the Society's publication of his book, *Understanding Medications*.
It traces its origin from the fact that fellow residents in the retirement community
where he now lives expect him, as the "only medicinal chemist among them . . .
to express expert opinions on topics ranging from space flight and atomic fission
and fusion to the meaning of various ailments." The resulting volume's organization reflects the author's stated objective to satisfy and stimulate the curiosity of
educated lay people about drugs.

The first chapter describes historical beginnings: early records of natural drugs,
remedies prevalent in medieval times, and early modern medicines, such as digi-
talis and various opiates. Chapters follow that address, respectively, the naming
of drugs, biomedical research and the role of the pharmaceutical industry in drug
development (and why drugs are expensive), modern drug discovery, and medication use/abuse. Next, discussion turns to specific drug classes, replete with interesting history regarding their evolutionary development and clear explanations
of pertinent physiological/pharmacological principles, follows.

A well written glossary rounds out this modestly sized book—which would
have benefited from an equally well-done index. As it stands, the index is regrettably lean, omitting many desirable access points to the wealth of isolated facts
otherwise hidden in the text's discursive style and presentation. For example, the
definition of detail men and women, embedded in the section on drug names, is
virtually lost to the reader seeking quick re-look-up, because it lacks an index
entry. Somewhat mitigating this drawback to accessibility is Burger's disclaimer
that *Understanding Medications* is not meant to be a household compendium. In
truth, it requires, indeed deserves, reading from start to finish (rather than piecemeal consultation) to savor its full value.

9.28 Wolfe SM, Hope RE. *Worst Pills Best Pills*. 2nd ed. Washington, DC:
Public Citizen's Health Research Group, 1993.

Subtitled "The Older Adult's Guide to Avoiding Drug-Induced Death or Illness," *Worst Pills Best Pills* lists 119 pills you should not use and 245 safer alternatives. Wolfe and Hope go on to explain the risks and benefits of 364 medications commonly used to treat the elderly. Indexed by both brand and generic names, the volume is appropriately printed in larger type and out-sized overall format to anticipate the needs of this patient group. *Worst Pills Best Pills* cites reputable references and offers defensible conclusions drawn from them, but its somewhat inflammatory, exhortative style may undermine the authors' stated intention of encouraging patient-doctor dialogue and prevention of over-prescribing.

9.29 Brown EH, Walker LP. *The Informed Consumer's Pharmacy. The Essential Guide to Prescription and Over-the-Counter Drugs*. New York: Carroll & Graf, 1990.

Although Brown and Walker open their book by counseling consumers to consult the *PDR*, the remainder of their introductory essays, when dealing with other controversial or debatable topics, reflect well-informed objectivity and are supported by bibliographic references. The chief drawback to this contribution to the consumer drug literature is that discussion addresses broad therapeutic and pharmacological classes of medications, omitting separate drug monographs. The authors rely on tables to relate their general discussion to specific brand names that consumers are likely to use as starting points in investigation.

Fortunately, *The Informed Consumer's Pharmacy* is well indexed, with much needed cross references from proprietary designations to appropriate tables, which show best selling drugs in various categories. FDA effectiveness ratings are included in the listing of cough remedies. Other tabulations address caffeine content in popular foods and drinks, recommended immunizations, sodium and potassium levels found in a selection of common foods, fiber content, drugs that cause photosensitivity, and brand name drugs not available as generics. A Special Topics section covers trends in self-testing, vitamins and mineral supplements, food-drug interactions, and drugs and the elderly.

9.30 Silverman H, ed. *The Pill Book—The Illustrated Guide to the Most-Prescribed Drugs in the United States*. 8th ed. New York: Bantam Books, 1998.

The Pill Book has been published as both a trade and mass market paperback and claims that more than four million copies of previous editions have been sold. Despite the alarm signals this boast may set off, the text is compiled by a Doctor of Pharmacy (PharmD) and is sensibly organized by generic name, with cross references from brand names. Excellent color plates are a redeeming feature in this resource, notwithstanding the dubious introductory matter that accompanies them ("could even save your life"), misguidedly implying that if a drug's appearance does not match the photographs, it may have been incorrectly dispensed.

Such sensationalism is wholly inappropriate to the subject matter. However, unlike most such visual identification guides (exasperatingly confined to products that already have their names clearly marked on the dosage form), *The Pill Book*'s photos actually cover tablets and capsules potentially more difficult to identify, such as those little green pills with only MP and the number 25 etched on them. Another helpful section suggests twenty practical questions to consider asking a physician or pharmacist, such as: What should I do if I forget a dose?

9.31 Herbert VH, Subak-Sharpe GJ, eds. *The Mount Sinai School of Medicine Complete Book of Nutrition*. New York: St. Martin's Press, 1990.
9.32 Herbert V, Subak-Sharpe GJ, eds. *Total Nutrition: The Only Guide You'll Ever Need—from the Mount Sinai School of Medicine*. New York: St. Martin's Press, 1995.

The Mount Sinai School of Medicine Complete Book of Nutrition includes material on food-drug interactions, along with a section on What's in Your Food featuring chapters on protein, carbohydrates, fats and cholesterol, and food additives. Other chapters discuss nutrition at various life stages (pregnancy, infancy and childhood, adolescence, old age), eating disorders, vegetarianism, food allergies, diabetes, nutritional needs of athletes, as well as nutrition and arthritis, skin, and hair. This book offers practical advice on restaurant eating for the calorie- and nutrition-conscious consumer, on food shopping and labeling, and on food storage and preparation.

Its successor, *Total Nutrition*, presents information in three major sections. Part I provides basic background material and assistance in differentiating between macro- and micro-nutrients. Part II examines age and gender-related issues. Part III focuses on chronic and acute illnesses. *Total Nutrition* also includes sample menus, numerous illustrations, and more than 200 tables.

9.33 Navarra T, Lipkowitz MA. *Encyclopedia of Vitamins, Minerals and Supplements*. New York: Facts on File, 1996.

The *Encyclopedia of Vitamins, Minerals and Supplements* presents objective information in everyday language concerning nutritional options, taking care to relay positive, negative, and neutral views. For example, it discusses alternatives to better known vitamins, as well as substances used in traditional Chinese, Ayurvedic (traditional Hindu), native American, and other herbal or homeopathic medical regimens. Entries in its dictionary arrangement offer explanations of concepts and conditions, such as absorption and acne, side by side with information regarding specific substances. Monographs for the latter provide data on toxicity, teratogenicity, dosage, drug interactions, and U.S. recommended daily allowance (RDA).

Nine appendices include 1) the food pyramid, 2) a glossary, 3) a nutrition chronology (history), 4) drug and nutrient interactions, 5) an RDA chart, 6) a position statement from the American Dietetic Association, 7) complete transcription of the Dietary Supplement Health and Education Act of 1994 (the scope of which is explained in the *Encyclopedia*'s foreword), 8) discussion of food labeling changes resulting from the Nutrition Labeling and Education Act of 1990 (effective May 1994), and 9) information on illnesses and injuries associated with the use of selected dietary supplements. The concluding bibliography cites both professional level and popular sources. Another bonus is a detailed index. Although its vocabulary aims at a well educated audience, the *Encyclopedia of Vitamins, Minerals and Supplements* would be a useful addition to library collections serving the general public.

9.34 Winter R. *A Consumer's Guide to Medicines in Food—Nutraceuticals That Help Prevent and Treat Physical and Emotional Illness*. New York: Crown, 1995.

A very different writing style and tone will be found in *A Consumer's Guide to Medicines in Food—Nutraceuticals*, exemplified by a chapter entitled "Why now purple cow?" Despite occasional lapses into language seemingly intended to provoke curiosity or laughter, Winter appears to offer sound, well-referenced advice and informed discussion of nutraceuticals. The author begins by explaining that this term was coined by DeFelice to give a wide-ranging field of scientific inquiry an identity, because "it extends from what chimpanzees eat when they don't feel well to creating superfoods through biotechnology." A nutraceutical is defined as any substance that may be considered a food, or part of a food, and that provides medical or health benefits, encompassing both the prevention and treatment of disease.

Falling under this semantic umbrella is an understandably diverse group of products: e.g., processed foods such as special cereals, herbal extracts, dietary supplements, and genetically engineered "designer" foods. Also called "prescriptive foods," nutraceuticals are not officially recognized as a distinct drug group under U.S. law. In Japan, Winter explains, they are known as FOSHU (foods for specified health use) and licensed by the government to make health claims. This book supplies information on food sources of nutrients and backs up discussion of nutraceuticals' potential benefits, as well as risks, with superscripted numbered references. The resulting bibliography belies its rather consciously coy packaging by assembling a helpful list of reputable sources. An appendix also lists U.S. government recommendations for nutrients.

9.35 Ody P. *The Complete Medicinal Herbal*. New York: Dorling Kindersley, 1993.
9.36 Bremness L. *Herbs*. Eyewitness Handbook Series. New York: Dorling Kindersley, 1994.

Ody's *Complete Medicinal Herbal* resembles a modest coffee table book, with its numerous colorful illustrations. Nonetheless, it includes a bibliography of reliable sources, although citations are, regrettably, not keyed to individual entries in the main portion of this volume. The author draws upon both Eastern and Western herbal traditions (European, Chinese, Ayurvedic) in compiling information on more than 250 remedies for common ailments. The *Herbal* opens with a brief historical overview, followed by a catalog of 120 botanicals listed alphabetically by Latin name and accompanied by pictures, a description of their medicinal applications, and cautions regarding use. A separate how-to section furnishes tips on harvesting and drying herbs, and on preparation of infusions, tinctures, syrups, unfused oils, creams, ointments, powders, capsules, compresses, and poultices. The final section, Home Remedies, groups entries by ailments, such as aches and pains or respiratory disorders.

Herbs, from the Eyewitness Handbook Series, would be an appropriate companion volume for a consumer collection, with more than 1,500 color photographs of 700 species and a separate section on healing herbs. Indexed by both common and scientific name, entries are arranged alphabetically within sections dedicated to general types of plants (e.g., trees, shrubs, herbaceous perennials, fungi). Illustrations are thoroughly annotated, providing a verbal description of significant characteristics and information on natural habitat. This beautiful little book does not, unfortunately, supply any references to the primary literature. Instead, it offers a "photo-encyclopedic approach" to the identification of botanicals and their chief uses, including aromatherapy, beauty treatment, and medical applications.

9.37 Juhn G. *Understanding the Pill. A Consumer's Guide to Oral Contraceptives*. Binghamton, NY: Pharmaceutical Products Press, 1994.

Another publication dealing with a frequently requested specialty topic is *Understanding the Pill*. Despite the fact that oral contraceptives are one of the few categories of prescription products for which a patient package insert (PPI) must be distributed when these drugs are dispensed in the United States, many questions on managing side effects and noncontraceptive uses of "the Pill" are not answered in the federally mandated PPI. Juhn explains how birth control pills work, differentiates among different types of medication (forms and levels of estrogen and progestin, 21- or 28-day schedules, RU486), and discusses risks and benefits in clear, easy-to-understand language (unlike the Pill package insert). Use of oral contraceptives for treatment of menstrual problems and these agents' other noncontraceptive actions earn an entire chapter's discussion in this book, as do alternative methods of birth control, and recurring questions (and answers) about the Pill. A glossary defines common gynecological terms, and a bibliography lists additional resources evaluated by the author.

9.38 Ferko AP, Barbieri EJ, DiGregorio GJ. *Warning: Drugs in Sports*. Philadelphia: Medical Surveillance, 1995.

The purpose of *Warning: Drugs in Sports* is to provide basic information about misuse of drugs by some athletes to enhance their individual performance and the potential dangers to which these individuals may be exposing themselves. The authors are pharmacology and medical faculty at Hahnemann University and the Medical College of Pennsylvania. Appropriate and inappropriate use of drugs, how drugs work in the body, an overview of drugs in sports, and major drugs of abuse (cocaine, marijuana, alcohol) are topics covered in introductory chapters, followed by brief monographs on individual substances. Substance entries, arranged by nonproprietary name, list common brand names, drug class, approved therapeutic use, illicit use by athletes, possible adverse effects resulting from improper use, and whether or not the drug is banned by the International Olympic Committee or the U.S. Olympic Committee.

The index to this slim volume provides access to substance monographs with both brand and generic name listings. Although an attempt has been made to identify additional sources of information in a separate section, the bibliography is somewhat sparse, including one pharmacology textbook, the *Physicians' Desk Reference* (6.10), *Drug Facts and Comparisons* (6.2), and a diverse list of thirty-six journal titles ranging from *Amino Acids* to *Adolescence*, and *Ergonomics* to the *New England Journal of Medicine*. The chief strength of *Warning: Drugs in Sports* is its highly focused scope. By concentrating on relaying basic information in everyday language, the authors have produced a practical manual for non-health-science professionals who must cope with an increasingly prevalent problem.

Consumer Drug Information on the Internet

Health is one of the hottest topics on the Internet, and consumer interest has spawned a surfeit of Web sites running the gamut from the reputable to the ridiculous. The U.S. government attempts to lend a helping hand in sorting out choices with its *HealthFinder* (http://www.healthfinder.gov) gateway. It includes a section on finding and evaluating online sources that is likely to be of more interest to information professionals than to the general public. For example, one option is a three-page Web site evaluation form available from Emory University's Office of Health Promotion.[12] Another *HealthFinder* link leads to a lengthy White Paper prepared for the Health Information Technology Institute of Mitretek Systems.[13] This document proposes a set of criteria that could be used by the general public to assess the quality of health information on the Internet.

A few additional references may be helpful to consumers seeking general guidelines on evaluating Web sites. Warning that medical data on the Net "ranges from rigorously peer-reviewed research to the electronic equivalent of the National Enquirer," McKenna has compiled a useful chart of evaluation tips for the general public.[14] Stephen Barrett, albeit less dispassionately, lists "Signs of a 'Quacky' Web Site" as part of his own contribution (see *QuackWatch* below). Renner[15] offers a medical doctor's perspective in two installments written for

Reuters Internet Health Watch. He outlines criteria used in his own reviews, with examples of what to look for when weighing content, credibility, off-site links, technical implementation, and ease of use.

There is nothing particularly novel in factors identified as key indicators of quality on the Web, compared to hardcopy attributes discussed in Chapter Five. Accuracy, timeliness, origin, documentation, and credibility are as important in judging online resources as in critiques of hardcopy publications. There are, however, major impediments to assessments of Internet publications, most of which center around non-disclosure. Whether intentional or unintentional, omission of pertinent information about a site's sponsor and contributing authors is a common occurrence. The URL is sometimes an indicator of nonprofit versus commercial status and academic versus home hobbyist origin, but clues such as these are not necessarily predictors of credibility.

Author or editor names can be extremely difficult to track down, as can their credentials. On one pharmacy subject hub examined for possible inclusion here, it was possible only to deduce that the author graduated from a school of pharmacy (evidenced by a commencement photo provided) and that she liked cats (another photo). No name or employment history was available. Even in a subject hub, this coyly casual approach detracts from the potential value of its content. When a Web resource contains more than one-line hotlinks, examining authority becomes critical. Anonymity is automatically suspect, and humility definitely misplaced, in the context of conveying scientific data.

Determining update frequency of Web sites is another challenge. Technology enables providers to change dates automatically. A site may be dead, so to speak, but offer few vital signs to diagnose its moribund state. Selected portions may, in fact, be updated, while the home page calendar remains fixed. Nondisclosure of data sources is also all too common, particularly in consumer-oriented publications. The prevailing sentiment appears to be that the general public is uninterested in back-up bibliography, so why bother? The result is a frustrating lack of information on which to base estimates of worth.

As annotations below will reveal, another criterion important in Web site evaluation is design. Is the source logically organized and easy to navigate? Does the interface provide adequate cues/clues to help consumers sort out what they need? For example, browsable indexes are useful assistants in a discipline where spelling is notoriously difficult. Access to brand names is also extremely desirable in consumer drug information sources. Most drug compendia focus, understandably, on active ingredients identified by nonproprietary (generic) names. Therefore, a bridge between brand and generic terminology needs to be provided. This is particularly important in sources that present information in records covering entire pharmacological categories (a time-saving, but arcane, practice to avoid in disseminating knowledge to lay readers).

Here, then, is a listing of the better sources of consumer drug information on the Web as of January 1999. *USP Dispensing Information—Volume 2: Advice for the Patient* (9.1) is ubiquitous, so differences in user interfaces require careful consideration when comparing sites, along with other extras found at a given URL.

InteliHealth—U.S. Pharmacopeia Dispensing Information
 ➪ http://ipn.intelihealth.com

Search capabilities offered to consumers for accessing *USP DI Advice for the Patient* are more forgiving than *InteliHealth*'s interface constructed for Volume 1 (see Chapter Six). Either brand or generic names can be submitted to the search engine, and separate alphabetical indexes of each type of name are also offered for browsing. *InteliHealth* makes two other USP databases available, as well: *Patient Education Leaflets* and *Medicine Charts* (photographs of dosage forms). Other bonuses at this site are the Condition Center, which uses the *Johns Hopkins Encyclopedia* as its source, and *InteliHealth*'s well-annotated list of links to other consumer health URLs.

Onhealth Resources
 ➪ http://www.onhealth.com/ch1/resource

IVI Publishing's *Onhealth* resource menu includes the USP Drug Database (again, that's *USP DI Advice for the Patient*), fact sheets for various medical conditions, an overview of alternative medical practices, and an index to common names of 140 herbs. *USP DI* is accessible via a browsable index that mingles both brand and generic names for easy use. Structured entries include separately displayable sections devoted to precautions, possible interactions, proper use and storage, major side effects, and other frequently asked questions. Extras here: *Onhealth* herbal monographs identify the scientific plant name, include a general description, and discuss target ailments, precautions, and OTC ready-made, as well as home-made, preparations.

MedicineNet—The Pharmacy
 ➪ http://www.medicinenet.com

Clicking on *The Pharmacy* in the left-hand frame of *MedicineNet*'s home page opens up an alphabetic index that includes both brand and generic names. Links from each index entry lead to a "Forum" for the drug, where information from all sections of this multilevel site is assembled in a structured menu. It begins with a link to the main drug monograph, whose content is supplied by a network of U.S. Board-certified physicians and allied health professionals (including two PharmDs). A second option in the Forum is to view data on related diseases and treatments. "The Doctor's Responses" are the last menu choice, where pertinent FAQs regarding the target drug are available for display. Another selection that sometimes also appears on the Forum results page is Related News & Updates. For example, if a new side effect has been reported recently, this fact would be discussed in the accompanying text. The interface on *MedicineNet* is a bit unusual, but easy to follow. The quality of consumer drug monographs is also unusual, but a welcome change from standard *USP DI* fare.

E-Pharmacy by Eckerd: OTC Resource Center
⇨ http://www.e-pharmacy.com/HTML/health_info/otc/index.html

The *Consumer Guide to Over-the-Counter Drugs* published by Eckerd Drugs is one of the best ready-reference sourcebooks on the Internet. Each separately accessible section addresses choosing the proper OTC product for a given condition. Topics covered include colds or allergic rhinitis, pain or fever relief, antacid/antiulcer products, antidiarrheals or laxatives, sleep-aids or stimulants, ophthalmic medications, antiemetics or emetics, antibacterials or antifungals, hemorrhoidal products, and vitamin, mineral, and herb supplements. Sections begin with guidelines for self-diagnosis (If you have . . . take . . .). Basic physiology is reviewed, along with explanations of how different categories of drugs act in the body. Tables conclude each section, listing common single source (brand) or multisource (generic/brand) OTC drugs, dosage forms available, and ingredients.

Two tables in the dietary supplements segment of the *Guide* are particularly noteworthy. One lists medicinal herbs considered safe, their uses, and precautions. A second identifies medicinal herbs considered unsafe, "So-called Uses," and side effects. In many respects, Eckerd's *Consumer Guide* is similar to the *Handbook of Nonprescription Drugs* (6.6) published by the American Pharmaceutical Association. This site could be as useful to health science professionals as it is to consumers; the reading level and general tone aims at a fairly high level of education and communication skills.

FDA Consumer Information—Drug Database
⇨ http://www.fda.gov/cder/consumerinfo

Staff of the FDA's Center for Drug Evaluation and Research prepare brief consumer-oriented monographs based on approved package insert information. They summarize the basics about new and innovative drugs approved since January, 1998. All drugs covered in the still tiny database at this URL are listed by brand name in the left-hand frame. Only twenty-six products are listed as of January, 1999. Full professional package inserts are hotlinked from consumer monographs—which would appear to undermine the purpose of creating patient leaflets in everyday language.

Another hidden gem among the multitude of choices offered elsewhere on the FDA site is a pamphlet entitled *Nonprescription Medicines, What's Right for You?* It is the attractive outcome of a joint project of the FDA and the Nonprescription Drug Manufacturers Association. The URL is http://www.fda.gov/opacom/what'sright. Refer to Chapter Sixteen for a detailed description of other *FDA Home Page* content, including additional material appropriate for consumers.

Dr. Koop's Community: The Pharmacy and *The Medicine Cabinet*
⇨ http://www.drkoop.com/drugstore

Visitors can invoke a browsable index of specific brand or generic names simply by entering a single letter (alphabetical character) into the search form on this Web page. However, not every drug shown on the resulting list has information associated with it, which is disconcerting, once a selection has been made. It is only after a query fails that you're likely to take seriously the small check-off box on the entry form labeled: "Only search drugs that have a drug information page." The question is, why would anyone want to search for names where no information would be provided? The interface has other quirks related to over-reliance on frames that make it awkward to use. Nevertheless, drug leaflets, once found, are well written and attractively presented. They are supplied by Multum Information Services.

Dr. Koop's Pharmacy also includes a drug interaction searching module. This program enables entry of multiple suspected agents for cross-checking. Drug interactions documented are graded by severity, and include drug-food effects. *The Medicine Cabinet* section of *Dr. Koop's Community* offers information on vitamins and minerals and guidelines for medication safety. Under the heading "Your Medicine Cabinet," a list of recommended drugs to have on hand is crosslinked to a medical encyclopedia with information on drug classes, such as uses, cautions, and side effects. A glossary supplies quick definitions of common pharmacy terms and drug-related vocabulary.

Mediconsult—General Drug Information
⇨ http://www.mediconsult.com/general/drugs

USP Advice for the Patient is the source reached through the search form at this URL. The interface will accept either brand or generic names and even condition keywords. However, queries often lead to general drug class monographs from *USP DI*, a possible way to perplex patients. Offsetting this flaw is additional drug information available in *Mediconsult*'s Educational Material section, where a variety of conditions are covered. One selection offered for display under most of these conditions is an excellent counseling aid entitled *Prescription Medicines and You*. This publication originates from a collaboration of the National Council for Patient Information and Education and the Agency for Health Care Policy and Research.

Medication Info Search
⇨ http://www.cheshire-med.com/services/pharm/med-form.cgi

The Cheshire Medical Center (Keene, NH) provides consumer-oriented drug information originating from First DataBank (suppliers to *Medscape*). The search form accepts brand or generic names, drug class terms, or disease/condition keywords. More unusually, it also enables Boolean logical combinations (asthma

AND . . .). Queries can, as in *USP DI*, lead to monographs covering drug classes. For example, in response to verapamil, results included an entry for calcium channel blockers and additional references to other monographs where verapamil was mentioned as an interacting agent. This characteristic could confuse consumers. Another way to retrieve medication information at this site is to scan an alphabetic index of generic and class names, cross referenced to brands. However, cross referencing is not reciprocal, i.e., there are no separate entries in this index for brands.

Healthtouch Online Drug Information

⇨ http://www/healthtouch.com/level1/p_dri.htm

Healthtouch Online Drug Information includes data on more than 7,000 prescription and over-the-counter medications, briefly highlighting common indications, self administration and storage instructions, and possible side effects. The source of these data is Medi-Span®. The database is searchable by brand or generic name.

MediSpan Drug Information Database from The Wellness International Network

⇨ http://www.stayhealth.com/medispan/index.html

The *Medispan Drug Information Database* includes very basic and brief patient information, embellished with dosage form images for some selections. Entries list sources of drugs (that is, companies) marketing the medication under a brand or generic name. The database can be searched by either type of name, with the alternative of browsing an integrated A–Z index to both trade and nonproprietary terms, as well.

Philadelphia Online—Health Philadelphia

⇨ http://health.phillynews.com/pharmacy/search.asp

Like *InteliHealth, Onhealth*, and *Mediconsult*, the Philadelphia site draws on the resources of the *U.S. Pharmacopeia* to provide consumers with reliable information about their prescriptions. The hardcopy counterpart is, again, *Advice for the Patient*. The interface here is slightly more intimidating than that constructed by others, requiring users to distinguish between generic or brand names when choosing which of two separate alphabetic indexes to browse. A second screen displays all matches found (single drug monographs, combinations, or those constructed for broad therapeutic classes), again asking the user to make selections from hotlinks that can be somewhat daunting to the uninitiated (e.g., See Angiotensin-converting Enzyme (ACE) Inhibitors, Systemic). Nonetheless, once reached, the information provided is identical to that offered in the hardcopy text or on the other USP-derived databases cited in this section.

Mayo Clinic Health Oasis Medicine Center

⇨ http://www.mayohealth.org/usp/common/index.htm

The *Medicine Center*'s menu includes the *USP Drug Guide* (a.k.a. *Advice for the Patient*), general drug information, and reference articles. The *USP* interface is comparatively poor, offering access by an index to generic names only. There are also no cross references from names covered in larger drug class monographs. For example, captopril cannot be found in Mayo's index to *USP DI*, because this drug is one of many folded into a mega-monograph on ACE inhibitors. Consumers can hardly be expected to cope with this user-hostile barrier. The General Drug Information option in the *Medicine Center* is a much more straightforward route to high quality consumer-oriented guides, such as pages devoted to avoiding medication mishaps, communicating with your healthcare provider, storing drugs, and interpreting expiration dating. Under the *Medicine Center*'s heading for Reference Articles is an impressive library of drug-related features from the *Mayo Clinic Health Letter*.

Medscape Drug Search from First DataBank
⇨ http://www.medscape.com/misc/formdrugs.html
Medscape Patient Information
⇨ (http://Patient.medscape.com/Home/Patient/PatientInfo.html

The best thing about Medscape's *Drug Search* is its scope: 20,000 drug products are covered in the *National Drug Data File* (*NDDF*) from First DataBank. The interface enables searching by brand or generic names, as well as disease/condition terms. The drawback to direct access by consumers is that the main portion of *NDDF* monographs is intended for use by health science professionals. However, as an aid to medication counseling, every *NDDF* entry includes a separate patient education monograph that can be displayed and printed for dissemination to clients. Under the *Medscape Patient Information* URL, visitors will find a menu of conditions, such as AIDS, allergies, blood diseases and disorders, etc. Text supplied is derived from government, association, and commercial publishers, including the National Eye Institute, *U.S. Pharmacist* magazine, the Micromedex *CareNotes*™ system, and patient information cards from *Hippocrates*.

Health-Center.com: Pharmacy
⇨ http://www.healthguide.com/english/pharmacy

Health-Center.com provides overviews of classes of medications, supported by bibliographic references. Categories addressed include: ADHD, antianxiety, antidepressant, mood stabilizer, antipsychotic, hormone, pain, and Parkinson's Disease medications. Under an icon labeled Other Medications, important counseling issues are discussed, such as things to tell your doctor, ways to remember your medication, and common questions about prescriptions. The content of this *Health-Center.com* area was developed by Clinical Tools, Inc., with research funding from the U.S. National Institute of Mental Health.

Drug INFONET Patient Package Inserts
⇨ http://www.druginfonet.com/ppi.htm

Drug INFONET provides direct links to PPIs supplied by five manufacturers. The collection can be accessed by browsing a list that includes brand, generic, manufacturer, and therapeutic class names. Only sixteen products are currently covered.

Virtual Drugstore—Vimy Park Pharmacy
⇨ http://www.virtualdrugstore.com/druglist.html

Visitors will find a table cross referencing common conditions to drug generic and brand names on the opening screen of the *Virtual Drugstore*. Clicking on a specific drug name leads to a patient monograph for the active ingredient. It, in turn, includes a hotlink to the drug class. Drug class entries list hotlinks to monographs for other drugs in the same category. Monographs usually include one or two references for further reading. Material offered at this site has been researched and written by Marie Berry, a lawyer and pharmacist working in Winnipeg, Manitoba.

RxHealth.com Drug and Disease Information Service
⇨ http://www.rxhealth.com

This site is provided by licensed Canadian pharmacists and limits its scope to patients with asthma, cardiovascular disease, diabetes, migraine or cluster headaches, or sexually transmitted diseases. For each category of ailment, drug information offers an overview of classes of drugs used in treatment, with an emphasis on background needed to increase compliance.

PediWeb
⇨ http://solar.rtd.utk.edu/~esmith/pedi.html

PediWeb is a pharmacy pediatrics page originating from the University of Tennessee's residency program for PharmD pediatric specialists. This attractively presented site includes sections for news, articles, reviews, and other links, plus a useful Parents Corner.

Columbia University College of Physicians & Surgeons Complete Home Medical Guide
⇨ http://cpmcnet.columbia.edu/texts/guide

Chapter 34 in Columbia's outstanding *Complete Home Medical Guide* is devoted to the Proper Use of Medications. Topics addressed include filling the prescription, the dosing schedule, forms of medications, side effects and drug allergies, drug interactions, traveling with drugs, drug classifications, and the home medicine chest. There is also a helpful list of abbreviations. Another portion of the *Guide* to note is Appendix A, devoted to commonly prescribed drugs. It consists of a table listing drugs by generic name, followed by brands, common side effects, drug interactions, and precautions.

PharmWeb—Patient Information
  ⇨ http://asclepius.ic.gc.ca/pwmirror/pwz/pharmwebz.html

Better known as a subject hub for pharmacy professionals, *PharmWeb* does include a small library of helpful educational materials. A section on how to use medicines focuses on self-administration instructions for ear, eye, or nose drops, eye ointment, pessaries or vaginal cream, suppositories, malaria tablets, and using a nebulizer. The text is based on patient information leaflets supplied by the U.K. National Pharmaceutical Association. Another *PharmWeb* series of consumer pages is a guide to treatment of common ailments, with coverage of athletes foot, cold sores, coughs, eye conditions, hayfever, migraine, mouth ulcers, vaginal thrush (candidiasis), and foot care for corns or bunions.

Avoiding Food and Drug Interactions
  ⇨ http://www.foodsafety.org/sf/sf162.htm

Linda Bobroff, an Assistant Professor at the University of Florida's Institute of Food and Agricultural Sciences, provides a consumer-oriented, but well referenced and lengthy, introduction to this important topic. It includes an overview of basic types of interactions and discussion of drug effects on nutritional status, food effects on drug absorption and utilization, and potential effects of sodium and alcohol. A helpful table organizes information for quick reference under the column headings: If You Take . . . , It's Wise to Avoid . . . , Because. . . .

Pharmaceutical Research and Manufacturers of America
  ⇨ http://www.phrma.org/publications/brochure/leading/lead10.html

PhRMA publishes an excellent *Health Guide Series* of booklets and also makes them available for immediate display on its Web site. Topics covered include heart attacks, breast cancer, strokes, prostate problems, menopause and osteoporosis, depression and mental illness, HIV/AIDS, Alzheimer's disease, cancer treatments, and getting the most from your medicines. Another set of patient-oriented publications issued online by PhRMA are overviews of diseases or special populations. Each summarizes key epidemiological data, as well as audits what's in the R&D pipeline for the target condition or group. This *New Medicines in Development Series* currently includes titles focusing on AIDS, biotechnology, cancer, heart disease and stroke, mental illnesses, neurologic disorders, new drug approvals, older Americans, and women.

Pharmacy and You—American Pharmaceutical Association
  ⇨ http://www.pharmacyandyou.org

APhA's new consumer home page includes brief explanations on topics such as pharmacists' licensure, education, and patient medication records. A Health Information section currently offers guidelines for coping with coughs and colds, chronic pain, epilepsy, and fever in your child. Under the heading About Your

Medicine is a meaty menu of useful advisories, including a guide to educating children about medicines, avoiding medication errors, asking pharmacists about nonprescription medicines, and reviewing the household medication inventory. A section labeled Facts About Patients is chock-a-block with statistics about prescription and OTC drug use, as well as consumer beliefs and practices related to medication use. *Pharmacy and You* also compiles a nationwide directory of poison control centers.

Pharmacy Times Patient Education Focus
⇨ http://www.pharmacytimes.com/pated.html

The retail trade magazine *Pharmacy Times* has assembled five pamphlets at this URL. Although intended for use by community pharmacists to print out and offer as handouts in the prescription pickup area, they can just as easily be accessed on the Web by patients themselves. Topics covered include diet aids, poison prevention, OTC medications and pregnancy, a parent's guide to infant formula, and poison ivy, oak, and sumac.

How to Read the Prescription
⇨ http://www.ns.net/users/ryan/rxabrv.html

Ryan Seo, a pharmacist at Sutter Medical Center in Sacramento, California, has created a key to common medical abbreviations used in written prescriptions.

Herbal Medicine and Dietary Supplement Sites for the Consumer

The use of herbal medicines in the United States has increased by 380% since 1990, according to Eisenberg's latest landmark study of trends in alternative medicine use.[16] In 1997 alone, an estimated fifteen million U.S. adults took herbal remedies and/or high dose vitamins concurrently with prescription medications. Since this figure represents roughly one in five prescription users, it's obvious that many consumers will be surfing the Web for information on botanicals, nutraceuticals, and related therapies. Internet coverage of ethnobotanical uses is particularly noteworthy, as is the scope of sites dedicated to identifying harmful or poisonous plants.

At the same time, separating the riches from the rubble is an ongoing challenge. The list of resources annotated in this section is, admittedly, quite selective (thorough coverage would require another book). Additional, more professionally oriented, herbal home pages are discussed in Chapter Twelve in the section on Pharmacognosy. Because the line between the professional and the popular in this subject area is by no means distinct, several titles featured under Pharmacognosy could also be equally useful to consumers. Fee-based sources of bibliography on medicinal plants can be found in Chapter Fourteen.

Algy's Herb Page
⇨ http://www.algy.com/herb/index.html

Somewhat frivolous at first glance (e.g., sections on gardening, cooking, and a seed exchange), *Algy's Herb Page* does include reputable material relevant to alternative medicine under its Apothecary icon. Unfortunately, it is easy to be diverted into segments devoted to recent Herb Talk bulletin board postings before finally tracking down more substantive material hidden under Links. Here, the page under Medicinal Herbs is the best selection. It begins with a series of full-text articles focusing on precautions, including an index of poisons and warnings about over-the-counter herbal remedies. Among items listed under Preparation is a Common Name Index, accessible by more than 800 terms, and ultimately linking to Grieve's *Modern Herbal*. Algy's annotated list of hotlinked databases includes click-on pointers to articles about individual plants, links to condition-specific articles, and a route to an Herbal Encyclopedia that enables browsing of symptoms or condition keywords to locate cross references to herbs that have been used to treat them.

Mrs. Grieve's A Modern Herbal
  ⇨ http://www.botanical.com/botanical/mgmh/mgmh.html

First published in 1931 by Mrs. M. Grieve, the database covers more than 800 plants. Lengthy monographs address medicinal, culinary, and cosmetic uses. Each entry lists synonyms, part used, habitat, physical description, cultivation, constituents, and preparation, along with folklore applications. Supportive bibliographic references are, unfortunately, few and far between. In addition to a browsable common plant name index, the file can be approached through a keyword search engine accessing the 860 pages of text. This Web page also offers separate indexes of recipes (29 plants) and poisons (44 plants). The remainder of *Botanical.com*'s site is largely dedicated to unannotated hotlinks to related Web resources.

Acupuncture.com
  ⇨ http://www.acupuncture.com/

This excellent Web site extends its scope beyond acupuncture to encompass herbology, Qi Gong, Chinese nutrition, Tui Na and Chinese massage, and diagnostics. Information for consumers includes well written explanations of each type of therapy and a listing of specific conditions where they are used. A directory of practitioners covers thirty-three countries, with entries for the United States subdivided by state, for the United Kingdom by country, and for Canada by province. "Marketplace" selections lead to reviews of books and software, product manufacturers or distributors, educational opportunities, and insurance companies that cover acupuncture.

Student Resources include a list of schools and colleges, associations, and a state-by-state guide to acupuncture laws (as of 1995). The section devoted to practitioners is equally informative. It offers discussion of clinical acupuncture points, treatment protocols, and underlying principles. A bibliography of traditional Chinese medical (TCM) journals features hypertext links, when available. A directory of professional organizations and a segment devoted to CEUs and seminars are other options. Under "Politics That Affect TCM," the news section is particularly noteworthy for its quality and timeliness.

MotherNature.com (formerly *Mother Nature's General Store*)
⇨ http://www.mothernature.com/

As its former title indicates, the original purpose of *MotherNature.com* was online shopping. The catalog taps into wares of more than 400 manufacturers of 30,000 health products. These include vitamins, nutritional supplements, minerals, bath & body preparations, herbs, homeopathic medications, aromatherapy, teas, and sports nutrition products. Along the way, however, *MotherNature.com* has evolved into a major consumer health education resource. For example, vernacular plant/herb name searches in the mail order catalog lead to a selection of products on the market containing the specified ingredient. In addition to noting product availability, search results include cross references to articles found elsewhere at this site. Monographs for individual herbs identify parts used and geographic distribution, health conditions in which the herb might be supportive, historical or traditional uses, active constitutents, normal dosage, and side effects or interactions. Color photographs enhance each entry and bibliographic references are always included.

An electronic *Health Encyclopedia* can also be consulted at *MotherNature.com*, independent of any ordering activity. Researched and written by a team of healthcare professionals (all of whose résumés are disclosed), the *Encyclopedia* is a treasure trove of high quality consumer health information. It includes a section on Health Concerns with 125 modules to choose from, each offering a description of the condition and a critical review of dietary supplements that may be helpful. All *Encyclopledia* entries provide references to peer reviewed primary literature. Other major subdivisions in this impressive e-book address nutritional supplements (239 entries), herbs and botanical extracts (150), homeopathic remedies (148), drug-herb/other supplement interactions for 100 of the most commonly prescribed drugs, and dozens of diet and other alternative therapies.

Another *MotherNature* bonus is a series of *Consumer Guides*, accessible from the Store Front menu. These publications are designed to help the general public make informed purchasing decisions. For example, the *Consumer Guide to Herbs* examines the issue of concentration versus potency and discusses various dosage forms available. Additional *Consumer Guides* are offered for vitamins, minerals, and supplements. As if this weren't enough, *MotherNature* also provides a Reading Room icon that leads to a classified archive of articles drawn from numerous sources, as well as back issues from *MotherNature*'s own online *Health Journal*.

Health WWWeb™—Integrative Medicine, Natural Health and Alternative Therapies
⇨ http://www.healthwwweb.com/

The Links Directory can be approached through thirty-one subject categories, most of which are devoted to broadly defined modalities such as herbs and botanical medicine, homeopathy, nutrition, and pharmacology. Hotlinked entries lack annotations, but do include full URLs for future reference, if the contents were transferred to paper. The integrative philosophy reflected in the site's title is also evident in its Web source list, where pertinent traditional online databases (*CAB Abstracts, EMBASE*) are cited side-by-side with smaller, Internet-only specialty resources.

Health WWWeb is more than a pathfinder to other sites. Its Resource Guide section includes a geographically classified international directory of licensed practitioners. Under the heading Health Information and Tools for Wellness, there is a collection of introductory articles on acupuncture, herbal dosing, and related topics. Monographs (with bibliographic references) on nine herbal medicines found in this section come from the *IBIS*™ (*Integrative Body Mind Information System*) database. *Health WWWeb*'s diet and nutrition section includes specific diets and background on popular remedies, but claims far outnumber supportive references to the primary literature here.

Natural Health Village
⇨ http:www.naturalhealthvillage.com

As a targeted news source for all types of alternative therapies, this home page is practically unparalleled in quality and merits frequent visits. Its Town Hall section provides an e-mail directory of U.S. Senate and House members and features informed discussion of pending federal legislation, such as the Access to Medical Treatment Act. Special reports offered under Town Hall include NIH's *Unconventional Cancer Treatments*, AMA's Council on Scientific Affairs *Report on Alternative Medicine*, and the *Report of the Special Committee on Health Care Fraud* from the Federation of State Medical Boards. Under Learning Center, users will find a free copy of *Alternative Medicine: Expanding Medical Horizons*, available for downloading in segments that can be selected from a detailed table of contents. The Learning Center also offers a medium size list of links to other sites, classified by subject, with brief annotations to assist in prescreening resources.

For current awareness, check out the Media Watch within the Learning Center, as well as *Natural HealthLine*® newsletter coverage. Each biweekly issue is well worth scanning in its entirety, with news of forthcoming and just completed conferences, legislative developments at the state level (as well as worldwide), commentary on pertinent television and radio programs, and notices of new books, Web pages, and other resources. Information is culled from scientific journals and business publications and replete with helpful hypertext links to primary sources. Back issues of *Natural HealthLine* are available through August 1996, accessible through the Site Index.

QuackWatch
⇨ http://www.quackwatch.com/

Fraud buster Stephen Barrett, MD, has assembled here a formidable collection of editorials and advice to encourage intelligent health decision making on the part of consumers. On the positive side, consumer protection books, magazines, and newsletters considered to be valuable are identified, along with helpful doctor-patient communication tips and "Signs of a 'Quacky' Web Site." A detailed table of contents makes the site easy to navigate, although a search engine has also been implemented to find all mentions of a specific topic in documents accessible via the home page. Separate sections are devoted to questionable products and services, misleading advertisements, "Golden Duck Media Awards" for credulous coverage, and "nonrecommended" sources of advice (naming specific books, individuals, organizations, periodicals, and publishers). Segments promised in the future are "Web Sites to Avoid" and "Prudent Use of Health Information on the Internet."

Barrett's take-no-prisoners style and sometimes sweeping indictments (e.g., "Ayurvedic Mumbo-Jumbo," "Homeopathy: The Ultimate Fake") may raise some eyebrows, but a visit to this URL is undoubtedly a useful antidote to much that is available elsewhere on the Internet concerning alternative health care. Access to two full length books is a bonus: the 300-page *Unconventional Cancer Treatments* issued by the U.S. Office of Technology Assessment in 1990 (filterable through a search engine, with a detailed table of contents for prescreening) and a 130-page *Dictionary of Metaphysical Healthcare* (J. Raso, 1997). The latter offers descriptions, pronunciations, and synonyms for 1,169 alternative medical methods, accessible from a browsable alphabetical index, and supported by a bibliography and general glossary of terms. In addition, detailed table of contents listings are shown for issues of the *NCAHF Newsletter* dating from January 1993 forward, supplemented with links to full-text articles from the National Council Against Health Fraud.

McMaster University's Health Care Information Resources—Alternative Medicine
⇨ http://www-hsl.mcmaster.ca/tomflem/altmed.html

McMaster's twenty-four pages of links are accompanied by descriptive annotations intended for consumers. Sites are organized into categories, beginning with general resources, and continuing on to twenty-five specific alternative medical methods or systems, including aromatherapy, flower remedies, herbal therapy, homeopathy, Kombucha tea, naturopathy, and shark cartilage. Introductory notes also point to a set of links to Web sites that specialize in discussion of healthcare fraud, available in a separate McMaster bibliography labeled "Illness." Best feature: several Canadian sites overlooked elsewhere are identified here, along with pertinent French-language home pages originating in both Canada and France. Worst feature: evaluative commentary tends to be uniformly glowing.

University of Pittsburgh—The Alternative Medicine Homepage
➪ http://www.pitt.edu/~cbw/altm.html

Maintained by Charles B. Wessel of the Falk Library of the Health Sciences at
the University of Pittsburgh, this large directory of Internet sites is an excellent
starting point for further Web crawling. Not only is the list satisfyingly lengthy,
it includes extremely helpful descriptive annotations, many of which explain the
basic tenets of the therapy targeted by a given site.

Tufts University Nutrition Navigator
➪ http://navigator.tufts.edu/index.html

A project of the Center for Nutrition Communication at Tufts' School of Nutrition Science and Policy, this Web database compiles and rates an awe inspiring
array of Internet sources. Separately marked sections identify those appropriate
for a health professional audience, educators, journalists, and the general public.
A search form offers keyword access to the entire collection. Results of queries
consist of a relevance ranked list of site titles, each of which also bears a numeric
rating based on expert assessment of its overall content and usability. Hyperlinks
from results lead to the full text of Tufts' reviews. Individual review pages consistently identify site sponsor, type of organization (government, academic, commercial, etc.), intended audience, date reviewed, and scores for accuracy and
depth of information. Scores for nutrition accuracy weigh factors such as the scientific evidence presented, how well the information is referenced, and if it is
current.

Structured reviews of this type are rare on the Internet. The usual drawback to
sites requiring detailed editorial input are limited scope or size, slow growth, and
infrequent updates. None of these flaws is detectable here. New sites are added
on a monthly schedule, and reviews already present are revised or refreshed on a
quarterly schedule. The collection is large and diverse, encompassing more than
275 reviewed Web resources.

Sympatico HealthyWay: Health Links—Alternative Medicine Directory
➪ http://www1.sympatico.ca/healthyway/DIRECTORY/B1.html

Sympatico's *Health Links* directory also offers structured and timely reviews
of Web sites. Its scope extends beyond diet and nutrition to include acupuncture/
acupressure, aromatherapy, herbology, homeopathy, oriental medicine, and other
alternative medicine systems. Clicking on any of these categories from the main
menu found at this URL leads to a list of reviewed sites, complete with ratings,
audience, and content notes. Full reviews can then be displayed as follow up.
Lists of unreviewed sites and articles or FAQs are also available in each category.
Under herbology, for example, Sympatico assembles twenty reviewed resources,
nineteen unreviewed, and nine hotlinks to articles on topics such as plant pharmacy, herbal dosing methods and philosophies of prescribing, and side effects,

safety, and toxicity of medicinal herbs. A *HealthWay Magazine* also published at this site (accessible from Sympatico's health home page) often features useful articles on nutritional supplements and related hot topics.

Aids to Medication Counseling

Sources designed to assist healthcare professionals in counseling patients on their medications can also be appropriate selections for patient education libraries. One of the best examples is the American Pharmaceutical Association's *Handbook of Nonprescription Drugs* (6.6). Although intended to enhance pharmacists' competence in communicating with consumers about self-medication options, its format and writing style are sufficiently accessible to make it a good choice for direct consultation by patients.

Portions of the *PDR for Ophthalmology* (6.12) are also dedicated to advice for patients. Notes included in *Psychotropic Drugs: Fast Facts* (6.34) remind medical staff of what patients and their families need to know about medications prescribed, such as administration in relation to meals, how to deal with forgetting a dose, and how to cope with immediate side effects. Therapeutic drug compendia intended for nurses often supply practical advice on patient or family education. Sources with substance-specific annotations regarding patient communication include *Nurses Drug Facts* (6.62) and the *PDR Nurse's Handbook* (6.66). However, publications wholly dedicated to assisting care-givers in the often difficult task of counseling patients on their medications will augment brief coverage of the topic found elsewhere.

9.39 *Medication Teaching Manual: The Guide to Patient Drug Information.* 7th ed. Bethesda, MD: American Society of Health-System Pharmacists, 1998.

The American Society of Health-System Pharmacists' *Medication Teaching Manual* offers 600 easy-to-photocopy monographs with coverage of 1,700 products, including the top 200 prescribed medicines in the United States. These ASHP materials, written at the consumer level, are intended to supplement and reinforce oral instructions to patients, and include otherwise hard-to-find information about cancer chemotherapy drugs (60 monographs) and home infusion medications (83 entries). Monographs in the seventh edition have been updated to comply with guidelines for format and content proposed by the U.S. government in 1997. Appendices offer tips on coping with nausea, mouth discomfort, and other unpleasantly prevalent side effects, as well as advice to patients on improving nutrition. The *Medication Teaching Manual* also includes an English-to-Spanish conversion chart that translates dosage instructions, commonly needed phrases, and prescription orders. A separate *Manual de Enseñanza de Me-*

dicamentos en Español is also published by ASHP. The sixth edition, issued in 1995, contains 500 concise entries written in Spanish.

9.40 *Patient Drug Facts*. St. Louis, MO: Facts & Comparisons, 1989–. Quarterly.

Patient Drug Facts (formerly *Professional's Guide to Patient Drug Facts for Improved Patient Counseling*) consists of adaptations of monographs from the respected publication *Drug Facts and Comparisons* (6.2), but concentrates on medications most frequently prescribed or purchased. Single copies of entries for any one of the 450 drugs, representing information on more than 6,000 Rx and OTC products, can be freely reproduced and distributed to practitioners and patients. An unusual bonus is that uses cited include both FDA-approved and unlabeled indications. Another extra is an IBM-compatible software program on diskette that is bundled with subscriptions to the quarterly looseleaf volume. This program can be used to produce customized (to the patient, as well as to the dispensing pharmacy) single-page handouts in layman's language (8th-grade reading level).

The hardcopy *Patient Drug Facts* groups monographs by therapeutic class, offering tabbed sections devoted to nutritionals, cardiovasculars, gastrointestinals, etc. An alphabetical index provides cross references from brand and generic names. Product listings at the beginning of the volume show dosage forms and strengths commonly marketed and indicate when generic availability is an option. Appendices compile a list of necessary household medicines, a useful quick reference guide to drug names that look or sound alike, a directory of poison control centers, a list of normal laboratory values, and a list of oral dosage forms that should not be crushed. A Color Locator Guide to 900 drugs groups photographs by color, to assist in rapid visual identification of tablets and capsules.

9.41 Griffith HW. *Instructions for Patients*. 5th ed. Philadelphia: W.B. Saunders, 1994.

9.42 *Patient Counseling Handbook*. Washington, DC: American Pharmaceutical Association, 1998.

Griffith's *Instructions for Patients* is not limited to drug information. Three-hole-punched instruction sheets, designed for photocopying and redistribution, cover more than 250 regimens, disorders, and diseases, including special diets.

The APhA's *Patient Counseling Handbook* is based on *USP DI Volume 1* (6.5), extracting information on more than 700 commonly prescribed drugs. Every monograph includes separately labeled sections: "For the Pharmacist" and "For the Patient." An index provides access by both brand and nonproprietary names. This publication specifically addresses patient counseling requirements mandated under OBRA legislation passed in 1990 (see Chapter Four) and includes a checklist to assist the pharmacist in this process.

9.43 *USP DI Patient Education Leaflets*. Rockville, MD: U.S. Pharmacopeial
Convention, 1982–.
9.44 *Spanish Counseling Companion*. Rockville, MD: U.S. Pharmacopeial
Convention, 1992.

Other spinoffs from *USP DI* are *Patient Education Leaflets*, which can be ordered as separate, preprinted publications or in personalized format with an organization's name and address added as a heading. A further customized option allows purchasers to add a listing of brand and generic drugs included in their formulary and pictogram illustrations for patient instructions. Leaflets contain information abstracted from *Advice for the Patient*, furnished in either a full (full sentences) or abbreviated easy-to-read (printed in larger type with simplified text) versions. Many are also available in Spanish. The *Spanish Counseling Companion* assembles 200 of the most requested leaflet titles, translated into Spanish, in one looseleaf binder. (For additional quick-reference sources of patient instructions in other languages, see multilingual guides in Chapter Ten.)

9.45 *Nonprescription Drug References for Health Professionals*. Ottawa: Canadian Pharmaceutical Association, 1996.

The Canadian Pharmaceutical Association's *Nonprescription Drug References for Health Professionals* (*NDR*) is designed to help practitioners answer questions about OTC drugs and other self-treatment options. It opens with an overview of consumer counseling issues and discussion of special patient groups. Chapters that follow deal with major nonprescription drug classes, including homeopathic, herbal, and nutritional products, as well as medical devices. Most chapters include highlights that can be photocopied for patients. Previously titled *Self-Medication Reference for Health Professionals*, this handbook could be usefully complemented with information compiled in two direct-to-consumer publications from the CPhA: *Understanding Canadian Nonprescription Drugs* and *Understanding Canadian Prescription Drugs* (see Additional Sources at the end of this chapter).

9.46 Mason P. *Nutrition and Dietary Advice in the Pharmacy*. Oxford: Blackwell Scientific Publications, 1994.

Nutrition and Dietary Advice in the Pharmacy is written for pharmacists to assist them in offering practical advice on healthy eating and food safety and in counseling patients on products commonly sold in community settings, such as weight loss aids, infant formulas, baby foods, and dietary supplements. Special attention is also given to supporting patients maintained on enteral and parenteral nutrition at home. In addition, Mason offers guidance on helping customers understand the importance of diet in management of conditions such as hypertension and in meeting the special nutritional needs encountered in pregnancy, the elderly, athletes, and cultural minorities.

Particularly noteworthy is a chapter on cultural diversity, which brings together information on ethnic groups that will be useful to any health science professional in daily contact with the general public. For example, information about each group covered in this chapter includes the naming system, traditional form of address, predominant religion, and language. It discusses ethnic group dietary patterns (consumption, or lack thereof, of meat, fish, dairy products), nutritional problems likely to arise from these established dietary practices, and how to recognize when members of the ethnic group may require alternatives to oral medications, such as during ritually-related periods of fasting. Because this book originates in Great Britain, ethnic groups discussed are those most prevalent in that country (e.g., Asian, Afro-Caribbean).

Geography also limits the selection of products listed in the appendix, which includes a directory of manufacturer names and addresses and a table of brand name multivitamins and mineral supplements (none of which is separately indexed). Nonetheless, Mason transcends cultural and geopolitical boundaries by providing practical pointers for professionals in a unique position to influence consumer behavior where informed intervention is increasingly needed: nutrition and dietary practices affecting health status.

9.47 *Home Care Resource Book*. Bethesda, MD: American Society of Hospital Pharmacists, 1993.

The *Home Care Resource Book* is a compilation of materials from other American Society of Hospital Pharmacists (now Health-System Pharmacists) publications, with the intent of bringing together into one convenient package information useful to home care practitioners. It includes, for example, the newly approved "Guidelines on the Pharmacist's Role in Home Care" and the Society's "Technical Assistance Bulletin on Quality Assurance for Pharmacy-Prepared Sterile Products." It also assembles a collection of extracts drawn from the *International Pharmaceutical Abstracts* database (14.8), presented in seven categorical sections: anti-infectives, antineoplastics, cardiovasculars, gastrointestinals, pain management, total parenteral nutrition, and "miscellaneous." The latter category provides citations to literature on vascular devices (catheters and care), infusion control devices, medical equipment, nutrition support, patient education, cost and reimbursement, and drug use evaluation.

The majority of abstracted references in drug therapeutic category sections address issues related to stability and compatibility. Sixty-seven individual drug monographs, adapted from counterparts in the fifth edition of ASHP's *Medication Teaching Manual* (9.39), have been revised for the *Home Care Resource Book* into more patient-oriented entries and are also printed in a larger, easier-to-read typeface. Though largely derivative of information that can be found elsewhere, this *Resource Book* is likely to be a good investment for both pharmacy and nursing libraries and individual practitioners, gathering pertinent material into one time-saving and informative volume.

9.48 Karig AW, Hartshorn EA. *Counseling Patients on Their Medications.* Hamilton, IL: Drug Intelligence Publications, 1991.

Karig and Hartshorn's series of drug counseling monographs employ medical abbreviations and are not written in lay language. *Counseling Patients on Their Medications* would, therefore, be a poor choice for direct consumer access. Information compiled is midway between a professional package insert and patient education leaflets, both in writing style and in degree of mediation/interpretation (or lack thereof). Organized into chapters dedicated to individual therapeutic classes, drugs entries within each chapter are arranged alphabetically by generic name. An index provides cross references from generic and brand names, the latter including both U.S. and selected Canadian trademarks.

References

1. Improper use of medication can lead to serious problems. *National Association of Chain Drug Stores Web page* at http://www.nacds.org/resources/rxmonth.html.

2. Sullivan SD, Kreling DH, Hazlet TK. Noncompliance with medication regimens and subsequent hospitalizations: A literature analysis and cost of hospitalization estimate. *J Res Pharm Econ* 1990;2(2):19–33.

3. Cardinale V. A conversation on compliance. *Drug Topics* 1993 Mar;137(6):38–45.

4. *Action plan for the provision of useful prescription drug information.* http://www.nyam.org/keystone.

5. Holmer AF. Direct-to-consumer prescription drug advertising builds bridges between patients and physicians. *JAMA* 1999 Jan 27;281:380–382.

6. DTC ad effect on consumer regard for physician advice is problematic—FDA. *The Pink Sheet* 1998 Sep 14; record # 39129, *F-D-C Reports Online.*

7. Prevention Magazine. *National survey of consumer reactions to direct-to-consumer advertising.* Emmaus, PA: Rodale Press, 1998.

8. Katz WA. *Introduction to reference work.* 5th ed. Basic information sources v. 1. New York: McGraw-Hill, 1987:237.

9. Kare A, Kucukarslan S, Birdwell S. Consumer perceived risk associated with prescription drugs. *Drug Inf J* 1996;30:467.

10. La Rocco A. The role of the medical school-based consumer health information service. *Bull Med Libr Assoc* 1994 Jan;82:50.

11. Barry C. Publicly-available information on marketed products. In: Pickering WR. *Information sources in pharmaceuticals.* London: Bowker-Saur, 1990:277.

12. Teach L. *Health-related Web site evaluation form.* Atlanta: Emory University, 1998. http://www.sph.emory.edu/WELLNESS/instrument.html

13. *Criteria for assessing the quality of health information on the Internet.* McLean, VA: Mitretek Systems, 1997. http://www.mitrtek.org/hiti/showcase/documents/criteria.html

14. McKenna MAJ. Health watch: Online researchers should be wary about some medical data. *Atlanta Constitution* 1995 Mar 1:B3.

15. Renner JH. In my humble opinion. *Internet Health Watch* at http://www.reutershealth. com/ihm and http://www.reutershealth.com/ihw/imho/column.html.

16. Eisenberg DM et al. Trends in alternative medicine use in the United States, 1990– 1997. *JAMA* 1998 Nov 11;280:1569–1575.

Additional Sources of Information

Baker LM. Physician-patient communication from the perspective of library and information science. *Bull Med Libr Assoc* 1994 Jan;82:36–42.

Book BB. *Understanding Canadian nonprescription drugs*. Ottawa: Canadian Pharmaceutical Association, 1993.

Bruning N, Weinstein C. *Healing homeopathic remedies*. New York: Dell, 1996.

Brushwood DB, Simonsmeier LM. Drug information for patients: duties of the manufacturer, pharmacist, physician and hospital. *J Leg Med* 1986;7:279.

Brushwood DB, Simonsmeier LM. Drug information for patients, part III: the physician's and the hospital's legal duty. *Consult Pharm* 1988;3:161–166.

Burton Goldberg Group. *Alternative medicine: The definitive guide*. Puyallup, WA: Futura Medical, 1993.

Collinge W. *The American Holistic Health Association complete guide to alternative medicine*. New York: Warner Books, 1996.

Consumer health and nutrition index. Phoenix, AZ: Oryx Press, 1985–. Quarterly.

Cosgrove TL. Planetree health information services: public access to the health information people want. *Bull Med Libr Assoc* 1994 Jan;82:57–63.

Cummings S, Ullman D. *Everybody's guide to homeopathic medicines*. Los Angeles: Tarcher, 1991.

Feuerman F, Handel MJ. *Alternative medicine resource guide*. Lanham, MD: Medical Library Association and Scarecrow Press, 1997.

Graedon J, Graedon T. *The people's pharmacy*. New York: St. Martin's Press, 1998.

Hafner AW. A survey of patient access to hospital and medical school libraries. *Bull Med Libr Assoc* 1994 Jan;82:64–66.

Hollon MF. Direct-to-consumer marketing of prescription drugs creating consumer demand. *JAMA* 1999 Jan 27;281:382–384.

Jacobs J, ed. *The encyclopedia of alternative medicine: A complete guide to complementary therapies*. Boston: Charles E. Tuttle, 1996.

Jadad AR, Gagliardi A. Rating health information on the Internet: Navigating to knowledge or to Babel? *JAMA* 1998 Feb 25;279:611–614.

Jonas WB, Jacobs J. *Healing with homeopathy: The complete guide*. New York: Warner Books, 1996.

The medical advisor: The complete guide to alternative and conventional treatments. New York: Time-Life, 1996.

Ody P. *Home herbal*. New York: Dorling Kindersley, 1995.

Rees AM, ed. *Developing consumer health information services*. New York: Bowker, 1982.

Silberg WM, Lundberg GD, Musacchio RA. Assessing, controlling, and assuring the quality of medical information on the Internet. *JAMA* 1997 Apr 16;277:1244–1245.

Sinclair BJ. *Alternative health resources; A directory and guide.* West Nyack, NY: Parker Publishing, 1992.

Smith DL. *Understanding Canadian prescription drugs.* Ottawa: Canadian Pharmaceutical Association, 1992.

Ullman D. *The consumer's guide to homeopathy.* New York: Putnam, 1995.

Webber G. Patient education: a review of the issues. *Med Care* 1990 Nov;28:1089–1103.

Wyatt JC. Commentary: measuring quality and impact of the World Wide Web. *Brit Med J* 1997 Jun 28;314:1879–1881.

10

Product Identification: Imprint Indexes and Foreign Drug Sources

Sources discussed in Chapter Three will answer many, but not all, drug identification questions. Two specific types of product inquiries usually require consultation of additional resources, 1) product identification from a description or observation of a dosage form and 2) foreign drug identification. Because specialized translation aids are often needed to answer questions about non-U.S. drugs, the third section in this chapter reviews multilingual guides. These guides can also assist in medication counseling of non-English-speaking patients.

Drug Identification from a Description or Observation of a Dosage Form

One study of 1,209 drug information requests reported that half of a total of 115 unanswered questions involved identification (ID) from a verbal description of a dosage form.[1] Bobbink[2] demonstrated the utility of tablet and capsule imprints in answering more than 200 telephone calls received during a year-long period in a single poison control center. Such questions arise when unconscious or otherwise uncommunicative patients are admitted to the hospital with unidentified drugs in their possession, often in unmarked containers. Concerned parents, or caretakers of elderly patients, are also the instigators of many such inquiries, as are law enforcement and regulatory personnel seeking to determine if drugs seized are illicit, counterfeit, or defective. The Poison Prevention Packaging Act, by mandating child-proof closures, inadvertently contributes to the problem, when frustrated patients transfer medications from their original packaging into easier-to-open containers. Generic substitution laws also generate visual identification inquiries (Has substitution occurred, or is this a dispensing error?).

It is ironic that pictorial inserts such as those provided in the *PDR* or the *Red Book* rarely include drugs difficult to identify by other means, i.e., by the brand or company names printed on the dosage forms themselves. The small white tablet scored on one side, with a numeric code or logo on the other, is far more frequently the subject of inquiry. Sources that index imprints and provide access to product identification information by color, size, and shape are much more valuable than the much touted and often poorly reproduced photographs included in many commercial compendia.

10.1 *IDENTIDEX*. Englewood, CO: Micromedex, 1978–. Quarterly.

The most extensive (and expensive) index of dosage form imprints available today has been compiled by Micromedex, the publishers of *POISINDEX* (8.10). A natural outgrowth or extension of the world's most comprehensive poisoning information resource, the *IDENTIDEX®* database backs up its listing of imprints with information on tablet and capsule color and shape. Its scope encompasses both prescription and OTC products, trademarked and generic drugs, U.S. and non-U.S. medications, and a selection of "street" drugs. For all but the latter, manufacturer telephone numbers are provided. Logo descriptions, when applicable, are also included. When dosage form attributes, such as color and shape, differ in earlier formulations from those of the currently marketed product, these data are also noted. *IDENTIDEX* is one of many optional subfiles available as part of customizable subscriptions to the CCIS (Computerized Clinical Information System) databank, marketed in both CD-ROM and Intranet networking versions.

10.2 *DrugPics*. San Bruno, CA: First DataBank. Quarterly.

DrugPics is a database of 3,000 drug images sold on CD-ROM as an enhancement module for use in conjunction with First DataBank's suite of electronic products, which include the *NDDF* (*National Drug Data File*). High resolution digitized photographic images in color show front and back views of solid dosage forms, with particular attention to significant markings, such as scoring or logos. Examples can be previewed on First DataBank's Web site at http://firstdatabank. com/drug/index.html.

10.3 *Drug Image Database*. San Bruno, CA: Medi-Span. Quarterly.
10.4 *Drug Imprint Database*. San Bruno, CA: Medi-Span. Monthly.

Both the *Drug Image Database*™ and *Drug Imprint Da*tabase™ are machine-readable files that can only be used if linked with an electronic National Drug Code file containing eleven-digit NDCs. Images are sold on CD-ROM, and the imprint module is distributed on diskettes, data cartridges, or magnetic tape. Descriptions provided by Medi-Span (a sister company of First DataBank) in their *Drug Imprint Database* identify coating, color, shape, and scoring of 2,500 solid dosage forms. Selected liquid dosage form attributes, also included, describe color, clarity, and flavor of products. Product overviews are available at http://www.firstdatabank.com/drug.

10.5 *TICTAC*. London: The Stationery Office, 1990–. Annual, updated quarterly.

Developed by the staff at the Toxicology Unit of St. George's Hospital Medical School in London, *TICTAC* is a CD-ROM resource for dosage form identification. Entries for more than 13,000 products encompass a variety of solid forms, including tablets, capsules, and transdermal patches. Both prescription and OTC, human and veterinary medications are covered, as well as illicit drugs, herbal preparations, homeopathic remedies, and imported (non-U.K.) products. The CD-ROM database interface enables searching on any combination of characteristics, such as color, shape, scoring, and logo. Entries for individual products, once found, provide narrative descriptions, manufacturer data (address, telephone numbers), and information on legal product status (if any) within the United Kingdom. Structural formulas and more than 25,000 digitized color images of actual dosage forms greatly enhance *TICTAC*'s utility.

Annual subscriptions entitle purchasers to quarterly CD-ROM update replacement discs. Subscribers are also able to access the *TICTAC* Web site for news flashes, new product information, and links to other relevant Internet sites.

10.6 *Chemist and Druggist Directory*. Tonbridge, England: Benn Business Information Services, 1968–. Annual.

The *Chemist and Druggist Directory* compiles an impressive tablet and capsule identification guide for British products (some of which are also marketed in the United States). Black-and-white drawings of many imprints and logos are included, cross referenced to a color-coded key that resembles a paint selection catalog. Products are also listed verbally by color, with a description of their other characteristics (scoring, logo, coding) tabulated. All index entries are keyed to manufacturers' addresses and telephone numbers in the United Kingdom. Because of the tendency of patients to hoard old medicines, this tablet and capsule identification guide includes indexing for many discontinued products.

The *Chemist and Druggist Directory* includes many other useful sections unrelated to dosage form identification. Its alphabetic directory of companies includes addresses, telephone/fax/telex numbers, a selective product listing, and, for many (but not all) manufacturers, names and titles of executive personnel and number of employees. Other sections of the *Directory* identify multiple establishment retail drug outlets and associations or organizations of interest. The latter listing is broad ranging (and broad minded) in scope, including information on organizations such as New Approaches to Cancer, the Northern Ireland Bio-Engineering Centre, the Office of Fair Trading, the Phobics Society, and the Scottish Pharmaceutical Federation. The *Directory*'s Buyers Guide covers chemists' sundries, equipment and supplies, veterinary remedies, and garden products, all accessible through one integrated alphabetical index.

Unlike its U.S. counterpart, the *Red Book* (3.15), this annual publication makes no attempt to identify all pharmaceutical products available or to provide detailed packaging and pricing data. A brand name index lists selected products, their use or application, and manufacturer. The *Chemist and Druggist Directory* also contains a geographic listing of larger hospitals and their pharmacy personnel, giving titles, degrees, and other qualifications. Transcriptions of important U.K. legislation and regulations conclude the volume, including the 1971 Misuse of Drugs Act controlled substance schedules, the Poison Act, lists of approved products and ingredients, drug controls in the Republic of Ireland, Law for Retailers, and a section on value-added tax.

10.7 Jellin J. *Ident-A-Drug Reference*. Washington, DC: American Pharmaceutical Association, 1998.

10.8 Swim JR. *Generic Drug Identification Guide*. 3rd ed. Abilene, TX: Drug Information Service Co., 1990.

The *Ident-A-Drug Reference* indexes 7,800 Rx and OTC tablet and capsule imprints. Each code is cross referenced to a generic name, physical description, and manufacturer. The *Generic Drug Identification Guide* is divided into four sections, the first of which is an index to imprints, in numeric order. Codes are followed by generic name, strength, dosage form, shape, color, and company name. Section II offers an identification guide accessible by generic name, cross referencing each name to an imprint code. Section III cross references nearly 4,000 generic names to brand names, and Section IV provides brand to generic name indexing. The *Guide*'s appendix contains a listing of drug manufacturer identification codes (NDCs), addresses, and phone numbers. Other reference material appended includes a directory of poison control centers, a key to common medical abbreviations, equivalent weights and measures, normal laboratory values, a list of medications that should not be crushed, and information regarding drug administration in relation to food consumption.

10.9 *National Drug Code Directory*. Rockville, MD: Bureau of Drugs, U.S. Food and Drug Administration, 1969–. Annual.

Because smaller U.S. generic drug manufacturers sometimes use their NDC company number (see Chapter Two) as an imprint, the *National Drug Code Directory* is occasionally useful in answering dosage form identification requests. Quarterly updates to the *Directory* are accessible on the *FDA Home Page* on the Internet (see Chapter Sixteen). The *American Drug Index* (3.6) also provides a helpful section of NDC company designations, updated annually.

Given the paucity of information available and the tendency of patients and their families to store unused medications indefinitely, be prepared for no more than a 50% success rate in answering physical identification queries. Many questions will also remain unanswered because they involve probable "street" drugs, illicitly manufactured and unlikely to be indexed.

Photographic Inserts in Drug Compendia

Despite reservations expressed at the beginning of this section regarding the value of photographic plates now inserted in many drug product guides discussed in previous chapters, it may be useful to review which compendia include them:

AARP Pharmacy Service Prescription Drug Handbook (9.6)
The AMA Guide to Prescription and Over-the-Counter Drugs (9.5)
The American Druggist's Complete Family Guide to Prescriptions, Pills, and Drugs (9.7)
The American Pharmaceutical Association's Guide to Prescription Drugs (9.8)
Compendium of Pharmaceutical and Specialties (10.20)
Mosby's GenRx (6.3)
Nurses Drug Facts (6.62)
Patient Drug Facts (9.40)
PDR Family Guides (9.24–9.26)
PDR Generics (6.8)
PDR Nurse's Handbook (6.66)
Physicians' Desk Reference (6.10)
Physicians' Desk Reference for Nonprescription Drugs (6.9)
The Pill Book (9.30)
The Red Book (3.15)
USP DI Volume 1—Drug Information for the Health Care Professional (6.5)
USP DI Volume 2—Advice for the Patient (9.1)
The USP Guide to Medicines (9.4)

"The Medicine Chart," originating in *USP DI* and replicated in *Mosby's GenRx*, arranges photos by generic names of products depicted. A companion index offers cross references to page locations from both brand and generic names. Imprint codes follow product entries in this index. Fortunately, a separate index to Medicine Chart photos provides direct access by imprint code.

In contrast, Medical Economics publications (*PDRs* and *The Red Book*) arrange their photographic sections by manufacturer name, making visual identification unnecessarily difficult. The *Physicians' Desk Reference for Nonprescription Drugs* offers pictures of packages more often than actual dosage forms, thus openly disclosing its commercial intent. *PDR Generics* does include indexing of imprint codes, but entries are not cross referenced to the photo section. Identification marks of products depicted in the latter are accessible only by visually scanning more than 1,500 photographs. *The Pill Book* organizes photos by brand name.

As might be expected, the consumer-oriented *AMA Guide*, AARP *Handbook*, and *American Druggist's Complete Family Guide* offer easy-to-use (but limited in scope) photo sections, sensibly arranged by color and size. Facts and Comparisons' aids to medication counseling, *Patient Drug Facts* and *Nurses Drug Facts*, both organize their visual identification sections by color, as well.

FDA Regulation of Imprints

The number of visual identification questions about approved U.S. drugs may be reduced as a result of revised FDA regulations regarding imprinting that became effective in September 1995. Product-specific codes/markings are now required on all solid oral OTC and prescription drugs, biologics, and homeopathic medicines authorized for interstate commerce, including pre-1938 grandfathered remedies. IND drugs, radiopharmaceuticals, and extemporaneously compounded medications intended for a single patient's use are exempted. Requirements can also be waived, on a case by case basis, for drugs whose physical characteristics make imprinting impossible. To minimize commercial disruption and undue expense to manufacturers, the rule does not mandate use of a national uniform coding scheme, such as the NDC system already in existence. Instead, company logos and other symbols are still considered acceptable markings, as long as the imprint, together with a product's color, shape, and size, is sufficient to identify it. Inclusion of alphanumeric characters is entirely voluntary.

When proposing these regulations, the FDA estimated that 70% of OTC drugs and 90–95% of all prescription drugs in interstate commerce were already imprinted, and that most existing markings complied with what was proposed. In fact, twenty-three states had previously enacted statutes requiring imprinting of prescription drugs, and Washington state had added mandatory marking of OTC products to its regulations. Robertson[3] reviews thirty years of legislative steps leading to the final rule. Since experience with this status quo has already shown that visual identification problems are not necessarily alleviated by imprinting, revised federal regulations may have little impact, unless information on symbols used, registered with the FDA, is compiled and publicly disseminated.

Even if such publication were undertaken, lack of uniformity in coding creates accessibility nightmares. How to index a combination of pictorial and alphanumeric material in an applications oriented, reasonably easy-to-use source is the challenge. *Trademarkscan*, a commercial database available online and in CD-ROM format, has developed a system for dealing with comparable material, enhanced with graphic display capabilities. Transcribing visually observed characteristics (such as size, color, image content, and printed characters) into readily searchable and predictably uniform data elements will be the first task of any publisher who undertakes the imprint project. Producing a useful hardcopy index to such data is nearly a practical impossibility.

Computer-assisted access to the database, if created, would certainly help solve visual identification problems. But, how to make it available at a less-than-punitive price, considering the undoubtedly high costs of development and maintenance, could prove to be a problem far more difficult than determining what that little white tablet, scored on one side and imprinted 0123 on the other, is. Many drug information professionals would settle for a complete and well organized printed index to codes alone, provided that sorting (sequencing) standards adopted follow traditional character-by-character rules long established in filing systems.

Foreign Drug Identification Sources

Due to the comparatively stringent regulations affecting drug approval in the United States, many manufacturers conduct drug research in other countries and prepare products for marketing abroad prior to submissions to the FDA. This, coupled with an increasingly mobile patient population, including immigrants and tourists returning from (or preparing for) travel abroad, may account for the high incidence of requests for data about foreign (non-U.S.) drugs reported in many information centers.

Analysis of requests received at one such center over a forty-month period showed that *Martindale* (6.1) answered 59% of foreign drug information queries, while *Unlisted Drugs* (3.8) answered 38%, *The Merck Index* (3.5) accounted for 20%, and *Index Nominum* (3.7) answered 22%.[4] Beginning a search in such international compendia saves time and usually yields at least a nonproprietary name and country of origin. Yet, information providers faced with an unusual number of foreign drug information requests may need to augment their reference collections with resources beyond those discussed thus far. More detailed product and prescribing information is available in many of the resources annotated in this section.

Preliminary Inquiries

Before beginning work on any drug identification request, it's wise to determine the source of the name to be investigated. Has the inquiry originated from a prescription, a journal article, or conversation with colleagues or patients? The source of the name may affect the reliability of its spelling in the initial request. It may also indicate whether the drug is currently on the market, or still under investigation.

Knowing what questions to ask before rushing to the reference shelf saves frustration. Some facts available to the requester are, all too often, not disclosed without prompting. For example, what evidence is available that indicates this is a foreign drug? Where and when was the medication last prescribed or dispensed? It's not uncommon for a pharmacist to call a drug information center for help in identifying drug X, without mentioning that he or she is reading the name from a prescription form with an address at the top. If country of origin cannot be determined, can a language be identified? Is a manufacturer also indicated?

If a prescription is the source of the inquiry, it's important to find out what dosage and strength are given. The same drug at different dosage levels may have different indications. What dosage form is described (tablet, capsule, liquid, suppository, injectable)? Sometimes these data will require translation before identification can proceed (see Multilingual Guides in this Chapter). Dosage form plays a critical role in establishing a domestic equivalent. A compound administered as a topical ointment, for example, may be used for an entirely different indication than when it is administered in oral form. Its pharmacokinetics and bioavailability will be affected by the form in which it has been ordered to be dispensed.

Is the intended therapeutic use known? In identification/equivalency questions, the agent may have been used for a different indication than some of its domestic chemical "equivalents." Thus, a true equivalent would be a drug approved for the appropriate indication and producing the same effect, whether or not it is chemically equivalent.

Circumstances may be such that it not always possible or feasible to obtain answers to these preliminary questions before proceeding with the literature search. But it is essential to be aware of the importance of such factors, in order to provide a response that is sufficiently informative for requesters to fulfill their own information needs.

Historical and Commercial Trends Influence Resource Selection

Political and historical trends exercise a strong influence on commerce. Major explorer nations and empire builders of the past often maintain economic ties with colonized countries long after formal government links have ceased. For example, a question about a drug last dispensed in southeast Asia or in Africa may well be answered by consultation of a French drug compendium. Economic and cultural ties resulting from former colonization also dictate that many drugs purchased abroad can be identified in British sources. Current commercial trends will also influence collection development. Who are the major drug producing nations today? Where are the majority of successful multinational firms headquartered? Which countries consistently lead the pack in introduction of new molecular entities? Answers to these questions will show that, beyond U.S. sources, best bet acquisitions will be those that specialize in identifying drugs on the market in Germany, France, and Japan.

10.10 *Rote Liste*. Frankfurt: Editio Cantor, 1935–. Annual.
10.11 Fricke U, Klaus W, eds. *Neue Arzneimittel*. Stuttgart: Wissenschaftliche Verlag, 1953–. Annual.

Rote Liste is the most comprehensive directory of pharmaceuticals available in Germany and, because of that country's dominance in the international drug market, this resource will help identify many products available elsewhere in the world. Annual editions list more than 5,500 chemically defined medicinals, nearly 500 botanical formulations and a comparable number of homeopathic products, as well as more than 250 "organ preparations." *Rote Liste* contains information on a total of approximately 9,800 dosage forms of 7,500 products from 400 suppliers and includes pricing information. Often referred to as the German-language *PDR*, this drug directory is far more all-inclusive in scope than the U.S. *Physicians' Desk Reference*. It covers more than 3,600 prescription remedies, including at least 300 marketed outside of pharmacies.

Individual product listings, arranged by eighty-seven pharmacological/therapeutic codes, are terse forms of labeling/package insert data. Each entry gives drug brand name, manufacturer, dosage, form, composition, concentration, indications, packaging, and price. A separate (green-edged) section lists drugs and specific warnings regarding use in pregnancy and lactation. Red pages provide overdose and toxicity treatment information and a directory of poison control centers throughout Europe. Another (orange-edged) section lists "street" drugs, with specific precautions, and also identifies products with a high alcohol content.

A separate section provides a company-by-company listing of products and a hotline telephone number for each. In addition to access by manufacturer and by pharmacological class, *Rote Liste* includes a brand name, a generic name, and an indications index. A keyword index to the pharmacological coding scheme is also provided, with numerous cross references. Appendices compile law and government data, such as narcotics dispensing regulations and a directory of human and veterinary health agencies. Appendices also include emergency protocols for severe anaphylactic reactions and extensive information regarding vaccines (for children, adults, travelers, etc.).

Because of its thorough indexing, *Rote Liste* is fairly easy to use. The chief challenge for the non-German user is meticulous translation of package inserts. German-English medical dictionaries rarely contain all terms needed. Specialized pharmaceutical, botanical, and other vocabulary often requires consultation of other sources (see Multilingual Guides in this Chapter). Many German drugs that become the subject of inquiry in the United States are combination products and often contain unusual plant and animal extracts.

Neue Arzneimittel is a well known collection of monographs on new drug entities introduced on the German market. It is published annually to provide an in-depth review of developments during the previous year. Information is presented in the context of pharmacological classes, comparing new agents with older alternatives. Chemical structures, tables, and other figures illustrate drug category discussions, which are further enhanced with bibliographies. An overview section included in each edition tabulates all drugs newly introduced in Germany, including those containing previously known ingredients. This annual round-up lists brand or generic name, manufacturer, active ingredients, dosage form, concentration, *Rote Liste* class, and analogous preparations. When more information is needed on new drugs (particularly background bibliography, which will transcend translation difficulties), *Neue Arzneimitel* can be helpful. Comparable, and complementary, sources in English include *Drugs of the Future* (15.6), *Drugs of Today*, and *The Year's Drug News* (all three from publisher J.R. Prous).

10.12 *Dictionnaire Vidal*. Paris: OVP Editions du Vidal, 1914–. Annual.
10.13 Median J et al, eds. *Guide National de Prescription des Medicaments*. Paris: Office de Vulgarisation Pharmaceutique, 1987–. Annual.

Political and historical trends place the French-language *Dictionnaire Vidal* next in order of overall utility for identification of non-U.S. drugs. At 2,000 pages, it is noticeably less bulky than *Rote Liste* (3,000 pages), but nonetheless provides a complete directory to pharmaceuticals and related products marketed in France. The opening section lists poison control centers, centers of pharmacovigilance, and abused substances and prohibited doping methods. The second, blue-edged portion of *Dictionnaire Vidal* provides cross references to brand names from generic (DCF) names. Preparations with only one active ingredient are identified in roman type; brand names of combinations appear in italics. Yellow pages that follow list products by "familles thérapeutiques."

The main portion of the volume is devoted to product monographs in alphabetical order by brand name, providing basic package insert data such as composition, strength, indications, precautions, adverse reactions, dosage, available forms and packages, prices, and manufacturer. One unusual feature is that each entry gives the year when the monograph was last reviewed by the French Drug Commission. Entries for radio-opaque contrast agents and blood products end this white-page product listing. The fourth, salmon-edge section describes selected medical devices, disinfectants, dietetic products, toiletries, test kits, and mineral waters. Accompanying the latter are entries for thermal resorts and spas. Green pages provide a directory of establishments (drug manufacturers and products). *Dictionnaire Vidal* is updated three times a year, with supplements issued in January, May, and October. A separately bound companion pamphlet compiles data on interactions, tabulated by compound class, and indexed by generic name and synonyms.

The *Guide National de Prescription des Medicaments*, subtitled "Le Vidal Thérapeutique," is more clinically oriented than the more obviously commercial (and more comprehensive) *Dictionnaire Vidal*. It organizes prescribing information into twenty-eight pharmacological or therapeutic categories, beginning each section's discussion with a broad overview of the family of compounds. Descriptions of properties they share in common follows, including indications, contraindications, precautions, and adverse effects. Commentary on the class concludes with entries for specific drugs, in which abbreviations for common properties discussed earlier in the section appear, when applicable, and an abstract reviews prescribing issues. More than 8,000 prescription drugs dispensed on the French market are cited in the *Guide National*. Appendices list new drugs, products discontinued since the last edition, a vaccination calendar, pharmaceutical laboratories, and brief directories of centers for HIV testing, drug abuse monitoring, and treatment of poisoning or alcoholism.

Two non-English Internet sources of ready-reference drug information for products on the market in Germany and Switzerland are identified in Figure 10.1. Alta Vista's translation support service could be used to assist in navigating these Web sites (see also Figure 10.2).

10.14 *Japan Pharmaceutical Reference (JPR). Administration and Products in Japan.* 3rd ed. Tokyo: Japan Medical Products International Trade Association, 1993.

10.15 *Japan Drug Guide* 1980–1995. Tokyo: Technomic, 1995.

10.16 Teshima K. *The Japanese Standards for Herbal Medicines.* Tokyo: Yakuji Nippon, 1993.

Published every four years, the *Japan Pharmaceutical Reference* compiles product information from manufacturers and includes a directory of companies. It is arranged alphabetically by proprietary name. Product entries include a selection of names used outside Japan, full descriptions of action and use, and bibliographic references. English-language package inserts for 285 ethical drug products from fifty-nine manufacturers are reproduced in the third edition. An index by Standard Commodity Classification for Japan (SSCJ) provides therapeutic class access; nonproprietary names are also indexed. In addition, the 1993 edition of *JPR* compiles statistics on the Japanese pharmaceutical industry, presented

Figure 10.1   Two Non-English Sources of European Drug Information on the Internet

---

- *Gelbe Liste Online*
  ⇨ http://195.27.173.69/wconnect/glwin/suchen.htm

  The Gelbe Liste, also known as "The Yellow Book," provides information about the 30,000 medicinal preparations on the market in Germany. Entries consist of package inserts, in German, augmented with pricing data. The Web database is updated monthly and can be searched by drug preparation (brand) name, medicine material (ingredients), or manufacturer.

- *Sanphar*
  ⇨ http://www.sanphar.ch

  Sanphar, an association of the Swiss pharmaceutical industry, offers a product information database with entries showing price, manufacturer, and composition for medications on sale in Switzerland. The interface is available in German or French.

Figure 10.2   Subject Specialty Multilingual Guides on the Internet

---

- *Glossary of Technical and Popular Medical Terms in Eight European Languages*
  ⇨ http://allserv.rug.ac.be/~rvdstich/eugloss/language.html

The *Glossary of Technical and Popular Medical Terms in Eight European Languages*, accessible free-of-charge on the Internet, could prove helpful when hardcopy resources are unavailable. Compiled by the Heymans Institute for Pharmacology, separate indexes are provided in Danish, German, Spanish, French, Italian, Dutch, Portuguese, and English. Each word or expression indexed is followed by its technical or popular equivalent and is preceded by two icons that refer, respectively, to the "multilingual lemma collection" and an English-language glossary. Clicking on the first produces a list of corresponding scientific and everyday language terms in all languages covered. The second icon leads to a definition in English. It is anticipated that definitions in other languages will be available in the future.

- *Spanish for Pharmacists*
  ⇨ http://www.nacds.org/resources/spanish.html.

The National Association of Chain Drug Stores offers an excellent guide to Spanish for pharmacists, available for immediate full-text display at the URL shown. Tables cross reference terms from English to Spanish and include pronunciations for the latter. Days of the week, months of the year, and numerous time of day or duration/interval keywords and phrases are compiled, as are terms for body parts, conditions, categories of medication, dosage forms, and essential verbs (chew, decrease, dilute, gargle, rub, inhale, etc.). Side bars give practical examples of translating prescription directions.

- *Essential Spanish for Pharmacists and Pharmacy Technicians*
  ⇨ http://www.pharmacyspanish.com.

A continuing education package consisting of hardcopy manuals and audio tapes is described in detail, with free previews of content, at this site. The multilingual CE module, available for a fee, is co-authored by Stephen and Mireya Whitaker and produced in association with the Texas Tech School of Pharmacy.

- *Spanish for the Pharmaceutical Profession*
  ⇨ http://www.cpha.com

The California Pharmacists Association distributes two ACPE-approved continuing education programs, both described at the URL given here. Volume 1 of *Spanish for the Pharmaceutical Profession* covers basic conversation in Spanish relevant to pharmacy practice. Volume 2—*Labeling Guide and Conversational Development* continues with skills building exercises to communicate medication instructions verbally and translate package insert and labeling information.

- *Alta Vista—Translation*
  ⇨ http://babelfish.altavista.com/cgi-bin/translate

Alta Vista's translation service is not geared to any specific subject specialty, but is designed for conversion of Web pages from one language into another. This could prove useful when visiting the growing number of non-English-language sites offering drug information. The service will translate plain text or Web (HTML) pages from French, German, Italian, Portuguese, or Spanish into English—or vice versa.

---

in time series covering 1975–1990. Data include pharmaceutical production by therapeutic category, new drugs approved, national healthcare expenditures, and death rate by major causes. Introductory material offers an overview of government regulations regarding drugs, group practices, drug abuse, and dissemination of drug information (i.e., package inserts and labeling).

The *Japan Drug Guide* is the successor to the *Japan Drug Index* and was first published in 1990. It compiles, in English, information on products currently available on the ethical market in Japan, as well as a selection of those under development. Data are accessible by company name, therapeutic class, or product name. Brief listings include name, originator, licensee, marketer, therapeutic classification, launched date or experimental stage of development, and pricing, when applicable. A total of 1,873 pharmaceuticals are covered, indexed by 4,437 synonyms, including many research codes. A separate listing shows the number of drugs per company and their status. Much (indeed, more) of the information on investigational agents this volume contains can be located and updated by searching *Pharmaprojects*, *IMSworld R&D Focus Drug Updates*, or other drugs-in-development directories online (see Chapter Fifteen). However, for products already on the market in Japan, the *Guide* can be a useful starting point in identification inquiries.

Although not, strictly speaking, a drug identification source, *The Japanese Standards for Herbal Medicines* could be helpful in handling phytomedical queries. Official monographs, in English, summarize government standards for quality, purity, and assay of eighty-three preparations listed in the *Japanese Herbal Medicine Codex* and 165 botanicals covered in the *Pharmacopoeia of Japan*. Appendices offer English-language translations of pertinent portions of the Japanese pharmacopeia, including tests for crude drugs and general rules/notices applicable to botanical pharmaceuticals imported to, or manufactured in, Japan.

10.17 *L'Informatore Farmaceutico*. 3 v. Milan: Organizzazione Editoriale Medico-Farmaceutica, 1940–. Annual.

10.18 *Repertorio Farmaceutico Italiano*. 6th ed. Milan: Centro Editoriale Documentazione sul Farmaco, 1992.

Migratory and immigration patterns make acquisition of Italian drug information sources a priority in many information centers. *L'Informatore Farmaceutico* is a virtual encyclopedia of drugs and related products marketed in Italy and in other European countries. Volume 1 focuses on listing what U.S. practitioners would consider standard pharmaceuticals (dubbed "medical specialties" in this source), providing indexes by active ingredients, brand names, therapeutic groups, and anatomic/therapeutic classification. Volume 2 is devoted to borderline or miscellaneous products (what *Martindale* has referred to as "ancillary substances"), accessible by brand name and by anatomic/therapeutic classification. A separate yellow section identifies 20,000 homeopathic medications. Green pages list medicinal herbs by their common names and provide cross references to Latin nomenclature. Volume 3 is a directory of manufacturers and suppliers. Encyclopedic in bulk as well as in scope, *L'Informatore Farmaceutico* is a valuable addition to foreign drug identification collections. OTC remedies covered in Volume 2 are often difficult to find elsewhere. Annual subscriptions include a companion, pocket-size drug reference manual.

Repertorio Farmaceutico Italiano offers more information about each listed drug than does *L'Informatore*, but it identifies fewer products overall. Limited to "medical specialties" (i.e., omits many homeopathic, nutritional, and other non-standard or OTC pharmaceuticals), *Repertorio* compiles prescription drug package inserts (in Italian). Entries are arranged alphabetically by brand name, followed by a pink-edged index to nonproprietary names, a blue-edged listing by therapeutic class, and a final directory of manufacturers, with addresses, telephone/fax/telex numbers, and product lists. This 1,830-page Italian drug compendium is a useful complement to the broader ranging, but less informative, *L'Informatore Farmaceutico.*

10.19 *Diccionario de Especialidades Farmaceuticas*. Mexico City: Ediciones PLM, 1944–. Annual.

Information centers in the southwestern region of the United States may find it helpful to acquire the *Diccionario de Especialidades Farmaceuticas*. The popularity of Mexico as a vacation destination for travelers from throughout the world means that medications on the market in that country tend to migrate to many other locations. Because therapeutic drug marketing is less regulated in Mexico than elsewhere, particularly with regard to the distinction between prescription and nonprescription sales, products legitimately imported by individuals may become the subject of inquiries from U.S. healthcare providers. The *Diccionario* is a Spanish-language guide to more than 3,500 products available in Mexico. Information is typical of that provided in package inserts elsewhere. Color coded indexes offer access by therapeutic class (blue), active ingredients (yellow), and companies ("laboratories," pink). Monographs for nutritional/dietetic products and diagnostics are also included in this 1,500-page directory. Ediciones PLM, the publishers of the *Diccionario*, have recently been purchased by Medical Economics, producers of the *PDR*.

10.20 *Compendium of Pharmaceuticals and Specialties*. Ottawa: Canadian Pharmacists Association, 1960–. Annual.
10.21 *Compendium of Nonprescription Products*. 5th ed. Ottawa: Canadian Pharmacists Association, 1998.

Close commercial ties with Canada, reinforced by recent trade agreements and simple proximity to the United States, are strong arguments for acquisition of that nation's best known drug dictionary. The *Compendium of Pharmaceuticals and Specialties* (*CPS*) is the PDR of Canada, but is a much more comprehensive directory of prescription and related products than its U.S. counterpart. Its Therapeutic Guide, on pink pages, lists drugs under sixteen general anatomical groups based on the World Health Organization's anatomic/therapeutic classification scheme. Each drug group listing is subdivided into specific therapeutic, pharmacological, and chemical categories. Green pages provide an alphabetical index of brand and nonproprietary names, incorporating U.S. brand designations derived from the previous year's *USP DI* (6.5). Yellow pages compile addresses and telephone numbers of Canadian pharmaceutical manufacturers and distributors.

The largest, white-paper section of *CPS* is devoted to more than 1,500 pages of monographs for 3,000 drugs, medical devices, and vitamins, interleaved with advertisements. Coverage expanded to include human blood and blood components in 1998. A lilac colored section, introduced in 1995, focuses on clinical information. Recent additions here are a directory of health organizations and a section on antineoplastic drug therapy. Blue pages offer a miscellaneous assortment of reference material, including information for the patient, drug regulations, clinical guidelines, patient monitoring information, a directory of resource agencies and literature, and data on nonmedicinal ingredients. An increasing focus on providing patient education materials is reflected in the *Compendium*'s inclusion of more than 200 drug monographs in everyday language, printed with wider margins to facilitate photocopying. Numerous tables address typical quick-reference needs: alcohol-containing and alcohol-free products and comparable compilations for gluten, sulfite, and tartrazine, drug-drug and drug-food interactions, and immunization schedules for infants and children. Another popular feature of the *CPS* is the ubiquitous (in *PDR*-like publications) Product Recognition Section, where color photographs of products selected by manufacturers are included.

The *Compendium of Pharmaceuticals and Specialties* can be purchased in CD-ROM format, as well as the hardcopy version described here. Further prescribing information on many drugs marketed in Canada will also be found in the *USP DI Volume 1* (6.5, which indexes both U.S. and Canadian brand names), but the *CPS* is a better choice for product identification. Data submitted to the Canadian Pharmacists Association since the latest annual edition of the *Compendium* are available free of charge through the *CPhA Home Page* on the Internet at http://www.cdnpharm.ca. Newly approved entities, new indications, and new dosage forms are all featured in Web updates. Users can scroll through indexes of brand, manufacturer, or generic names, as well as therapeutic classes, to locate recently released product information.

The *Compendium of Nonprescription Products* (*CNP*) provides professionally oriented monographs for OTC remedies marketed in Canada. This CPhA publication also includes more than sixty tables listing available formulations and their ingredients. Its Patient Information section discusses signs and symptoms and summarizes both pharmacological and nondrug options for treating them.

10.22 *British National Formulary*. London: The Pharmaceutical Press, 1981–, Semiannual.

10.23 Nathan A. *Non-prescription Medicines*. London: The Pharmaceutical
       Press, 1998.

Presented in a small, soft-bound handbook format for quick-reference use, the
British National Formulary (*BNF*) is intended to offer guidance in prescribing,
dispensing, and administering medicines. Unlike the U.S. *National Formulary*
(11.8), this book is not intended to establish official standards for the manufacture of drugs that it identifies. Instead, it organizes information into chapters devoted to therapeutic classes and groups discussion of medications by the body
systems they affect. Drugs are listed by generic (BAN) name, followed by proprietary preparations available in the United Kingdom and information on forms,
strengths, dosage, and prices.

Appendices address a potpourri of topics, including interactions, IV additives,
"borderline" (nondrug) products, and precautionary labeling. *BNF 36*, issued in
September 1998, incorporates a Dental Practitioners' Formulary and a separate
Nurse Prescribers' List. The volume concludes with an index of manufacturers
and a general index. Updated every six months, the *BNF* is the product of a Joint
Formulary Committee of the British Medical Association and the Royal Pharmaceutical Society of Great Britain. As such, its content reflects current best practice, as well as legally authorized uses of all medicines on the U.K. market.

Non-prescription Medicines is a new imprint from The Pharmaceutical Press,
the official publishing arm of the Royal Pharmaceutical Society. More than thirty
chapters are packed into fewer than 200 pages in this concise reference guide.
Each chapter focuses on a common minor ailment, reviewing its causes and treatment options among OTC compounds available in the United Kingdom. Structured, formulary-like monographs are listed by nonproprietary name and include
information on administration and dosage, precautions, contraindications, and interactions. Entries end with lists of brand name preparations and manufacturers.
Rounding out each chapter are summaries of Product Selection Points and suggestions for the most appropriate products that the community pharmacist could
recommend.

10.24 Bazaz MC et al, ed. *Indian Pharmaceutical Guide*. New Delhi: Pam-
       posh, 1963–. Annual.

The *Indian Pharmaceutical Guide* is especially helpful in identifying many
homeopathic and herbal preparations that make their way into the United States.
Product listings (in English) provide information on composition, packaging, and
prices and are indexed by both generic name and company. The *Guide* also
serves as a directory to the pharmaceutical industry in India, compiling relevant
laws, as well as names and addresses of organizations and institutions, chemists
and druggists, and manufacturers and distributors. Cosmetic manufacturers are
also listed.

10.25 *Australian Prescription Products Guide*. 2 v. Hawthorn, Victoria: Aus-
       tralian Pharmaceutical Publishing, 1959–. Annual.

The *Prescription Products Guide* compiles package inserts for more than 3,000 products approved for marketing in Australia. Incorporating a nonprescription product guide from the 19th edition forward (1990), the *P.P. Guide* includes briefer monographs for unapproved remedies and related items, as well. It compiles information on medicinal plant extracts, nutritional products, and other therapeutic alternatives. The alphabetical list of Rx preparations identifies single-entity (one active ingredient) medications under brand names and combination products under the generic name of each constituent (Australian Approved Names, with cross references from other nonproprietary designations).

The *P.P. Guide* also contains pharmacological and therapeutic indexes and compiles a directory of manufacturers, importers, and distributors, giving full addresses and telephone/fax/telex numbers. Additional reference material includes an explanation of use-in-pregnancy categories, a cumulative list of discontinued products dating from 1986, drug regulations, directories of poison and drug information centers and patient support organizations, and drug interactions data. The latter section includes discussion of mechanisms, selected bibliographic references, and a quick-reference table of clinically significant interactions. Another table lists drug combinations which do not interact, also accompanied by references. An online version of the *Australian Prescription Products Guide* is now available on the Internet at http://appco.com.au/appguide/default.htm (user registration required).

10.26 *MIMS Australia.* St. Leonards, Australia: MediMedia. Annual, with bimonthly updates.
10.27 *MIMS OTC.* St. Leonards, Australia: Multimedia. Annual, with bimonthly updates.

MIMS Australia compiles package inserts for 2,300 Rx and OTC drug products, classified by therapeutic category. Entries represent official prescribing information approved by the Therapeutic Goods Administration (TGA), the Australian counterpart of the FDA. The annual volume also includes a tablet and capsule identification guide and is available in both hardcopy and CD-ROM format. Bimonthly updates require a separate subscription and consist of abbreviated monographs for newly introduced products.

MIMS OTC incorporates most products covered in *MIMS Australia* annual and bimonthly editions, but extends its scope to include more herbal preparations and therapeutic devices. The OTC directory provides abbreviated product information (compared to full *MIMS Australia* entries) for most nonprescription pharmaceutical products and other therapeutic goods (e.g., dressings, baby formulas) commonly available in Australian pharmacies. It is marketed in both hardcopy and CD-ROM editions (see http://www.mims.com.au).

A *MIMS Disease Index* is also available from the same publisher. With discussion of diagnosis, management, and treatment for 170 common conditions,

MedMedia's *Disease Index* bears some resemblance to *Conn's Current Therapy* (6.15) in its approach to differentiating various therapeutic options.

10.28 Muller NF, Dessing RP. *European Drug Index*. 3rd ed. Amsterdam: Amsterdam Medical Press, 1994.

First published in 1990, the *European Drug Index* has gradually expanded its scope to include products on the market in nineteen countries, including Austria, Belgium, the Czech Republic, Denmark, Finland, France, Germany, Italy, the Netherlands, Norway, Poland, Portugal, Spain, Switzerland, Sweden, and the United Kingdom. This edition extends coverage to Bulgaria, Greece, and Hungary. English-language monographs begin with a brand name, followed by manufacturer, dosage forms, strength, and generic names of active ingredients. Each entry concludes with an anatomic/therapeutic classification code and reference to the product's country of origin. The drug classification scheme is one developed by the Nordic Council on Medicines, collaborating in recent years with the WHO Centre for Drug Statistics Methodology. It offers access by fourteen major anatomical groups, further subdivided into narrower therapeutic subgroups. Drugs are categorized by site of action, indication, and chemical characteristics, based on the same principles as the EPhMRA system discussed in Chapter Two and illustrated in Chapter Fifteen. The chief value of this compendium is brand name access to products from many nations, although information provided is somewhat cryptic when therapeutic equivalency is at issue. It is usually necessary to follow up in other directories listed in this section that offer full package inserts.

A bonus that the *European Drug Index* offers is a dictionary of dosage form terms in Danish, Dutch, Finnish, French, German, Greek, Italian, Norwegian, Spanish, and Swedish, with English-language counterparts. This cross-reference guide could prove to be extremely helpful when translating labeling in foreign-language drug compendia or when preparing to search the *IMSworld New Product Launches* or *Products Monographs* databases online (15.18–15.19).

10.29 Schlesser JL, ed. *Drugs Available Abroad*. Detroit, MI: Gale Research, 1991.

Drugs Available Abroad compiles information on prescription products obtainable in Australia, Canada, the Caribbean, Central America, Mexico, Scandinavia, South Africa, and Western Europe. Subtitled "A guide to therapeutic drugs available and approved outside the U.S. (but not approved by FDA)," the implied intent of this publication appears to be similar to that of an earlier book entitled: *Orphan Drugs—Your Complete Guide to Effective, Tested Medications Outside the U.S. and Their Availability*, now outdated. This impression is reinforced by prefatory material describing procedures for exporting or importing unapproved drugs.

Drug monographs are arranged alphabetically by generic name (USAN preferred, INN when no USAN has been assigned). Each includes information on where the product is available, its release date, synonyms (including lab codes), brand name and manufacturer, how it is supplied, indications, and recommended dosage. A summary of precautions, contraindications, interactions, and adverse effects follows, along with information on U.S. status (whether the drug is currently—as of 1991—being tested for FDA approval). What drugs, if any, are already available in the United States to treat the same conditions are also identified. Five separate indexes provide access by drug name (7,000 generic and brand entries), drug action, clinical indications, company, and country-in-use. Appendices include a directory of 1,800 manufacturers and a listing of regulatory authorities. The latter provides a country-by-country overview of drug approval requirements and protocols or procedures. It's important to note that *Drugs Available Abroad* is somewhat limited in scope, covering approximately 1,000 products. Data are derived from the *Ringdoc* database and its successor, the *Derwent Drug File* (14.10), as well as foreign drug compendia such as those cited earlier in this section of the *Guide*.

Multilingual Guides: Help for the Xenophobe

Nine of the foreign drug identification sources discussed in the previous section are published in languages other than English, as their annotations have indicated. Translations of package inserts can be challenging even to those fortunate few whose linguistic ability extends beyond "menu" French, Spanish, or German. Standard bilingual medical and scientific dictionaries typically do not provide adequate assistance in deciphering specialized vocabulary used in inserts, which may include botanical, zoological, and pharmaceutical terminology. The *European Drug Index*'s (10.28) multilingual guide to drug dosage forms, cross referencing keywords in ten languages to their English-language counterparts, will be helpful in translating prescriptions and labeling. WHO's parallel listings of generic drug names in Latin, English, French, Russian, and Spanish in its periodic publication of *International Nonproprietary Names* (3.2) could also be useful. Unfortunately, however, it lacks permuted (rotated) indexing; alphabetical entry is by Latin name only. Acquiring one or two of the following much more extensive guides is recommended for information centers facing an unusual number of foreign drug identification requests.

10.30 Sliosberg A, ed. *Elsevier's Medical Dictionary*. 2nd ed. Amsterdam: Elsevier, 1991.

10.31 Sliosberg A, ed. *Elsevier's Dictionary of Pharmaceutical Science & Techniques*. 2 v. Amsterdam: Elsevier, 1980.

10.32 Spilker B, ed. *Medical Dictionary in Six Languages*. New York: Raven Press, 1995.

10.33 Dorian AF, ed. *Elsevier's Dictionary of Chemistry, Including Terms from Biochemistry, in English, French, Spanish, Italian, German*. Amsterdam: Elsevier, 1983.
10.34 Kryt D, ed. *Dictionary of Chemical Terminology in Five Languages*. Amsterdam: Elsevier, 1980.
10.35 Steinbichler E. *Steinbichler's Lexikon für die Apothekenpraxis in Sieben Sprachen*. Frankfurt: Govi Verlag, 1963.

None of these dictionaries provide definitions of terms. Instead, they show equivalent keywords in several languages. The two Elsevier multilingual guides edited by Sliosberg list equivalents in English, French, Italian, Spanish, and German. Latin cross references are also included in volume 2, subtitled *Materia Medica*, of *Elsevier's Dictionary of Pharmaceutical Science and Techniques*. It is especially useful in translating terms for substances of vegetable or animal origin used in human and veterinary pharmaceuticals. Volume 1 provides pharmaceutical technology terms.

Spilker's *Medical Dictionary in Six Languages* offers translation assistance by identifying 7,500 commonly used words and phrases in English and giving their counterparts in French, Italian, Spanish, German, and Japanese. Abbreviations are also listed in a separate section. Languages covered in *the Dictionary of Chemical Terminology*, edited by Kryt, are English, French, German, Polish, and Russian. *Steinbichler's Lexikon* is a seven-language cross-reference guide for pharmaceutical practice. Rotated indexing of German, French, Spanish, Italian, Greek, Russian, and English terms assists access. The *Lexikon* concludes with a collection of commonly used (and needed) phrases, with entry points (left-hand column listings) provided solely in German. However, this compilation of phrases is not so extensive that it cannot be scanned to locate needed information, such as dosage and administration instructions.

10.36 Carriere G, ed. *Dictionary of Surface Active Agents, Cosmetics, and Toiletries*. Amsterdam: Elsevier, 1978.
10.37 *Multilingual Dictionary of Narcotic Drugs and Psychotropic Substances under International Control*. New York: United Nations, 1993.

The *Dictionary of Surface Active Agents* cross references English, French, German, Spanish, Italian, Dutch, and Polish terms. The *Multilingual Dictionary of Narcotic Drugs and Psychotropic Substances* provides Arabic, Chinese, English, French, Russian, and Spanish equivalents and includes bibliographic references.

The older imprint dates on many of the references in this section may distress practitioners accustomed to equating recent with better. The fact is, language guides such as these do not date quickly, and there are very few publications of this type. Indeed, some are currently out of print. However, many are still available in library reference collections or obtainable through second-hand booksellers. Some may even turn up in gifts to libraries bequeathed by grateful users or alumni. Such treasures often languish unused and unappreciated in large collections until someone points out their potential value in reference work.

Drug information professionals may also find it helpful to have other types of multilingual guides on hand in preparation for an entirely different type of inquiry. English-speaking pharmacists and physicians working in areas with a non-English-speaking patient population may request assistance in translating idiomatic phrases needed for labeling, written instructions, and other patient education and counseling aids. Help is available (but well hidden) in the pharmacy practice journal literature.

10.38 Strauss S, Blumberg M. Multilingual Guide for Pharmacists. *Pharm Times* 1970 Aug;36:49–53 and 1970 Sep;36:54–63.
10.39 Thomas J. Foreign Language Labels. *Aust J Pharm* 1977 Aug;58:461–466 and 1977 Sep;58:555–562.
10.40 Language Equivalents of Common Medical Directions. *Aust J Pharm* 1977 Oct;58:609–610.
10.41 Spanish for Pharmacists. *Tex Pharm* 1984 May;53:35.
10.42 Julia AM, Garcia SV, Breckinridge MF. Spanish Labeling Guide. *Drug Intell Clin Pharm* 1983 Jul-Aug;17:580–590.

Strauss and Blumberg compile Spanish, French, Greek, and German words or phrases for parts of the body, colors, numbers, and a pharmacy phrase book of "95 Often Used Sentences" in their two-part article published in *Pharmacy Times*. Thomas translates twenty common prescription directions from English into eighteen other languages, including Latvian, Bulgarian, Estonian, Russian, Slovene, and Ukrainian, in addition to those covered by Slavens (10.45). A follow-up anonymous article in the *Australian Journal of Pharmacy* offers translations from English into Motu (New Guinea) and Pidgin (10.40). Additional labeling guides and patient instructions have been published to help pharmacists better communicate with Hispanic patients (10.41–10.42).

10.43 Bartilucci AJ, Durgin JM. *Language Guide for the Clinical Pharmacist*. New York: St. John's University Press, 1971.
10.44 Strauss S. *Patient Dosage Instructions: A Guide for Pharmacists*. 3rd ed. Ambler, PA: IMS America, 1975.

Bartilucci and Durgin's short *Language Guide* booklet lists sixteen common questions a pharmacist may need to ask a patient and fifteen questions a patient may ask a pharmacist. Chinese, French, German, Italian, Polish, Spanish, and Yiddish equivalents are given. In *Patient Dosage Instructions*, Strauss also provides an introduction to the provision of multilingual pharmacy service.

From 1972 to 1976, the *Canadian Pharmaceutical Journal* published a sixteen-part series of bilingual guides to label instructions, compiled by Slavens. To avoid redundancy, abbreviated citations to installments in this series are included here under one reference number.

10.45   Slavens RR. Common Portuguese Label Instructions. *Can Pharm J* 1972 Dec;105:390–391.

———Common Italian Label Instructions. 1973 Feb;106:48–49.

———Common French Label Instructions. 1973 May;106:146–147.

———Common Lithuanian Label Instructions. 1973 Aug:106:254–255.

———Common Czech Label Instructions. 1973 Oct;106:316–317.

———Common Spanish Label Instructions. 1974 Jan;107:14–15.

———Common Danish Label Instructions. 1974 Apr;107:22–23.

———Common Polish Label Instructions. 1974 Jun;107:176–177.

———Common Hungarian Label Instructions. 1974 Oct;107:326–327.

———Common Norwegian Label Instructions. 1974 Dec;107:402–403.

———Common Dutch Label Instructions. 1975 Mar;108:16–17.

———Common German Label Instructions. 1975 Jul;108:246–247.

———Common Croato-Serbian Labels. 1975 Sep;108:318–319.

———Common Turkish Label Instructions. 1975 Dec;108:410–411.

———Common Swedish Label Instructions. 1976 Feb;109:50–51.

———Common Finnish Label Instructions. 1976 Apr;109:104–105.

Finally, several sources discussed in previous chapters include Spanish-language consumer-oriented material: *The Red Book* (3.15), *Nurse's Drug Facts* on CD-ROM (6.62), *Mosby's Patient GenRx* (9.11), ASHP's *Medication Teaching Manual* (9.39), and the USP *Spanish Counseling Companion* (9.44). Multilingual guides on the Internet are featured in Figure 10.2.

References

1. Snow B. Foreign drug information retrieval. *Med Ref Serv Q* 1982;1(3):44.

2. Bobbink S, Williams D, Robertson WO. Use of drug imprints. *Vet Hum Toxicol* 1986 Apr;28:160.

3. Robertson WO. Imprinting solid medication forms: status update. *Vet Hum Toxicol* 1995 Feb;37:78–79.

4. Snow B: 43.

Additional Sources of Information

Chemist and Druggist Guide to OTC Medicines for Pharmacists and Pharmacy Assistants. 13th ed. Tonbridge, England: Miller Freeman, 1998.

Cummings S, Ullman D. *Everybody's guide to homeopathic medicines.* Los Angeles: Tarcher, 1991.

Fletcher HJ, Scotland C, Moody M. Computerized OTC advice in four languages. *Int Pharm J* 1992;6:30–34.

Names of 89 essential oils in English, Latin, French, German, Dutch, Spanish and Italian. *Soap Perfum Cosmet* 1971 Apr;44:243–246.

11

Industrial Pharmacy

Pharmaceutical information needs in industry include many of the topics covered thus far, depending on the individual requester's area of responsibility. Reference collections in corporate libraries must, however, accommodate the added dimension of technical development and actual production of dosage forms. Questions posed by drug company personnel may require consultation of the literature related to pharmaceutics, biopharmaceutics, or pharmaceutical technology. The science of pharmaceutics focuses on physical and chemical factors that influence formulation and manufacturing, involving tests on preparations for dissolution data, filtration, pH, ionization, crystallization, solubility, surface action, etc. Biopharmaceutics examines the effects of formulation on drug action within the body. Biopharmaceutic studies correlate physical-chemical properties, as well as particle size, coating, and route of administration, with drug bioavailability, pharmacokinetics, and bioequivalency. Pharmaceutical technology topics extend inquiries regarding formulations into production issues, such as sterilization and contamination, preservatives, vehicles, equipment, packaging, closures, and quality control. Drug stability investigations, discussed in Chapter Seven in relation to *in vitro* incompatibilities, are frequently the subject of industrial pharmaceutical scientists' queries. Questions regarding assay or analysis of drugs (i.e., quantitative or qualitative testing of pharmaceutical preparations for content, impurities, or detection of counterfeits) can also be anticipated.

Archer[1] provides an excellent overview of information needs in industry related to technical development and production of drugs. He cites basic chemistry and toxicology sources to support personnel working on process development, who must determine the best means for preparing chemical entities in bulk, safely and economically. *Beilstein*, *The Dictionary of Organic Compounds*, and Fieser and Fieser's *Reagents for Organic Synthesis* are examples of sources required to answer questions posed by organic chemists.

It is in the area of analytical development and quality assurance that the requisite bibliography shifts to publications that fall within the scope of this *Guide*. *Clarke's Isolation and Identification of Drugs* (8.17–8.18), discussed earlier as a sourcebook in analytical toxicology, is equally essential in collections supporting analytical chemists in industry. Other basic reference material on pharmaceutics will also be needed.

11.1 Beckett AH, Stenlake JB. *Practical Pharmaceutical Chemistry*. 4th ed. 2 v. London: Athlone Press, 1988.

11.2 Brittain HG, ed. *Analytical Profiles of Drug Substances and Excipients*. New York: Academic Press, v. 1–, 1972–. Annual.

11.3 Lund E, ed. *The Pharmaceutical Codex: Principles and Practice of Pharmaceutics*. 12th ed. London: The Pharmaceutical Press, 1994.

Beckett and Stenlake's *Practical Pharmaceutical Chemistry* is a textbook to support courses on analysis, with volume 1 dedicated to introductory basics and volume 2 devoted to more advanced topics, with particular attention to physical techniques of analysis. *Analytical Profiles of Drug Substances* puts techniques to practical use in monographs that include a description, physical properties, information on synthesis, stability/degradation, and methods of analysis for individual compounds. Each annual volume profiles fifteen to twenty substances, augmenting chemical data provided in its monographs with information on metabolism, biopharmaceutics, pharmacokinetics, and toxicity, backed up with bibliographic references. A title change in 1993 (v. 21) added excipients to coverage, and the original series editor Florey was succeeded by Brittain in the following year. Compiled under the auspices of the American Association of Pharmaceutical Scientists, this series is intended to supplement official drug compendia.

The Pharmaceutical Codex addresses the principles and practice of pharmaceutics in a broader context. Section 1 describes the characteristics, formulation, and preparation of different types of dosage forms, such as oral solids or inhalation products. Physicochemical aspects are dealt with in chapters on solution properties, suspensions, emulsions, and aerosols. Section 2 focuses on subjects associated with product design, development, and presentation, including stability and packaging. Section 3 provides information on the preparation and supply of medicines, discussing design criteria applicable to production facilities, processes, and validation. Section 4 examines pharmaceutical microbiology, sterile processing, and contamination control. Section 5 brings together material on electrolyte replacement, nutrient fluids, and dialysis solutions. Nomenclature is the topic featured in Section 6, closing out Part I. Part II of *The Pharmaceutical Codex* includes pharmaceutical data on specific drug substances, presented in monograph format.

11.4 Cunniff PA, ed. *Official Methods of Analysis of AOAC International*. 16th ed. 2 v. Gaithersburg, MD: AOAC International, 1998.

AOAC (formerly the Association of Official Analytical Chemists) is an independent organization devoted to promoting methods validation and quality measurements. *Official Methods* contains more than 2,400 collaboratively tested and peer reviewed procedures. Volume I covers methods for analysis of drugs, including drugs in animal feed. Separate sections address cosmetic analysis and veterinary toxicology. Volume II focuses on analysis of specific types of foods, with vitamins and other nutrients, color additives, direct and indirect food additives, natural toxins, infant formulas, and medical diets all singled out as individual headings. This AOAC publication is available in looseleaf printed format, to accommodate insertion of ongoing additions and revisions, and on CD-ROM.

11.5 Ghosh MK. *HPLC Methods of Drug Analysis.* Heidelberg: Springer-Verlag, 1992.

Ghosh's *HPLC Methods of Drug Analysis* is a concise compilation of information on the chemical properties of drugs and on high pressure liquid chromatography methods for their analysis. This laboratory manual describes approximately 1,300 HPLC methods for analysis of drugs and drug components from raw materials, finished pharmaceuticals, or biological samples. Information is organized under 232 headings, listed by INN. Although each entry includes a CAS RN, chemical name, and the "three most common proprietary names" used worldwide, there is no master index offering access by this alternative nomenclature. Access is, unfortunately, limited to a single generic name for each substance covered.

11.6 *Basic Tests for Pharmaceutical Substances.* Geneva: World Health Organization, 1986.
11.7 *Basic Tests for Pharmaceutical Dosage Forms.* Geneva: World Health Organization, 1991.

WHO's *Basic Tests for Pharmaceutical Substances* is intended to help field workers verify the identity of drugs when confusion arises because labeling and physical attributes do not provide adequate confirmation, or when gross degradation, adulteration, or contamination is suspected to have occurred during storage and transport. The 321 substances covered represent the majority of medications included in the WHO *Model List of Essential Drugs.*[2] Tests listed for each drug do not require fully qualified pharmacists or chemists to conduct them, and reagents and necessary equipment are purposefully kept to a minimum. Drug monographs are organized alphabetically by INN and simply list identification and degradation tests recommended for each pharmaceutical substance. No synonyms are provided in monographs or included as cross references in the index, which may forestall rapid access by intended users. For example, there is no index entry for *acetaminophen* that would lead readers to the relevant monograph for *paracetamol*.

Basic Tests for Pharmaceutical Dosage Forms, also published by the World Health Organization, provides instructions for rapid screening tests to verify the identity of 150 drugs in common use, whether formulated in tablet, capsule, solution, lotion, or other forms. Once again, the emphasis is on compiling practical procedures aimed at ensuring quality control through detection of degradation or adulteration, either unintentional or as a result of tampering or counterfeiting. Methods described require only readily available reagents and equipment and could be used by hospital pharmacists, customs inspectors, warehouse personnel, and others who must confirm the identity and integrity of purchased drug materials.

Official Compendial Standards

Industrial pharmacy information centers must include a core collection of pharmacopeias. Developed in response to concerns over consistency in the ways medicines were compounded, pharmacopeias establish official standards of identity, strength, purity, and quality for drugs in the issuing or sponsoring country. Meeting compendial standards is a prerequisite to marketing a drug in the political jurisdiction responsible for their publication.

11.8 *United States Pharmacopeia, The National Formulary 1995–USP 23/NF 18*. Rockville, MD: U.S. Pharmacopeial Convention, 1994.

11.9 *Pharmacopeial Forum*. v. 1–. Rockville, MD: United States Pharmacopeial Convention, 1975–. Bimonthly.

First published in 1820, the *United States Pharmacopeia* (*USP*) did not achieve primary official status until the enactment of the first major U.S. drug law, the Pure Foods and Drug Act, in 1906. Although it was cited in legislation as early as 1848, in the Drugs and Medicines Act, the *USP* shared this distinction with a number of European pharmacopeias also in circulation at that time.

The history of the *USP* is somewhat unusual, in that it originated in the private sector and remains to this day a production of a nongovernment institution, the United States Pharmacopeial Convention. The "Convention" designation reflects the fact that this national pharmacopeia was conceived as a collaboration and cumulation of contributions from three separate geographic districts, each of which sent delegates from medical societies and schools to the initial meeting in 1820. The product of their work was a 272-page book written in Latin and English, covering 217 drugs then in common use. The instructions it contained showed that many drugs could be collected from nature and prepared as simple mixtures. With the intent of covering only medicinals whose merit was well established and understood, contributing physicians proposed new editions every ten years. Primary responsibility for development of *USP* monographs was gradually delegated to chemists and pharmacists, who introduced simple laboratory tests and assays to set standards for strength and purity. These appeared for the first time in *USP VI* (1880).

The selective coverage and infrequent publication schedule of the *United*

States Pharmacopeia led the APhA to begin publishing *The National Formulary* (*NF*) in 1888, to provide standards for drugs not included in the *USP*. Both compendia were recognized as legal authorities in the 1906 Act and continued on concurrent ten-year publication cycles until 1940, when the need for more frequent (five-year) editions was recognized. In 1974, the United States Pharmacopeial Convention purchased *NF* from the APhA and assumed responsibility for issuing both volumes. The two appeared for the first time under one cover in the 1979 edition, with the *USP* portion dedicated to monographs for active ingredients and the *NF* section containing entries for other ingredients (i.e., excipients). Before the merger, the *USP* had begun, in its eighth edition, to include recommended dosage and dispensing information in its monographs. Even after the spin-off of *USP DI* (6.5) from the *USP-NF* in 1980, the quantity of data in the combined compendia necessitated issue of *USP-NF* in two volumes in 1983 and three volumes in 1989 (now also available on CD-ROM).

USP 23/NF 18, effective in 1995, relays official standards in more than 3,400 drug monographs and 250 entries for excipients/additives. It also includes general chapters on tests, assays, and reagents (indicators and indicator test papers, buffer, colorimetric, and volumetric solutions). Coverage is based on a substance's medical value and extent of use. Accordingly, nutritional supplements (vitamins, minerals, enteral products) have been added in recent years, and a dozen monographs on veterinary drugs represent the initial installment in a projected series of entries scheduled to expand in scope. Also new in this edition is a chapter on sterile drug products for home use. An International Harmonization icon now identifies monographs shared in common with European and Japanese pharmacopeias.

Since 1975, the *Pharmacopeial Forum* has published drafts and discussion related to new or revised monographs between editions of the *USP*. The *Forum* also publishes newly designated USANs (officially recognized nonproprietary names) on a bimonthly basis. Routine monitoring of this newsletter enables scientists to preview and participate in the development of drug standards and to propose adoption of evolving analytical methods. Between editions of *USP/NF*, new or revised monographs, once finalized, are issued in periodic supplements. For example, the *Ninth Supplement* (1998) contained nine new botanical monographs.

It's important to remember that the *USP-NF* does not cover all products on the market in the United States and that the presence of a monograph in this publication is not necessarily an indicator of U.S. market availability. Admission criteria for compendial inclusion expanded in 1997. Monographs for substances that are used extensively in compounding or commerce will be prepared, regardless of FDA approval status or lack of recognition in *USP DI*. Furthermore, some of the existing standards have been developed as a service to authorities in other countries where the *USP* is legally recognized and applied. Eight Spanish-language editions, published between 1908 and 1958 (*USP XV*), bear witness to its adoption as a government standard in many Central and South American countries.

Another distinction to note when consulting the *USP-NF* is that between product conformance and strict compliance with compendial specifications regarding test methodologies. Manufacturers may use non-*USP* methods to analyze their products, as long as the method employed will ensure that the product ultimately meets standards as described in *USP,* which conformance must be demonstrated through testing by FDA personnel using *USP-NF* methods.

11.10 *Homeopathic Pharmacopoeia of the United States.* Washington, DC: Homeopathic Pharmacopoeia Convention of the United States, 1989. [reprint of 1964 edition]

Subsequent legislative amendments have not altered the legal status of *The Homeopathic Pharmacopoeia of the United States,* which, along with the *USP* and *National Formulary,* was officially recognized in the 1938 FDC Act (sponsored by Senator Royal Copeland, a homeopathic physician) as a reference standard. It was first published in 1897; the latest (seventh) edition was issued in 1964 and reprinted in 1988. Its main use today is by practicing homeopathists and government agencies responsible for ensuring that authorized standards are met.

11.11 *European Pharmacopoeia.* 3rd ed. Sainte-Ruffine, France: Maisonneuve, 1997. Updated with annual, cumulative supplements.

Since its 1974 adoption by eight signatory states, the *European Pharmacopoeia* (*EP*) has become the official source of drug standards for twenty-seven nations, nineteen of which participate in its production.[3] Countries where the *EP* takes precedence include:

Austria	Italy
Belgium	Luxembourg
Bosnia-Herzegovina	The Netherlands
Croatia	Norway
Cypress	Portugal
Czech Republic	Slovakia
Denmark	Slovenia
Finland	Spain
France	Sweden
Germany	Switzerland
Greece	Turkey
Iceland	United Kingdom
Ireland	Yugoslav Republic of Macedonia

EP monographs, once adopted by a unanimous vote of delegates to the European Pharmacopoeia Commission responsible for their preparation, supersede any prior entries in the national or regional pharmacopeias still published by many of these countries. The third edition compiles 1,200 monographs for bulk drug substances and 250 entries establishing official chemical and biological analytical methods and reagents. The 1999 *Supplement to the European Pharmacopoeia*, the first to be published on a cumulative basis (incorporating both 1998 and 1999 updates), increased *EP* coverage to 1,450 harmonized European monographs. Between annual supplements, the *Pharmeuropa* newsletter, first issued in 1988, provides information on proposed revisions and additions (comparable to the *Pharmacopeial Forum*, 11.9).[4]

The process of selecting drugs to be covered, determining test methodologies and specifications for formulations, and agreeing upon wording and style of *EP* entries is a lengthy one, prompting many participating nations to continue developing their own compendia as interim standards while awaiting Commission concurrence. At the same time, enforcement authority has always remained the responsibility of individual countries, whether ensuring manufacturers' compliance with *EP* or with local pharmacopeial standards. Hence, companies doing business in many European markets will need to verify conformance not only with *European Pharmacopoeia* monographs, but also with other official compendia, when available. Bear in mind, also, that the *EP* does not publish detailed dosage form monographs, whereas national or regional authorities may do so.

11.12 *The International Pharmacopoeia.* 3rd ed. 4 v. Geneva: World Health Organization, 1979–1994.

The International Pharmacopoeia (*IP*) lacks the legal authority for harmonization that the *European Pharmacopoeia* carries, but can, nonetheless, be a useful acquisition in industrial pharmacy collections for companies intending to market drugs in Third World countries. Since its first edition in 1952, *IP* entries have sought to accommodate the economic and technological realities of developing nations, where quality control laboratories are unlikely to be fully equipped to perform many of the tests set forth in the *USP*. In sponsoring the development of *International Pharmacopoeia* monographs, WHO's emphasis has remained on providing basic methods to verify drug identity and to detect seriously compromised quality in therapeutic products due to decomposition, degradation, or adulteration that may occur under less than ideal storage or transport conditions (see also 11.6–11.7).

Volume 1, published in 1979, covers forty-two general methods of analysis. Descriptions of each are followed by recommended procedures for techniques classified as physical, chemical, biological, pharmacognosy, and miscellaneous. Thereafter, *IP* monographs focus on quality specifications for essential drug substances: 126 in Volume 2 (1971), 157 in Volume 3 (1988), and 24 in Volume 4 (1994). Monographs for finished dosage form preparations were first published by WHO in the 1994 volume of *The International Pharmacopoeia* (39 capsules, tablets, injections, and powders for injections). This fourth volume also provides, for the first time, separate quality specification entries for excipients.

11.13 *British Pharmacopoeia.* 3 v. London: Her Majesty's Stationery Office, 1998. Annual.

Because the *British Pharmacopoeia* (*BP*) has traditionally exerted a strong influence on other nations' drug quality control programs, it is another candidate for core industrial collection status. In common with the *USP*, the *BP* is frequently cited as a standard for dosage form, as well as bulk drug, standards by other countries in stating their requirements for imported medications. Volume I covers drug substance monographs, and Volume II provides comparable entries for formulated preparations, including blood products, immunologicals, radiopharmaceuticals, and surgical materials. Monographs for corresponding products covered in the *European Pharmacopoeia* (11.11) are also incorporated into this edition of the *British Pharmacopoeia.* Where appropriate, these have been enhanced to identify UK relevance by adding lists of *BP* preparations.

The hardcopy 1998 *British Pharmacopoeia* is accompanied, for the first time, by a CD-ROM that makes the complete text fully searchable and includes graphics for display and printing. Another bonus is that subscriptions now include the latest *British Pharmacopoeia-Veterinary*, both as a separate printed volume and integrated as a part of the full-text CD-ROM. Annual publication of both human and veterinary standards volumes will begin in 1999. Between editions, subscribers will have access to interim updates and revisions on the *BP* Web site at http://www.pharmacopoeia.co.uk. Additional resources planned at this site are a daily news service and links to other relevant URLs.

Biopharmaceutics Guides

Dosage form design and its relationship to bioavailability is the focus of biopharmaceutics research. Publications annotated here represent but a few of the recent contributions to reference bibliography needed to support drug delivery investigators.

11.14 Ansel HC, Popovich NG, Allen L. *Pharmaceutical Dosage Forms and Drug Delivery Systems.* 6th ed. Baltimore: Williams & Wilkins, 1994.

Ansel, Popovich, and Allen's *Pharmaceutical Dosage Forms and Drug Delivery Systems* is considered a definitive textbook on the topic and was formerly entitled *Introduction to Pharmaceutical Dosage Forms.* Influential factors in dosage form design are discussed in detail, including selection of nontherapeutic ingredients, product formulation, and good manufacturing practice. Separate chapters address solids, solutions and suspensions, injectables, topical product design, aerosols, suppositories, and transdermal drug delivery systems. Liberally illustrated with photographs, figures, and tables, this book also includes suggestions for follow-up reading and a glossary.

11.15 Lieberman HA, Lachman L, Schwartz JB, eds. *Pharmaceutical Dosage Forms: Tablets.* 2nd ed. 3 v. New York: Marcel Dekker, 1989–1990.

11.16 Avis KE, Lieberman HA, Lachman L, eds. *Pharmaceutical Dosage Forms: Parenteral Medications.* 2nd ed. 3 v. New York: Marcel Dekker, 1992–1993.

11.17 Lieberman HA, Rieger MM, Banker GS, eds. *Pharmaceutical Dosage Forms: Disperse Systems.* 2nd ed. 3 v. New York: Marcel Dekker, 1996–1998.

Pharmaceutical Dosage Forms is another highly-regarded textbook series published in three three-volume sets covering tablets, parenteral medications, and disperse systems. These include information of interest not only to pharmaceutical scientists in industry, but also useful as reference material for professionals in other fields, such as healthcare practitioners or legal investigators seeking technical background. For example, the final parenteral volume, issued in 1993, provides chapters on quality assurance and testing procedures, records and reports, and pertinent federal regulations. Its scope has been extended in this second edition to incorporate more information on medical devices used in parenteral drug delivery, adding material on biological control tests for device materials and updating information on regulations in light of the Safe Medical Devices Act of 1990 and developments in device control in the European Community. *Disperse Systems* volumes, the latest installment in the series, provide detailed information on specialized products such as emulsions, liposomes, polymers, surfactants, and other pharmaceutical excipients.

11.18 Welling PG, Tse FLS, Dighe SV, eds. *Pharmaceutical Bioequivalence.* New York: Marcel Dekker, 1991.

Pharmaceutical Bioequivalence organizes contributions from twenty-five scientists into sixteen chapters comprising three major subdivisions: 1) bioequivalence and its determination, 2) species differences and pharmacodynamic models, and 3) perspectives of regulatory agencies worldwide with regard to bioequivalence testing. Given the controversial and complex nature of this key factor in dosage form design and the eminence of its authors, this book is a good choice for industrial pharmacy reference collections. (Refer to Additional Sources for further biopharmaceutics selections.)

Resources to Support Formulation Development

Considering that the current U.S. drug law (FDC Act of 1938) was precipitated by deaths associated with excipient-related toxicity (diethylene glycol used as a vehicle for sulfanilamide), it is not surprising that information required for formulation development focuses, to a large extent, on finding safe and appropriate nontherapeutic ingredients to ensure delivery of active drug substances in the quantity and at the rate of release and bioavailability intended. Nontherapeutic agents intentionally included in drug formulations are generally known as excipients, but may also be referred to in the literature as additives, vehicles, bases, or pharmaceutical adjuvants or "necessities." These ingredients are not necessarily inactive or inert. They include diluents, fillers, flavors, preservatives, stabilizers, surfactants, binders, lubricants, and comparable categories of substances used to assist in efficacious drug delivery to the patient. Reilly[5] furnishes an excellent introduction to such "Pharmaceutical Necessities." *Remington's* (6.52), *The Merck Index* (3.5), *Martindale's* (6.1), and *RTECS* (8.33, 14.28) all include excipients in their coverage.

The physical and chemical properties of the therapeutic drug substance, as well as the circumstances surrounding its intended use (e.g., hospitalized or ambulatory outpatients, route of administration) exercise the strongest influence on excipient selection, but other decisive factors include commercial availability, economical production in bulk, esthetic acceptability, and freedom from contamination. Drug formulation scientists need access to information on excipients that will assist in identifying the best substances to accomplish various functions (e.g., acidification, sweetening) without interacting or interfering with other drug ingredients or triggering adverse effects in patients.

11.19 Wade A, Weller PJ. *Handbook of Pharmaceutical Excipients*. 2nd ed. Washington, DC: American Pharmaceutical Association, 1994.

By systematically describing the chemical and physical properties of candidate ingredients, Weller and Wade, in their *Handbook of Pharmaceutical Excipients*, provide a respected aid to selection of suitable substances for formulation. Published jointly by the APhA and the Pharmaceutical Society of Great Britain, the second edition of the *Handbook* adds fifty-eight new monographs to revisions of the 145 supplied in the original 1986 volume. Both organizations have unofficially assumed responsibility for augmenting information compiled in the *National Formulary* (11.8), which, until recently, confined its selective coverage to those substances found in approved NDAs, in widespread use, and administered systemically.

Handbook data include boiling point, bulk and tapped density, compression characteristics, hygroscopicity, flowability, melting point, particle size distribution, refractive index, specific surface area, and solubility, i.e., properties that can have fundamental effects on bioavailability, bioequivalence, and stability of formulations. Scanning electron microphotographs (SEMs) are also included for many substances. This edition has added information on the safe use of excipients, surveying the literature for adverse reactions associated with substances covered (see also *Adverse Reactions to Drug Formulation Agents*, 7.18). Some entries offer mini-monographs describing related substances, and others describe a large class of substances with similar uses and properties, such as suppository bases.

Twenty-two data elements organize information conveyed in each entry into a uniform and easy-to-use format: nonproprietary name, synonyms, chemical name and CAS registry number, empirical formula and molecular weight, structural formula, functional category (e.g., tablet binder), applications in pharmaceutical formulation or technology, description, pharmacopeial specifications, typical properties, stability and storage conditions, incompatibilities, method of manufacture, safety, handling precautions, regulatory status (generally recognized as safe-GRAS), pharmacopeias where cited, related substances, comments, specific bibliographic references, general references, and monograph author(s).

Nonproprietary names listed include *BP* (11.13), *EP* (11.11), and *USP-NF* (11.8) nomenclature. For nonpharmacopeial substances, other standard names are used, such as USAN. The *Handbook*'s index is thorough and practical, cross referencing from chemical, nonproprietary, and brand names, as well as "applications" terms, such as wetting agents, cationic surfactants, or preservatives. Appendix I is a directory of suppliers, presented in two separate listings, one by excipient name and another alphabetically by company name, grouped into four sections by geographic location: U.K., rest of Europe, USA, and other countries. Appendix II in the *Handbook of Pharmaceutical Excipients* is devoted to information on laboratory methods.

11.20 Ash M, Ash I. *Handbook of Pharmaceutical Additives.* Washington, DC: American Pharmaceutical Association, 1996.

11.21 Smolinske SC. *Handbook of Food, Drug, and Cosmetic Excipients.* Boca Raton, FL: CRC Press, 1992.

Weighing in at 1,132 pages, the *Handbook of Pharmaceutical Additives* supplements the scope of Wade and Weller's compendium. Its international coverage assembles entries for 3,500 brand name products and 2,500 chemicals that function as pharmaceutical additives. This volume also cross references products into seventy-five functional classifications, such as alkalizing agents or lubricants. In addition, the Ash *Handbook* provides a worldwide directory of 600 manufacturers.

The CRC *Handbook of Food, Drug, and Cosmetic Excipients* is narrower in scope, presenting detailed monographs for seventy-seven of the more than 8,000 excipients in use. Each entry lists the substance's regulatory classification (e.g., emulsifying agent, suspending agent), synonyms, available formulations, industrial products, animal toxicity data, human toxicity (immediate and delayed hypersensitivity), with commentary on clinical relevance. Monographs conclude with bibliographic references and feature tables of representative pharmaceutical products where the excipient is an ingredient, listing both brand names and manufacturers. The author notes that this information has been compiled through consultation of the *Physicians' Desk Reference* (6.10), *POISINDEX* (8.10), and *Drug*

Facts & Comparisons (6.2). Smolinske's introduction outlines the U.S. regulatory history and labeling requirements for each type of excipient (food, drug, or cosmetic). The index in this source is limited to cross references from alternative names, omitting application and potential use entries found in both the Wade and Ash handbooks cited above.

11.22 *Food Chemicals Codex*. 4th ed. Washington, DC: National Academy Press, 1996.
11.23 Lewis RJ. *Food Additives Handbook*. New York: Van Nostrand Reinhold, 1989.
11.24 Igoe RS, Hui YH, eds. *Dictionary of Food Ingredients*. 3rd ed. New York: Chapman & Hall, 1996.

One way to avoid lengthy and expensive testing required if entirely new (to regulatory authorities) drug excipients are selected is to survey substances already approved for use in foods and the information available concerning their potential toxicity or adverse reaction potential (see also 8.36–8.37). The *Food Chemicals Codex* compiles requirements for identification, specifications, test methods, and analysis data into more than 700 monographs. The *Codex* is recognized by the FDA as defining "appropriate food grade" and by government authorities in Australia, Great Britain, and New Zealand in determining the eligibility of substances for classification as GRAS (generally recognized as safe). Vendors of products containing ingredients meeting *Codex* specifications can use the initials FCC on labeling to indicate compliance. This important source covers more than 800 food grade substances, including additives, food processing aids, dextrose, and frustose.

Lewis' *Food Additives Handbook* discusses not only direct additives, but also packaging material components, pesticides added during processing (as well as those remaining as residues on food), and selected animal drugs with residue limitations in finished foods intended for humans.

The *Dictionary of Food Ingredients* covers more than 1,000 commonly used food additives, including natural ingredients, FDA-approved artificial or synthetic additives, and compounds used in food processing. Entries define functionality, chemical properties, and applications. A diskette-based version of the *Dictionary* provides cross links between similar ingredients, as well as facilitating quick look-ups by name and function or application (e.g., emulsifier, acidulant). Both hardcopy and machine-readable editions reprint the U.S.-approved listing of food ingredients from the *Code of Federal Regulations*.

11.25 Clydesdale FM. *Food Additives: Toxicology, Regulation, and Properties*. Boca Raton, FL: CRC Press, 1996.
11.26 Warner C. Molderman J, Fazio T, Sherma J. *FDA Food Additives Analytical Manual*. 2 v. Gaithersburg, MD: AOAC International, I-1983, II-1987.

Clydesdale's *Food Additives* compilation transcribes information from the Priority-Based Assessment of Food Additives (PAFA) database maintained by the FDA's Center for Food Safety and Applied Nutrition. It includes chemical toxicity data summaries based on evaluative surveys of the primary literature. Each entry is presented in a standardized format for quick reference. The *Food Additives Analytical Manual* (also known as FAAM) provides laboratory methodologies for determining compliance with FDA regulations. Separate chapters address individual additives or an entire class of pertinent compounds. Coverage includes both direct and indirect additives, as well as animal drugs.

11.27 Burdock GA. *Encyclopedia of Food and Color Additives*. 3 v. Boca Raton, FL: CRC Press, 1996.

The *Encyclopedia of Food and Color Additives* brings together a formidable amount of information, with monographs on 2,500 ingredients arranged alphabetically. Entries describe, in everyday language, what each additive is (molecular formula, physical/chemical properties) and where it originates. For naturally occurring substances, this includes family, genus, and species of origin, as well as geographic location. Regulatory notes for each additive cite GRAS status, *CFR* references, and restrictions on amount used, permitted applications, or processing, when applicable. Uses listed show how the FDA has classified the substance among thirty-two designated functions (e.g., antioxidants, texturizers). An index to the three-volume *Encyclopedia* provides access to all entries by CAS registry number and multiple synonyms. The latter include official FDA or PAFA terminology, IUPAC nomenclature, and common or folklore names for natural products. Both current and previously used CAS numbers have been compiled, as well.

11.28 Marmion DM. *Handbook of U.S. Colorants*. 3rd ed. New York: John Wiley & Sons, 1991.

Following passage of the 1938 Food Drug Cosmetic Act, the FDA defined three categories of color additives. FD&C colorants are certified for use in foods, drugs, and cosmetics in general. D&C dyes are considered safe in drugs and cosmetics, either ingested or used in direct contact with mucous membranes. "Ext D&C" colors are classified as safe only in products intended for external application. Tables in Marmion's *Handbook of U.S. Colorants* annotate approved uses and restrictions, as well as provide cross references to *Colour Index*[6] numbers and FDA official names.

Presented in three parts, the *Handbook* begins with background on the history of color additive regulation in the United States. Part I also supplies lists of currently permitted colorants (as of 1990). Each listed entry is accompanied by a description, properties, and areas of use. Part II focuses on colorant analysis, outlining procedures to meet purity requirements. Part III is a self-described "potpourri," including information on resolution of mixtures and analysis of commercial products. The resolution section addresses the needs of analytical chemists in determining the amounts and identity of individual colorants in mixtures and offers an annotated bibliography of references to specific procedures. Analysis of commercial products is also supported with an annotated bibliography, citing sources of methods to analyze general product groups, such as baked goods, beverages, or drugs. This edition of Marmion's *Handbook* also extends its scope to include colorants permitted in medical devices, such as those found in surgical sutures, surgical cements, and contact lenses.

11.29 *International Cosmetic Ingredient Dictionary and Handbook.* 7th ed. 3 v. Washington, DC: Cosmetic, Toiletry, and Fragrance Association, 1997.

Some ingredients employed in cosmetics may also have a more easily identifiable safety record than entirely novel compounds under consideration as candidate excipients in drug formulations. For this reason, reference materials related to cosmetics are often in demand in pharmaceutical industry collections. Publications from the Cosmetic, Toiletry, and Fragrance Association (CTFA) are the best known sources. The *International Cosmetic Ingredient Dictionary and Handbook* considers laws of countries other than the United States. Developed for the purpose of encouraging uniform labeling and identification of ingredients, it lists more than 9,000 INCI (International Nomenclature Cosmetic Ingredient) names, along with 37,000 chemical synonyms and brand designations. Entries represent submissions from more than thirty-one countries worldwide and 630 suppliers of raw materials. This publication is recognized in national laws and regulations of many nations as the primary source for uniform names required in labeling of cosmetics, toiletries, and other personal care items marketed within their borders. It is also considered a comprehensive list of source data, composition, and chemistry of raw materials used in cosmetics. However, it's important to remember that this *Dictionary* does not represent an "approved list" certified or endorsed by the CTFA or by any individual government.

Monographs in the *International Cosmetic Ingredient Dictionary* give INCI name, CAS registry number, empirical formula, definition or structure, information sources (various compendia), technical names (includes common names, trivial names, CAS chemical names in inverted and noninverted format, INN, USAN, brand names). Entries now also integrate material published heretofore in a separate CTFA *Handbook*, with the objective of assisting users in understanding the purpose of an ingredient in a formulation and comparing it with other compounds found in the *Dictionary*. Accordingly, monographs compile information on composition, function, chemical class, and, when available, product categories in which the ingredient has been reported as used in formulations. The FDA Voluntary Reporting Program is the source of these category data. OTC drug categories pertinent to the cosmetic industry are included as "functions": antiacne preparations, anticaries agents, antimicrobials, antiperspirants, drug astringents, external analgesics, oral healthcare drugs, skin bleaching agents, skin protectants, sunscreens, and vaginal drugs.

Indexing includes a list of INCI nomenclature, cross referenced from chemical or brand names. *Colour Index* numbers are integrated into this section. A separate CIR index is an alphabetical list, by INCI names, of substances covered in the Cosmetic Ingredient Review in the United States. Another useful index lists compounds authorized as Category I active ingredients in U.S. OTC drug products. Other index listings identify, respectively, EC approved ingredients and those authorized in Japan. Additional cross referenced lists offer access by CAS RNs, EINECS numbers (European Inventory of Existing Commercial Chemical Substances), and empirical formulas. The suppliers index in this volume is actually an alphabetical directory of manufacturers cited in the *Dictionary*, compiling complete addresses, telephone, and fax numbers.

Purchase of the three-volume hardcopy publication currently includes a CD-ROM version of this and other CTFA titles, complete with cross-searchable links. The machine-readable database transcribes the complete text of the *International Cosmetic Ingredient Dictionary and Handbook*, the *CTFA List of Japanese Cosmetic Ingredients*, the *CTFA International Color Handbook* (11.30), *Cosmetic Ingredient Review (CIR) Final Reports*, the *International Buyers Guide*, and Titles 16 and 21 of the *U.S. Code of Federal Regulations* (4.25).

11.30 *CTFA International Color Handbook*. 2nd ed. Washington, DC: Cosmetic, Toiletry, and Fragrance Association, 1992.
11.31 *CTFA Compendium of Cosmetic Ingredient Composition*. 4 v. Washington, DC: Cosmetic, Toiletry, and Fragrance Association, 1990.

The *CTFA International Color Handbook* is designed to assist regulatory and technical personnel in selecting permissible color additives in accordance with national requirements worldwide. It brings together pertinent regulations from forty-nine countries and provides a comparative analysis of their similarities and differences to U.S., EU, and Japanese regulations.

In the *Compendium of Cosmetic Ingredient Composition*, the emphasis shifts to chemical and physical specifications for hundreds of raw materials, not just colorants. Many of these ingredients are components in personal care products, a category of consumer goods containing some OTC drugs and devices. The four-volume set includes a *Specifications* handbook that lists names and chemical definitions of ingredients, cross referenced to specifications and testing methodologies to determine them. A separate *Methods* volume compiles descriptions of nearly 200 procedures, with complete apparatus requirements and detailed equations for calculating test results. The remaining two volumes in the *Compendium* assemble informative descriptions of more than 400 personal care product ingredients.

11.32 *Cosmetic Bench Reference*. Wheaton, IL: Allured Publishing, 1998.

The *Cosmetic Bench Reference* (*CBR*) has appeared in several guises over the years. It began in 1957 as the hard-cover *International Encyclopedia of Cosmetic*

Material Trade Names. From 1982 through 1987, the *CBR* appeared in the August issue of *Cosmetics & Toiletries. CBR* is a good guide to international brand names, which are integrated into the master list of ingredients as cross references to preferred CTFA names. Entries include CAS RN, CTFA CIR status, as well as indicators of whether final safety reports or scientific literature reviews are available for cited ingredients. A particularly useful feature is a separate listing of materials by function (definitions of functions are included). Coverage of mixtures, along with single chemical entities, further reinforces the utility of the *Cosmetic Bench Reference* as an aid in choosing excipients needed. Premixed components can help formulators find potential shortcuts to more economical formulations. The *CBR* also compiles a directory of manufacturers and other suppliers of ingredients.

11.33   Braun DB. *Over-the-Counter Pharmaceutical Formulations.* Park Ridge, NJ: Noyes Publications, 1994.

Another shortcut to formulation development and choice of excipients is examination of ingredients in comparable products already on the market. Braun's *Over-the-Counter Pharmaceutical Formulations* offers a classified guide to composition, with nineteen chapters dedicated to various therapeutic categories of products. Each chapter consists of two parts, the first presenting detailed composition data on representative brand name preparations, and the second relaying information on starting or prototype formulations contributed by forty-one suppliers of raw materials for OTC drugs. This reference source contains the composition of 559 brand name drugs produced by sixty-four manufacturers. General or prototype formulations add 270 alternatives to the total of 829 OTC formulations provided. Two appendices are directories of pharmaceutical manufacturers and of raw materials suppliers. Companies, brands, and active ingredient names are all access points in this volume's index. OTC drug classes covered include acne treatments; antacids/antiflatulants; antidiarrheals; antiemetics; antifungals/bacterials; antiperspirants; antipruritics; asthma treatments; cold and allergy products; contraceptives; dandruff, seborrhea, and psoriasis therapies; external analgesics; hemorrhoidal products; internal analgesics, antipyretics, and menstrual products; laxatives; ophthalmic drugs; sedatives and stimulants; sunscreens; and vitamins and minerals.

11.34   Flick EQ. *Cosmetic and Toiletry Formulations.* 2nd ed. Park Ridge, NJ: Noyes Publications, v.1–, 1989–.
11.35   Flick EQ. *Cosmetics Additives, An Industrial Guide.* Park Ridge, NJ: Noyes Publications, 1991.

The 1,800 entries in Volume 1 of Flick's *Cosmetic and Toiletry Formulations* are also organized into separate sections devoted to general categories of products, followed by directory information. Each formulation entry lists raw materials used, percent by weight of each, suggested formulation procedure, and source of data (company or organization that supplied the formula). Brand names of ingredients are cross-referenced to generic designations and to company names in an alphabetic ingredient directory following the fourteen formulation chapters. A directory of supplier addresses concludes the volume. Subsequently issued volumes in this series are actually supplements published in 1992, 1995, 1996, and 1998 duplicating the product category/directory section arrangement, but adding more than 2,000 formulations not found in Volume 1. *Cosmetic and Toiletry Formulations* includes listings for antiperspirants and deodorants, beauty aids, creams, fragrances and perfumes, insect repellents, lotions, shampoos, soaps, and baby, bath and shower, hair care, shaving, and sun care products.

Cosmetics Additives, An Industrial Guide, from the same author and publisher, is basically a directory of ingredient suppliers. Entries for eighty-four manufacturers and distributors are arranged alphabetically by company name. Each company's listing includes product names and numbers, with brief descriptions of the properties and applications of each ingredient or additive. The *Industrial Guide* concludes with an index to the 4,000 brand names covered and a directory of supplier addresses.

Sourcebooks in Pharmaceutical Technology

Guides to manufacturing processes and general reference works addressing a broad spectrum of topics related to pharmaceutical technology will round out the basic industrial pharmacy collection.

11.36 Sittig M, ed. *Pharmaceutical Manufacturing Encyclopedia.* 2nd ed. 2 v. Park Ridge, NJ: Noyes Publications, 1988.

The *Pharmaceutical Manufacturing Encyclopedia* has been compiled with the intent to accelerate the introduction of generic drugs after patent expiration of brand name products. Editor Sittig also foresees opportunities for innovative chemists to develop processes that go beyond original patent claims and offer a legal route to extending a product's shelf life. Entries in this *Encyclopedia*, arranged alphabetically by generic name, give details for the manufacture of 1,295 pharmaceuticals (available as of 1988) marketed as brand name products somewhere in the world. Information is derived from pertinent U.S. and U.K. patents. In addition to patent-derived process data, product entries also cite references to the primary literature related to the drug's synthesis and pharmacology. Two indexes offer access by brand name and by any of 2,000 names for raw materials used in the manufacture of products covered.

11.37 Swarbrick J, Boylan JC, eds. *Encyclopedia of Pharmaceutical Technology.* New York: Marcel Dekker, v. 1–, 1988–.

Due to its broad ranging scope, the *Encyclopedia of Pharmaceutical Technology* should be considered a core collection title in libraries serving not only the pharmaceutical industry, but also chemical and pharmacy education. Well written monographs contributed by recognized subject experts from the United States and Europe address a variety of topics related to drug discovery, development, regulation, manufacturing, and commercialization. For example, entries include essays on bioabsorbable polymers, bioavailability of drugs and bioequivalence, the economics of pharmaceutical research and development, expiration dating, gamma radiation sterilization, gastrointestinal absorption of drugs, and gels and jellies. Monographs on orphan drugs, new drug applications, nonprescription drugs, medical devices, and liability aspects of drugs and devices cited in Chapter Four demonstrate the potential utility of this source. The basic A–Z set of seventeen volumes was completed in 1997. Volume 18, issued in 1998, is a supplement adding entries on a spectrum of subjects that illustrate, once again, the *Encyclopedia*'s outstanding contribution to the reference literature. Additions include essays on hydrogels, ultrasonic nebulizers, transdermal drug delivery systems, WHO and the harmonization of regulatory requirements for medical products, and pharmaceutical patents and the Waxman-Hatch Act.

11.38 DeSain C. *Drug, Device and Diagnostic Manufacturing.* 2nd ed. Buffalo Grove, IL: Interpharm Press, 1992.

Subtitled "The Ultimate Resource Handbook," DeSain's *Drug, Device and Diagnostic Manufacturing* is an eclectic compilation of definitions, basic explanations of concepts and processes, and bibliographies of recommended reading. An appendix of information sources includes government agencies; associations, institutes, and laboratories; journals, newsletters, and periodic reports; publishers; agency research centers; continuing education providers; and financing information resources. Although directory entries are complete, bibliographic citations to reference books are not. Titles, publishers, and (occasionally) authors are given, but no other data.

The breadth of topics covered and common sense approach to providing concise answers to industry-related questions mitigate, somewhat, flaws in bibliographic citation style. Chapters address manufacturing facility operations, documentation systems and documentation control, quality assurance, process validation, and similar issues. Case studies illustrate how individual companies deal with operational challenges and describe situations that have led to problems. Organizations marketing products to the pharmaceutical industry will find these thumbnail sketches useful in characterizing norms and learning more about internal procedures. Sections devoted to funding and financing and the cost of R&D are particularly useful in this regard. *Drug, Device and Diagnostic Manufacturing* covers an unusually diverse selection of subject matter and would be a good introductory reference source for startup companies, individuals newly hired in the industry, and organizations with something to sell to them.

References

1. Archer M. Technical development and production information. In: Pickering WR, ed. *Information sources in pharmaceuticals*. London: Bowker-Saur, 1990:113–143.

2. *The use of essential drugs. Model list of essential drugs.* 8th list. Geneva: World Health Organization, 1995.

3. European Pharmacopoeia—"a living European institution." *Scrip* 1989 Jul 12;1428:6.

4. Pharmeuropa's first issue published. *Scrip* 1988 Oct 10;1356:3.

5. Reilly WJ. Pharmaceutical necessities. In: Gennaro AR, ed. *Remington's pharmaceutical sciences*. 19th ed. Easton, PA: Mack Publishing, 1995:1380–1416.

6. Society of Dyers and Colourists, American Association of Textile Chemists and Colorists. *Colour index*. 3rd ed. 9 v. Bradford, England: Society of Dyers and Colourists, 1971–.

Additional Sources of Information

Aulton ME. *Pharmaceutics: the science of dosage form design*. New York: Churchill Livingstone, 1988.

Balsam MS, Sagarin E. *Cosmetics: science and technology*. 2nd ed. 3 v. New York: Kreiger, 1992.

Banker GS, Rhodes CT, eds. *Modern pharmaceutics*. 3rd ed. New York: Marcel Dekker, 1996.

Bauer K, Garbe D, Surburg H, eds. *Common fragrance and flavor materials*. 3rd ed. New York: John Wiley & Sons, 1997.

Biological substances: international standards and reference reagents 1990. Geneva: World Health Organization, 1991.

Brooks G, ed. *Biotechnology in healthcare: An introduction to biopharmaceuticals*. London: The Pharmaceutical Press, 1998.

Burdock GA. *Fenaroli's handbook of flavor ingredients*. Boca Raton, FL: CRC Press, 1994.

Burger's medicinal chemistry and drug discovery. 5th ed. 5 v. New York: Wiley, 1995–1997.

Carstensen J. *Drug stability, principles and practices*. 2nd ed. New York: Marcel Dekker, 1995.

Chien YW, ed. *Novel drug delivery systems*. 2nd ed. Drugs and the pharmaceutical sciences, v. 50. New York: Marcel Dekker, 1991.

CTFA list of Japanese cosmetic ingredients. 3rd ed. Washington, DC: Cosmetic, Toiletry, and Fragrance Association, 1997.

Evaluation of certain food additives and contaminants. Technical report series no. 859. Geneva: World Health Organization, 1995.

Florence AT, ed. *Materials used in pharmaceutical formulation*. Boston: Blackwell Scientific Publications, 1984.

Foye WO, Williams D, Lemke TL, eds. *Principles of medicinal chemistry*. 4th ed. Baltimore: Williams & Wilkins, 1995.

Japanese Pharmaceutical Excipients Council. *Japanese pharmaceutical excipients 1993.* Tokyo: Yakuji Nippon, 1994.

Japanese Pharmaceutical Excipients Council. *Supplement to Japanese pharmaceutical excipients.* 3rd ed. Tokyo: Yakuji Nippon, 1998.

Japanese standards of pharmaceutical ingredients 1991 and supplement. Tokyo: Yakuji Nippon, 1992.

Karsa DR, Stephenson RA, eds. *Excipients and drug delivery systems for pharmaceutical formulations.* Boca Raton, FL: CRC Press, 1995.

Kreuter J, ed. *Colloidal drug delivery systems.* Drugs and the pharmaceutical sciences, v. 66. New York: Marcel Dekker, 1994.

Lieberman R, Mukherjee A, eds. *Principles of drug development in transplantation and autoimmunity.* Austin, TX: R.G. Landes, 1996.

Martin AN. *Problem solving, physical pharmacy IV.* Philadelphia: Lea & Febiger, 1993.

McGinty JW. *Aqueous polymeric coatings for pharmaceutical dosage forms.* 2nd ed. New York: Marcel Dekker, 1997.

Mitra AK, ed. *Ophthalmic drug delivery systems.* Drugs and the pharmaceutical sciences, v. 58. New York: Marcel Dekker, 1993.

Ranade VV, Hollinger MA, eds. *Drug delivery systems.* Boca Raton, FL: CRC Press, 1995.

Reiger MM, Rhein LD, eds. *Surfactants in cosmetics.* 2nd ed. New York: Marcel Dekker, 1997.

Ridgway K, ed. *Hard capsules: Development and technology.* London: The Pharmaceutical Press, 1987.

Romanowski P, Schueller R. Your primer of technical terms and chemical jargon; a "dictionary" of the terms you may encounter in the formulation lab. *Cosmet Toiletries* 1995 Mar;110(3):44–49.

Schirmer RE. *Modern methods of drug analysis.* 2nd ed. 2 v. Boca Raton, FL: CRC Press, 1991.

Senzel AJ, ed. *Newburger's manual of cosmetic analysis.* 2nd ed. Gaithersburg, MD: AOAC International, 1977.

Tableting Specifications Manual. Washington, DC: American Pharmaceutical Association, 1995.

Toxicological evaluation of certain food additives and contaminants. WHO food additives series no. 35. Geneva: World Health Organization, 1996.

Tyle P, ed. *Specialized drug delivery systems; manufacturing and production technology.* Drugs and the pharmaceutical sciences, v. 41. New York: Marcel Dekker, 1990.

Waggoner WC. *Clinical safety and efficacy testing in cosmetics.* New York: Marcel Dekker, 1989.

12

Special Topics

Sources discussed in previous chapters will answer the majority of drug information questions originating from health science professionals. Hardcopy bibliography to support inquiries that occur less frequently is the focus of this chapter. Examples of such inquiries include 1) pharmacognosy, 2) veterinary drugs, and 3) the history of pharmacy. Discussion of additional pharmacognosy resources available online is included in Chapter Fourteen.

Pharmacognosy: The Literature of Natural Drugs

Pharmacognosy literature deals with descriptive pharmacology of crude drugs derived from nature (i.e., plants, animals, bacteria, fungi, marine organisms). The study of folk medicine (ethnopharmacology) has spurred much research in the discipline. When the same or similar species are found to be used for comparable purposes in culturally and geographically unrelated communities, scientific investigations into efficacy often yield promising new compounds. The potential scope for investigation is enormous; more than 80% of plant species have yet to be screened for chemical/biological activity.[1] No textbook on the history of pharmacy is without mention of the use of plant- and animal-derived remedies from ancient times. Indeed, until the 1920s the practice of pharmacy was limited, for the most part, to the preparation of such extracts. It was not until the introduction of sulfa drugs in the 1930s that medicine began to rely more and more on synthetic organic chemicals in therapy.

It has been estimated that more than half of the 250 largest pharmaceutical companies are conducting research into phytotherapeutics.[2] Houghton[3] attributes this revival of interest in plant-derived medicinals to several factors, including the undisputed clinical efficacy of many natural products, such as vincristine and taxol. Compounds isolated from plant material have frequently served as molecular templates (models) for designing more effective synthetic drugs (e.g., alkaloids of curare). They have also proved to be inexpensive sources of "feedstock" molecules readily transformed into drugs. Production of some oral contraceptives, for example, is made possible by the processing of steroidal components in yams or sisal.[4] Such success stories add impetus to research efforts, along with increased recognition of the urgent need to salvage important ethnobotanic information before it is lost, due to disappearing cultures and destruction of natural habitats.

Furthermore, botanicals are good business. According to the World Health Organization, 80% of the global population relies on plant-based drugs for health care. In the United Kingdom and North America, at least 25% of the active components in currently prescribed medicines were first identified in higher plants.[5] In Germany, France, Italy, Austria, and Switzerland, phytomedicines are an integral part of conventional medical therapy. The U.S. market for botanicals is calculated to be only one-third the size of that in Europe.[6] Yet, U.S. consumer out-of-pocket expenses for herbal products in 1997 alone were estimated at $5.1 billion.[7] Companies that specialize in production of herbal remedies have experienced an annual sales growth of 12–15%, a much higher rate than seen in sales of conventional OTCs.[8]

Renewed public interest in natural medicine is also reflected in pharmaceutical information queries. In addition to dietary supplements, herbal teas and cigarettes may be the subject of inquiry, and reference material on medicinal plants in general is currently in demand. Many pharmacognosy questions are likely to mirror major issues and concerns regarding drugs used in nonorthodox medicine, which have been cogently summarized by De Smet.[9] For example, relatively little is known about possible drug interactions or lab test modifications when orthodox and natural remedies are taken concurrently, although *Meyler's Side Effects of Drugs* (7.1, 7.2) has begun to compile pertinent bibliography. Effects of over consumption may also lead to inquiries, as well as requests for bibliography on potential contaminants in herbal medicines.

Identifying product ingredients is a first step before adequate literature research on adverse effects can be conducted. Unfortunately, this is not always an easy task, as was compellingly illustrated in a 1992 survey of nutritional supplements published in *JAMA*.[10] Results cite numerous unusual or unidentifiable ingredients among the 235 substances listed in labeling for 311 products on the market in the United States. In a subsequent search of the scientific literature, the authors were unable to locate toxicity data for 139 of compounds named (59% of the sample). These data emphasize the need for sources that focus on natural product ingredients. In addition, aids to visual identification of plants are likely to be required, both to forestall erroneous identification of self-collected botanical material and to assist in *post hoc* investigation of mishaps.

Martindale's (6.1) contains many references to herbal medications and their uses (past and present). Earlier editions of the *United States Dispensatory*[11] are worth tracking down for the excellent documentation of historic uses they can provide. The first twenty editions (1833–1960), published under the title *Dispensatory of the United States of America*, offer encyclopedic coverage of botanicals, supported by background bibliography. (See also the *Dictionary of Protopharmacology*, 12.58.) Biotoxin resources discussed in Chapter Eight will answer many questions about poisonous or injurious plants and animals (8.48–8.56). A few selections from the popular (consumer-oriented) pharmacognosy bibliography are cited in Chapter Nine, *The Honest Herbal* (9.19) and APhA's *Practical Guide to Natural Medicines* (9.20) being the most noteworthy. Additional popular and professional resources are listed at the end of this chapter. Selection is based on their potential ability to answer frequently asked questions. Publications annotated in more detail below represent only a small sample of reference material available.

Textbooks

12.1 Evans WC, ed. *Trease and Evans' Pharmacognosy*. 14th ed. London: W.B. Saunders, 1996.

12.2 Robbers JE, Speedie MK, Tyler VE. *Pharmacognosy and Pharmacobiotechnology*. Baltimore: Williams & Wilkins, 1996.

12.3 Bruneton J. *Pharmacognosy, Phytochemistry, Medicinal Plants*. New York: Springer Verlag, 1995.

Among professional works, *Trease and Evans' Pharmacognosy*, first published in 1934, heads the list as a definitive introductory textbook on the topic. It includes extensive background material on plant morphology, anatomy and taxonomy, herbal medicine, pharmacology, phytochemistry and chromatography, and commercial production of natural products. In monographs organized by chemical type (e.g., alkaloids, saponins, steroids, phenolics), plant-derived pharmaceuticals singled out for discussion encompass tumor inhibitors, opiate analgesics, cardiac glycosides, corticosteroids, anthraquinone laxatives, and volatile oil carminatives. New in this edition are chapters dedicated to coloring and flavoring agents, antihepatotoxic and hypoglycemic agents, and antiprotozoal drugs derived from plants, as well as biologically active compounds from marine sources. The text covers the contribution of plants to both orthodox and complementary systems of medicine, expanding its scope in the 14th edition to include essential oils used in aromatherapy, plants used in African traditional medicine, and Chinese herbs used in the United Kingdom. Both the editor and contributors are acknowledged experts in their field, who have richly supplemented their discussion with references to further reading.

For many years, Tyler's *Pharmacognosy* was also a standard textbook used in pharmacy school curricula in the United States. After nine successive editions

(1921–1988), a new text issued with a modified title signals changes in the scientific discipline. With pharmacobiotechnology added to its coverage, this publication acknowledges innovations in drug discovery and development from natural products. At the same time, chapters seen in previous versions of the text, each devoted to a class of chemicals important in phytopharmaceuticals, are replicated and expanded. Complex polysaccharides, glycosides, lipids, terpenoids, steroids, phenylpropanoids, alkaloids, and proteins and peptides are dealt with in turn. What's new in *Pharmacognosy and Pharmacobiotechnology* are concluding chapters devoted to antibiotics, biologics, and immunomodulators.

Chemistry is the primary emphasis in Bruneton's contribution to the literature of pharmacognosy. Discussion begins with a section devoted to compounds of primary metabolism, such as carbohydrates, proteins, and enzymes. Part II of *Pharmacognosy, Phytochemistry, Medicinal Plants* focuses on phenolics, acetates, and shikimates, including tannins, flavinoids, and anthrocyanins. Part III compiles chemical data on terpenoids and steroids of botanical origin. In Part IV, alkaloids come under scrutiny. With its thorough review of the chemical basis of herbal pharmacology, Bruneton's work qualifies as a core reference for researchers and advanced students, rather than an introductory text.

Official Compendia

As was noted in Chapter Eleven, the *USP/NF* (11.8) has stepped up production of standard-setting monographs for botanicals in recent years. However, many popular herbal preparations currently on the U.S. market have yet to be addressed in official compendia originating in this country. This may account for the high degree of interest in standards evolving in Western Europe, where phytomedicinals have long been an integral part of therapeutic options.

12.4 Brumenthal M et al., eds. *The Complete German Commission E Monographs: Therapeutic Guide to Herbal Medicines.* Boston: Integrative Medicine Communications, 1998.

In 1978, the German Federal Health Agency established an independent panel of experts to collect information on botanical remedies sold in German pharmacies and evaluate the evidence regarding their safety and efficacy. Known as Commission E, the panel produces brief monographs that either approve or disapprove specific herbal drugs for nonprescription use. Each evaluation takes into account history of use, chemistry, pharmacological studies in animals, human clinical studies, when available, and even subjective assessments by patients and physicians, based on clinical experience. Accordingly, the resulting monographs have been eagerly awaited by scientists and medical practitioners worldwide. Tyler (12.9), for example, has referred to this body of work as "the most accurate information available."

The American Botanical Council commissioned translations of *Commission E*

Monographs into English, which has led to the 685-page resource cited here published by Integrative Medicine Communications. It includes monographs for 380 herbs and fixed combinations, 190 of which show evidence of proven safety and efficacy. Details regarding approval status, composition (plant family, plant part, primary chemical constituents), uses, mechanism of action, dosage and maximum duration of administration for safe use, side effects, interactions with conventional drugs, and contraindications are included for each botanical, with entries listed by common English name, followed by Latin pharmacopeial and German names. Separate therapeutic indices enable access to approved herbs by 150 indications authorized in Germany, by pharmacological action, by side effect keywords, or by contraindications terminology. Unapproved herbs are indexed by pharmacological action, side effects, and (in an addendum) contraindications. Chemical and taxonomic cross-reference indices have also been constructed for this English-language edition of the *Commission E Monographs*.

Other extras in the volume include excerpts from pertinent European regulations, with portions of the German and European pharmacopeias transcribed, as well as extracts from European Economic Community Standards for Quality of Herbal Remedies. Appendices provide 1) a key to abbreviations and symbols, 2) weights and measures, 3) German Federal Gazette (*Bundesanzeiger*) citations, 4) a list of European Scientific Cooperative on Phytotherapy (ESCOP) monographs, 5) an inventory of relevant WHO monographs, 6) a glossary, and 7) a master index.

12.5 *ESCOP Monographs on the Medicinal Uses of Plant Drugs.* Exeter, Devon, England: European Scientific Cooperative on Phytotherapy, 1990–.

The European Scientific Cooperative on Phytotherapy is a quasiofficial group formed in 1989 as an umbrella organization of national associations devoted to advancing knowledge in the area of botanically-derived drugs. Harmonization of regulatory status is its chief goal. To accomplish this, ESCOP is compiling proposals for European Monographs summarizing the medicinal uses of plant drugs and evaluating their safety. The first five of these were submitted to the Committee for Proprietary Medicinal Products (CPMP) in 1990, followed by ten more in 1992. Since then, their format has changed to comply with guidelines for Summary of Product Characteristics (SPC) documentation subsequently adopted by the European Union. SPCs are an important part of applications to market medicinal products for human use in any of the EU member states. Once authorized, SPCs become the information base from which product data sheets (labeling, professional package inserts) are derived.

Hence, *ESCOP Monographs* issued from 1993 forward give more emphasis to clinical data and pharmacological properties, including pharmacodynamics, pharmacokinetics, and preclinical safety evaluations. It should be noted that these published summaries are not the precise equivalents of SPC proposals submitted to regulatory authorities, because they omit details regarding the specific products under consideration. However, *ESCOP Monographs* do provide compilations of scientific data on plant drugs, resulting from a thorough review and critical evaluation of the available literature and other clinical evidence of safety and efficacy. Their content will supplement and complement *Commission E* standards, which is why a list of them is a valuable addition to appendices in the English-language edition described in the previous entry (12.4). A complete inventory of genus-species (cross referenced to common names) covered in *ESCOP Monographs* published thus far is also available at http://www.ex.ac.uk/ phytonet/pubs.html. Five fascicules, each containing ten monographs, are currently available.

12.6 *British Herbal Pharmacopoeia*. 2nd ed. Bournemouth, Dorset, England: British Herbal Medicine Association, 1996.
12.7 Bradley P, ed. *British Herbal Compendium*. v. 1. Bournemouth, Dorset, England: British Herbal Medicine Association, 1992.

These two British Herbal Medicine Association publications have not been formally adopted as official regulatory standards, but are, nonetheless, likely to prove helpful to manufacturers of phytomedicines. First published in 1990, the *British Herbal Pharmacopoeia* contains monographs outlining quality standards for 169 herbs commonly used in the United Kingdom for the preparation of botanical drugs. Thin-layer chromatographic techniques for comparative identification of botanicals are the chief focus of *BHP* entries, to provide quality control guidelines for physical specification of plant raw materials introduced into commerce. Monographs also include descriptions of powdered materials and brief reference to therapeutic actions.

The *British Herbal Compendium* is designed to complement the *BHP* by summarizing research findings on the therapeutic efficacy and safety of 84 plant drugs covered in the *British Herbal Pharmacopoeia* published in 1990. Monographs in the *Compendium* consist of sections on constituents, therapeutics, regulatory status, and references. Information included under constituents considerably augments *BHP* content by providing structural formulas, whenever possible, and citing assay methodologies.

Because many of the phytomedicinals covered in the *British Herbal Compendium* are regulated as foods or nutritional supplements, rather than drugs, the regulatory status portion of monographs distinguishes between the two. Not only is the official status in the United Kingdom defined for each plant drug, but also its regulatory position under Belgian, French, German, U.S., and EU law. Citations to pharmacopeial monographs for given drugs already available in the official compendia of various nations within Europe are listed, as well as references to pertinent *USP/NF* (11.8) standards.

Similarly meticulous is documentation compiled to support information summarized in the therapeutics section of each monograph. References to numerous scientific journal articles and books will serve as good startup bibliographies when further research is contemplated. When original text cited is not in English, language is noted, as is the presence of an English-language abstract, when available. A final, fifth section is added to many monographs in the *British Herbal Compendium*. It consists of translated excerpts of therapeutic information drawn from applicable published regulatory guidelines in effect in Belgium, France, or Germany. These three European countries are singled out because they are actively engaged in national assessments of plant drugs on a generic, rather than product-by-product, basis.

12.8 *Research Guidelines for Evaluating the Safety and Efficacy of Herbal Medicines*. Geneva: World Health Organization, 1993.

Standardization and regulation of research are issues that must be addressed before botanicals can be more fully integrated into primary health care. The World Health Organization has been active in fostering discussion of these issues and in development of quality control specifications as reference points for national regulatory authorities. *Research Guidelines for Evaluating the Safety and Efficacy of Herbal Medicines* represents a consensus of criteria reached by seventeen experts in pharmacology, biochemistry, and traditional medicine. In Part One of this book, the special properties of herbal medicines are outlined from the point of view of designing research protocols acceptable in the scientific, as well as legal and regulatory, community. Part Two sets out detailed guidelines, including recommended methods of investigation for preclinical studies and Phase I-IV clinical trials. Part Three presents specific recommendations for research: e.g., how to establish the identity and quality of plant materials and preparations, methodologies for pharmacodynamic studies, and standards for toxicity testing.

Clinical Reference Sources

Unlike textbooks of pharmacognosy or official compendial standards for herbal drugs, clinical reference sources offer more immediately practical guidance to healthcare practitioners seeking information on safe and effective use of natural products.

12.9 Tyler VE, Robbers JE. *Herbs of Choice. The Therapeutic Use of Phytomedicinals*. 2nd ed. Binghamton, NY: Pharmaceutical Products Press, 1998.

Herbs of Choice is a good example of this type of publication. In it, Tyler and Robbers have compiled valuable information on the pharmacology, therapeutics, and toxicology of common phytomedicinals. Organized in chapters dedicated to disorders associated with ten body systems (e.g., digestive system problems, respiratory tract), discussion evaluates scientific evidence of safety and efficacy (or lack thereof) for more than 100 herbs likely to be encountered in self-medication by patients. The second edition adds entries for herbs that have become popular since the original 1994 volume. It also updates discussion of available clinical data to reflect a flurry of research into efficacy and mode of action.

12.10 Newall CA, Anderson LA, Phillipson JD. *Herbal Medicines, A Guide for Healthcare Professionals*. London: The Pharmaceutical Press, 1996.

Published under the auspices of the Royal Pharmaceutical Society of Great Britain, *Herbal Medicines, A Guide for Healthcare Professionals* assembles evidence regarding the quality, safety, and efficacy of 141 herbs already present in remedies commonly sold by pharmacies in the United Kingdom. Monographs, arranged alphabetically by vernacular plant name (e.g., Golden Seal, Cowslip), summarize available scientific information with the intent of providing practitioners with sufficient facts to advise the general public on rationale and safe use. Appendices cover potential drug-herbal interactions and, in nineteen separate listings, group together herbs with specific actions, such as laxative, diuretic, hypotensive, allergenic, or irritant ingredients.

12.11 *PDR for Herbal Medicines*. Montvale NJ: Medical Economics, 1998.

Published in collaboration with Phytopharm Consulting, the new *PDR for Herbal Medicines* relays "prescribing information" for more than 600 herbs in common use in the United States. Entries include descriptions of each plant and compounds derived from it, a summary of pharmacological effects, documented indications, other uses, applicable precautions and contraindications, overdose information, modes of administration, and dosage. Supportive bibliography has been derived from the *German Commission E Monographs* (12.4).

12.12 Brendler T, Gruenwald J, Jaenicke C, eds. *Herbal Remedies*. 2nd ed. Washington, DC: American Pharmaceutical Association, 1997.

Herbal Remedies is a CD-ROM resource with coverage of more than 600 plants. Entries compile scientific and common names, plant family and basic botanical information, and geographic origin. Habitats are shown on a world map and color photos accompany the majority of monographs. Data on more than 670 botanical drugs include ingredients and active constituents, specifications for extraction and forms of administration, pharmacology, uses, side effects, interactions, and toxicity. The CD-ROM also provides a glossary of botanical and medicinal terms.

12.13 Wichtl M, Bisset NG, eds. *Herbal Drugs and Phytopharmaceuticals, A Handbook for Practice on a Scientific Basis*. Boca Raton, FL: CRC Press, 1994.

Herbal Drugs and Phytopharmaceuticals assembles detailed monographs on 181 medicinal plants selected for inclusion based on a survey of German pharmacies. This beautifully presented, large format reference book includes color prints of the actual "crude drug" form (dried plant part used medicinally) and color photographs of plants growing in their natural habitat. Arranged by Latin names, entries begin by bringing together alternative nomenclature (a selection of French, German, and English names) and citing references to pharmacopeial standards, when applicable. Each monograph identifies medicinally active constituents (often with chemical structures), indications, side effects, commercially available forms of phytomedicines, exporting countries, and regulatory status. Information on authentication using macroscopical, microscopical, and chromatographic techniques emphasizes diagnostic features of the crude drug which are essential for reliable identification. Discussion also mentions likely adulterations and storage requirements. Wichtl, translated from German into English by Bisset, clearly distinguishes between phytochemicals whose efficacy has been substantiated and those where only empirical folk evidence exists. Abstracts of *Commission E Monographs* (12.4) are included. The full text of package inserts (translated again, when necessary) is included in monographs for plants available as licensed drugs. A combined subject index offers access by alternative names and indication keywords.

12.14 Weiss RF. *Herbal Medicine*. Beaconsfield, England: Beaconsfield Publishers, 1988.

Weiss' *Herbal Medicine* is a translation of the sixth German edition of *Lehrbuch der Phytotherapie*, which aims to present only clinically significant and scientifically validated uses of phytomedicinals. Introductory chapters provide an overview of the terminology and history of herbal medicine, discussing the role of empiricism (and its drawbacks) in establishing proof of efficacy for plant-derived drugs. Written by a medical doctor for use by fellow physicians, this book includes detailed guidelines for prescribing, dependent on clinical diagnoses. Organized by body systems (e.g., digestive, cardiovascular, respiratory, urinary), discussion focuses on the medicinal actions of a variety of plants and herbal preparations, with suggested prescriptions, details of dosage, application, and precautions. Information on botanical features and occurrence is also included, with many entries illustrated by line drawings. Bibliographic references are cited throughout this work, with a preference, as might be expected, for German-language source materials. The index to *Herbal Medicine* enables access by both common and scientific plant names and by conditions or indications.

12.15 Ross IA, ed. *Medicinal Plants of the World*. Totowa, NJ: Humana Press, 1998.

In *Medicinal Plants of the World*, Ross features twenty-seven major plant species widely used in medical formulations available commercially around the globe. A separate chapter on each plant summarizes available scientific data on chemical constituents, pharmacological activities, and clinical experience. Information supplied includes how each plant is used therapeutically in different countries. Color photos, detailed botanical descriptions, and listings of common names worldwide will assist in identification. Further investigation will also be assisted by the substantial bibliography of 1,585 references compiled in this 448-page compendium.

12.16 Der Marderosian A, Liberti L. *Natural Product Medicine. A Scientific Guide to Foods Drugs Cosmetics.* Philadelphia: G.F. Stickley, 1988.

Broader in scope than several other sources cited in this section, *Natural Product Medicine* nonetheless shares the same purpose: to provide health science professionals with authoritative background material. The authors are both associated with publication of *The Lawrence Review of Natural Products* (12.17). Their first nine chapters describe natural products by chemotaxonomic class and mechanism of action (e.g., CNS stimulants). Discussion includes the pharmacological activity of various food substances and potential drug interactions, as well as covering diseases induced by naturally occurring dietary compounds, and herbal teas (benefits and hazards). Other chapters in the first section of the book describe the clinical impact of poisonous plants and animals; consequences of interactions between Rx, OTC, and natural medicines; and the clinical implications of health foods.

The second half of the volume consists of well-referenced monographs for individual natural products judged by the authors as being of greatest clinical importance. Each entry brings together information on nomenclature, taxonomy, history, chemistry, pharmacology, and toxicology and is designed to answer such questions as: What active compounds have been isolated from this product? What evidence is there to substantiate or disprove its medical use? Is this product safe? Appendices include a good startup bibliography of additional pharmacognosy resources and a useful glossary.

12.17 *The Lawrence Review of Natural Products.* St. Louis: Facts and Comparisons, 1980–. Monthly.

Established in 1980, *The Lawrence Review of Natural Products* issues three to five brief reviews of selected products per month, each produced on separate looseleaf sheets in a standardized monograph format. As a rule, monographs present information in nine sections: scientific (Latin) names, common names, botany or description of source, history, chemistry, pharmacology, toxicology, summary, and references. Characterized by lucid prose and sound scientific assessments, these reviews are an inexpensive and popular source of basic pharmacognosy data. The looseleaf format has evolved into a cumulative Monograph System, which compiles more than 200 previously published *Lawrence* product reviews that, once purchased, can be kept up-to-date by annual subscription. Filing updates is simple, requiring insertion of new sheets into the alphabetical sequence, where monographs are arranged by a common product name identified in their upper right-hand corner. Each is clearly dated and indicates whether it replaces a previous monograph issued at an earlier date. Subscriptions to the Monograph System include a semiannual subject index, issued in June and December, which lists monograph topics in bold face, along with the date of their most recent update, and provides additional keyword access by scientific and common names.

12.18 *American Herbal Products Association's Botanical Safety Handbook: Guidelines for Safe Use and Labeling.* Boca Raton, FL: CRC Press, 1997.

The *American Herbal Products Association Botanical Safety Handbook* contains more than 600 entries, alphabetized by Latin binomial. Dubbed "safety monographs," each outlines safe use and precautions, including specifics related to prior health conditions, pregnancy, and breast feeding. Appendix 1 in the *Handbook* provides profiles of active herbal constituents. Appendix 2 focuses on known herbal actions or functions, such as emetics, stimulants, or photosensitivity agents. Appendix 3 lists herbs by labeling classifications such as: external use only or not to be used in pregnancy. Bibliographic references and a plant index conclude the *Botanical Safety Handbook*. Given its origin, this source could prove useful to manufacturers of herbal products. However, as with many brief guides on the topic now appearing on the market, the intended audience is unclear. Holistic practitioners and consumers could also be potential users.

Identification Resources

It's often difficult to classify pharmacognosy ready-reference tools for the purpose of collection development. Many aids to identification, for example, provide basic therapeutic information, as well as regulatory status. However, resources annotated in this section tend, in general, to be designed for quick consultation to derive substance/plant lists that match user-defined criteria and to glean basic nomenclature and chemical data before further bibliographic research is initiated.

12.19 Leung AY, Foster S. *Encyclopedia of Common Natural Ingredients.* 2nd ed. New York: John Wiley & Sons, 1995.

Since publication of the first edition in 1980, Leung's *Encyclopedia of Common Natural Ingredients* has achieved the status of a reference classic, due to its coverage of frequently requested substances and well organized, lengthy monographs. This new edition, with a scope increased to more than 500 ingredients, includes many herbs that have grown in popularity since their omission in the initial volume. What has not changed is the quality and organization of its content. Arranged by common name, entries include a general description of the compound, information on chemical composition, a summary of pharmacological or biological activities, uses (pharmaceutical, cosmetic, food, folk medicine), commercial preparations, and regulatory status. Information supplied for the latter is no longer limited, as was the case in the first edition, to GRAS designation or *USP/NF* inclusion. Other applicable FDA regulations, if any, are cited, as well as *German Commission E Monographs* (12.4).

A brief bibliography concludes each *Encyclopedia* monograph. Individual references are keyed to previous discussion with superscripted numbers, ensuring that every fact presented is easily related to relevant citations. Leung's Chinese heritage is an underlying benefit to this work, which is able to draw upon both classic and modern Chinese texts and more than fifty journals inaccessible to many scholars of Western pharmacognosy. A new section devoted to Chinese cosmetic ingredients (more accurately, twenty-three Chinese herbs used in cosmetic products in the United States and elsewhere) demonstrates this advantage. The index offers user-friendly access by both common and scientific names, as well as therapeutic and anatomical keywords (e.g., abdominal pain, abortion, abscesses-folk remedies for, skin).

12.20 *Dictionary of Natural Products.* 7 v. London: Chapman & Hall, 1994.

The seven-volume *Dictionary of Natural Products* is a good starting point for identification of naturally derived compounds perhaps falling outside the scope of Leung's *Encyclopedia* and other sources listed in this section. Five printed indexes facilitate access to the main alphabetical arrangement of entries by 1) name, 2) species, 3) type of compound, a cross reference list that employs 500 headings classifying substances by structure, e.g., "pyrrolizidine alkaloid," 4) molecular formula, in Hill notation, and 5) CAS registry number. Since data on closely related compounds are often combined in the same *Dictionary* monograph, it's important to consult the indexes to avoid overlooking relevant entries. Bibliography accompanies each monograph, supporting systematically organized discussion of the featured product's synthesis/isolation and properties, as well as hazards. Chemical structures are also provided. Supplementary volumes have been issued in hardcopy since 1995 (volume 8 forward). Semiannual updates are an advantage of the CD-ROM version of *The Dictionary of Natural Products*, now also available from Chapman & Hall.

12.21 Harborne JB, Baxter H. *Phytochemical Dictionary. A Handbook of Bioactive Compounds from Plants.* London: Taylor & Francis, 1993.

The *Phytochemical Dictionary* generally restricts its coverage to products of higher plants that are either biologically active (including those whose chief distinction is toxic, rather than therapeutic, potential) or economically valuable. These include more than 3,000 flavoring substances, natural sweeteners, poisons, carcinogens, and coloring agents. Information is presented in five parts reflecting chemical classification: carbohydrates and lipids, nitrogen-containing compounds (excluding alkaloids), alkaloids, phenolics, and terpenoids. Individual chapters deal with subclasses within these general groups. Entries for plant constituents are listed by "trivial" (common) name. Monographs include synonyms, class of compound, major sources (plant name and family, with frequency of occurrence), chemical structure (graphic diagram), molecular weight and formula, biological activity, and use by humans. Although source citations are omitted from individual substance entries, a bibliography of general encyclopedias and other references is provided in the introduction to each section. The *Phytochemical Dictionary*'s index cross references from synonyms for compound names, but not plant names.

12.22 Duke JA. *CRC Handbook of Medicinal Herbs*. Boca Raton, FL: CRC Press, 1985.

12.23 Duke JA. *Handbook of Biologically Active Phytochemicals and Their Activities*. Boca Raton, FL: CRC Press, 1992.

12.24 Duke JA. *Handbook of Phytochemical Constituents of GRAS Herbs and Other Economic Plants*. Boca Raton, FL: CRC Press, 1992.

In the *CRC Handbook of Medicinal Herbs*, Duke marshals folklore and fact side by side in monographs for 365 folk medicinal species, including "those of dubious salubrity." Arranged alphabetically by botanical name, entries also cite common or colloquial names of plants featured and compile notes from the literature on uses, folk medicinal applications, chemistry, and toxicity. In addition, they are accompanied by line drawings. Four lengthy tables are a particularly attractive feature of this book. Table 1 correlates all 365 species with their toxicity ratings and price data (as of 1983). Table 2, entitled "Toxins: Their Toxicity and Distribution in Plant Genera," lists LD_{50}, LC (lethal concentration), or TD (toxic dose). Table 3 focuses on higher plant genera and their toxins, and Table 4 lists pharmacologically active phytochemicals. Although notes included in individual monographs are drawn from a core list of seventy-six references, a background bibliography of 353 sources enhances the *Handbook of Medicinal Herbs*, as does its detailed index of plant names and indications.

Given this good precedent, Duke's *Handbook of Biologically Active Phytochemicals and Their Activities* falls short of expectations. This 1992 contribution issued by the same publisher consists of a succession of cryptic entries citing name, action, plant source, LD_{50}, and, when available, effective or inhibitory concentrations or doses. Frequent abbreviations, although explained in the introduction, reinforce the impression of a rote formula-like, and rather sparse, approach. Nonetheless, this compilation covers most, if not all, GRAS herbs, many medically important foods, and 500 "strictly medicinal" plants. All told, its scope encompasses 1,000 plants and 3,000 compounds. The generally-recognized-as-safe list is also the basis of selection in Duke's *Handbook of Phytochemical Constituents*, the title of which is somewhat misleading. Instead of a handbook, this publication is simply a listing of constituents, with no textual accompaniment other than a general introduction.

12.25 Glasby JS. *Dictionary of Antibiotic-Producing Organisms*. Chichester, England: Ellis Horwood, 1992.

12.26 Glasby JS. *Dictionary of Plants Containing Secondary Metabolites*. London: Taylor & Francis, 1991.

Glasby is a recognized authority on antibiotics (see also 3.14). The *Dictionary of Antibiotic-Producing Organisms* compiles information on fungal and bacterial species that have been investigated, as well as a small number of plant and marine organisms which produce antibiotics. Bibliographic references accompany each organism's monograph and often include citations to patent applications (always a bonus). The volume concludes with an index to antibiotics. Glasby's *Dictionary of Plants Containing Secondary Metabolites* lists plants alphabetically by genus-species. Indexing offers the alternatives of approaching material by compound class, chemical names, or simplified generic names (more than 19,000 compounds are listed). References included in each monograph cite pre-1988 literature on the isolation of compounds, structure, and physiological properties.

12.27 Lewis DA. *Anti-inflammatory Drugs from Plants and Marine Sources*. Agents and Actions Supplements, v. 27. Berlin: Birkhauser Verlag, 1989.

Anti-inflammatory Drugs from Plants and Marine Sources begins with a section devoted to providing background on pathophysiology and pharmacology of broad drug classes and an assessment of their anti-inflammatory activity (pharmacological screening). Section II divides discussion of drugs derived from plants and animals into their respective chemical classes (e.g., alkaloids, flavinoids). Section III covers extraction of active constituents and tissue culture, as well as the topic of diet and arthritis. Each chapter includes suggested readings and other references. The undoubted value of the subject content in this supplement to *Agents and Actions* is undercut, somewhat, by difficult-to-read photoreproduction from an obviously homegrown, word processed manuscript. Another drawback is that the appendix simply lists medicinal plants and marine species covered in the volume, but does not provide page references. The two indexes that are provided list medicinal compounds by generic names and drug class terms, and general subject terms.

12.28 D'Amelio FS. *Botanicals: A Phytocosmetic Desk Reference*. Boca Raton, FL: CRC Press, 1998.

In *Botanicals: A Phytocosmetic Dictionary*, D'Amelio brings together information on the most common herbal derivatives used in cosmetics worldwide. After the opening chapter's overview of folkloric use of herbs and their constituents, discussion turns to forms of extracts, plant identification, and common terminology. Methods of identification and extraction are highlighted, including infrared spectroscopy, gas liquid chromatography, and thin layer chromatography. The percolation process and production of decoctions and infusions are among other topics covered, as well as properties of essential oils, aromatherapy, hair care botanicals, marine natural products, and Indian and Oriental herbs used in cosmetics. A botanical quick reference chart, a Japanese botanicals cross reference list, and a glossary are value-added features in the *Phytocosmetic Desk Reference.*

12.29 Penso G. *Index Plantarum Medicinalium Totius Mundi Eorumque Synonymorum.* Milan: Organizzazione Editoriale Medico-Farmaceutica, 1983.
12.30 Penso G. *Lexicon Plantarum Medicinalium.* Milan: Organizzazione Editoriale Medico-Farmaceutica, 1991.

In *Index Plantarum Medicinalium,* Penso aims to fulfill a need identified by a World Health Assembly in 1978, whose participants requested that WHO compile an international inventory of plants used medicinally. Sources employed to accomplish this monumental task included national pharmacopeias and formularies, as well as published journal literature and legislation. The result is a 1,026-page list of plants, arranged by genus-species. Entries include synonyms, listed alphabetically, with an associated author name, when available. Countries where the plant is used medicinally are also identified by a code (ninety-one nations). With more than 21,000 botanical names and synonyms, including Ayurvedic and Unani designations, the *Index Plantarum Medicinalium* is an unusually eclectic nomenclature source.

The Lexicon Plantarum Medicinalium, a much shorter (193-page) compendium, is intended to assist translation of plant names. Main entries are confined to Latin (Linnaean) terms. Each is followed by its English, German, Spanish, French, Italian, and Russian vernacular counterparts. Fortunately, these terms are also provided as cross references in the alphabetically arranged *Lexicon.* Plants listed are those most widely used medicinally and available on the market.

Regional and Ethnobotanical Bibliography

The literature of pharmacognosy contains many examples of publications whose purpose is to document ethnobotanical traditions in various cultures and geographic regions. Selections are as fascinating and diverse as the cultures they represent.

12.31 Ba Y, Keli P, eds. *Colour Atlas of Chinese Traditional Drugs.* Beijing: Science Press, 1987 (reprinted 1989).
12.32 *Medicinal Plants in China.* Manila: WHO Regional Office for the Western Pacific, 1989.

Given the resurgence of public interest in non-Western medical traditions, books on Chinese drugs are much in demand. The *Colour Atlas of Chinese Traditional Drugs* is intended for popular use, according to its introduction, but information provided will also be of interest to scientific professionals. It describes drugs, as well as the plants, animals, and minerals from which they are derived. Individual entries identify chemical constituents and clinical uses, with instructions for preparation also included. Very good color photographs are the most unusual feature of this book, showing both living plants and drugs prepared from them, in crude form (i.e., roots, leaves). The drawback is the arrangement of monographs, which is supposedly according to the number of strokes of the first Chinese character of each drug's name. The index by English name will not help resolve navigation problems, because nomenclature listed is a translation of the Chinese phonetic name for the crude drug (e.g., Zongban, Biazu). Fortunately, a second index is also provided, with Latin names (of plants, animals, crude drugs) used as entry points. The *Colour Atlas of Chinese Traditional Drugs* describes 178 drugs and related compounds, 166 of plant origin and twelve derived from animals. It is stunningly enhanced with 653 color photographs.

Compiled by the Institute of Chinese Materia Medica and the China Academy of Traditional Chinese Medicine, *Medicinal Plants in China* focuses on 150 commonly used species. Arranged alphabetically by botanical (Latin) name, monographs list synonyms, including both English and Chinese names. Entries identify parts of plants used medicinally, appearance, habitat, distribution, indications, and dosage. Color photographs show both live plants *in situ* and crude drug parts. Separate indexes offer access to botanical names in Chinese phonetic (Pinyin) alphabet and in Chinese Han characters.

12.33 Huang KC. *The Pharmacology of Chinese Herbs*. 2nd ed. Boca Raton, FL: CRC Press, 1998.

12.34 Zhu CH. *Clinical Handbook of Chinese Prepared Medicines*. Brookline, MA: Paradigm Publications, 1989.

12.35 Hsu HY et al. *Oriental Materia Medica, A Concise Guide*. Long Beach, CA: Oriental Healing Arts Institute, 1986.

Following an interesting historical overview of Chinese traditional medicine, Huang organizes information on *The Pharmacology of Chinese Herbs* into chapters focusing on body systems where their therapeutic value shows potential. For example, monographs for botanicals with possible application in heart disorders are included in the cardiovascular chapter. Individual entries for 473 herbs are listed under an English-language name transliterated from Chinese and identify the genus-species (in Latin) from which they originate. Structural formulas are included, along with a brief summary of chemical composition, pharmacological action, toxicity, and therapeutic use. Separate indexes to herb names and general subject terms are supplemented with an appendix listing Chinese equivalents of English-language names.

As its title foretells, the *Clinical Handbook of Chinese Prepared Medicines* is treatment oriented. After reviewing the history of their manufacture and quality control regulations, Zhu discusses prepared medicine formats, both in traditional, as well as modern, Chinese medicine. A third preparatory chapter covers general guidelines for administration, including combining prepared formulations, general contraindications, and precautions. Part II is the heart of this *Handbook*, providing individual entries for the most commonly used and clinically significant prepared medicines available in the United States. Arranged by therapeutic use, monographs list the source (text or physician generally credited with having first introduced the formula), composition, format, and administration of each drug, including the manufacturer name, product name, dosage forms available, and recommended regimen. Although, where appropriate, Western medical disease categories are discussed in conjunction with traditional indications, the *Handbook* is intended as a clinical reference guide for practitioners already familiar with the basic tenets and guiding symptomatology of traditional Chinese medicine.

In referencing "channels entered," drug profiles in *Oriental Materia Medica* also assume, to a certain extent, some familiarity with traditional practices. The introduction to this volume does offer a brief history and overview of the topic. The 768 monographs that follow are organized by applications, such as sudorifics, purgatives, and febrifuges. Each entry lists names, origin, essence and flavor, channels entered, traditional uses, actions, chemical constituents, pharmacology (very briefly stated), and dosage. Reference material includes a bibliography and a glossary of Western disease names. There are five indexes in all: common names, scientific and pharmaceutical names, Chinese names in Pinyin transliteration and in Wade-Giles transliteration, and Japanese names in Hevon transliteration.

12.36 Maciocia G. *The Practice of Chinese Medicine: The Treatment of Diseases with Acupuncture and Chinese Herbs.* New York: Churchill Livingstone, 1994.

As its subtitle indicates, herbal remedies share the stage with acupuncture in *The Practice of Chinese Medicine*. Both have, after all, been used concurrently since the first recorded writings about the discipline (206 B.C.). Accordingly, in each chapter of this book, the author follows up discussion of differential diagnosis of a featured medical condition with guidelines on acupuncture points and Chinese herbal formulas for treatment. Conditions selected as chapter topics (thirty-four in all) include general symptoms, such as headaches, sinusitis, cough, chest pain, as well as specific conditions: e.g., Parkinson's, nephritis, asthma, allergic rhinitis. Case studies which accompany discussion of differential diagnosis will assist readers in understanding traditional theories without prior knowledge of their specialized terminology. Equally useful is Maciocia's brief summary of the parallel Western medicine differential diagnosis at the end of each chapter, as well as the author's prognoses of Western therapeutic outcome when Chinese medical treatment is included. The use of both herbs and acupuncture in conjunction with, and concurrent to, Western medicines, is realistically examined. Examples include inhalational therapy for asthma and anticholinergics or levodopa for

Parkinson's, both of which present no conflicts with Chinese herbal prescriptions and acupuncture.

12.37 *Medicinal Plants in Viet Nam.* Manila: WHO Regional Office for the Western Pacific, 1990.

12.38 Duke JA, Vasquez R. *Amazonian Ethnobotanical Dictionary.* Boca Raton, FL: CRC Press, 1994.

Medicinal Plants in Viet Nam is a joint publication of the World Health Organization and the Institute of Materia Medica Hanoi. Arranged alphabetically by Latin binomial, 200 monographs give local and English-language names for plants featured, physical descriptions, flowering period, distribution, parts used medicinally, chemical composition, and therapeutic uses. Color drawings accompany entries, but no references to the literature are included. Indexes provide access by English, Vietnamese, and scientific (Latin) names.

Duke's *Amazonian Ethnobotanical Dictionary* is organized in much the same manner, but succinct comments on medical uses do serve the stated purpose of communicating folklore, albeit unverified in scientific literature. As is seen in other works by this noted author (12.22–12.24), poisonous or toxic plants are invariably identified. In addition to cross references from common to scientific names, the *Dictionary* includes an index to indigenous medicinal uses (e.g., abortifacient, abscess, alopecia, altitude sickness)

12.39 Iwu MM. *CRC Handbook of African Medicinal Plants.* Boca Raton, FL: CRC Press, 1993.

12.40 Ghazanfar SA. *Handbook of Arabian Medicinal Plants.* Boca Raton, FL: CRC Press, 1994.

The *CRC Handbook of African Medicinal Plants* provides an introductory overview of botanical materia medica used in African traditional medicine practiced by at least one of more than 2,000 different tribes. An opening section catalogs medicinal plants and their uses, identifying parts contributing to preparations. Detailed pharmacognosy information is confined to coverage of 152 major herbs, for which individual monographs compile common names, synonyms, African name(s), and habitat or distribution. Entries also identify chemical constituents, their pharmacological activity, and medical applications. Bibliography cited is drawn from more than 870 publications. Two indexes offer access either by species/plant family or by subject keywords. Tables cross reference plants to specific conditions that they are used to treat.

The *Handbook of Arabian Medicinal Plants* begins with an explanation of traditional systems of medical treatment in the Middle East, highlighting beliefs regarding diagnosis, bone setting, cupping, cauterization, and use of heat therapy. Each of the 260 monographs that follow, arranged by Latin name, lists vernacular names, plant description, distribution, chemical composition, and information on medicinal uses. Illustrated with line drawings, entries include author commentary and supportive bibliographic references resulting from a survey of the chemical literature published from 1982 through 1993. An appendix correlates medical conditions with plants used to treat them in Bahrain, Kuwait, Oman, Qatar, Saudi Arabia, Yemen, and the United Arab Emirates.

12.41 Kindscher K. *Medicinal Wild Plants of the Prairie*. Lawrence, KS: University Press of Kansas, 1992.

12.42 Moore M. *Medicinal Plants of the Desert and Canyon West*. Santa Fe, NM: Museum of New Mexico Press, 1989.

In returning to home ground, the U.S. researcher into ethnobotany will find no less exotic fare. Kindscher's *Medicinal Wild Plants of the Prairie* is primarily a history of the traditions and beliefs that have surrounded the medical use of plants indigenous to the region. The author documents applications of 203 species, 172 as used therapeutically by Indians, and the remainder as employed by settlers (1830–1930) and their physicians. Material is organized in alphabetic order by botanical name. Entries for the forty-three plants most widely used are divided into sections devoted to Indian use, Anglo-folk use, medical history, and recent scientific research. Although not intended as a medical guide or "herbal," this book does refer to previous listings of the plants, when applicable, in the *USP* or *NF* (1882–1965). Black-and-white drawings are included, as well as maps showing the geographic distribution of species cited. Kindscher also provides a glossary; a detailed index by plant names, medical indications, and tribes; and numerous references to pertinent primary literature.

In Moore's *Medicinal Plants of the Desert and Canyon West*, the emphasis is less on history and more on actually preparing and using botanicals. Unfortunately, illustrative material is very sparse, including only a few line drawings and fewer color plates, so that would-be self-healers could run the risk of misidentification. Monographs do describe the appearance and habitat of species selected for inclusion, and maps are provided. Entries offer tips on cultivation, collection, and preparation. Obviously intended for the consumer, the overall arrangement is by common name used in the West, with a brief section devoted to formulas for treating various ailments, ranging from hemorrhoid ointment, to mastitis therapy, to flypaper. Although no references accompany individual plant listings, a selective bibliography for further background reading is supplied, along with a therapeutic use index and an index to plants by alternative names.

12.43 Johnson T, ed. *CRC Ethnobotany Desk Reference*. Boca Raton, FL: CRC Press, 1998.

Johnson offers a quick inventory of claimed attributes and historical uses throughout the world of 28,000 plant species. Concise, uniformly structured monographs list Latin name, common names, taxonomic family, geographic range, action/application, active constituents, indigenous use(s), body part or system treated, habitat, and bibliographic references. Sources used to construct the

CRC Ethnobotany Desk Reference include U.S. government ethnobotany databases available on the Internet (see next section), as well as a core bibliography of reference works. Johnson's own Web site, *HerbWeb*, provides a selection of sample monographs from the CRC compilation, accessible via a browsable index to common names and illustrated with line drawings.

Internet Sources of Ethnobotanical and Phytomedicinal Information

Most material available on the Internet in this subject area is geared toward herbalism, rather than pharmacognosy. It's difficult to draw a straight line between the two viewpoints, but herbalists tend to be involved in the preparation and promotion of plant-derived remedies, rather than in pharmacological investigation of crude drug materials. Some would characterize this as a holistic approach, contrasted with the emphasis on isolated plant constituents and underlying natural product chemistry seen in pharmacognosy literature. Both disciplines share an interest in ethnobotany and folk medicine as a source of empirical evidence and impetus for further research. Accordingly, the selection of Web sites described in this section is a decidedly diverse mixture ranging from government-sponsored databases to hobbyist home pages. The URLography begins with three subject hubs, continues on to descriptions of eight substantive databases, and concludes with annotations for a medley of other informative sites chosen for their quality and potential utility to readers of this book. Criteria used in evaluation have been enumerated elsewhere.[12]

Botanical Medicine Resources on the Web
⇨ http://cpmcnet.columbia.edu/dept/rosenthal/Botanicals.html

The Rosenthal Center for Complementary and Alternative Medicine's home page is maintained by Jackie Wooten, a name familiar to many in alternative medicine circles. Botanical medicine is one of several specialized, fully annotated subject hubs available at Rosenthal's Web site. Categories compiled are mailing lists (listservs), databases, online journals, herb sites, illustrations or virtual gardens, and education, training, political, and regulatory sources.

Internet Directory for Botany: Economic Botany, Ethnobotany
⇨ http://www.helsinki.fi/kmus/botecon.html

A well maintained site from the Botanical Museum, Finnish Museum of Natural History in Helsinki, the *Directory*'s categories include ethnobotany, herbal medicine, and poisons. Hundreds of links are compiled, and many are accompanied with helpful descriptive annotations.

Medicinal Plant Databases
⇨ http://www.inform.umd.edu/PBIO/Medicinals/pharmacognosy.html

This subject hub, created by Michael Tims at the University of Maryland, provides one-line (title only) links to a host of sites listed under separate categories for pharmacognosy, herbalism, chemistry, molecular modeling, medical resources, and specific plants/conditions. Caution: it's a slow loader, due to an animated opening graphic.

CAM Citation Index—National Center for Complementary and Alternative Medicine
⇨ http://altmed.od.nih.gov/nccam/resources/cam-ci

The National Center for Complementary and Alternative Medicine, created by a Congressional mandate in October 1998, hosts the *CAM Citation Index* at its U.S. government-sponsored Web site. This database is simply a searchable subset of 90,000 bibliographic references derived from *MEDLINE* (1966–1997). The interface enables keyword searching, but browsing by major *MeSH* (14.2) topical headings to retrieve citations is also an option.

Dr. Duke's Phytochemical and Ethnobotanical Databases
⇨ http://www.ars-grin.gov/duke

This Web site introduces a new and better interface to the *Phytochemical, Ethnobotany,* and *Medicinal Plants of Native America* databases also accessible through the Probe search engine from the USDA (see separate entries elsewhere in this section). Plant name searches yield chemicals and activities or folk medicinal uses. Queries involving named chemicals lead to plants containing them or activities of the substances searched. "Activity" keywords can produce results itemizing either plants or chemicals. This site also offers a list of bibliographic references used and the *Tico Ethnobotanical Dictionary.*

Ethnobotany Database
⇨ http://probe.nalusda.gov:8300/cgi-bin/browse/ethnobotdb

International in scope, the *Ethnobotany Database* correlates known folk medicinal practices with geographic location and plant nomenclature data in more than 80,000 entries. Both browse and query functions have been built into the USDA-hosted Probe search engine, enabling access by plant names, country, applications (uses), or combinations thereof. Regrettably, the search form is complex and poorly documented.

HerbMed
⇨ http://www.amfoundation.org/herbmed.htm

HerbMed is a database of evidence-based information, resulting from a survey of scientific data, on the use of herbs for health. Newly released in 1998, the keyword-searchable file currently contains monographs for only twenty-one plants. Each entry summarizes evidence of clinical activity and mechanisms of action, backed up with hotlinks to bibliographic references derived from *MED-*

LINE (14.1) and U.S. patents. Warnings, preparations, and mixtures are other sections typically included in each lengthy monograph. *HerbWeb* is hosted by the nonprofit Alternative Medicine Foundation (Bethesda, Maryland).

The International Bibliographic Information on Dietary Supplements Database (IBIDS)
⇨ http://www.nal.usda.gov/fnic/IBIDS

IBIDS is produced by the Office of Dietary Supplements of the U.S. National Institutes of Health, in conjunction with the Food and Nutrition Information Center of the National Agricultural Library (USDA). It includes bibliographic citations, accompanied by abstracts (when available), related to vitamins, minerals, and selected herbal and botanical supplements. At its initial release in 1998, IBIDS material was derived solely from *MEDLINE* (14.1), *AGRICOLA*, and *AGRIS*, three other databases with a broader scope. The subset represented in this new electronic resource is expected to be augmented in the future with references from ten other online databases, subject to an agreement with their suppliers and a continuing NIH-industry partnership with The Dialog Corporation. Additions are planned from *AMED* (14.15), *EMBASE* (14.4), *IPA* (14.8), *ExtraMED*, *MANTIS*, *PASCAL*, *PsycINFO*, and other food technology and biological literature indexes.

IBIDS currently covers publications from 1986 to the present and focuses on compiling information related to the top fifty botanicals identified by the European Union (also best sellers on the U.S. market). A complete list of keywords used to derive the database, as well as journals covered, can be viewed at this Web site. The search engine offers general keyword and field-specific query options and many sophisticated logical combinations. The subject scope of *IBIDS* is impressive, encompassing the use and function of supplements, the role of supplementation in metabolism, chemical composition, food fortification, and the growth and production of botanical products employed as supplements.

Medicinal Plants of North America
⇨ http://probe.nalusda.gov:8300/cgi-bin/browse/mpnadb

Medicinal Plants of North America is based on a two-volume book of the same name published in 1986 by the University of Michigan's Museum of Anthropology. Since that time, its scope has been enlarged to include foods, dyes, fibers, and other uses of plants (see *Native American Ethnobotany*). More than 17,000 records document medicinal applications of 2,000 botanical species by any of 123 Native American groups. The file is searchable by plant (common name, family, genus, taxon), tribe, and use.

Native American Ethnobotany Database
⇨ http://www.umd.umich.edu/resources/bydept2/besci/anthro/
about_ethnobot.html

This database is a substantially enlarged version of *Medicinal Plants of North America* (searchable elsewhere via the USDA). This updated edition by the same author (Daniel E. Moerman, University of Michigan) includes foods, dyes, fibers, and other uses of plants in 47,000 entries. It covers uses of 4,029 species by any of 291 Native American groups. An easy-to-use search form permits Boolean combinations, if desired. Response is quick and leads to brief records identifying genus, family, tribe, medicinal use, and the precise bibliographic reference (book or journal) where the information was obtained. A new hardcopy book based on this Web site's contents has been published by Timber Press (Portland, Oregon, 1998), entitled *American Indian Ethnobotany.*

Phytochemical Database
⇨ http://probe.nalusda.gov:8300/cgi-bin/browse/phytochemdb

The *Phytochemical Database* is a product of a collaboration between well known phytoscientist James Duke and Stephen M. Beckstrom-Sternberg (see also *Ethnobotany Database* and *Medicinal Plants of North America*) A compilation of plant chemical data, it is searchable by pharmacological or toxic activity keywords, substance name, assay and result terminology, and common plant name or family, genus, and taxon.

Cyberbotanica
⇨ http://biotech.chem.indiana.edu/botany/

Cyberbotanica is a home page maintained by Lucy Snyder of Indiana University's Biotech Project. The focus is on plants as cancer treatments. It opens with a chart listing ten botanicals by common and scientific name, cross referenced to the medical compounds they have produced and to brand names, when applicable. Hypertext links from plant names lead to descriptions and natural history information. Clicking on medical compounds directs users to consumer-oriented biochemical and pharmacological information. Both types of entries are now backed up with bibliographic references (largely limited to general sources such as *The Merck Index* or *PDR*). Hyperlinked lists of other botany and chemotherapy WWW sites are short, but do include descriptive annotations. *Cyberbotanica* is supplemented with tables listing more than seventy other anticancer botanicals under investigation and twelve plant chemicals.

EthnoMedicinals Home Page
⇨ http://walden.mo.net/~tonytork/

Anthony R. Torkelson, site author, is a research scientist at G.D. Searle and author of *The Cross Name Index to Medicinal Plants* (CRC Press, 1996). His list of pharmacognosy books and other references, enhanced with links to Internet locations, could be of interest in collection development, as would be a listing of favorites from his own library. The remainder of this home page is entirely composed of links to other sources, classified under the headings Botany, Magic, and

Pharmacy; Pharmacognosy; Ethnobotanical Information; and Potpourri. New additions in 1998 are a list of links, briefly annotated, for Foods as Medicines, and, under Plant Talk, exemplary entries for eleven medicinal plants. These brief monographs include common names in various languages, natural habitat, ethnobotanical uses, and symptoms treated.

Henriette's Herbal Homepage
 ⇨ http://sunsite.unc.edu/herbmed/

Both culinary and medicinal plant uses are included in the scope of Henriette Kress's compendium, which bears many of the stigmata of hobbyist home pages (e.g., a typo in the very first line). Albeit couched in a breezy style, material presented is often informative and potentially useful outside the confines of the popular herbalist community. For example, a large plant nomenclature database provides cross references from Latin names to Finnish, Swedish, English, German, and French counterparts. Available for downloading in targeted language segments, its scope encompasses more than 8,000 Latin names representing about 6,000 plants. Medicinal herb FAQs have also been constructed for a long list of individual plants, as well as for specific medical conditions, different "schools" of herbal healing (Western, Ayurvedic, homeopathic, Bach flower, and traditional Chinese), and processing methods (distilling, tinctures, oils, balms, liniments).

Herb Research Foundation
 ⇨ http://www.herbs.org/index.html

The best feature of this attractively designed site is its online newsletter under the News & Views icon. Here, you will find timely coverage of herbal news summarized from the popular media, as well as sections devoted to scientific developments, reviews of research in progress, and highlights of events affecting the herbal industry and worldwide political context. Under a separate Hot Page icon, another *HRF* bonus is informative fact sheets, dubbed "Greenpapers," about individual herbs and herbal topics. The same Hot Page icon leads to a directory of links to other Web sites.

The Herbal Bookworm
 ⇨ http://www.teleport.com/~jonno/index.shtml

Jonathan Treasure's small (alas) collection of reviews is extraordinarily well done, providing readers with a thorough evaluation by an author who knows what he is talking about. Unfortunately, only seven reviews (albeit lengthy) are currently available. Treasure has, however, recently introduced "Shorts," a section devoted to minireviews and ratings. Another intriguing segment of this site is the Readers Page, where various ranked lists of resources have been compiled. "All Time Top 10" and "Top Ten Recent" compilations show results of polling professional herbalist mailing list members. "Bottom of the Barrel" shows titles not recommended by the same group. Counter-balancing these admittedly opinionated selections is a list of *Herbalgram*'s current top ten best sellers (two of which are, interestingly enough, on the previous "Bottom" list). *The Herbal Bookworm* could be a good site for both personal and professional collection development.

HerbNET

⇨ http://www.herbnet.com/

Don't be put off by the commercial look and feel of this site's opening page. It is sponsored by the Herb Growing and Marketing Network. Beneath the hype is a solid core of useful information attractively presented. Under Associations, many entries are annotated, and all bear posting dates. Under Press is a series of book reviews, a list of pertinent periodicals online via the Internet, and a directory of other journals that could be helpful in collection development. "Potpourri" is the place to find a subject-classified, annotated directory of other Web sites and listservs. *HerbNET*'s *Magazine* is a little on the light side (many recipes), but does regularly feature good monographs under "Medicinal Herb of the Month." Full-text access to monthly back issues is offered through June 1998.

HerbWeb

⇨ http://www.herbweb.com

Created by Tim Johnson, this site's overall structure changes with disconcerting frequency (at least four times over a 12-month period), requiring relearning to locate favorite portions. The icon for Herbs offers access, through a browsable index to common names, to excerpts from the *CRC Ethnobotany Desk Reference* (12.43). Selection of a given plant name leads to a one-page illustrated monograph describing action, indigenous uses, and native habitat and range, supported by bibliographic references. Another pertinent portion of this home page, labeled Johnson's Encyclopedia, is a classified directory of off-site links. A third option on *HerbWeb*'s main menu is Visionary Plants. Links listed here focus on phytofugitive uses of substances such as amanitas, cannabis, khat, mescaline, opium, and psilocybin. Many lead to what appear to be the author's own experiences in using the named plants. Dubbed "Entheobotany" (presumably from the Greek *enthetikos* = fit to put in), this portion of *HerbWeb* is unusual, to say the least.

Kohler's Medizinal Pflanzen

⇨ http://www.mobot.org/MOBOT/research/library/kohler

Hermann A. Kohler's *Medizinal Pflanzen* was published in 1887. Illustrations by L. Mueller and C. F. Schmidt from the three-volume set have been digitized at this site and made accessible by scientific name. Although slow-loading, the 300 detailed drawings are magnificent. Original copies of the book now reside at the Harvard Botanical Museum and the Missouri Botanical Garden.

Medical Herbalism

⇨ http://medherb.com/

Only one complete sample issue (Spring 1994) of *Medical Herbalism* is available for immediate display free-of-charge. Detailed tables of contents can be browsed for back issues from October 1989 forward, with an option to order individual copies. Judging from these examples, the newsletter provides a quarterly roundup of recently published clinical research with meaty abstracts or extracts from the professional medical literature, in addition to lengthier feature articles. An interesting item in the sample issue currently displayed is a list of "Top Herbs in Medical Practice" resulting from a 1993–94 survey (89 respondents). Offered for comparison is a list of best selling herbs compiled in 1921 by a distributor of botanical products. The *Medical Herbalism* home page also provides a classified directory of links to other sites, including medical and scientific journals, plant pharmacy sources, and research databases. Annotated selections show a successful effort to quality-filter entries.

Raintree
  ⇨ http://rain-tree.com/

The product of a group of companies that advocate preservation of the Amazon rainforest by promoting use of sustainable and renewable botanic sources, the *Raintree* home page includes a large section on plants. It can be approached through one of four alphabetical lists: common and botanical names, plant properties and actions, medical disorders and actions, or recorded ethnobotany uses. Illustrated monographs are supported by references to the primary scientific literature. The site has recently been enhanced with links to current clinical abstracts (obtained through *PubMed*) and browsable by common plant names. More cross-linking between the plant monograph and clinical reference sections would be desirable. A separate "Articles Published" section on the home page currently compiles only 17 items, most from popular media sources, and a Clinical Trials section includes only one reference. Visitors to this site will also find links to photo galleries of plants. Other links to alternative medicine and herbal Web resources sometimes, but not always, include annotations.

Southwest School of Botanical Medicine
  ⇨ http://chili.rt66.com/hrbmoore/HOMEPAGE/HomePage.html

Michael Moore's home page is well known in botanical circles and is a vehicle for providing his publications in downloadable format (see 12.42). Other classic works on "eclectic medicine" and materia medica are also offered as ASCII text or Acrobat files. Medicinal plant images are a major focus—hundreds of photographs, color illustrations, engravings, and pen-and-ink drawings can be viewed, if desired. A recent enhancement to this site is a collection of research journal abstracts, culled during the past ten years, on 148 different genera. Another mid-1997 addition is a database listing known chemical constituents for more than 250 plant medicines. The latter information has been compiled from *Napralert*

(14.42) and Duke's phytochemical and ethnobotanical databases (see previous entries in this section).

Veterinary Drugs

Even libraries dedicated to human medicine need access to information on veterinary drugs. Why? Resources can be useful in supporting laboratory animal care. In addition, products approved for veterinary use have sometimes migrated, illicitly or intentionally, into human therapy. A need to identify drugs intended for animal use also arises when accidental exposures occur. The tendency on the part of consumers to hoard old medicines does not exempt unused portions of veterinary prescriptions for their companion animals. In limited drug information collections, identification facilities afforded by *The Merck Index* (3.5), *Martindale* (6.1), or the *USP Dictionary* (3.1), all of which cover selected veterinary products, should be sufficient. *Unlisted Drugs* (3.8) also indexes animal drugs. Drug information centers and larger medical libraries will benefit from acquiring one or two of the following specialized compendia.

12.44 *Veterinary Pharmaceuticals and Biologicals—1999/2000.* 11th ed. Lenexa, KS: Veterinary Medicine Publishing, 1998. Biennial.

First published in 1982, *Veterinary Pharmaceuticals and Biologicals* (*VPB*) is probably the best known source of veterinary drug information in the United States. Essentially a practice-oriented catalog of nearly 4,000 animal care products from 230 manufacturers, this publication is sometimes dubbed "the veterinary *PDR*" and is, in fact, issued by a subsidiary of Medical Economics. Its four introductory sections compile extensive background material for healthcare providers, including Veterinary Medical Association guidelines for supervising the use and distribution of prescription drugs and FDA Compliance Guides on "extralabel" indications, uses in food-producing animals, and drugs approved for humans, but used in animal medicine.

The main product information portion of *VPB* organizes entries into six sections covering pharmaceuticals, therapeutic diets and nutritional supplements, biologics, diagnostic aids and supplies, parasiticides and insecticides, and disinfectants. Animal Aids rounds out the selection, with a potpourri of shampoo, bath, deodorant, antibacterial, antichew, and flea control products. Entries for medications are, essentially, package inserts, many of which supply background on pharmacology and include pertinent bibliographic references. Where *VPB* departs from its metaphorical counterpart (the *PDR*) is in attempting to provide listings for all FDA/USDA-approved drug products, even if the only information that can be communicated is what these agencies publish at the time of authorization, i.e., brand name, manufacturer, active ingredients, and indications. The volume's alphabetical index incorporates both brand and generic names into one unified list.

The *VPB* also includes extensive appendices that address veterinary drug pharmacology, interactions, incompatibilities, and lab test interferences. Charts summarize information on important biologics and vaccines, anthelmintics and parasiticides, drug withdrawal times in animals, and selected dosages in laboratory animals. Acknowledging that most veterinarians providing patient care maintain an in-house inventory of frequently used products (the "practice formulary"), Appendix 6 offers a starter list of useful drugs and dosage information. Two state-by-state directories of veterinary diagnostic labs and animal product distributors bring the total number of pages in this massive tome to 1,550. A *VPB Supplement* is issued for the years between biennial editions.

12.45 Bishop Y. *The Veterinary Formulary*. 4th ed. London: The Pharmaceutical Press, 1998.

The Veterinary Formulary was first published in 1991 under the auspices of the British Veterinary Association. It has the same basic purpose as its counterpart for human drugs, *The British National Formulary* (10.22)—promoting safe, rational, and effective prescribing. The result is an impressively professional, information packed compendium that covers not only U.K.-approved products, but also preparations from nine other countries, including Australia, Eire, France, Germany, Italy, The Netherlands, Norway, Sweden, and the United States. It identifies drugs used to treat or control various types of infections, those with known action on specific body systems (e.g., gastrointestinal, cardiovascular, respiratory), and medications that affect nutrition and body fluids. Other sections deal with production enhancers, vaccines and immunological preparations, and herbal medicines (newly added in the fourth edition).

Organized by generic name (BAN or INN), more than 700 monographs provide information needed for prescribing and conclude with references to any of 2,000 U.K. proprietary preparations. European, Australian, and U.S. alternatives are also cited. Entries itemize species for which the preparations are licensed, dose forms, strengths, and withdrawal periods. A concluding index to the 656-page volume integrates disease terms, indications, and drug names. Two features are bonuses that would translate well across geographic borders: 1) information is included on a selection of 500 medicines licensed only for use in humans, but known to be commonly used in animal practice, and 2) off-label indications and dosage of veterinary drugs are also discussed. Both types of entries are clearly marked to avoid confusion.

Background reference material assembled in *The Veterinary Formulary* is extensive. The volume begins with general guidance on prescribing, divided by animal species, with special population conditions discussed in separate sections: e.g., hepatic impairment, pregnancy, lactation, or neonates. Management of poisoning was added in the second edition. Coverage extends to invertebrates (including bees), exotic species (reptiles, birds, ostriches), and less common companion animals (e.g., fish). As in the *VPB*, appendices list interactions and incompatibilities.

By including the new British Veterinary Code of Practice on Medicines, *The Veterinary Formulary* demonstrates its commitment to providing legislative, as well as practical prescribing, information. The text highlights legal aspects of prescribing animal drugs in the United Kingdom, including recordkeeping and labeling requirements, and rules governing animals in competition (racehorses, polo ponies, greyhounds, racing pigeons). A concluding index of manufacturers is really a directory of addresses and telephone/fax numbers of companies whose products are cited and of other organizations associated with British veterinary practice.

12.46 Rossoff IS. *Handbook of Veterinary Drugs and Chemicals.* 2nd ed. Taylorville, IL: Pharmatox Publishing, 1994.

According to its author, the first edition of the *Handbook of Veterinary Drugs* (1975) was the subject of legal action by the FDA, due to its discussion of off-label uses. Despite this context of controversy, Rossoff has assembled a formidable amount of detailed dosage and use information under 2,100 headings, building on many years' experience as a practitioner and reportedly drawing on the content of 24,000 primary sources. *Handbook* entries are arranged alphabetically by generic name or, in the case of mixtures and common combinations, by vernacular name (e.g., *A-C-E mixture* for anesthesia = ethyl alcohol + chloroform + ether). A master index to alternative names provides cross references from chemical names, lab codes, and brands, encompassing many non-U.S. brand designations.

Drug monographs summarize uses, warnings, adverse effects, and interactions, but omit bibliographic references. The author carefully notes when the FDA has prohibited use in food-producing animals. Dose data are especially extensive, covering large and small animals, domesticated and wild, laboratory subjects (e.g., frogs, mice), fowl, and farm animals. An extensive therapeutic use and cross reference index integrates entries for drug classes, actions (pre-anesthesia), uses (hoof lesions, abscesses), interactions, and adverse effects. Consultation of this combined index shows, for example, an entry for abortifacients, followed by drugs used to induce abortion, those that cause it as an untoward effect, and those that can be used to prevent threatened abortion (all clearly distinguished from one another).

12.47 Adams HR, ed. *Veterinary Pharmacology and Therapeutics.* 7th ed. Ames: Iowa State University Press, 1995.

Adams' *Veterinary Pharmacology and Therapeutics* is a textbook. Its sections are dedicated to drug categories, arranged by site of action (e.g., CNS, cardiovascular) or conditions (microbial diseases, neoplasia). Additional segments are devoted to drug/chemical residues in edible tissues of animals and legal control of animal drugs in the United States. Many chapters include extensive monographs on major drugs, discussing both approved and off-label indications, and supported by thorough bibliographies. Chemical structures, numerous tables, and a selection of black-and-white photographs ensure that the massive (more than 1,100-page) text is attractively presented. A single index encompassing drug brand and generic names, animal species, medical conditions, and other subject concepts assures its accessibility.

12.48 Fraser CM, ed. *The Merck Veterinary Manual.* 7th ed. Rahway, NJ: Merck & Co, 1998.

First published in 1955, *The Merck Veterinary Manual* is subtitled "A handbook of diagnosis, therapy, and disease prevention and control for the veterinarian." Accordingly, Part I deals with diseases of common domestic animals, large and small, and is divided into fourteen sections by body system. Part II focuses on behavior; III on clinical values and procedures; IV on fur, laboratory, and zoo animals; and V on management, husbandry, and nutrition. Part VI, Pharmacology, opens with discussion of basic concepts in pharmacotherapeutics and continues on to systemic drugs, presented in anatomic categories. A "chemotherapeutics" segment is confined to the use of antimicrobial agents, organizing material by chemical or pharmacological class. Anti-inflammatory agents, immunotherapy, antineoplastics, antiseptics and disinfectants, and growth promoters are presented in turn, with tables frequently used to summarize treatment facts for quick reference.

Remaining parts of the *Manual* are devoted to, respectively, poultry, toxicology, and zoonoses (diseases of animals capable of afflicting man). A table in the toxicology section identifies ornamental plants toxic to companion animals. Were it not for these numerous charts and an excellent index, much of the value of the enormous amount of material crammed into *The Merck Veterinary Manual* would be lost in its densely printed small pages.

12.49 *IVS—Index of Veterinary Specialties.* St. Leonards, Australia: Medi-Media. Annual, with three supplements.

The *Index of Veterinary Specialties* is published by the producers of *MIMS Australia* (10.26). The annual hardcopy edition includes product monographs for 2,000 veterinary products marketed in Australia. Arranged by twenty-one therapeutic categories, entries are indexed by brand name, nonproprietary name, and action or indication. A separate index provides access to animal medications by manufacturer name. *IVS* is also available on CD-ROM, updated semiannually.

12.50 Gfeller RW, Messonnier SP. *Handbook of Small Animal Toxicology and Poisonings.* St. Louis: Mosby-Year Book, 1998.

The *Handbook of Small Animal Toxicology and Poisonings* focuses on diagnosis and emergency care of toxicoses in dogs and cats. Entries for toxic chemicals (including drugs) and toxic plants are arranged in alphabetical order in separate sections. Each bears a symbol for quick reference to what type of treatment to initiate. This feature, being somewhat cryptic, could undermine the utility of this source in busy practice settings. However, an index provides rapid access to *Handbook* contents by incorporating terms for toxicants, treatments, and clinical signs.

Several Internet sites offer access to additional animal drug information. The *FDA Home Page*, for example, links to the Center for Veterinary Medicine's fully searchable database of approved NADAs, to complete summaries of safety and effectiveness (SS&Es), and to adverse drug event reports (refer to Chapter Sixteen for further details). Additional sources for veterinary therapeutics are identified in Figure 12.1.

12.51 Boschert K, ed. *NetVet: Mosby's Veterinary Guide to the Internet*. St. Louis: Mosby, 1998.

Mosby's Veterinary Guide to the Internet is a hardcopy spinoff of the popular *NetVet* Web site maintained by Boschert. Part I provides an overview on how to get started on the Internet, intended for veterinary professionals. Part II compiles reviews of 450 sites selected by Boschert and evaluated by veterinary librarians and practitioners. More than 2,000 bookmarks on an accompanying diskette are sure to give purchasers a jumpstart on finding the best resources online. Subsequent updates are scheduled for downloading four times a year from a special page at Mosby's Web site. Examples of reviews that appear in *NetVet: Mosby's Veterinary Guide to the Internet* can be viewed at http://www1.mosby.com/Mosby/netvet.

Information on the History of Pharmacy

The history of pharmacy is closely linked with the history of medicine. In Great Britain, the profession of apothecary evolved during the 1600–1700s as a separate group of medical practitioners who would care for patients unable to afford the high fees demanded by university educated physicians of the time. As apothecaries gradually became more accepted as the equivalent of modern day general practitioners, a separate group of individuals, known as chemists and druggists, began to assume the time-consuming responsibilities of mixing and compounding medications for apothecaries.

When the fledgling profession migrated across the Atlantic during colonization, changes were inevitable. The need for formal education on the spot was recognized soon after the American Revolution. The first U.S. medical school to include "pharmacy" in the title of one of its faculty was the Medical School of the College of Philadelphia, in 1789. Official licensing of pharmacists who were not also physicians began in 1816. It was not until 1821 that the first independent

Figure 12.1   Free Internet Sources of Veterinary Drug and Therapeutics Information

- *NetVet*
    ⇨ http://netvet.wustl.edu/vet.htm

    The *NetVet* site on the Internet is an enormous subject hub compiled by Ken Boschert, contributor to the book of the same name (12.51). Career, education, organizations, meetings, directory, e-lists, publications, images, government, and commerce are main menu options, along with two extra choices for Specialties and Electronic Zoo. Veterinary Specialties is a classified list, equivalent to twenty-three printed pages, of one-line (title only) hypertext links to Web resources focusing on any of thirty subject areas in animal health, including alternative medicine, anesthesiology, biotechnology, nutrition, pharmacology, and toxicology. The Electronic Zoo portion of this pathfinder broadens the scope to encompass additional animal resources. Here, icons provide links to resources devoted to amphibians, birds, cats, cows, dogs, ferrets, fish, horses, invertebrates, marine mammals, pigs, primates, rabbits, reptiles, rodents, small ruminants, wildlife, and zoo animals. Libraries of animal images, sounds, and fiction round out the enormous collection. *NetVet* is enlivened throughout with dynamic, and often entertaining, graphics. This is definitely a five star Web launch pad.

- *"Virtual" Veterinary Center—Martindale's Health Science Guide*
    ⇨ http://www-sci.lib.uci.edu/HSG/Vet.html

    Another huge subject hub, this time with annotations, Martindale's "Virtual" Veterinary Center includes categories for dictionaries and glossaries, literature and patent searching, online journals, veterinary schools and curricula, textbooks, databases, images, biosciences, clinical sciences, care and use of laboratory animals, diagnostic testing, and vaccination schedules. Picklists of species are integrated into this site to assist in selection of genetics resources and tutorials on diseases and parasites.

- *World-Wide Web Virtual Library: Animal Health, Well-Being, and Rights*
    ⇨ http://www.tiac.net/users/sbr/animals.html

    This large subject hub begins with general sites, such as *NetVet*, covering many types of animals. Part 2 lists specialized titles with a focus on one type of animal, identifying forty-one categories starting with armadillos, badgers, bats, and bears and ending with seals, shrews, skunks, snakes, tigers, turtles, and wolves. Part 3 gathers hotlinks to miscellaneous documents and images. Unfortunately, no annotations accompany individual entries to assist in prescreening.

- *EpiVetNet*
    ⇨ http://epiweb.massey.ac.nz

    EpiVetNet is that rare commodity, a veterinary epidemiology resource. It is a subject hub maintained by Dirk Pfeiffer at Massey University in New Zealand. Categories covered include calculators and statistics guides, textbooks, organizations, software, and general veterinary sites, in addition to epidemiology.

- *AltVetMed—Complementary and Alternative Veterinary Medicine*
    ⇨ http://www.altmedvet.com

    An informative site with articles provided by two DVMs as a public service, *AltVetMed* includes a U.S. and Canadian membership directory for the American Holistic Veterinary

Medical Association. It also supplies information about the Academy of Veterinary Homeopathy and other pertinent associations. Lists compiled of books and periodicals cover both human and animal alternative medical topics, as do directories of Internet mailing lists, private networks, newsgroups, and hotlinked Web sites (without annotations). Fulltext articles address a variety of topics of interest to pet owners, such as allergic skin disease, arthritis, dental care, epilepsy, flea control, flower remedies and herbs in veterinary medicine, homeopathy, acupuncture, and vaccination decisions. A Pet Food Advisory discusses ingredients and choosing a good food and lists manufacturers of products with no artificial ingredients or preservatives.

- *Veterinary Emergency Drug Calculator*
  ⇨ http://www.cvmbs.colostate.edu/clinsci/wing/emdrughp.html
  The *Veterinary Emergency Drug Calculator* is designed to help in the management of severe emergencies in dogs and cats. Modules cover dosage in cardiopulmonary arrest, ventricular arrhythmias, hypoglycemia, shock, and maintenance volumes of crystalloid fluids. Only entry of body weight in pounds is needed in either calculator to determine from drug/condition charts the correct quantities of medication and other details of administration. Wayne Wingfield, a DVM at Colorado State University, is the author.

- *Veterinary Abbreviations & Acronyms*
  ⇨ http://www.library.uiuc.edu/vex/vetdocs/abbs.htm
  This reference aid bases its selection of terms on abbreviations and acronyms found in the *Merck Veterinary Manual* (12.48), supplemented with many other sources to fill in the blanks left by standard abbreviations dictionaries.

- *Poisonous Plants*
  ⇨ http://hammock.ifas.ufl.edu/txt/fairs/18132
  Botanist David Hall presents brief monographs for fifty-nine plants that pose significant hazards to animals in the southern United States, making them accessible by an A–Z common name list. Each entry includes a description and identifies season(s) of greatest risk, symptoms of poisoning, active principle involved, and parts of the plant containing poison. Treatment information accompanies some, but not all, descriptions. Another selection at this site is a list of poisoning symptoms cross referenced to possible causal plants. A third option is a Poisonous Plants Glossary. This Web site is maintained by the Florida Cooperative Extension Service of the University of Florida.

- *Poisonous Plants Home Page*
  ⇨ http://phl.vet.upenn.edu/~triplett/poison/index.html
  Richard Davies and Robert Poppenga, faculty members at the University of Pennsylvania, are the organizers of this School of Veterinary Medicine site. Forty-nine plants are currently covered in monographs that include color photographs and descriptive, but little or no treatment, information. Entries are accessible by two separate indexes of common and Latin names. A glossary of selected botanical terms is another main menu selection.

- *Cornell University Poisonous Plants Web Page*
  ⇨ http://www.ansci.cornell.edu/plants/plants.html
  Still under development in January 1999, this home page is a small subject hub with links to other sites focusing on plants poisonous to livestock and pets, as well as a readyreference aid containing textual documents. The document collection includes an alpha-

betical listing of botanical names by genus and species, a description of types of poisons present, an inventory of animals commonly affected, and a brief article entitled "Medicinal Plants for Livestock—Beneficial or Toxic?" Dan Brown of the Cornell College of Veterinary Medicine is the team leader behind the collaborative Web project.

- *Illustrated Buyers Guide to Veterinary Equipment and Supplies*
  ⇨ http://www.vetmedpub.com
  More than 200 products are listed, including computer software, dental equipment and supplies, diagnostic/monitoring equipment, kennel and grooming supplies, laboratory equipment, medical/surgical supplies, and operating/recovery room equipment.

---

educational institution in the western hemisphere dedicated to the profession was founded: the Philadelphia College of Pharmacy. The establishment of the American Pharmaceutical Association in 1852 in Philadelphia is generally considered to mark widespread recognition of U.S. pharmacy as a healthcare occupation separate from medical doctors.

Nonetheless, much reference material on the history of medicine will also be relevant to the history of pharmacy. Fortunately, the founding of the American Institute of the History of Pharmacy in 1941 spurred publication of several specialized resources in this subject area. The Institute sponsors the development of the majority of reference material related to the evolution of pharmacy in the United States, of which the following are only a few examples. Figure 12.2 identifies several excellent sources available on the Internet.

12.52 Sonnedecker G. *Kremer's and Urdang's History of Pharmacy*. 4th ed. Madison, WI: American Institute of the History of Pharmacy, 1986.

Kremer's and Urdang's History of Pharmacy is the standard textbook on the topic and is equally appealing as recreational reading. Part One reviews pharmacy's early antecedents in Babylonia, Egypt, and Greco-Roman culture. Part Two traces the emergence of the profession in selected European countries. Part Three is an overview of pharmacy's historical milestones in the United States, including chapters on the growth of associations, birth of legislative standards, development of professional education, and establishment of a literature. Numerous appendices offer a diverse collection of fascinating material, such as a list of representative drugs used by American Indians, a chronological table of founding dates for state pharmacy associations in the United States, and comparable chronologies documenting the passage of state pharmacy laws and establishment of schools of pharmacy. Another appended section is devoted to pharmacy history appreciation groups and a worldwide listing of museums. Appendix 6 compiles bibliographic historical notes on the pharmacy literature. The glossary comprising Appendix 7 is really a succession of brief pharmacohistorical notes, providing background on individuals (e.g., Abbott, Wallace, Calvin), as well as subject related terminology, such as "quintessence" (as used by Paracelsus), "show

Figure 12.2 History of Pharmacy on the Internet

- *The History of Pharmacy*
  ⇨ http://www.lindsaydrug.com/newhist.htm
  The Lindsay Drug Company, a community pharmacy in Troy, New York, has created a beautiful site enhanced with images and text based on Cowen and Helfand's *Pharmacy, An Illustrated History* (12.57).

- *The History of Pharmacy in Pictures*
  ⇨ http://barbital.phar.wsu.edu/history
  Washington State University's history page includes both text and pictures taken from Bender's *Great Moments in Pharmacy* (Parke, Davis, 1965). Set aside time when visiting this URL; its many images take a long time to load, but it's well worth the wait.

- *Virtual Tour of the History of Pharmacy Museum—University of Arizona*
  ⇨ http://www.pharm.arizona.edu/museum/index.html
  The *Virtual Tour* is fascinating, informative, and full of unique photographs accompanied by a lively textual narrative.

- *PharmInfoNet Gallery*
  ⇨ http://pharminfo.com/gallery/glly_mnu.html
  The *PharmInfoNet Gallery* includes stunning photographs of antique apothecary jars from the Philadelphia College of Pharmacy and Science, a selection of engravings from Barton's *50 Medicinal Plants Indigenous to the United States* (1832), and a few other images of vintage pharmacy realia.

- *History of Pharmacy: A Guide to Sources*
  ⇨ http://www.simmons.edu/~tudesco/pharmacy
  Simmons College hosts the best subject hub on the topic, created by Sarah Tudesco of the Massachusetts College of Pharmacy Library. Categories include a bibliography of print resources, plus annotated hotlinks to Internet topical sites, related associations, museums, and an illustrated page of "Fun Pharmacy Facts."

- *Links to Sites Related to the History of Pharmacy—American Institute of the History of Pharmacy*
  ⇨ http://www.pharmacy.wisc.edu/aihp/links.html
  AIHP provides its own brief list of links to related resources.

- *Royal Society of Chemistry Historical Image Collection*
  ⇨ http://www.rsc.org
  The Royal Society of Chemistry's historical collection includes more than 8,000 images, 2,000 of which have been scanned into digital form. Original portraits, individual photographs, glass lantern slides, photomicrographs, cartoons and caricatures, and illustrations from books are all directly searchable free of charge, with copies available for a fee. Images of contemporary scientists are part of the scope of this intriguing collection. The RSC's library also offers an historical chemistry information service to tap into its catalog of 3,000 books spanning the sixteenth through nineteenth centuries.

---

globes," and the like. Black-and-white photographs and numerous other illustrations add to this volume's timeless appeal.

12.53 *Pharmacy in History.* Madison, WI: American Institute of the History of Pharmacy, 1959–. Quarterly.
12.54 *Pharmaceutical Historian.* Edinburgh, Scotland: British Society for the History of Pharmacy, 1967–. Quarterly.

The American Institute of the History of Pharmacy's bibliography also includes an excellent quarterly journal, *Pharmacy in History*, which is indexed in *International Pharmaceutical Abstracts* (14.8), *Historical Abstracts*, and *America: History & Life*—but not in *MEDLINE* (14.1). *Pharmaceutical Historian* is its British counterpart.

12.55 Griffenhagen G, Stieb EW. *Pharmacy Museums and Historical Collections in the United States and Canada.* Madison, WI: American Institute of the History of Pharmacy, 1988.

Griffenhagen and Stieb's *Pharmacy Museums and Historical Collections* organizes its listings by state and city, separating U.S. and Canadian sites. Brief descriptions identify collections ranging in size and importance from "four cases of apothecary jars, scales, weights, measures" hidden in a university hallway to completely preserved retail shops. The first specialized museum in the United States, organized by the Philadelphia College of Pharmacy in 1821, is no longer listed.

12.56 Parascandola J. *The Development of American Pharmacology.* Baltimore: Johns Hopkins University Press, 1992.

Chief of the History of Medicine Division at the U.S. National Library of Medicine, Parascandola has compiled a comprehensive history of the evolution of a scientific discipline in *The Development of American Pharmacology*. Rooted in materia medica and linked with the education of medical practitioners, pharmacology as we know it today results from the work of Abel, whose name appears in the subtitle of this book. A concluding bibliographic essay by its author highlights other useful sources of information.

12.57 Cowen DL, Helfand WH. *Pharmacy, An Illustrated History.* New York: Abrams, 1990.

Replete with reproductions of posters, photographs, paintings, and other realia from the renowned collection of Helfand, *Pharmacy, An Illustrated History* is that rare combination of an attractive and, at the same time, instructive book. Eleven chapters follow the origins of the practice of pharmacy from ancient times through the Industrial Revolution, and on into the twentieth century. Exhaustively indexed, the *Illustrated History* also includes a 17-page list of sources for further study.

12.58 Estes JW. *Dictionary of Protopharmacology. Therapeutic Practices, 1700–1850*. Canton, MA: Science History Publications, 1990.

Estes traces the derivation of the term "protopharmacology" to 1975, when the word was coined to describe the study of drugs used before modern academic pharmacology (i.e., pre-1849). He explains that this study was almost exclusively empirical—that is, based on physicians' observations—in contrast to modern day methods, which focus on sites and modes of action in intact animals or isolated tissues. The *Dictionary of Protopharmacology* is designed to assist researchers into historical medical practices in understanding therapeutic terms that appear in English-language texts written from 1700 through 1850. Estes's fascinating compilation will even help identify some proprietary preparations of the time, such as Peter's Pills, Oil of Peter, and Permont Water. Definitions sometimes include references to modern journal literature, to provide background on, for example, the use of Ricini Oil as a cathartic. The *Dictionary of Protopharmacology* would be an excellent reference for an historical novelist, especially a mystery writer (not a few of whom telephone medical libraries for information).

References

1. Stehlin D. Harvesting drugs from plants. *FDA Consum* 1990 Oct;24(8):20–23.

2. Fellows LE. Pharmaceuticals from traditional medicinal plants and others; future prospects. In: Coombes JD, ed. *New drugs from natural sources*. London: IBC Technical Services, 1992:93.

3. Houghton PJ. Biologically active compounds; detection and isolation from plant material. *Cosmet Toiletries* 1994 Jun;109(6):39–47.

4. Pharmaceuticals from plants: great potential, few funds. *Lancet* 1994 Jun;343(8912):1513–1519.

5. Balandrin MF, Klocke JA, Wurtele ES, Bollinger WH. Natural plant chemicals: Sources of industrial and medicinal materials. *Science* 1985;228:1154–1160.

6. Marwick C. Growing use of medicinal botanicals forces assessment by drug regulators. *JAMA* 1995 Feb;8:607.

7. Eisenberg DM et al. Trends in alternative medicine use in the United States, 1990–1997. *JAMA* 1998 Nov 11;280:1569–1575.

8. Mitchell S. Healing without doctors. *Am Demographics* 1993 Jul;15:48.

9. De Smet PAGM. Drugs used in non-orthodox medicine. In: *Meyler's side effects of drugs*. 12th ed. New York: Elsevier, 1992:1209–121.

10. Philen RM, Ortiz DI, Auerbach SB, Falk H. Survey of advertising for nutritional supplements in health and body building magazines. *JAMA* 1992 Aug;268:1008–1012.

11. Osol A, Pratt R. *The United States Dispensatory*. 27th ed. Philadelphia: Lippincott, 1973.

12. Snow B. Internet sources of information on alternative medicine. *Database* 1998 Aug;21:65–73.

Additional Sources of Information

Pharmacognosy

Andrews T. *A bibliography on herbs, herbal medicine, natural foods, and unconventional medical treatment.* Littleton, CO: Libraries Unlimited, 1982.

Angier B. *Field guide to medicinal plants.* New York: State Mutual Books, 1992.

Artuso A. *Drugs of natural origin: Economic and policy aspects of discovery, development, and marketing.* Binghamton, NY: Haworth Press, 1997.

Attaway DH, Zoborsky OR, eds. *Marine biotechnology: Pharmaceutical and bioactive natural products.* v. 1– New York: Plenum, 1993–.

Baldwin CA, Anderson LA, Phillipson JD, Spencer MG. Drug information—herbal concern. *Pharm J* 1987 Oct;239:R13-R14.

Bianchini F, Corbetta F. *Health plants of the world. Atlas of medicinal plants.* New York: Newsweek Books, 1977.

Boericke W. *Materia medica with repertory.* St. Louis: Fomur International, 1982.

Cannell RJP, ed. *Natural products isolation.* Methods in Biotechnology, v. 4. Totowa, NJ: Humana Press, 1998.

Chaudhury RR. *Herbal medicine for human health.* Geneva: World Health Organization, 1991.

Craker LE, Simon JE. *Recent advances in botany, horticulture, and pharmacology.* 4 v. Binghamton, NY: Food Products Press, 1986–1991.

Crellin JK, Philpott J. *Herbal medicine past and present.* 2 v. Durham, NC: Duke University Press, 1989.

Devon TK, Scott AI. *Handbook of naturally occurring compounds.* New York: Academic Press, 1972–.

Dhawan BN. Methods for biological assessment of plant medicines. In: Wijesekera RO, ed. *The medicinal plant industry.* Boca Raton, FL: CRC Press, 1991:77–84.

Duke JA. *Handbook of medicinal herbs.* Boca Raton, FL: CRC Press, 1985.

Duke JA. *Medicinal plants of the Bible.* Buffalo, NY: Trado-Medic Books, 1983.

Foster S, Duke JA, eds. *A field guide to medicinal plants: Eastern and central North America.* Peterson field guide series. Boston: Houghton Mifflin, 1990.

Israel R. *The natural pharmacy product guide.* Garden City, NY: Avery Publishing, 1991.

Jacob W, Jacob I, eds. *Medicinal plants in the Biblical world.* Pittsburgh, PA: Rodef Shalom Press, 1990.

Johnston ST, Wordell CJ. Homeopathic and herbal medicine: considerations for formulary evaluation. *Formulary* 1997 Nov;32(11):1166–1168,1171–1173.

Kaufman PB. *Natural products from plants.* Boca Raton, FL: CRC Press, 1998.

Kinghorn AD, Balandrin MF, eds. *Human medicinal agents from plants.* ACS symposium series, v. 534. Washington, DC: American Chemical Society, 1993.

Krochmal A, Krochmal C. *A field guide to medicinal plants.* New York: Random House, 1984.

Lewis WH, Elvin-Lewis MPF. *Medical botany. Plants affecting man's health.* New York: Wiley-Interscience, 1982.

List PH, Schmidt PC. *Phytopharmaceutical technology.* Boca Raton, FL: CRC Press, 1989.

MacDonald G. *A dictionary of natural products: Terms in the field of pharmacognosy.* 2nd ed. Medford, NJ: Plexus Publishing, 1997.

Maisch JM. *A manual of organic materia medica: drugs from natural sources.* New York: Gordon Press, 1992.

McCarthy S. *Ethnobotany and medicinal plants bibliography: January 1990-June 1991.* Upland, PA: Diane Publishing, 1993.

McCarthy S. *Ethnobotany and medicinal plants bibliography: July 1991-July 1992.* Upland, PA: Diane Publishing, 1993.

Millspaugh CF. *Medicinal plants: an illustrated and descriptive guide to plants indigenous to and naturalized in the United States which are used in medicine.* 2 v. New York: Gordon Press, 1980. [reprint of 1892 ed]

Moldenke HN, Moldenke AL. *Plants of the Bible.* New York: Dover, 1986.

Pettit GR, Hogan F, Herald C. *Anticancer drugs from animals, plants and microorganisms.* New York: Wiley, 1994.

Phillipson JD, Ayres DC, Baxter H. *Chemistry and pharmacology of natural products* [series]. New York: Cambridge University Press, 1989–.

Polunin M. *The natural pharmacy.* New York: Collier Books, 1992.

Tang W, Eisenbrand G. *Chinese drugs of plant origin: Chemistry, pharmacology, and use in traditional and modern medicine.* New York: Springer-Verlag, 1992.

Thompson MF, Sarojini R, Nagabhushanam R, eds. *Bioactive compounds from marine organisms, with emphasis on the Indian Ocean.* Brookfield, VT: Ashgate Publishing, 1991.

Wagner H, Bladt S, Zgainski M. *Plant drug analysis.* 2nd ed. New York: Springer-Verlag, 1995.

Weinstock CP. Medicines from the body. *FDA Consum* 1987 Apr;21:6–11.

Werbach MR, Murray Mt. *Botanical influences on illness: A sourcebook of clinical research.* Tarzana, CA: Third Line Press, 1994.

Zohary M. *Plants of the Bible: A complete handbook to all the plants with 200 full-color plates taken in the natural habitat.* London: Cambridge University Press, 1983.

Veterinary Drugs

Allen DG, Pringle JK, Smith DA. *Handbook of veterinary drugs.* 2nd ed. Philadelphia: Lippincott-Raven, 1998.

Barragry TB. *Veterinary drug therapy.* Philadelphia: Lea & Febiger, 1994.

Brander GC et al. *Veterinary applied pharmacology and therapeutics.* 5th ed. Philadelphia: W.B. Saunders, 1991.

Craigmill AL, Sundlof SE, Riviere JE. *Handbook of comparative pharmacokinetics and residues of veterinary drugs.* Boca Raton, FL: CRC Press, 1994.

Hardee GE, Baggot JD, eds. *Development and formulation of veterinary dosage forms.* 2nd ed. New York: Marcel Dekker, 1999.

Muir WW, Hubbell JAE, Skarda R. *Handbook of veterinary anesthesia.* 2nd ed. St. Louis: Mosby, 1994.

Nyberg CR, Porta MA, Boast C. *Laboratory animal welfare: A guide to reference tools, legal materials, organizations, federal agencies.* Twin Falls, ID: BN Books, 1994.

Plumb DC. *Veterinary drug handbook.* 2nd ed. Ames: Iowa State University Press, 1994.

Prescott JF, Baggott JD, eds. *Antimicrobial therapy in veterinary medicine*. Ames: Iowa State University Press, 1993.

Riviere JE, Craigmill AL, Sundlof SF. *CRC Handbook of comparative pharmacokinetics and residues of veterinary antimicrobials*. Boca Raton, FL: CRC Press, 1991.

Sirois M. *Veterinary clinical laboratory procedures*. St. Louis: Mosby, 1994.

History of Pharmacy

Bender G, Parascandola J, eds. *American pharmacy in the colonial and revolutionary periods*. Madison, WI: American Institute of the History of Pharmacy, 1977.

British Society for the History of Pharmacy: Martindales and their book. *Pharm J* 1992;248:787–788.

Gambardella A. *Science and innovation; The U.S. pharmaceutical industry during the 1980s*. New York: Cambridge University Press, 1995.

Helfand WH. *The picture of health: Images of medicine and pharmacy from the William H. Helfand collection*. Philadelphia: University of Pennsylvania Press, 1991.

Higby G. Panel discussion: Historical literature of American pharmacy. *Pharm Hist* 1992;34:74–94.

Higby GJ, Stroud EC. *The history of pharmacy: A selected annotated bibliography*. Bibliographies on the History of Science and Technology, v. 25. New York: Garland, 1995.

King NM. *Selection of primary sources for the history of pharmacy in the United States*. Madison, WI: American Institute of the History of Pharmacy, 1987.

Liebenau J, Higby GJ, Stroud EC, eds. *Pill peddlers: Essays on the history of the pharmaceutical industry*. Madison, WI: American Institute of the History of Pharmacy, 1990.

Parascandola J, Keeney E. *Sources in the history of American pharmacology*. Madison, WI: American Institute of the History of Pharmacy, 1983.

Riddle JM. *Quid pro quo; Studies in the history of drugs*. Brookfield, VT: Ashgate Publishing, 1992.

Scarborough J. Text and sources in ancient pharmacy. *Pharm Hist* 1987;29:81–84.

Smith MC. *Pharmacy and medicine on the air*. Metuchen, NJ: Scarecrow Press, 1989.

Sonnedecker G. Beginning of American pharmaceutical journalism. *Pharm Hist* 1991;33:63–69.

Ukens C. Bard and pharmacy: Shakespeare knew a thing or two about the practice. *Drug Topics* 1993;137(Suppl 3):44.

Wilson T. Pharmacy in fiction and film. *Int Pharm J* 1989;3:210–212.

13

Business Directories and Statistical Data Sources

The bulk of business information required for market research and competitive intelligence can, and should, be accessed through interactive online systems or, at the very least, in machine-readable format. Vast quantities of data are available only electronically by computer, because their timeliness would otherwise be severely compromised and, due to sheer volume, their potential utility would be difficult to exploit fully in printed form. This chapter will, therefore, be comparatively brief, confining discussion to sources that are, for the most part, published only in hardcopy. Such sources include retail trade directories; buyer's and product guides; statistical compilations of pharmacy services, operations, and manpower data; and directories of pharmacy faculty and educational programs. Although an introductory guide to drug sales and utilization reference publications is included here, additional background on this topic is offered in Chapter Fifteen's discussion of market research and competitive intelligence sources online.

Resources to Determine U.S. Product Availability

Perhaps ironically, relatively few of the drug compendia discussed in previous chapters can be used to determine if a product is on the market in the United States. To provide this capability, a resource must 1) index U.S. brand names, cross referenced to manufacturers, 2) be updated at least once a year, and 3) identify as many products as possible, including both single-entity and combination formulations, as well as prescription and over-the-counter medications. Figure 13.1 lists hardcopy publications that meet these criteria. Best bets are flagged to indicate which sources offer more comprehensive coverage, but no single reference can ever be judged truly definitive in this regard.

It should be noted that not all products in the *American Drug Index* are cur-

Figure 13.1   Resources to Determine U.S. Product Availability

Title	Reference #	Manufacturer Directory	Price
AHFS Drug Information	6.4	√	
♦ American Drug Index	3.6	√	
♦ Drug Facts and Comparisons	6.2	√	Cost Index
♦ Mosby's GenRx	6.3	√	√
The Orange Book	4.42		
PDR	6.10	√	
PDR for Nonprescription Drugs	6.9	√	
♦ PDR Generics	6.8	√	√
♦ Red Book	3.15	√	
USP DI	6.5		√
USP Dictionary	3.1	√	
Veterinary Pharmaceuticals and Biologicals	12.44	√	

♦ = Best bets (i.e., most comprehensive)

rently on the market, but if an *ADI* entry refers to package size and dosage form strength, the drug is likely to be available. Similarly, if brand names accompany *USP Dictionary* (USAN) entries, this is an indication (but not a guarantee) of market availability. Most entries in Figure 13.1 that are not flagged are relatively selective in the scope of their brand name indexing. For example, *The Orange Book* omits grandfathered drugs and those still undergoing DESI review. The *PDR* and *AHFS Drug Information* are even more limited in coverage, with entries representing only a selection of products on the market today.

Company or Service Directories and Buyer's Guides

In clinical practice settings, company directories included in drug compendia such as *Martindale* (6.1), *Mosby's GenRx* (6.3), the *Physicians' Desk Reference* (6.10), *American Drug Index* (3.6), and the *Red Book* (3.15) are usually sufficient to answer quick reference inquiries regarding manufacturer identification and location. Remember, also, that the annual *Chemist and Druggist Directory* (10.6) includes a manufacturer and product listing for companies in the United Kingdom, including number of employees and names of executive personnel. However, information centers supporting market research will need to extend their scope to include a collection of separately published directories offering access not only to pharmaceutical manufacturer listings, but also to suppliers of services to the industry.

13.1 *Scrip Directory of European Pharmaceutical Companies*. Richmond, Surrey, UK: PJB Publications, 1987–. Annual.

The *Scrip Directory of European Pharmaceutical Companies* compiles names, addresses, and telephone/fax numbers for more than 3,800 manufacturers located in any of forty-four Eastern and Western European nations and is arranged alphabetically by country. Appendices include a country-by-country listing of industry associations and of regulatory authorities. A comparable arrangement is used in presenting information on 2,000 companies and organizations in the *European Animal Health Directory*, published by PJB. Parallel sources include: the *Scrip Directory of Pharmaceutical Companies in Australasia and the Far East* (3,000 companies, fifteen countries); *Scrip Directory of Pharmaceutical Companies in North, South and Central America* (2,700 companies, forty countries); *Scrip Animal Health Directory for the Americas* (1,680 companies); and *Scrip's Rest of the World Directory of Pharmaceutical Companies*, with coverage of 3,600 companies in any of sixty countries in Africa and the Middle East, as well as India, Pakistan, and Bangladesh.

13.2 *World Pharmaceuticals Directory/93*. 5th ed. Chatham, NJ: PharmacoMedical Documentation, 1994.

The *World Pharmaceuticals Directory* is a cumulative compilation of companies with product entries in *Unlisted Drugs* (3.8). It is issued irregularly, usually every two to three years. The fifth edition, published in September 1994, covers *ULD* volumes issued from 1949 through 1993, listing more than 8,800 manufacturers and industrial or academic research organizations from any of fifty-six countries. The *Directory* provides a key to mnemonic codes used in *Unlisted Drugs* product monographs, cross referenced to full organization names and followed by a cumulative listing of drug names and their *ULD* citations. A separate corporate name and address directory is more conveniently arranged by full company name, making this volume useful for ready-reference consultation other than for its intended purpose of providing manufacturer name access to *Unlisted Drugs*.

13.3 *Euro-Pharma Guide to the European Pharmaceutical Industry*. 2nd ed. Hamburg: B. Behr's Verlag, 1994.

The *Euro-Pharma Guide to the European Pharmaceutical Industry* supplies entries for 2,472 companies located in any of seventeen countries, including the Czech Republic, Slovakia, Poland, Hungary, Norway, Finland, Sweden, and the United Kingdom. Additional listings, confined to firms located in Germany, identify eighty-six contract manufacturers and 129 service companies. Services indexed include testing laboratories, medical information systems, executive search firms, medical translations, and employee training. The main directory portion of the volume is arranged geographically, with companies listed alphabetically by name within each country's section. Company entries include mailing address, telephone and fax numbers, description of product range, number of employees, and annual turnover in U.S. dollars. Some, but not all, entries also identify chief executives and list subsidiaries. A separate section in the *Euro-Pharma Guide* indexes executives (7,717) and their positions in companies listed. A directory of industry associations, organized by country, is also included. The multipart index ending the volume offers access by product range keywords (e.g., aldosterone antagonists, anesthetics, antiallergic drugs) and by company name.

13.4 *Pharmaceutical Marketers Directory.* Boca Raton, FL: CPS Communications, 1977–. Annual.

Compiled by the publishers of *Medical Marketing & Media*, the *Pharmaceutical Marketers Directory* includes separate sections for 1,500 healthcare companies, 300 advertising agencies, and 800 publications where advertising is accepted. A section entitled Production Promotion Summaries lists healthcare manufacturers with their agencies of record and identifies marketing management personnel keyed to the products that they handle. These summaries include the previous year's journal-spending figure (for advertising) by each company. A large classified section of the directory will help locate firms by advertising specialties and other services, such as telemarketing, meetings and exhibits, audiovisual and graphics production, printing and lithography, packaging and labeling, executive search consultants, public relations, market research, and direct mail database management.

13.5 *OPD Chemical Buyers Guide.* New York: Schnell Publishing, 1913–. Annual.

13.6 *Chem Sources USA.* Ormond Beach, FL: Directories Publishing, 1958–. Annual.

13.7 *Chem Sources-International.* Ormond Beach, FL: Directories Publishing, 1987–. Biennial.

The *OPD Chemical Buyers Guide* and *Chem Sources* publications list suppliers of bulk chemicals for laboratory or industrial use. The *OPD* directory, popularly known as the "Green Book," is published annually as part of a subscription to *Chemical Marketing Reporter*. It includes addresses and telephone numbers for more than 1,400 suppliers of 18,000 chemicals, as well as related service vendors. The latter include chemicals distribution and chemical traffic firms. More than 150 entries identify suppliers of storage, containers, and packaging materials and services; 300 carriers and packagers are also listed. Another useful section compiles references to chemical company catalogs, brochures, and data sheets.

One drawback is that the number and variety of advertisements interspersed with *OPD* directory entries sometimes interfere with its functionality in quick lookups. Another problem that sometimes arises in using this type of buyers guide is chemical nomenclature. Although cross references from many alternative names are included, further research is sometimes required before appropriate entries can be located. *Chem Sources* directories are now available online, which has greatly enhanced their accessibility. Their scope and features are highlighted in Chapter Fifteen (15.27, 15.28).

13.8 *Medical Device Register.* 2 v. Montvale, NJ: Medical Economics, 1982–. Annual.
13.9 *Health Devices Sourcebook.* Plymouth Meeting, PA: ECRI, 1979–. Annual.

These two directories focus on providing product and supplier information for medical devices. Overlap between the two sources is by no means complete; each contains data not found in the other. The *Medical Device Register*, from the publishers of the *PDR* and the *Red Book*, consists of two volumes, the second of which contains supplier profiles (11,000 manufacturers and distributors). Each profile includes number of employees, ownership, method of distribution, sales volume, revenue, and net income. Key executives are listed, along with contact information and a product list. Volume 1, the Product Directory, indexes more than 90,000 items, cross referencing them to manufacturers and to their FDA device category classification. Product specifications and prices (when available) are also included. Separate indexes provide access by 6,500 device category keywords and by brand names. A *Mid-Year Supplement* to the *Medical Device Register* is available for separate purchase, as is an *International Edition* covering sixty countries, 6,000 suppliers, and 23,000 products. *Health Devices Sourcebook*, produced by a highly respected, non-profit independent research organization, is most easily accessible in online or CD-ROM format (refer to Chapter Fifteen, 15.25, for a detailed description).

13.10 *GEN Guides to Biotechnology Companies.* Larchmont, NY: Mary Ann Liebert, 1995–. Annual.
13.11 *The Biotechnology Guide U.S.A.* Research Triangle Park, NC: Institute for Biotechnology Information, 1997.
13.12 Coombs J, Alston YR. *The Biotechnology Directory 1998.* New York: Stockton Press, 1998.

GEN Guides to Biotechnology Companies is a one-volume collection of fourteen directories. The 1999 edition includes guides to 1) biotechnology companies, 2) bioprocess engineering firms, 3) peptide and peptide instrumentation companies, 4) law firms, 5) venture capital companies, 6) biotechnology recruiters, 7) biotechnology consultants, 8) contract research organizations, 9) biotech attachés to foreign embassies, 10) state biotechnology centers and university bioprocessing facilities, 11) cell and tissue culture companies, 12) technology transfer centers, 13) advertising agencies, and 14) biotechnology software companies. Company listings provide details regarding ownership, founding date, market and business focus, capitalization, stock ticker symbol, R&D partnerships, marketing and licensing agreements, international ventures, facilities, number of employees, and products on the market, as well as those under development. Personnel listings identify executives in charge of research, marketing, regulatory affairs, and purchasing. Compiled each year by the editors of *Genetic Engineering News*, *GEN Guides* includes more than 4,000 directory entries and a cross-guide index by company name and location. The publisher has also issued this resource on CD-ROM.

The Biotechnology Guide U.S.A. from the Institute for Biotechnology Information is much more limited in scope, assembling data on more than 1,300 companies, including venture capital firms. Entries identify company founding date, number of employees, address and telephone/fax numbers, and names of top management staff. Other information typically provided includes financing data, R&D budget, revenue, technologies used, and products in development and on the market. A *State-by-State Biotechnology Directory* is also available from the same publisher. This companion volume is essentially a telephone book listing contact names and addresses for biotechnology centers, companies, and regulatory personnel at both the state and federal level.

The Biotechnology Directory from Stockton Press is published in association with the journal *Nature-Biotechnology*. It includes information on more than 9,000 companies, research centers, and academic institutions worldwide. Company Profiles list address and telecommunications details (phone, fax, e-mail, Web site URL), number of employees, and areas of research activity. Entries are arranged geographically by country, and the 1998 edition provides, for the first time, a state-by-state index. Part of *The Biotechnology Directory* is also a buyer's guide, listing more than 2,000 items.

13.13 *The Technomark Register of Contract Research Organisations (CROs) in North America*. Lawrenceville, NJ: Technomark Consulting Services, 1995.

The Technomark Register of Contract Research Organisations in North America is a 600-page directory to 275 CROs in the United States and Canada. Section I compiles details on more than 150 firms offering clinical research services, including drug registration and data management. Section II focuses on preclinical, toxicology, and analytical service providers (fifty in all). Section III covers a miscellany of specialized drug development support service firms: e.g., those involved in formulation development, computer and documentation support, or clinical trials supplies. A particularly attractive feature of this directory is its standardized, two-page-per-company, format, employing charts and other graphic material to assist in comparisons between CROs. Entries itemize a wealth of descriptive details, such as year of formation, annual revenues, ownership (public or private), subsidiaries and associated companies, physical area of total premises, number of staff, languages spoken, and names of executive personnel. Other directories from the same publisher include: *European Contract Research*

Organisations (with coverage of more than 450 CROs) and *The Technomark Register of Contract Packagers & Manufacturers in Europe*. New editions of each were published in 1995.

13.14 *Who's Who—CTFA Membership Directory*. Washington, DC: Cosmetic, Toiletry, and Fragrance Association, 1998. Annual.
13.15 *CTFA International Buyers' Guide*. Washington, DC: Cosmetic, Toiletry, and Fragrance Association, 1998. Annual.

The Cosmetic, Toiletry, and Fragrance Association's annual *Who's Who Membership Directory* is international in scope, with entries for more than 300 active members and an additional 300 associate member companies. The latter include manufacturers of raw materials used in cosmetics and personal care products, as well as pertinent trade and consumer magazine publishers. Entries include names and titles of key executives, complete mailing address, telephone and fax numbers, and a description of products and services.

The *CTFA International Buyers' Guide* is a worldwide listing of cosmetic raw materials and their suppliers. More than 9,000 nonproprietary (INCI) ingredient name listings are cross referenced to 57,000 brand and technical names and their manufacturers. Suppliers of packaging materials and services, testing facilities, consulting services, and private label manufacturers are included in the *Buyers' Guide* directory of more than 1,500 provider companies in any of thirty-five countries worldwide. This publication is also accessible free of charge on CTFA's Web site at http://www.ctfa.org.

There are, in fact, a multitude of company directories on the Internet—far too many to attempt a comparison here. Figure 13.2 identifies some of the targeted resources available today for locating company home pages. The best of these also include brief profiles, financial data, and recent press releases. All sources listed are available free of charge.

Membership directories of many other important industry associations (see Appendix D) are also available on the Internet. For example, the Association of the British Pharmaceutical Industry (ABPI) lists names, addresses, and telephone numbers of its members, enhanced with hotlinks to their Web sites (http://www.abpi.org.uk). PhRMA, the Pharmaceutical Research and Manufacturers of America trade association, offers its complete directory of member companies and international and research affiliates for immediate display in its annual report at http://www.phrma.org.

13.16 *Chemical Week-Buyers' Guide Issue*. New York: McGraw Hill, 1937–. Annual.
13.17 *DCI Directory Issue*. New York: Advanstar Communications, 1994–. Annual.

Special issues or supplements to industry journals often include valuable directories easily overlooked if shelved with other serials in a library collection. One

Figure 13.2   A Selection of Specialized Company Directories on the Internet

- *Bio Online—Biotechnology Companies and Resources*
  ⇨ http://search.bio.com/search
  Vitadata Corporation supplies company profiles for more than 300 firms at this site.

- *BioSpace*
  ⇨ http://www.biospace.com
  Profiles for 400 companies are supplemented with financial and investor resources at this URL. Synergistic Media Network, the publisher, also archives press releases about each company.

- *InterPharma*
  ⇨ http://www.interpharma.co.uk
  Maintained by Medical Database Limited, this directory covers 14,000 support service organizations, such as market research firms and consultancies, for the pharmaceutical industry.

- *Medical Device Link*
  ⇨ http://www.devicelink.com
  Entries for 5,000 suppliers and 300 consultants are assembled here, along with references to related articles published in *Medical Device & Diagnostic Industry* magazine. Its publisher, Canon Communications, is responsible for this site.

- *National Biotechnology Information Facility Company Register*
  ⇨ http://www.nbif.org/industry/register.html
  Companies can be located alphabetically by name or in indexes by geographic region.

- *The NetSci Yellow Pages*
  ⇨ http://www.netsci.org/Resources/Biotech/Yellowpages/top.html
  Network Sciences Corporation provides brief overviews of many pharmaceutical and biotechnology companies, including those privately held.

- *PharmaVentures Links Page*
  ⇨ http://www.worldpharmaweb.com/comps.htm
  The consulting firm PharmaVentures offers a gratis "directory of directories" for biopharmaceutical company information, with hypertext pointers to other company locators and search engines. Specific hotlinked entries include the top fifty healthcare companies, the top 100 biotech firms, and the top fifty drug delivery companies. CROs and Japanese pharmaceutical companies are other targeted areas.

- *ReCap—Signals*
  ⇨ http://www.recap.com/mainweb.nsf
  Recombinant Capital is well known for this database of pharmaceutical, device, and biotech company information. Company searches yield not only home page links, but also valuation graphs, analyst reports, stock quotes, recent SEC filings, and reviews of company news, such as alliances, contracts, and clinical trials.

familiar example is the annual *Buyers' Guide Issue* of *Chemical Week*. Another is the *Directory Issue* of the trade journal *Drug & Cosmetic Industry* (*DCI*), published every July. This information-packed source features sections devoted to "Who's Who" in the cosmetic and toiletries business, consulting and special service firms, and industry associations. Types of services indexed include advertising claim substantiation, biological testing, package testing, relocation of plants, contract packaging, and private formula manufacturers. Specialty manufacturers are listed by type of product, such as cleansing materials, brushes and applicators, and aerosols. Listings for drugs and pharmaceuticals contract firms are subdivided by dosage forms (e.g., capsules-hard gelatin, tablet coating). Machinery and equipment suppliers are also identified. In addition, the *DCI* issue compiles a raw material directory that will help locate suppliers of many natural products (herbs, plant extracts) and formulation aids, such as surface-active agents, surface-treated pigments, and the like.

13.18 "Global Resource Directory." *Pharmaceutical Technology International*. Annual (July-Aug issue).

13.19 "Directory." *Pharmaceutical Technology (USA)*. Annual (July-Aug issue).

13.20 "Buyers Guide and Resource Directory." *Medical Device Technology*. Annual (June or July issue).

13.21 "Who's Who in R&D Companies." *Cosmetics & Toiletries*. Annual (Jan issue).

The journals *Pharmaceutical Technology International* and *Pharmaceutical Technology (USA)* each publish annual resource directories with listings for important industry associations, schools of pharmacy, and companies. The global edition identifies key contacts in Europe, the United States, and Japan. The U.S. edition includes entries for federal agencies, state organizations, and industry publications. Both special issues also compile a buyer's guide featuring suppliers of chemicals and raw materials; packaging, clean room and laboratory equipment and supplies; computer hardware; and contract manufacturing, testing, and service companies. The "Buyers Guide and Resource Directory" published in the June or July issue of *Medical Device Technology* is a comparable listing of materials, manufacturing supplies, service companies, trade associations, and government regulatory bodies (by country).

The annual directory issue of *Cosmetics & Toiletries* is a who's who of companies that provide consulting, testing, and research and development services. This trade journal publishes other minidirectories on an irregular basis, periodically offering international listings of product development consultants, testing laboratories, and formulation or ingredients suppliers. It should be noted that journals cited in this chapter are all indexed in *International Pharmaceutical Abstracts* (14.8), which is an excellent resource for tracking down special directory issues in both trade and professional publications.

Retail Trade Directories: Chain and Independent Pharmacies

There is no all-in-one hardcopy directory of U.S. pharmacies. However, various publications address separate segments of the retail drug business.

13.22 *The Hayes Druggist Directory.* Newport Beach, CA: Edward N. Hayes, 1912–. Annual.
13.23 *The Hayes Independent Druggist Guide.* Newport Beach, CA: Edward N. Hayes, 1981–. Annual.
13.24 Murphy GR, ed. *Directory of High Volume Independent Drug Stores.* Tampa, FL: CSG Information Services, 1992–. Biennial.

Issued annually in March, *The Hayes Druggist Directory* lists all retail pharmacies in the United States, organized alphabetically by state and city. Entries include name, address, telephone number, and credit rating based on an assessment of a store's estimated financial strength. Each city's listing identifies the county name and total population. *The Hayes Independent Druggist Guide* limits its scope to community pharmacies with "5 or less [sic] stores" and is issued in September each year. Another Hayes compilation, *Top-Rated Independent Pharmacies*, lists stores with an estimated financial strength of $75,000 or more and credit ratings of A or B (high or good). Published twice a year, in March and September, it can be ordered in magnetic tape format or as preprinted mailing labels.

The *Directory of High Volume Independent Drug Stores* profiles more than 8,500 one-unit retailers, providing names of owners, presidents, head pharmacists, and general buyers. Company listings include sales volume and percentages, product lines carried, square footage, and year founded. This directory is also available in magnetic tape format.

13.25 *The Hayes Chain Drug Store Guide.* Newport Beach, CA: Edward N. Hayes, 1987–. Annual.
13.26 *NACDS Membership Directory.* Alexandria, VA: National Association of Chain Drug Stores. Annual.

The Hayes Chain Drug Store Guide is published each year in September and includes three sections: a chain headquarters listing, a geographic list of chain outlets, and an alphabetical listing of outlets. The *NACDS Membership Directory* is an alphabetical guide to chain drug companies' headquarters locations. In addition to mailing address and telephone/fax numbers, each entry includes names of executives and buyers, the total number of retail outlets, and the number of pharmacies. An international member section cites National Association of Chain Drug Stores members located in Argentina, Canada, Germany, Mexico, Panama, Puerto Rico, and Sweden. A domestic, state-by-state section identifies which members operate in each state. This directory also lists drug trade associations, state boards of pharmacy, state pharmaceutical associations, state retail associations, and accredited colleges of pharmacy.

13.27 *Drug Store Market Guide.* Mohegan Lake, NY: Melnor Publishing, 1981–. Annual.

13.28 *Directory of Drug Store and HBC Chains.* Tampa, FL: CSG Information Services, 1945–. Annual.

The *Drug Store Market Guide* lives up to its name by providing more information about NACDS members and other retail outlets. It includes a list of leading U.S. drugstore chains, ranked by retail sales during the previous year, and identifies number of stores in each chain. There is a comparable ranked list of leading drug wholesalers. Deep discounters are also ranked by number of locations (outlets). However, the bulk of this directory is dedicated to assembling detailed profiles of eighty-three major drug markets (geographic areas) in the United States, including share-of-market estimates, demographic statistics (total population, number of households), and retail sales projections for every county within each market area. The *Drug Store Market Guide* is divided into seven regional sections, each introduced with a map, summary of cities and markets covered, and a table showing total drugstore sales in the region compared to total U.S. figures. Within each municipality or market, further breakdowns are included, listing sales per capita and sales per household.

The *Directory of Drug Store and HBC* [formerly *HBA*] *Chains* compiles information on more than 1,800 chains (defined as companies having two or more retail locations). Collectively, they account for approximately 25,000 drug or health and beauty aid (HBA) stores. Entries identify sales volume, trading area (square footage), primary wholesaler, distribution centers, product lines carried, key executives, and buying/administrative personnel. This directory also includes 120 drug wholesale companies and their 240 divisions.

13.29 *Annual Register of Pharmaceutical Chemists.* London: The Pharmaceutical Press, 1998. Annual.

13.30 *Annual Register of Merchants' Premises.* London: The Pharmaceutical Press, 1998. Annual.

The Royal Pharmaceutical Society of Great Britain publishes two *Register* directories each year based on official licensure data. The *Annual Register of Pharmaceutical Chemists* provides an alphabetical list of all registered pharmacists in the United Kingdom. In the separate List of Bodies Corporate and a Register of Premises, it also identifies all corporations operating retail pharmacies, including hospital pharmacies that are registered. Organized by country, directory entries are presented in further geographic breakdowns by county and town. The *Annual Register of Merchants' Premises* is a directory of U.K. agricultural merchants and saddlers licensed as distributors of veterinary medicines.

Remember, also, that the annual *Chemist and Druggist Directory* (10.6) contains a geographic listing of larger hospitals in Great Britain and their pharmacy personnel, noting their titles, degrees, and other qualifications.

Sources of Drug Sales and Utilization Data

Sales and utilization data tend to command a high price. Companies seeking detailed, worldwide statistical collections must have deep pockets (as it were). Except for staff in market research departments of major corporations, few readers will be able to obtain access to many of the resources described in the next section. However, brief summary data on hot topics, such as top selling drugs or most prescribed medications, can be found in the journal literature and on a few Internet sites identified later in this chapter. A selection of government publications will also offer another inexpensive route to highly specialized drug utilization data.

Major Market Research Suppliers

One company's name is practically synonymous with drug sales and utilization data worldwide: IMS. Founded in Europe in 1957 under the name "Intercontinental Medical Statistics," IMS quickly established a reputation as a preeminent provider of market data needed by the pharmaceutical industry. Today, IMS Global Services maintains major data collection and analysis programs, including MIDAS and IMSPACT.

MIDAS (Multinational Integrated Data Analysis Service) collates sales audits of pharmaceutical markets around the world. National IMS offices gather information at a local level in more than sixty countries. Derived from actual records of sales (e.g., invoices) by wholesalers or pharmacies, audit data are, in effect, a census of pharmaceutical commerce. Individual country's sales data are the basis for detailed, customized reports prepared by IMS for corporate subscribers. Summaries are also issued in the *World Drug Market Manual-Countries* and *-Companies*, publicly available online for use by both subscribers and nonsubscribers (15.32, 15.22). "Pack and presentation" details for launched products (i.e., labeling, indications, dosage form, strength, packaged quantities, pricing) are presented in the *IMSworld New Product Launches* and *Product Monographs* databases (15.18, 15.19).

Extracts from MIDAS summary reports are available for free preview at the IMS Global Services Internet site (http://www.ims-global.com). A bar graph currently offered shows pharmaceutical sales volume (in U.S. dollars) in eleven leading markets worldwide. Another summary identifies the top ten products, based on worldwide sales, presented in a two-year time series. Top selling therapeutic categories during the past twelve months in thirteen leading countries are the subject of a third "Market Insight" link, and the top ten corporations are singled out in a fourth summary.

IMS also monitors hospital distribution channels in twenty-two countries and collects medical statistics related to prescribing and to treatment of diseases in thirty-one nations. IMSPACT is the outgrowth of these data collection activities in the U.S. market. It contains reports from seven audits conducted by IMS America: 1) *Pharmaceutical Markets, Drugstores*; 2) *Pharmaceutical Markets, Hospitals*; 3) *National Disease and Therapeutic Index* (*NDTI*); 4) *National Detailing Audit*; 5) *National Mail Audit*; 6) *National Journal Audit*; and 7) *National Prescription Audit*. Taken together, these reports provide detailed sales data, on a monthly basis, for both hospital and drugstore purchases, accessible by company (drug supplier), product (at the pack or presentation level), and therapeutic class. *NDTI* correlates usage of drugs with diagnoses. Promotional statistics available include the number of units and dollars spent on mail and journal advertising and medical sales representation. The *National Prescription Audit* gauges new prescriptions written and new and refill prescriptions dispensed.

Scott-Levin, a consulting firm founded in 1982, is equally well known within the pharmaceutical industry for its market research audits. Its *Physician Drug & Diagnosis Audit* (*PDDA*) reports on patient visits and resulting treatment regimens among 365,000 office-based U.S. physicians in twenty-nine medical specialty areas. From this base sample, Scott-Levin extrapolates national estimates of drug use for major diagnoses or diseases. *PDDA* also tracks patient drug requests, as well as drug switching and the reason for medication substitutions. Extensive physician demographic and patient characteristics data are collected in this audit, enabling correlation of these factors with prescribing practices.

Scott-Levin also monitors drug sales at the retail level in the United States. Its *Source*™ *Prescription Audit* (*SPA*) gathers statistics on medications actually dispensed at any of 34,000 retail pharmacies, including chains, independents, mass merchandisers, and food store outlets. This sample represents an estimated 70% of all dispensed prescriptions and is gathered electronically on a weekly basis, with trend data available back to January 1991. Another measure of marketplace dynamics reported by *SPA* is method of payment, such as Medicaid, HMO, PPO, or cash. Statistics on generic substitution, based on a sample of 900 pharmacies nationwide, are also captured electronically in the *Source Prescription Audit*.

Scott-Levin is also the producer of several annual reports much quoted in the industry press. For example, the firm has polled physicians, pharmacists, nurse practitioners, physician's assistants, and HMO pharmacy directors to rank pharmaceutical companies by key attributes indicative of overall corporate image. First issued in 1992, *Pharmaceutical Company Image* reports now appear biennially. Substantive extracts of survey results have been included in industry analysts' reports collected in the *Investext* (15.38) database online.

Various promotional audits are also conducted to gauge the effectiveness of leading pharmaceutical companies' selling practices. For example, since 1984, Scott-Levin has published an annual report on *Sales Force Structures and Strategies*. In this publication, the field sales organizations of the top forty companies in the U.S. drug industry are examined in detail, showing trends in sales force size, promotional priorities, and quality ratings of sales representatives by their customers. Sales call activity levels in the market of office- or hospital-based physicians are reported in a separately published *Personal Selling Audit (PSA)/ Hospital Personal Selling Audit (HPSA)*. In another subscription service called *PMEA-Rx Link*, Scott-Levin correlates physicians' prescribing behavior with their participation in pharmaceutical company-sponsored meetings and events These and other market research publications from Scott-Levin are catalogued at the Web site URL: http://www.scottlevin.com/services. The latest title added to the repertoire is a *DTC Advertising Audit* designed to measure the impact of direct-to-consumer advertising campaigns.

The Trade Press

Both Scott-Levin and MIDAS/IMSPACT services are available only to paid subscribers. However, summary data derived from the IMS *National Prescription Audit* are widely reported in the trade press. For example, *Pharmacy Times* publishes statistics from the *Audit* each year in its April issue. The *Pharmacy Times* report includes data for comparison of prescription volume during the two previous years. The top 200 brand name drugs, determined by nationwide ranking of new and refill prescriptions, are identified, along with their manufacturers and original market launch date. The twenty leading therapeutic classes are also listed, ranked by sales and ranked by number of prescriptions dispensed. A free online version of this report is available at http://www.pharmacytimes.com/ top200.html. It includes statistics on pharmaceutical company promotional expenditures for office visits, hospital detailing, journal advertising, and television ads over the past year.

Drug Topics (also in April) typically reports IMS *Audit* statistics on numbers of prescriptions by classes of drugs, identifying those therapeutic categories showing the largest gains. The *Drug Topics* list singles out the top ten retail drugs, as well as the fastest growing branded products, based on prescription activity. *Hospital Pharmacy*'s April issue highlights a different segment of the *National Prescription Audit*: the top twenty-five best selling (dollar volume) drugs to hospital pharmacies. The report points out changes in ranking from the previous year's tabulation and shows brand ranking within therapeutic categories. Remember, also, that *Mosby's GenRx* (6.3) flags top selling medications in the United States. Keyword index entries enable users to identify the top 100, 200, 300, and 400 lists.

American Druggist publishes results of its own top 200 survey of most frequently dispensed prescription drugs in February each year. The June issue reports findings of *American Druggist*'s prescription trends survey from a sample of retail outlets. Data include average price, dollar volume, ratio of third-party to self-pay prescriptions, amount of time spent by retail pharmacists in medication counseling, and numbers of prescriptions dispensed in chain versus independent pharmacies. *American Druggist* also began an annual survey in 1994 to estimate generic drug use in prescriptions filled at the retail level. Based on a sample of more than 700 pharmacists, most favored sources for generics are reported and the top fifty products are listed. *American Druggist* also periodically publishes a list of top selling OTC products.

Among these trade journals, *Drug Topics* stands out for its extension of sales data reporting to product categories other than prescription drugs. It can provide figures on consumer spending and market share for OTC medications, vitamins, home healthcare products, foods, cosmetics, hair and dental preparations, and household supplies typically sold in community pharmacies. For example, one issue of *Drug Topics* listed the top 100 brands, in terms of sales, of nonprescription drugs and health and beauty aids. (Remember, to locate recent reports from any of the journals mentioned in this section, consult *International Pharmaceutical Abstracts*, 14.8.)

Internet Sources

The Web site of another retail magazine publisher, Miller Freeman, is a good place to check for comparable data on health and beauty aids, as well as OTC pharmaceutical preparations, in the United Kingdom. Under the Features icon, market watch tables show the top ten products in each category, with sales figures cumulated for the past year. Under the Practice icon, a business statistics section reveals trends in pricing and costs for various toiletries and nonprescription remedies. URLs for this and related Internet sources cited throughout this chapter are compiled for quick reference in Figure 13.3.

Another rich source of drug sales and utilization data on the Internet is the National Association of Chain Drug Stores (NACDS). Facts and figures, summarized in bar graphs, pie charts, and beautifully formatted tables, include pharmacy retail sales in chains, independents, mass merchandisers, food stores, and mail order outlets. Both Rx and OTC drugs are covered, as well as sales of health and beauty aids. Rx volume is also reported for each type of retail outlet. These free Web-based reports are the result of a collaboration between IMS America and NACDS.

The "Facts and Figures" portion of the Pharmaceutical Research and Manufacturers of America home page on the Internet also contains many useful statistical tidbits. Detailed data on member companies' collective R&D expenditures and sales are gathered in PhRMA's *Annual Survey*, which can be viewed free-of-charge. Additional tables assemble numeric information from government and other nonmember sources (e.g., IMS) on topics such as per capita healthcare ex-

Figure 13.3   URLs for a Selection of Drug Sales and Utilization Sources

- *Managed Care Digest Series* (HMO and other group purchasing practices)
  ⇨ http://www.managedcaredigest.com
- *Miller Freeman dotpharmacy* (market trends for OTCs and HBAs)
  ⇨ http://www.dotpharmacy.co.uk/index.html
- *National Association of Chain Drug Stores* (retail industry facts and figures)
  ⇨ http://www.nacds.org/industry
- *National Center for Health Statistics* (National Ambulatory Medical Care Surveys)
  ⇨ http://www.cdc.gov/nchswww)
- *National Clearinghouse for Alcohol and Drug Information* (substance abuse data)
  ⇨ http://www.health.org
- *Pharmaceutical Research and Manufacturers of America* (industry profile & PhRMA facts)
  ⇨ http://www.phrma.org
- *Pharmacy Times* (top 200 Rx report)
  ⇨ http://www.pharmacytimes.com/top200.html

penditures, generic drugs' share of market, and the balance of trade in medical products. A "PhRMA Facts" segment links to one-page snapshots of key issues, often supplemented by graphs. For example, tallies of new medicines in development for children, women, AIDS, cancer, and other selected diseases are covered in separate PhRMA Facts sheets, accompanied by explanatory text. Another menu option, Backgrounders, leads to an array of minireports on hot topics such as generic drugs, prices and profits, and direct-to-consumer advertising. These reviews almost invariably supply statistics in support of the industry viewpoints that they advocate. The *PhRMA Home Page* also offers the full text of the Association's *Industry Profile* book, review of which would be a solid introduction to the U.S. market. A detailed table of contents and separate table of figures enables users to pinpoint portions likely to supply data needed.

U.S. Government Publications

In addition, drug utilization data of various types are collected by agencies of the U.S. government, most notably the National Center for Health Statistics (NCHS), which became part of the Centers for Disease Control (CDC) in 1987. Publications resulting from the National Ambulatory Medical Care Survey and the National Health Interview Survey, issued as part of the *Vital and Health Statistics* ["Rainbow"] *Series*, are of particular interest. Preliminary findings are often available in *Advance Data* reports, which are used as the means for early release of data from NCHS.

13.31 *National Ambulatory Medical Care Survey:* [year] *Summary.* Vital and

Health Statistics Series Advance Data Reports. Hyattsville, MD: National Center for Health Statistics. Annual.

Advance Data annual reports from the National Ambulatory Medical Care Survey are typically two to three years behind actual data collection. They summarize physician visits by patient and practice characteristics, diagnosis, and services provided. Tables present statistics on visits during which drugs were prescribed or used, number of medications ordered or provided, and "drug mentions," tallied by therapeutic class and for the top twenty generic names.

Subset reports are also prepared by NCHS and issued irregularly as part of the *Advance Data* series. For example, a report on *Office Visits to Neurologists* summarizes drug mentions by therapeutic category and top brand or generic names, enabling comparisons to data collected for visits to all physicians, regardless of specialty. Similar reports have been prepared regarding office visits to urologists, psychiatrists, dermatologists, pediatric specialists, internists, otolaryngologists, obstetricians and gynecologists, cardiovascular disease specialists, and general surgeons, all published as *Advance Data Reports*.

13.32 *National Hospital Ambulatory Medical Care Survey:* [year] *Emergency Department Summary.* Vital and Health Statistics Series Advance Data Reports. Hyattsville, MD: National Center for Health Statistics. Annual.

13.33 *National Hospital Ambulatory Medical Care Survey:* [year] *Outpatient Department Summary.* Vital and Health Statistics Series Advance Data Reports. Hyattsville, MD: National Center for Health Statistics. Annual.

An *Emergency Department Summary* is also issued each year (again, with a two- to three-year lag time in statistics reported). It includes data on the number of drugs provided and top twenty drugs mentioned, listed by generic name, as part of treatment furnished during hospital emergency department visits. The annual *Outpatient Department Summary* tabulates number of drugs prescribed during visits and number of drug mentions, by brand or generic name. Both outpatient and emergency department final and full data collection results are ultimately issued together on one CD-ROM disc as part of Series 13 of *Vital and Health Statistics*.

Summary data reports from all three national ambulatory medical care surveys are available for immediate display or downloading, free of charge, at the *NCHS Home Page* on the Internet. Graphs showing percentage of drug mentions by therapeutic class in physicians' office visits and emergency department visits can easily be located under the Data Warehouse icon. Another graph shows usage data on the twenty most frequently prescribed drugs in outpatient departments. Under the FASTATS icon, summary sheets are listed for alcoholism, use of contraceptives, immunization, illegal drug use, vitamin intake, and therapeutic drug use.

A separate summary of *Alcohol- and Drug-Related Visits to Hospital Emergency Departments*, based on the same national survey, is available in paper copy format (see Additional Sources at the end of Chapter Seven). A complementary publication, *Data from the Drug Abuse Warning Network (DAWN)* was discussed in Chapter Eight (8.43). Other NCHS publications focusing on pharmaceutically related topics can easily be located by consulting the *American Statistics Index* (online or hardcopy). *Advance Data Reports* are available, for example, on use of medical device implants, vitamin and mineral supplements, fluoride-containing dental care products, controlled drugs in office-based ambulatory care, and contraceptives.

In addition to drugs sales and utilization data, information on expenditures may be needed. *Health, U.S.* (13.36), an NCHS publication cited in the next section as a source of professional manpower data, also reports on public health agency and personal health expenditures by U.S. residents each year, broken down by type, including hospital care, physician services, and prescriptions.

Other Statistical Sourcebooks

Hundreds of data sets addressing a multiplicity of anticipated information needs are compiled annually in *Parexel's Pharmaceutical R&D Statistical Sourcebook*.

13.34 *Parexel's Pharmaceutical R&D Statistical Sourcebook.* Waltham, MA: Parexel, 1995–. Annual.

Topics covered include R&D spending trends, drug and biologic development costs, and statistics on products in development, which are tallied for a spectrum of therapeutic classes. Both international and domestic (FDA) regulatory statistics are assembled, showing average new drug application review times and otherwise hard-to-find information, such as the number of agency-imposed clinical holds. Parexel also analyzes data on genomics and high-throughput screening in order to measure the impact of these new technologies on drug development today. Consulting the *R&D Statistical Sourcebook* should be a first stop in answering most questions related to pharmaceutical industry performance benchmarks, such as drug discovery and ultimate launch success rates and time-to-market statistics.

13.35 Hartzema AG, Mullins CD, eds. *Pharmaceutical Chartbook.* 2nd ed. Binghamton, NY: Pharmaceutical Products Press, 1995.

It's difficult to know where to classify a unique resource like the *Pharmaceutical Chartbook*. It includes visual depictions of a variety of factors important to the industry, particularly those affecting drug distribution. This book is essentially a collection of graphs—usually bar graphs—charting trends. Separate sections of the collection are devoted to population demographics, drug utilization data, drug costs, reimbursement, pharmaceutical development and production, human resources, policy changes (laws), and summary statistics on manufacturers, wholesalers, and distributors. Sources of data for each chart, meticulously referenced, are astonishingly diverse: e.g., the U.S. Senate Special Committee on Aging, the FDA, the National Center for Health Care Statistics, the Department of Commerce, the National Wholesale Druggists Association *Operating Survey*, the *Lilly Hospital Pharmacy Survey*, state boards of pharmacy, the Health Insurance Association of America, IMS America, and the Bureau of the Census. This compilation of nearly 200 visual aids could be a time saver in answering last minute requests for data to support presentations. However, the *Chartbook*'s omission of an index means that the detailed table of contents must be relied upon for location of relevant graphs and charts.

Pharmacy Services, Operations, and Manpower Data

Since 1987, the American Society of Health-System Pharmacists has conducted an annual survey of hospital pharmacy practice in the United States. ASHP gathers data on a variety of factors, such as drug costs, personnel cuts, patient focused services, use of technicians, computerization, formulary management, residency programs, drug distribution systems, ambulatory care services, and quality assurance programs. Results are published in the *American Journal of Health-System Pharmacy*.[1-3] Cotter and McKee have reported the outcome of comparable surveys in the United Kingdom.[4] The European Association of Hospital Pharmacists mailed 4,393 questionnaires to pharmacists in eighteen countries in 1995. The result, published the following year, tallies factors such as computerization, staffing levels, and service provision for extemporaneous compounding, IV admixture programs, formulary management, therapeutic drug monitoring, and drug information.[5]

Two major pharmaceutical companies have lent their names and funds to other compilations of statistical data related to pharmacy services. In its *Managed Care Digest Series™*, Hoechst Marion Roussel (HMR) publishes facts and figures about HMO's use of closed formularies, in-house versus external or mail-order pharmacies, drug utilization review (DUR) programs, prior authorization requirements to control physician prescribing, and drug purchasing practices. Calculations of pharmacy costs as a percentage of HMO operating expenses are also provided in each annual report, as is the percentage of prescriptions filled with brand name, versus generic, drugs. Sample tables of contents and summary slide presentations derived from each of four HMR titles published each year are available at http://www.managedcaredigest.com. The series of reports includes: *Institutional Digest, Medical Group Practice Digest, Integrated Health Systems Digest*, and *HMO-PPO Digest*. Another analysis of drug purchasing and prescription control practices is the *Novartis Pharmacy Benefit Report*.

The National Association of Chain Drug Stores surveys its membership each year to obtain data on factors such as selling space, number of employees, and salaries. This information is tabulated by retail channel (type of store) and published (along with sales data mentioned in the previous section) on the NACDS Web site at http:www.nacds.org/industry.

A feature often overlooked in the National Association of Boards of Pharmacy *Survey of Pharmacy Law* (4.31) is annual licensure statistics for registered pharmacists, broken down by practice settings. Several federal government reports also include manpower data.

13.36 *Health, U.S.* Washington, DC: National Center for Health Statistics, 1975–. Annual.

13.37 *Factbook: Health Personnel, U.S.* Rockville, MD: Bureau of Health Professions, 1993–. Biennial.

13.38 *Occupational Projections and Training Data.* Washington, DC: Bureau of Labor Statistics, 1971–. Biennial.

The massive *Health, U.S.* annual reports from the National Center for Health Statistics compile statistics on healthcare expenditures and revenue, facilities, services, manpower, and health status of the population. Data provided for trend analyses date back to 1970. Each edition contains information on employment in the health service industry by setting, and in hospitals by occupation. Immediately following this section is a tabulation of total and first-year enrollments in health occupations schools, broken down by profession. As noted previously, the portion of the report dedicated to healthcare costs and financing also reports expenditures for hospital care, physician services, and prescription drugs each year. The latest edition of *Health, U.S.* is available in PDF format for downloading free of charge at the NCHS Web site (http://www.cdc.gov/nchswww).

The *Factbook: Health Personnel, U.S.* is a new biennial document series, begun in 1993, that extracts data on labor supply and education of health professionals included in *Health, U.S.* The Bureau of Labor Statistics also issues a biennial report on occupational employment and educational and training completions. Data reporting in *Occupational Projections* typically lags behind collection by two years, but projections are included into the next century.

Reports are issued less frequently in the United Kingdom, where manpower surveys are conducted by the Royal Pharmaceutical Society and published in the *Pharmaceutical Journal.*[6] Statistics on full-time, part-time, and unemployed male and female pharmacists are typically presented, with breakdowns for different areas of employment, such as community, hospital, industry, wholesale, and teaching.

Directories of Pharmacy Faculty and Educational Programs

Although U.S. government documents cited (13.36–13.38) include general data on pharmacy education, two organizations can be relied upon for more systematic and detailed coverage of educational programs and teaching personnel: the American Association of Colleges of Pharmacy (AACP) and the American Council on Pharmaceutical Education.

13.39 *Roster of Faculty and Professional Staff.* Alexandria, VA: American Association of Colleges of Pharmacy,, 1989–. Annual.

Each year, AACP publishes a *Roster of Faculty and Professional Staff* employed at accredited schools of pharmacy in the United States. The directory is arranged alphabetically by state, and within each state, by institution name. Staff listings (both AACP members and nonmembers) include position, degrees, academic discipline, mailing and e-mail address, fax, and direct dial telephone number. A back-of-the-book index offers an integrated alphabetical name listing for more than 5,000 full- and part-time personnel. The *Roster* also includes staff listings for affiliated institutional member schools in Canada, Malaysia, the Philippines, Thailand, and Wales.

13.40 *Accredited Professional Programs of Colleges and Schools of Pharmacy.* Chicago: American Council on Pharmaceutical Education, 1985–. Annual.
13.41 *Approved Providers of Continuing Pharmaceutical Education.* Chicago: American Council on Pharmaceutical Education, 1984–. Annual.
13.42 *Graduate Programs in the Pharmaceutical Sciences.* Alexandria, VA: American Association of Colleges of Pharmacy, 1991–. Annual.

The American Council on Pharmaceutical Education also issues a directory of *Accredited Professional Programs* and, in a separate volume, a list of *Approved Providers of Continuing Pharmaceutical Education.* AACP focuses on advanced degree providers in its annual compilation of *Graduate Programs in the Pharmaceutical Sciences.* For comparative analysis of undergraduate degree programs and their admission criteria, refer to AACP's *Pharmacy School Admission Requirements.*[7]

A list of pharmacy technician education and training programs available in the United States and Canada has also been published periodically in the *Journal of Pharmacy Technology.*[8] The *Chemist and Druggist Directory* (10.6) lists schools of pharmacy in the United Kingdom. Worldwide lists of pharmacy schools and colleges are also available on the Internet (see Figure 13.4).

13.43 *Residency Directory.* 2 v. Bethesda, MD: American Society of Health-System Pharmacists, 1999. Annual.

The American Society of Health-System Pharmacists' *Residency Directory* identifies ASHP-accredited pharmacy practice residencies nationwide. Entries in Volume One describe each training site and highlight its special features, such as opportunities for advanced education in a given subject area. Volume Two includes standards and regulations governing ASHP accreditation, with special at-

Figure 13.4   Internet Directories of Pharmacy Schools and Continuing Education Sites

- *Pharmacy Continuing Education Sites Around the World*
  ⇨ http://info.cf.ac.uk/uwcc/phrmy/WWW-WSP/PhrmCEsites.html
  David. J. Temple at the Welsh School of Pharmacy (Cardiff) has compiled this alphabetical list by country. It includes CE programs originating in schools of pharmacy, as well as nonuniversity sources.

- *Pharmacy-Related Academic Institutions on the Internet*
  ⇨ http://www.pharmweb.net/pwmirror/pw8/pharmweb8.html
  PharmaWeb's hotlinked directory is organized by country. This URL also provides a search form for locating specific colleges, departments, or schools by name, city, or country in the International Pharmaceutical Federation (FIP) database. The latter includes contact names, mailing and email addresses, telephone and fax numbers, and URLs, when available.

- *Virtual Library: Pharmacy*
  ⇨ http://www.pharmacy.org/schools.html
  David Bourne of the University of Oklahoma maintains the *Virtual Library: Pharmacy* worldwide list of schools, colleges, faculties, and departments.

- *The World List of Schools of Pharmacy*
  ⇨ http://info.cf.ac.uk/uwcc/phrmy/WWW-WSP/SoPListHomePage.html
  Another directory maintained by David Temple at the Welsh School of Pharmacy, University of Wales, this country-by-country list of hypertext links can also be viewed as a list of URLs, if desired.

tention to programs in specialty areas of practice. These include oncology, critical care, infectious disease, pediatrics, nutritional support, psychopharmacy, or drug information residencies. Ohri and Pincus offer guidance on "digging up details on residency and fellowship programs."[9]

13.44 *Profile of Pharmacy Students*. Alexandria, VA: American Association of Colleges of Pharmacy. Annual.

Projections for pharmacy manpower are assisted by the AACP's *Profile of Pharmacy Students*. This annual report shows the number of Doctor of Philosophy (PhD), Doctor of Pharmacy (PharmD), and Bachelor of Pharmacy (BS) degrees conferred during the previous year. Gender, race, and ethnicity of graduates are summarized. Similar statistics are presented for enrolling students.

References

1. Reingold DJ, Santell JP, Schneider PJ, Arenberg S. ASHP survey of pharmacy practice in acute care settings: prescribing and transcribing—1998. *Am J Hosp Pharm* 1999 Jan 15;56:142–157.

2. Reeder CE, Kozma CM, O'Malley C. ASHP survey of ambulatory care responsibilities of pharmacists in integrated health systems—1997. *Am J Hosp Pharm* 1998 Jan 1;55:35–43.

3. Reeder CE et al. ASHP national survey of pharmacy practice in acute care settings—1996. *Am J Hosp Pharm* 1997 Mar 15;54:653–669.

4. Cotter SM, McKee M. Survey of pharmaceutical care provision in NHS hospitals. *Pharm J* 1997 Aug 16;259:262–268.

5. Delaney T. EAHP survey of hospital-based pharmacy services in Europe—1995. *European Hosp Pharm* 1996;2(3):92–105.

6. Survey of pharmacists 1988–1990. *Pharm J* 1991 May;246;621–625.

7. *Pharmacy school admission requirements.* Alexandria, VA: American Association of Colleges of Pharmacy. Annual.

8. Technician education and training programs. *J Pharm Technol* 1993 Jul-Aug;9;164–165.

9. Ohri LK, Pincus KT. Digging up details on residency and fellowship programs. *Am J Hosp Pharm* 1994 Nov;51;2786–2787.

Additional Sources of Information

Bundes-apotheken-register 1993/94. Stuttgart: Deutsche Apotheken Verlag, 1993.

Donohue TF, Sprouse CR. *Drug formularies and the pharmaceutical industry: Thriving in the managed care era.* Waltham, MA: Parexel, 1995.

Griffith NL, Schommer JC, Wirschung RG. Survey of inpatient counseling by hospital pharmacists. *Am J Hosp Pharm* 1998 Jun 1;55:1127–1133.

HIMA emerging market report. Washington, DC: Health Industry Manufacturers Association, 1996.

International health data reference guide. Hyattsville, MD: National Center for Health Statistics, 1994.

Ohri LK, Pincus KT. Computerized database for residency and fellowship programs. *Am J Hosp Pharm* 1993 Jun;50;1137–1138.

Pharmacists' directory and yearbook, 1998–1999. London: The Pharmaceutical Press, 1998.

Profile of pharmacy faculty. Alexandria, VA: American Association of Colleges of Pharmacy. Annual.

Raehl CL, Bond CA, Pitterle ME. 1995 National clinical pharmacy services study. *Pharmacotherapy* 1998;18(2):302–326.

Ross JA, Mauldin WP, Miller VC. *Family planning and population: A compendium of international statistics.* New York: The Population Council, 1993.

Rozek RP. Critique of the GAO report on differences in prices for prescription drugs between Canada and the United States. *J Res Pharm Econ* 1995;6;77–91.

Scrip's review of 1997. Richmond, Surrey, England: PJB Publications, 1998. Annual.

Statistical abstract of the United States. Washington, DC: U.S. Dept. of Commerce, 1878–. Annual.

Stonier PD. *Discovering new medicines—careers in pharmaceutical research and development*. Chichester, England: John Wiley & Sons, 1994.

Universal health care almanac. Phoenix, AZ: Silver & Cherner, 1993–. Quarterly.

Wyszewiarski L, Mick SS, eds. *Medical care chartbook*. Ann Arbor, MI: Health Administration Press, 1991.

Practicum 4

This practicum exercise will help you evaluate your ready-reference source selection skills and review information presented in Chapters Nine through Thirteen. Questions posed can be answered without actual reference to hardcopy sources. Suggested answers are included in Appendix E.

Directions: Assume that you have available for your use all of the sources cited in previous chapters. Unless otherwise indicated, your response to each question should consist of:
   a. a list of sources to be consulted, with order of priority indicated, and
   b. a brief explanation of the rationale behind your selection of resources and sequence of consultation.

1. Is there a U.S. equivalent of *Dopom* tablets, a combination OTC sleep aid last purchased in Europe by the patient?
2. A patient is admitted to the hospital with white tablets, imprinted "0260" and scored on one side, in his possession. Identify the tablets.
3. A market research company needs a list of community pharmacies in Rhode Island.
4. What was the prescription volume of antihypertensive medications in the United States in 1985, 1990, and 1995?
5. Where can a chemist obtain sulfonyldioxide?
6. What is the address of Tutag Pharmaceuticals?
7. Where can I find a list of U.S. pharmacy schools and their admission requirements?
8. Locate a commercial source for a tablet press (machine) in the Northeast.
9. What are the official guidelines for assaying ethylparaben?
10. What was the sales volume of prophylactics in community pharmacies each year from 1990 forward?
11. Where can I find recommendations for medicines that should be on hand in the average household?

12. Can you tell me which of these nonprescription products I'm considering contains ingredients that used to be available only by prescription?
13. We need to contact all academic librarians with responsibility for collections supporting pharmacy colleges.
14. Who can supply extracts from coneflowers and arnica, as well as "No leaf" and kukui nut oil, appropriate for use in cosmetic formulations?
15. Where will I find a drug photo identification aid that is arranged by color and size, rather than product name or company?
16. How many students are enrolled in doctoral programs in pharmacognosy in the United States, and how many have obtained degrees in this discipline in the past five years?
17. In what percentage of hospitals are IV admixture programs pharmacy-based? Are data available to show growth or decline in such services in the past decade?
18. Where can a consumer find a discussion of nutritional supplements, with a comparison of multivitamin products?
19. A patient planning an extended trip to Europe wants to know equivalents of Drug X marketed abroad.

14

Compiling a Bibliography with Online Resources

Using the reference tools discussed in previous chapters can save a great deal of time, because of their compilation and distillation of information previously published piecemeal over time and in a wide variety of primary sources. However, bound reference books quickly become dated, sometimes necessitating a follow-up search in more recent literature to check for any new reports that may affect the reliability of clinical data published in a monograph perhaps two or three years previously. Also, many ready-reference works cited earlier in this *Guide* provide limited documentation for the facts that they contain. The information provider may, then, be faced with assembling a bibliography of supportive references to augment citations included in tertiary sources.

When a more current or extensive bibliography is needed to answer a pharmaceutical query, consultation of abstracting and indexing services is the most efficient way to accomplish the task. Yet, due to economic and physical space constraints, even major resource libraries today rarely maintain hardcopy subscriptions to all secondary sources relevant to the subject area. Most information centers rely, instead, on CD-ROM or online access to selected indexes. Compact disc technology offers expanded on-site storage and in-house networking capabilities, as well as predictable pricing. Online access requires no local storage or maintenance, relying instead on telephone connections (e.g., for the Internet) to large repositories of machine-readable information stored elsewhere. Fees for *ad hoc* online usage are usually based on connect time and page or per-unit output charges. Ongoing high volume online database access can also be contracted at a flat or fixed cost on a semiannual or annual basis.

Other factors, beyond maintenance and cost, differentiate between these two most prevalent forms of subscribing to abstracting and indexing sources: 1) databases available, 2) timeliness of updates, and 3) search capabilities. Although the number of CD-ROM titles is steadily increasing, many more publications are available online. When a source is offered in either format, the CD-ROM version is usually updated less frequently. Most importantly, major online databanks provide more sophisticated and comprehensive search capabilities, such as simultaneous multifile access, whereby results from multiple sources can be consolidated, and duplicate references to the same journal articles cited in more than one index can be detected and eliminated.

However, both CD-ROM and online versions of literature indexes do share many enhancements to research capabilities. For example, printed secondary sources typically index by author name(s) and a limited number of publisher-assigned keywords to describe the subject matter of primary sources cited. In machine-readable form, secondary publications generally provide additional access points, such as publication date, language, journal name, and author affiliation or address. Although all of these elements may be present in the hardcopy service, only one can be used as an entry point to the material in manual lookups.

For example, a pharmacist may seek information on "possible respiratory effects of drug X in human adult males," and is particularly interested in locating studies reportedly conducted at three medical centers in the United States. In a hardcopy source such as *Index Medicus*, the pharmacist has the choice of looking under the drug name or under subject keywords such as "respiratory," "lung," or "pulmonary." The researcher must then scan multiple references listed under any one of these terms in a succession of annual volumes (and individual monthly updates for the current year) until relevant citations can be located.

In other words, hardcopy access requires users to coordinate multiple concepts manually and visually and to consult separate issues, when date of publication is unknown. In a machine-readable database, terms for all concepts (drug + lung + human + adult + male) can be entered in a single search request. Factors such as author location (e.g., named medical centers in the United States) are also indexed and directly accessible. The computerized interface will compile a list of citations indexed under each keyword entered and match the lists to locate those which contain the combination of terms (concepts, author addresses, etc.) that the searcher has specified. All of this is done in a matter of seconds, and only those references which match search requirements—i.e., a precoordinated bibliography—need be displayed.

In addition to facilitating coordination of multiple concepts and accelerating the retrieval process, another advantage of computerized access is that title and abstract textwords are usually also searchable, not just publisher-assigned index terms. This capability means that users unfamiliar with the vocabulary preferred by indexers will still be able to find relevant bibliography. The success of their query will be based on their ability to predict what words are used by authors when writing about the topic under investigation, rather than being based on prior knowledge of indexing protocols. Once a few pertinent items are retrieved, the user can examine descriptive keywords assigned by the database publisher and incorporate them into a subsequent search request to achieve more comprehensive results. Thus, subject access is considerably augmented in machine-readable databases compared to that offered in hardcopy counterparts. For this reason, familiarity with both online and CD-ROM resources has become a prerequisite to efficient literature retrieval in support of drug information service.

Discussion in this and succeeding chapters will focus on major secondary resources directly relevant to the pharmaceutical subject area and available online through vendors of computerized information most commonly used in medical libraries or corporate information centers in the United States: DataStar, Dialog, the National Library of Medicine's MEDLARS or ELHILL system, QUESTEL-ORBIT, Ovid Technologies, SilverPlatter, or STN International. Many databases are also available in CD-ROM format, but no attempt is made here to address the varying capabilities or content of individual resources offered on compact disc versus online, or to list all possible vendors of either CD-ROM or online databases cited.

Instead, the purpose of *Guide* descriptions is to provide an overview of the structure and content of each database, highlighting special features that influence database selection and potential utility in answering typical drug information queries. Following individual source descriptions are notes on practical applications, with selected search examples to illustrate possible strategies. Although entry protocols differ depending on the vendor chosen for local access, Dialog or DataStar samples shown should be easily translatable to other systems. Databases featured in this chapter are, for the most part, abstracting and indexing services designed to assist researchers in compiling bibliographies on specific topics within the general subject areas of pharmacology and therapeutics, adverse reactions and interactions, pharmaceutics, and pharmacognosy. Online aids to drug identification and location of alternative nomenclature conclude this introductory overview. (See Appendix B for additional resources.)

Pharmacology and Therapeutics Databases

Although there are many subject specialty databases available today, four files stand out in any compilation of health science resources, because they contain information on virtually every category of biomedicine: *MEDLINE, EMBASE, BIOSIS Previews*, and *SciSearch*. Familiarity with these omnibus files is essential to effective pharmaceutical information service.

MEDLINE

MEDLINE is the most well known biomedical indexing source, due to its early introduction in machine-readable format, its low cost made possible through U.S. government subsidy, and its undoubted quality.

14.1 *MEDLINE*. Bethesda, MD: National Library of Medicine, 1966–. Updated weekly. Available on DataStar, Dialog, MEDLARS, QUESTEL-ORBIT, Ovid, SilverPlatter, and STN; also on CD-ROM.

This database combines the content of three hardcopy titles: *Index Medicus*, *Index to Dental Literature*, and *International Nursing Index*. Journal references compiled from these printed indexes have been augmented, since 1975, with abstracts reproduced from primary sources (added to 66% of records 1975–). Literature published in any of more than seventy countries and forty languages is represented, but 75% of *MEDLINE* citations are to English-language sources; 38% are drawn from journals published in the United States. Approximately 3,600 journals are scanned for pertinent bibliography. Selected chapters from monographs were also indexed from 1976 through 1981.

Although it's easy to retrieve references online using "natural language" or "free text" techniques (i.e., user-selected terminology without reference to database user aids), research in *MEDLINE* will be more thorough and systematic if users first consult the list of *Medical Subject Headings* (*MeSH*) employed by indexers.

14.2 *Medical Subject Headings—Annotated Alphabetic List*. Bethesda, MD: U.S. National Library of Medicine. Annual.

National Library of Medicine (NLM) personnel choose from descriptive terms listed in *MeSH* to identify major concepts covered in primary sources cited. Because only *MeSH* descriptors are used to index subject matter in the database, the *Medical Subject Headings* volume functions as an authority list of controlled *MEDLINE* vocabulary. Consulting *MeSH* prior to going online can provide insight into indexing practices and valuable assistance to searchers. *MeSH* is referred to as a "thesaurus," since it not only lists *MEDLINE* headings, but also provides numerous cross references from synonyms or alternative keywords searchers may have in mind for a topic, directing them to the preferred terminology used in the database.

14.3 *Medical Subject Headings—Tree Structures*. Bethesda, MD: U.S. National Library of Medicine. Annual.

Pharmaceutical questions sometimes require searching broad topics, such as retrieving bibliography for all analgesics or all central nervous system effects, then adding in another subject factor. Trying to deduce all of the specific terms under which relevant items might appear in such cases is difficult. Fortunately, NLM publishes another user aid, the *Tree Structures*, which arranges subject headings in an outline format, grouping terms together when they are conceptually related. Using such a classification scheme facilitates broad concept retrieval, as will be illustrated in discussion of drug category searching later in this chapter.

Another special indexing feature in *MEDLINE* is subheadings. These topical qualifiers represent recurring, but usually secondary, concepts in information requests, such as adverse effects or diagnostic use (see Figure 14.1). They enable searchers to focus bibliographic output by coordinating qualifying terms with *MeSH* descriptors. For example, a strategy containing a drug's nonproprietary name is likely to retrieve citations not only to pharmacology and therapeutics material, but also chemical synthesis, analysis, and toxicity. To isolate references where pharmacokinetics of the drug are discussed, the PK subheading can be linked directly to its *MeSH* descriptor. The entry format for coordinating main headings with subheadings in *MEDLINE* varies from vendor to vendor (e.g., *drug(L)pk* on Dialog, *drug/pk* on MEDLARS, *drug with pk* on DataStar); consult your search system's user aids for further details.

Figure 14.1   A Selection of MEDLINE Subheadings for the Pharmaceutical Searcher

---

Drug/chemical qualifiers:

administration and dosage (AD)	economics (EC)
adverse effects (AE)	genetics (GE)
agonists (AG)	immunology (IM)
analogs and derivatives (AA)	isolation and purification (IP)
analysis (AN)	metabolism (ME)
blood (BL)	pharmacokinetics (PK)
cerebrospinal fluid (CF)	pharmacology (PD)
urine (UR)	poisoning (PO)
antagonists and inhibitors (AI)	radiation effects (RE)
biosynthesis (BI)	secretion (SE)
chemistry (CH)	standards (ST)
chemical synthesis (CS)	supply and distribution (SD)
contraindications (CT)	toxicity (TO)
deficiency (DF)	therapeutic use (TU)
diagnostic use (DU)	ultrastructure (UL)

Disease term qualifiers:

chemically induced (CI)	epidemiology (EP)
complications (CO)	etiology (ET)
diagnosis (DI)	mortality (MO)
drug therapy (DT)	prevention and control (PC)
economics (EC)	

Organisms/anatomical term qualifiers:

drug effects (DE)

Chemical Indexing in MEDLINE

MEDLINE's choice of drug and chemical terminology reflects a strong clinical orientation. Accordingly, simplified or generic names are generally preferred over chemical names, lab codes, or brand names. For drugs, U.S. Adopted Names (USAN—see Chapter Two) are the standard. When indexing drug preparations containing a combination of active ingredients, *MEDLINE* assigns descriptors for each of the active compounds. Brand or proprietary names are searchable only if included in the title or abstract reproduced from the primary source.

The rationale behind use of a controlled vocabulary in a database is predictability, from the user's point of view. By limiting indexers to a finite list of terms from which to choose when they describe the content of sources cited, a database publisher is able to offer the reassurance of uniformity and consistency not present in everyday (natural) language. Unfortunately, controlled vocabularies like *MeSH* do not readily accommodate change. For the sake of consistency, relatively few new descriptors are introduced each year. This restriction means that new drugs are not always easily identifiable in *MeSH* indexing.

For this reason, additional "uncontrolled" chemical terminology has been added to *MEDLINE* records since June 1980. Added terms include 1) Enzyme Commission numbers, 2) CAS registry numbers, and 3) names of substances that these numbers represent. Thus, substances named in a source article are easily identified in database entries, regardless of whether they have a *MeSH* controlled vocabulary descriptor or whether they have appeared in the title or abstract reproduced online. Other details about this indexing are significant. Unlike most other online databases, *MEDLINE* includes EC numbers in records even when the author has referred to an enzyme only by other names. If both an EC number and an RN are available as alternate codes for an enzyme, only the EC number is provided as an access point in the *MEDLINE* record.

Searchers should also be aware that *MEDLINE* indexers typically use the registry number of the parent compound when identifying salts or stereoisomers. For example, several pharmaceutical preparations contain *prednisolone* salts. However, references to *prednisolone sodium phosphate* (RN 125–02–0) or *prednisolone sodium succinate* (RN 1715–33–9) are indexed with the RN for the parent compound *prednisolone* (RN 50–24–8). Some *MEDLINE* citations also list registry numbers as "0" (zero), when NLM personnel have been unable to locate a code from in-house sources (see 14.39). Thus, users should beware of relying too heavily on RNs when searching chemical substances in *MEDLINE* and be prepared to supplement RN strategies with alternative terminology, such as nonproprietary or other names obtained from nomenclature sources.

EMBASE (Excerpta Medica)

Excerpta Medica, a division of the Elsevier publishing companies, provides international coverage of literature on human medicine and related disciplines in the form of hardcopy indexes, abstract journals, CD-ROM publications, and online databases. Material from more than forty hardcopy secondary literature sources is included in *EMBASE* online, which also contains many references (40%) not cited in printed counterparts.

14.4 *EMBASE.* Amsterdam, The Netherlands: Elsevier Science Publishers, 1974–. Updated weekly. Available on DataStar, Dialog, Ovid, Silver-Platter, and STN; also on CD-ROM.

Although based in the Netherlands, Excerpta Medica focuses on dissemination of medical information in English; 77% of database records are references to English-language sources, which are drawn from more than 4,000 journal titles published in any of 119 countries and thirty-nine languages. All abstracts and indexing terms are in English. As with *MEDLINE, EMBASE* concentrates on journal articles, although approximately 1,000 books per year were indexed from 1975 through 1980. Abstracts accompany 60% of records.

EMBASE offers unusually thorough indexing of the world's drug related literature. Toxicology, biophysics/bioengineering (including medical devices and drug delivery systems), psychiatry, forensic medicine, as well as environmental and occupational health, are also emphasized in coverage, with much data available in *EMBASE* not cited elsewhere online. A larger number of basic science journals are indexed in this file than in *MEDLINE*. More than 70% of its subject descriptors are devoted to drug and chemical nomenclature.

14.5 *EMTREE Thesaurus.* 3 v. Amsterdam: Excerpta Medica, 1999.

Indexing vocabulary is derived from the *EMTREE Thesaurus*, which consists of approximately 40,000 drug and medical preferred terms and cross references from 150,000 synonyms to preferred descriptors. Still more synonyms and cross references are included in online implementations of *EMTREE* than are available in the hardcopy edition. Thus, *EMTREE* online can provide valuable search assistance not only for using *EMBASE*, but can also contribute possible alternative terminology for use in search strategies in other online databases that do not have a controlled vocabulary (such as *SciSearch* or *TOXLINE*). For example, *EMTREE* online lists sixteen related terms for the drug *amfebutamone*, including two brand names, the developing company's research code, four different generic names used internationally, and two chemical names found in the literature. Such a wealth of nomenclature, specifically compiled to assist searchers, would not be found in *MEDLINE*'s thesaurus (*MeSH*).

EMBASE has developed a classification scheme similar in purpose to the *Tree Structures* in *MEDLINE*. When research on broad topics is required, pharmaceutical searchers will find the *EMTREE* hierarchical list (included in the three-volume user aid cited above) helpful in locating appropriate, conceptually related terms. Discussion of drug category searching later in this chapter will illustrate the utility of this powerful feature.

EMBASE also introduced "link" terms in 1988 to assist users in focusing on frequently requested secondary aspects of topics (see Figure 14.2). Similar in rationale to the topical subheadings in *MEDLINE,* link terms are available for many of the same concepts. For example, to retrieve citations to pharmacokinetics of a drug, PK can be used in *EMBASE* in exactly the same way as was illustrated in discussion of PK in *MEDLINE* (see above). Furthermore, PD expresses pharmacology in both sources, and AN identifies analytical studies. The *EMBASE* link term SI (side effect) is a direct counterpart to CI (chemically induced) in *MEDLINE.*

Note, however, that *EMBASE* separates the concepts of drug administration and drug dosage under AD and DO, while *MEDLINE* includes them under the single topical qualifier AD. *EMBASE* uses CR to index references to drug concentration in body fluids or tissues, while *MEDLINE* includes specific qualifiers for analysis in blood (BL), cerebrospinal fluid (CF), or urine (UR). DT (drug therapy) can be linked with drug terms in *EMBASE,* but the same abbreviation in *MEDLINE* can be applied only to descriptors for diseases or conditions. (TU for therapeutic use is the closest *MEDLINE* counterpart for DT as it is used in

Figure 14.2   EMBASE Link Terms

Drug term qualifiers:

adverse drug reaction (AE)	drug interaction (IT)
clinical trial (CT)	drug therapy (DT)
drug administration (AD)	drug toxicity (TO)
drug analysis (AN)	endogenous compound (EC)*
drug combination (CB)	pharmaceutics (PR)
drug comparison (CM)	pharmacoeconomics (PE)**
drug concentration (CR)	pharmacokinetics (PK)
drug development (DV)	pharmacology (PD)
drug dose (DO)	

Disease term qualifiers:

complication (CO)	etiology (ET)
congenital disorder (CN)	prevention (PC)
diagnosis (DI)	radiotherapy (RT)
disease management (DM)**	rehabilitation (RH)
drug resistance (DR)***	side effect (SI)
drug therapy (DT)	surgery (SU)
epidemiology (EP) etiology (ET)	therapy (TH)

*Introduced January, 1991
**Introduced January, 1997
***Introduced January, 1996

EMBASE, and is directly linkable with drug names.) Another notable difference between *MEDLINE* subheadings and *EMBASE* link terms is that the latter offer several extras for the pharmaceutical searcher, such as the ability to easily identify references to drug combinations (CB) or drug-resistant conditions (DR), to locate pharmaceutics studies (PR), or to isolate a substance discussed as an endogenous (EC), rather than exogenous, compound (a useful feature when coordinated with hormone descriptors).

Chemical Indexing in EMBASE

Generic names are preferred for indexing citations about established drugs. The *EMBASE* standard for pharmaceutical nomenclature is the World Health Organization's International Nonproprietary Name (INN—see Chapter Two). This editorial policy means that the name used for a drug in the *Physicians' Desk Reference* (6.10), *Drug Facts and Comparisons* (6.2), or *MEDLINE* may sometimes differ from that used in *EMBASE*.

Another difference compared to NLM indexing is that the preferred *EMTREE* descriptor for a combination preparation is a brand name. This policy facilitates retrieval of references to nonprescription drugs, among which combination products predominate. Generic or chemical name descriptors are also assigned to such citations, providing access points to each of the active ingredients in preparations discussed. Another bonus is that brand names and manufacturers are added to records when primary source authors mention such names in the original article text. The advantage this extra indexing offers is illustrated in search examples shown later for retrieving brand name comparisons.

CAS registry numbers and Enzyme Commission numbers are included as cross references to preferred terms in the *EMTREE* thesaurus online and are also directly searchable. However, as in *MEDLINE*, it's a good idea to supplement RN strategies with drug name synonyms for comprehensive recall.

BIOSIS Previews

Produced by BioSciences Information Service, *BIOSIS Previews* incorporates all material published in *Biological Abstracts* (1969–), *Biological Abstracts/ Reports, Reviews, Meetings* (*BA/RRM*, 1980–), and *BioResearch Index*, the predecessor of *BA/RRM* (1969–1979).

14.6 *BIOSIS Previews*. Philadelphia: BioSciences Information Service, 1969–. Updated weekly. Available on DataStar, Dialog, Ovid, SilverPlatter, and STN; also on CD-ROM.

Taken together, the three printed counterparts to the machine-readable database ensure ecumenical scope in coverage of life science literature. Each year, *BIOSIS* indexing encompasses more than 7,000 journal titles, books, theses, institutional and government reports, scientific book reviews, symposia, and conference proceedings. U.S. patents were also indexed selectively from 1986 through 1989. (Patent coverage continues in the *BioBusiness* database from the same publisher.) Items indexed are published in any of more than 100 countries and fifty-seven languages; 86% of citations are, nonetheless, references to English-language source material. Author abstracts were added to *BIOSIS* in 1976 and accompany 55% of records from that year forward.

Much broader in subject scope than *MEDLINE* or *EMBASE, BIOSIS Previews* estimates that at least half of its citations are relevant to human medicine. All core books and serials identified in the "Library for Internists"[1] are indexed in this database. The pharmaceutical searcher will find *BIOSIS* to be a major secondary literature source for locating bibliography on the early stages of drug development and on toxicology, pharmacology, and biotechnology. Pharmacognosy topics, as well as references to agrochemicals, environmental pollutants, occupational hazards, cosmetics, and food additives, are also well represented. The emphasis in *BIOSIS* is on research, rather than routine clinical practice, data.

Controlled indexing focuses on major subject concepts and taxonomic identification. An authority file online lists preferred keywords and phrases, as well as broader and narrower related terms. Beginning in 1999, *MeSH* disease descriptors will be added to database records.

Chemical Indexing in BIOSIS Previews

U.S. Adopted Names (USAN) are preferred in indexing drug related bibliography. CAS RNs were added in 1998. Enzyme Commission numbers, lab codes, brand names, and names for combination products are included as access points only when they are specifically mentioned in the original source being indexed. From 1969 through 1984, chemical names and other polysyllabic subject keywords in citation titles and descriptors were frequently segmented to assist searchers in retrieving significant word fragments. For example, *dimethylsulfoxide* might appear as *di methyl sulfoxide* or *dimethyl sulfoxide, neonate* as *neo nate, antineoplastic* as *anti neoplastic*. *BIOSIS* advises the use of alternate entry formats and multiple synonyms when searching subject concepts retrospectively.

A selection of controlled vocabulary terms will assist users in retrieving bibliography related to drugs and other chemicals within given classes. Known as "modifiers" or "affiliations," many of these keywords match the categories used in the *U.S. Pharmacopeia* (11.8) to describe pharmacological action or therapeutic use of a substance. Examples include:

abortifacient-drug
antianginal-drug
appetite-stimulant-drug
hematologic-drug

oxytocic-drug
pharmaceutical adjunct-drug
vitamin-drug

Consult the *BIOSIS* authority file online for a complete list of drug modifiers, and check vendor documentation for entry formats in online or CD-ROM systems.

SciSearch

The Institute for Scientific Information (ISI) publishes several secondary services of potential interest to pharmaceutical researchers, perhaps the best known being the *Current Contents* series. Various titles in this series are also available in the machine-readable database *Current Contents Search* (see Appendix B). However, another ISI database, *SciSearch*, offers the advantage of *Current Contents'* legendary timeliness, but with a greatly enhanced subject scope, value-added indexing, and more sophisticated search capabilities.

14.7 *SciSearch*. Philadelphia: Institute for Scientific Information, 1974–. Updated weekly. Available on DataStar, Dialog, and STN; also on CD-ROM.

The closest printed counterpart to *SciSearch* is *Science Citation Index*, issued bimonthly in four parts: the Source Index, the Permuterm Subject Index, the Citation Index, and the Corporate Index. The *SciSearch* database contains all four components, but differs in content from the hardcopy indexes in two ways: 1) indexing of books is not included online, but 2) additional citations derived from ISI's *Current Contents* series (*Clinical Medicine, Life Sciences*, and *Agriculture, Biology, Environmental Sciences* editions), not all included in the hardcopy *Science Citation Index*, do appear online in *SciSearch*. Furthermore, this database (dubbed *SCI Expanded* on the Web) began, in 1998, to index 2,000 more journals than are covered in print or CD-ROM editions. *SciSearch* also began incorporating abstracts in 1991; 64% of records added since that time have included author summaries reproduced from primary sources.

From the point of view of the pharmaceutical searcher, *SciSearch* offers several benefits. One is its breadth in subject scope. It is a multidisciplinary index to the literature of science and technology, offering access to 5,600 journal titles published in any of fifty countries and thirty-one languages (87% English). Users will find that this database covers many "fringe" or interdisciplinary topics less consistently surveyed in more specifically subject oriented publications. For example, research on medical devices, biometrics, or computer applications in medical care may be published in the specialty journals of several different disciplines (engineering, biomedicine, mathematics, pharmacy), many of which will be included in the *SciSearch* source list because of ISI's all embracing approach to the sciences. ISI's cover-to-cover indexing policy also benefits researchers concerned with possible omissions in bibliographies compiled from sources such as *MEDLINE, EMBASE,* or *BIOSIS Previews,* each of which has a more selective subject scope.

Indexing in *SciSearch* is unusual, in that it is largely computer generated. Two new types of subject descriptors were added in 1991: author keywords and "Key-Words Plus." Although author-provided descriptors reproduced from source journals are not always present in database records, KeyWords Plus accompany most references added since 1991. Generated through a computerized algorithm developed by ISI, KeyWords Plus are recurring words or phrases found in titles of articles used as cited bibliographic references or footnotes in the primary source documented in a *SciSearch* record. Although these titles are not displayed as part of the Cited Reference field online, they are analyzed and selectively excerpted for production of keyword indexing. Since a close relationship usually does exist between references cited by authors and the topic of articles where they are cited, KeyWords Plus can complement other access points.[2]

Bibliographies accompanying primary sources supply another unique search capability pioneered by ISI: cited reference searching. Using this feature, it is possible to locate articles that cite a given source, thus tapping into the "invisible college" in the scientific research community. Starting with a bibliographic reference for a work already known to be relevant, searchers can find related publications through citation indexing. For example, a cited reference strategy was used to update information presented in the introduction to Chapter Seven of this book. Using bibliography found in preparing the previous edition (e.g., references to seminal publications in the *Archives of Internal Medicine* and *JAMA* by Miller and Talley), it was easy to locate fifty-five more recent articles by other authors focusing on the epidemiology of adverse effects. Newer work in the sciences tends to cite older precedents, whether they reinforce or contradict results reported in the current publication. This phenomenon creates communities of researchers sometimes linked only by the literature networks that bibliographies accompanying their articles reveal. In the sample case study described here, tracking down cited references led to some publications that were not located in a subject keyword search, since the language used to describe drug-related events can be somewhat difficult to predict.

Tracing authors building upon the work of a core source is particularly helpful in exploring literature related to very new research areas, where terminology used by authors has yet to be standardized and is usually entirely absent in controlled vocabulary indexing. Again, cited reference strategies often uncover publications on the cutting edge that may elude searchers relying on keyword strategies alone.[3] For this reason, it's a good idea for authors to conduct citation searches periodically on their own work, to gauge its impact and often unforeseen applications in research completed by others.

Chemical Indexing in SciSearch

Direct subject access in *SciSearch* is confined to title and abstract words, descriptors provided by authors, and KeyWords Plus—none of which are predictable. Thus, no standards can be relied upon when searching pharmaceutical concepts in *SciSearch*. This lack of standardization means that natural language strategies are called for, i.e., extensive use of synonyms for drug names and imaginative second guessing about the ways source authors may have referred to topics under investigation.

International Pharmaceutical Abstracts

Although *International Pharmaceutical Abstracts* (*IPA*) lacks the size and breadth in scope to be characterized as an omnibus resource, its depth of indexing literature specifically related to the subject area merits a closer look. Virtually all pharmacy specialty journals published throughout the world are indexed in *IPA*. Although 60% of the 800 journal titles covered originate outside the United States, 87% of this database's references are to English-language source material. Literature published in any of more than twenty-five other languages is also represented. *IPA* indexes all U.S. state pharmacy journals and identifies all source articles that qualify for pharmacy continuing education credit.

14.8 *International Pharmaceutical Abstracts*. Bethesda, MD: American Society of Health-System Pharmacists, 1970–. Updated monthly. Available on DataStar, Dialog, Ovid, SilverPlatter, and STN; also on CD-ROM.

Section headings and scope notes included in Figure 14.3 reflect this file's thorough coverage of the literature of pharmacy. *IPA* in both CD-ROM and on-line format offers access to extensive bibliography about pharmaceutical concepts less well addressed in other medical databases, such as pharmaceutics, chronopharmacology, drug stability, pharmaceutical technology, and quality control in drug manufacture. *IPA* is the best source for locating studies about the effects of formulation on pharmacokinetics, physical/chemical properties, dosage form, or route of administration. *IPA* also indexes bibliography on topics such as pharmaceutical packaging, preservatives, flavorings, equipment, or vehicles. It compiles citations not found elsewhere on cosmetic formulation, pharmacognosy, and pharmacy practice issues, such as OTC medication counseling, hospital drug distribution systems, IV additive programs, and formulary development. In a study of online database indexing of pharmaceutical journals, 12% of *IPA*'s journal coverage was found to be unique (not duplicated in *MEDLINE, EMBASE, BIOSIS Previews*, or *CA Search*).[4]

Figure 14.3   International Pharmaceutical Abstracts Section Headings and Scope Notes*

Adverse Drug Reactions
> Unexpected or unintentional reactions when a medication is given in normal dose range and route of administration: e.g., reactions not listed as typical side effects, iatrogenic drug addiction, hypersensitivity, potentiation of dormant or other disease states.

Biopharmaceutics
> Effects of formulation, physical-chemical properties, particle size, and dosage form on the body or tissue: e.g., pharmacokinetic studies, *in vivo* dissociation time studies, absorption and adsorption, effect of sustained-release medications, generic and therapeutic equivalency studies, bioavailability, effect of route of administration on drug action if dosage-form-related.

Drug Analysis
> Assay or analysis for quantitative or qualitative testing; determination of content, impurities, counterfeit drugs.

Drug Evaluations
> Therapy or specific *in vivo* effects of established (noninvestigational or experimental) drugs: e.g., clinical cases, dosage amount comparisons, discussions of resistance, tolerance, placebo effects.

Drug Interactions
> *In vivo* drug-drug, drug-chemical, or drug-food interactions related to therapy or diagnosis; includes synergism, summation, potentiation, antagonism, competition, and interactions of drugs and radiation therapy.

Drug Metabolism and Body Distribution
> Includes excretion, endogenous physiological interactions, biotransformation, placental barrier and transfer, drugs present in lactation, pharmacokinetics, test or analysis of drugs in body fluids or tissue, effect of route of administration on drug availability and breakdown.

Drug Stability
> Decomposition of specific pharmaceuticals and *in vitro* incompatibilities: e.g., hydrolysis, effects of temperature, moisture, light, containers or packaging. Includes parenteral admixture incompatibilities.

Environmental Toxicity
> Toxicity due to environmental exposure or contact: e.g., occupational drug poisoning, zoonoses, pollutants, hospital-acquired infections.

History
> History of pharmacy and drug use, including drug discoveries, pharmacy law, pharmacy literature and art.

Information Processing and Literature
> Discussions of drug literature and drug information and its use, including data processing, automated recordkeeping, nomenclature issues, information transfer.

Institutional Pharmacy Practice
> Pharmacy practice in hospitals, extended care facilities, nursing homes, and other institutions. Includes discussion of pharmacist's role in compounding parenterals, in outpatient and inpatient care, and administrative control, drug distribution systems.

Investigational Drugs
Action in humans of drugs that are under investigation: i.e., not currently used in the United States.

Legislation, Laws and Regulations
Includes discussions of patents, standards, licensure, accreditation, taxation, recalls, liability cases, narcotic regulations.

Methodology
Means and methods of evaluating drug action in humans, animals, or biological systems: e.g., clinical study design, laboratory equipment, systems, procedures.

Microbiology
Pharmaceuticals and their effects on, or preparation from, microorganisms; microbiology important to pharmacy, e.g., *in vitro* antibiotic spectrum studies, resistance studies.

Pharmaceutical Chemistry
Includes references to synthesis, structure-activity studies, separation and purification, structure determinations.

Pharmaceutical Education
Includes residency programs, continuing education, academic education, as well as pharmacy technician training.

Pharmaceutical Technology
Manufacturing, formulas and formulation of pharmaceuticals, sterilization and contamination, packaging, quality control, preservatives, flavorings, vehicles, equipment, closures, hardness and disintegration tests, etc.

Pharmaceutics
Physical pharmacy or chemistry, rheology, nonroutine tests on pharmaceutical preparations: e.g., dissolution, filtration, pH studies, ionization, crystallization, solubility, and surface action studies.

Pharmacognosy
Isolation, extraction, or growth of plants producing drugs or drug products; study of pharmaceuticals derived from other natural sources, as well.

Pharmacology
References to mode or mechanism of drug action; general discussions other than clinical evaluations of drugs or diagnostic agents: e.g., establishing the biological activity of newly synthesized chemicals, activity due to structural relationships, site of action determinations, pharmacogenetics, drug screening, establishing route, dose, and dosage schedule.

Pharmacy Practice
Pharmacy in general, including discussions of the pharmacist's role in the community, compounding techniques, dispensing, labeling, prescriptions, pharmacy design, etc.

Preliminary Drug Testing
References to animal studies of experimental drugs still under investigation. Includes animal studies on new uses of established drugs, tissue cultures.

Sociology, Economics and Ethics
Effects of drugs, pharmacy, pharmaceutical practice or medicine in society and the economics and/or ethics involved in pharmacy: e.g., cost surveys, marketing, medication error studies, drug overuse or abuse, health care planning.

Toxicity
Toxicity, toxicology, poisoning, overdose, lethal dose studies of drugs or chemicals. Includes references to addiction, teratogenicity, habituation, withdrawal, antidotes, contraindications.

---

*Scope notes adapted from *IPA Users Guide.*

14.9 *IPA Thesaurus and Frequency List*. 8th ed. Bethesda, MD: American So-
    ciety of Health-System Pharmacists, 1997.

It's helpful to examine the *IPA Thesaurus* of subject terms for presearch strategy formulation. This user aid, which includes cross references from drug brand
names, lab codes, and chemical names, is also integrated into the *IPA* database
online for quick reference consultation during the course of a search. Controlled
indexing vocabulary reflects terminology used by clinical pharmacists, and the
content of abstracts provides data needed by professionals in the pharmaceutical
field. (See the sample record accompanying discussion of brand name comparisons later in this chapter, Figure 14.5).

Chemical Indexing in IPA

Drugs are indexed under U.S. Adopted Names (USAN). Investigational agents
not yet assigned a generic name are cited by lab codes referenced by source authors. Such codes take precedence over chemical names as preferred index terms,
when both appear in source documents. CAS registry numbers have been consistently assigned in database records and are preferred over EC numbers in enzyme
literature indexing. Using CAS RNs in online strategies will help searchers transcend nomenclature changes likely to occur in keyword indexing at various
stages in a drug's development. References to articles discussing pharmacological or therapeutic categories of drugs can be retrieved using the *American Hospital Formulary Service* (6.4) classification scheme. The *CTFA Cosmetic Ingredient Dictionary* (11.29) is also cited by *IPA* as a name authority.

Derwent Drug File

Formerly entitled *RINGDOC*, the *Derwent Drug File* (*DDF*) was available on a
subscriber-only basis until 1994. As a result, it is less well known outside the
pharmaceutical industry than many other databases cited here. Nonetheless, the
fact that this source was developed in private consultation with drug companies
indicates its potential utility.

14.10 *Derwent Drug File*. London: Derwent Information, 1964–. Updated
    weekly. Available on DataStar, Dialog, QUESTEL-ORBIT, and STN.

DDF selectively indexes 1,200 journal titles and many conference proceedings. Literature from more than forty countries, published in any of twenty-four
languages, is included. Each database record contains a detailed abstract written
by a Derwent subject specialist and is accompanied by extensive drug oriented
indexing designed to facilitate high precision searching. Subscribers continue to
have access to a separate version of the file, enhanced with extended abstracts
(1983–). The scope of both implementations is identical; *DDF* covers all aspects

of drugs, from design to post-marketing surveillance. It includes articles on drug analysis, biochemistry, pharmacology, adverse effects, clinical studies, disease treatment, toxicology, and drug comparisons.

It is possible to search on broad "Thematic Groups" of references (e.g., side effects, pharmacology, or therapeutics), narrower section headings (antiallergics, anesthetics, drug delivery), and specific controlled vocabulary descriptors. A 1994 *Derwent* reload introduced role terms, comparable to subheadings in *MEDLINE* or links in *EMBASE*, that can be used to qualify drug and disease descriptors. These include:

AE	side effect, toxicity
DI	drug interaction
DM	drug metabolism
PH	pharmacology
TR	treatment

Nonproprietary names (INN, USAN) are preferred drug indexing vocabulary, and CAS registry numbers are also searchable. A companion database, the *Derwent Drug Registry*, functions as a name authority file for *DDF*, compiling nomenclature data for more than 25,000 compounds into separate records, each of which contains the Derwent registry name (preferred descriptor), synonyms, CAS RN, pharmacological activity, and information regarding chemical substructure that enables searchers to locate drugs with similar ring configurations.

InPharma

Among the most timely and comprehensive current awareness sources published today, *InPharma* is an abstracting service for monitoring the clinical drug literature, with a focus on new findings in human pharmacology and therapeutics. Its printed newsletter counterpart is published weekly by ADIS Press, but the online database previews printed issues with daily updates.

14.11 *InPharma*. Auckland, NZ: ADIS International, 1983–. Updated daily. Available on DataStar, Dialog, and SilverPlatter; also on CD-ROM.

More than 2,300 biomedical journal titles are scanned each year for information on drug research and development and new product introductions. Other resources cited include press releases, company reports, and conference literature. Database records feature lengthy and evaluative summaries written by ADIS staff, augmented with controlled indexing taken from the *ADIS Drugs and Disease Thesaurus*. New product introductions are listed in *InPharma* on a weekly basis, identifying generic name, therapeutic use, brand name, manufacturer, and country where approved. Extensive bibliographies on current subjects of interest are also a regular feature.

LMS Drug Alerts Online

Another database produced by ADIS Press is based on a series of publications entitled *Literature Monitoring and Evaluation Service* (*LMS*)

14.12 *ADIS LMS Drug Alerts Online*. Auckland, NZ: ADIS International, 1983–. Updated monthly. Available on DataStar, Dialog, and STN; also on CD-ROM.

LMS Drug Alerts Online focuses on twenty-nine major therapeutic/topical areas, drawing its information from more than 2,300 major biomedical journals published worldwide each year. *LMS* sections include:

Affective Disorders	(1992–)
Alzheimer's Disease & Cognition	(1992–)
Antibacterials	(1985–)
Antifungals	(1998–)
Antithrombotics	(1993–)
Antivirals	(1989–)
Anxiety Disorders	(1992–)
Arrhythmias	(1983–)
Cancer Chemotherapy	(1988–)
Diabetes	(1990–)
Epilepsy & Seizure Disorders	(1992–)
Heart Failure	(1983–)
Hyperlipidaemia	(1989–)
Hypertension	(1993–)
Inflammatory Bowel Disease	(1998–)
Ischaemic Heart Disease	(1983–)
Men's Health	(1998–)
Nausea & Migraine	(1992–)
Obesity	(1998–)
Obstructive Airways Disease	(1986–)
Pain Control	(1996–)
Parkinson's Disease & Movement Disorders	(1992–)
Peptic Ulcer Disease	(1986–)
Pharmacoeconomics	(1994–)
Psychotic Disorders	(1992–)
Rheumatic Disease	(1983–)
Transplant Rejection	(1994–)
Vaccines	(1994–)
Women's Health	(1996–)

Each *LMS* database record consists of a highly structured and lengthy summary, invariably including the purpose of the study, an ADIS score rating the quality of trial design and reporting, editorial comment on the strengths and weakness of the study design, details of trial demographics (number of patients, age, gender), summary of methodology, and results. Drugs and regimen data are presented in easy-to-read tables (1990–), and results and side effects are also tabulated for quick review at a glance. Descriptors assigned to each record are drawn from the *ADIS Drugs and Disease Thesaurus*. Several secondary concept qualifiers, when coordinated with drug or disease main headings, help in fine-tuning *LMS* retrieval. Examples of qualifying terms consistently used include:

Drug-related	**Disease-related**
abuse	contributory factors
adverse reactions	diagnosis
antimicrobial activity	epidemiology
drug interactions	incidence
overdose	management
pharmacodynamics	pathogenesis
pharmacokinetics	prevention
therapeutic use	treatment

ADIS also routinely identifies study types, enabling searchers to limit output to *in vitro* studies, epidemiological surveys, incidence studies, and the like.

IDIS Drug File

The *Iowa Drug Information Service* (*IDIS*) has been providing access to core English-language clinical drug literature since 1966. Designed for use in drug information centers and hospitals providing clinical pharmacy services, it was originally produced in microform under the auspices of the University of Iowa College of Pharmacy. By extracting the indexing component from *IDIS*, the online database offers an automated interface to the full-text of articles included in subscriptions to the microform service.

14.13 *IDIS Drug File*. Iowa City: Iowa Drug Information Service, 1966–. Updated monthly. Available on DataStar, Ovid, and SilverPlatter; also on CD-ROM.

This database is relatively small, indexing 180 journals with a focus on drug therapy in humans. What sets it apart is extremely detailed indexing and, for microform subscribers, immediate access to the full text of sources cited. U.S. Adopted Names (USAN) are preferred in drug indexing, as well as *American Hospital Formulary Service* (*AHFS*, 6.5) classification by pharmacological action or therapeutic use. Disease descriptors are adapted from the *International Classification of Diseases, Ninth Revision, Clinical Modification* (*ICD-9*). *IDIS* is a good choice when a selective bibliography on a clinical topic is needed, particularly when a query involves specific types of side effects, route of administration, pharmaceutical incompatibilities, or pharmacokinetics.

The Iowa Drug Information Service home page on the Internet includes a complete bibliography of references to *IDIS* (1966 to date), many of which represent evaluations of the database and comparisons to other sources. The Web site also provides the full text of a helpful newsletter published for *IDIS* users. It offers valuable search tips and strategy guidelines for research on current clinical issues, scope notes for new indexing terms, and introductions to recently approved drugs. Although strategy guidelines assume access via CD-ROM, they are easily translatable to the online environment. The home page address is http://www.uiowa.edu.80/~idis/.

Other Pharmacology and Therapeutics Resources

For information related to acquired immune deficiency syndrome or HIV-related topics, *AIDSLINE* is the database of choice.

14.14 *AIDSLINE*. Bethesda, MD: U.S. National Library of Medicine, 1980–. Updated monthly. Available on DataStar, Dialog, MEDLARS, Ovid, SilverPlatter, and STN; also on CD-ROM.

Originally a subject oriented subset derived from *MEDLINE*, the online file has been enhanced with references to conference papers, government reports, monographs, and records from *HealthSTAR*, *CANCERLIT*, *CATLINE*, and *AVLINE* databases. Indexing protocols match those established in *MEDLINE*.

14.15 *Allied and Alternative Medicine*. Wetherby, W. Yorkshire: British Library, 1985–. Updated monthly. Available on DataStar, Dialog, and SilverPlatter.

The *Allied and Alternative Medicine* database (*AMED*) is one of the few online bibliographic sources totally dedicated to indexing the topic of complementary therapeutics. Approximately 350 medical journals are scanned for material related to herbalism, homeopathy, diet therapy, acupuncture, traditional Chinese medicine, and other alternatives to conventional medical care.

14.16 *CAB Health*. Wallingford, Slough, England: CAB International, 1973–. Updated monthly. Available on DataStar, Dialog, and SilverPlatter; also on CD-ROM.

Produced by what was once known as the Commonwealth Agricultural Bureaux, *CAB Health* recently replaced several separate CAB files, incorporating, for example, the Bureau of Hygiene and Tropical Diseases' *AIDS Database*. Material included in the relaunched (in 1995) *CAB Health* database includes bibliographic citations and abstracts from nine printed publications: *Abstracts on Hygiene and Communicable Diseases*; *Tropical Diseases Bulletin*; *Current AIDS*

Literature; *Helminthological Abstracts*; *Nutrition Abstracts & Reviews, A— Human & Experimental*; *Review of Medical and Veterinary Mycology*; *Review of Medical and Veterinary Entomology*; *Protozoological Abstracts*; and *Review of Aromatic and Medicinal Plants*. These sources are also included in a separate, larger database entitled *CAB Abstracts* (DataStar, Dialog, SilverPlatter, STN). *CAB Health* indexes 11,000 journal titles, as well as conference proceedings, books, and technical reports, surveying research from 130 countries.

14.17 *CANCERLIT*. Bethesda, MD: U.S. National Cancer Institute, 1963–. Updated monthly. Available on DataStar, Dialog, MEDLARS, Ovid, SilverPlatter, and STN; also on CD-ROM.

World renowned as a comprehensive index to oncology literature, *CANCER-LIT* is the obvious choice for questions requiring bibliography related to cancer chemotherapy. Formerly entitled *CANCERLINE*, this database covers all aspects of cancer therapy, including research on carcinogens (positive and negative data) and references to drugs used to treat common side effects of chemotherapy, such as nausea, anorexia, and hair loss. Since 1980, *MeSH* (*MEDLINE*) indexing vocabulary has been used; for searches to access literature published prior to that date, natural language strategies are recommended.

14.18 *Drug Information Fulltext*. Bethesda, MD: American Society of Health-System Pharmacists. Current information, updated quarterly. Available on DataStar, Dialog, Ovid, and SilverPlatter; also on CD-ROM.

Drug Information Fulltext (*DIF*) includes all information published in two ASHP hardcopy sources discussed earlier in this book: *AHFS Drug Information* (6.5) and the *Handbook on Injectable Drugs* (7.31). An average of 100 journal articles are reviewed for each of the drug monographs in *DIF*. The supportive reference bibliographies omitted from hardcopy *AHFS* monographs are included in *DIF* records online. The advantages of this feature are illustrated when *DIF* entries are compared with those in another online drug compendium with a similar purpose: *USP DI*.

14.19 *USP DI Volume 1: Drug Information for the Health Care Professional*. Rockville, MD: U.S. Pharmacopeial Convention. Current information, updated quarterly. Available on Dialog; also on CD-ROM.

USP DI Volume 1 is the online counterpart of the hardcopy publication of the same name, described in detail in Chapter Six (6.5). The database also includes introductory versions of drug monographs published in the monthly *USP DI Update* newsletter. However, unlike *Drug Information Fulltext*, the *USP DI*'s correspondence to its printed equivalent is not readily discernible to the first-time user. Instead of monographs on individual drugs, as found in the printed publication, records in *USP DI* online generally cover an entire category of drugs, bringing together information supplied in multiple printed entries. For example, prescrib-

ing and precautions data for lisinopril are embedded in a twenty-nine-page monograph covering systemic angiotensin-converting enzyme (ACE) inhibitors. The
same database record also includes information on benazepril, captopril, enalapril, fosinopril, quinapril and ramipril (other ACE inhibitors commercially available in the United States or Canada).

This approach undoubtedly reduces redundancy that separate drug entries
would create in a machine-readable compendium, but, at the same time, it increases the effort required of users to locate product-specific data in lengthy meg-
amonographs. On the other hand, side-by-side summaries of data on factors such
as absorption, half life, protein binding, or onset of action, listing values for each
drug in the category, encourages comparisons of therapeutic alternatives.

Entries in *USP DI Volume 1* meticulously note which indications are approved
and which (if any) are not included in U.S. or Canadian product labeling. Information on precautions summarizes results of animal studies to determine carcinogenicity, mutagenicity, effects on pregnancy and fertility, teratogenicity, and
breast feeding, including negative or inconclusive data. Drug interactions noted
are selected on the basis of their clinical significance, with effects on diagnostic
and physiologic test results systematically itemized. The portion of monographs
devoted to adverse effects points out which events signal the need for medical
attention and their rate of incidence. A Patient Consultation section in online records highlights selected text extracted from *USP DI Volume 2: Advice for the
Patient* (9.1, see also 14.33).

Users should be aware that brands, dosage forms, and strengths identified represent a selection of products available, rather than a comprehensive listing. For
example, only two brand names are given for lisinopril in *USP DI*, while six
brands are cited in *Drug Information Fulltext*. (The latter also shows manufacturer names for each brand, which information the *USP DI* omits.) Another major
difference between the two sources online is in bibliographic references supplied
to support facts conveyed in monograph entries. *USP DI* confines itself to citing
only a few journal articles per drug discussed. *Drug Information Fulltext* offers
extensive bibliographies for each drug, with each reference cited by number
within the body of preceding text to facilitate follow up on specific facts documented. The *USP DI*'s brief bibliographies are general and are not directly corre-
lated to textual discussion by bracketed or superscripted numbers. For example,
for lisinopril, *USP DI* compiles three references to the published literature; *DIF*
supplies a total of thirty-three, including manufacturer prescribing information,
consensus guidelines reached by professional groups regarding the treatment of
high blood pressure, and a long list of journal articles documenting evidence
from clinical trials.

14.20 *Lexi-Comp's Clinical Reference Collection.* Hudson, OH: LexiComp.
Current information, updated quarterly. Available on SilverPlatter.

Launched in 1998, *Lexi-Comp's Clinical Reference Collection* includes full
text drawn from eight hardcopy sources of fast facts. A module pooling drug data

from them all has been created for quick reference in the online database. Source publications include: the *Drug Information Handbook* (6.20), *Pediatric Dosage Handbook* (6.31), *Geriatric Dosage Handbook* (6.35), *Infectious Diseases Handbook* (6.46), *Poisoning & Toxicology Handbook* (8.2), *Laboratory Test Handbook*, *Diagnostic Procedures Handbook*, and *Anesthesia and Critical Care Handbook*.

14.21 *Pharm-Line*. London: Guy's Hospital, 1978–. Updated weekly. Available on DataStar and Dialog.

Pharm-Line is the result of a collaboration between Guy's and St. Thomas's Hospital Trust and the U.K. Drug Information Pharmacists' Group. Practicing pharmacists working in National Health Service hospitals contribute abstracts found in this database, which selectively indexes approximately 100 key English-language pharmacy and medical journals. The subject focus is on the clinical use of drugs and pharmacy practice. Topics covered include adverse effects and interactions, pharmacokinetics, drug stability and analysis, pharmacoeconomics, and formulary management.

14.22 *Physician Data Query Protocol File*. Bethesda, MD: U.S. National Cancer Institute. Current, updated monthly. Available on MEDLARS and Ovid; also on CD-ROM.

Part of a collection of *PDQ* databases devoted to cancer information (see also 14.35, 14.36), the *Physician Data Query Protocol File* contains details on more than 1,400 active and approved cancer treatment protocols. Clinical trials supported by the U.S. National Cancer Institute predominate, but additional records document other studies, when data are submitted by investigators. Entries compile information on protocol objectives, patient entry criteria, treatment regimen, dosage, and participating organizations. A *PDQ Backfile* database is also available, containing comparable information on clinical trials that are no longer accepting patients. The National Institutes of Health Web site offers a subset of the *PDQ* database, free-of-charge, at http://www.nih.gov/health/.

Influential Factors in Database Selection

There are many databases offering access to research oriented and peer-reviewed literature in biomedicine. Factors that will influence resource selection are often inherent in the question posed. For example, is finding a specific type of publication a necessary part of the answer? Are references to clinical trials needed, or practice guidelines, case reports, a conference paper? Perhaps a special subject population is the focus of the inquiry, such as pediatric or geriatric patients? Are routes of administration or dosage form pivotal to the topic under investigation? Or is locating references to the bioequivalence of brand name products the problem to be solved? Each of these different types of requests is typical in the pharmacology and therapeutics subject area. And each requires a different set of resources and access methodologies to deliver pertinent bibliography.

Clinical Trials

The best sources for locating bibliographic references to clinical trial results are *MEDLINE, EMBASE, BIOSIS Previews*, and *SciSearch*. Since 1991, *MEDLINE* has flagged citations with a special publication or document type indicator to facilitate access. Specific "phase" indexing was introduced in 1993, and "controlled clinical trial" was first singled out as a publication type in 1995. The good news is that clinical trial terms have now been assigned retrospectively back through 1985, and the National Library of Medicine has promised complete retrospective identification of trials as a document type back to 1966. The list of current *MEDLINE* options includes:

    clinical trial
    clinical trial, phase I
    clinical trial, phase II
    clinical trial, phase III
    clinical trial, phase IV
    controlled clinical trial
    multicenter study
    randomized controlled trial

It is not necessary to enter all of these phrases in answer to a request for bibliography on clinical trials of a given drug. Those describing specific types of trials are double-posted under the general term *clinical trial*, with the exception of references identified as *multicenter study*. Defined as a controlled study executed by two or more cooperating institutions, the latter is usually also of interest to practitioners requesting citations to trials. Thus, it's a good idea to OR together both publication types for a thorough survey of pertinent bibliography in *MEDLINE*. For example, a basic strategy to retrieve references to clinical trials of perindopril on DataStar would be: *perindopril and (clinical-trial or multicenter-study).pt*. Note that study type keywords usually require qualification to a specific segment of records (designated record elements, paragraphs, or fields in some software systems). In this example, clinical trial terms are limited to the publication type (PT) paragraph. Precise entry format will differ from system to system.

EMBASE introduced the phrase clinical trial or its abbreviation CT as a link term in 1988. This editorial enhancement means that searchers can link the phrase or its abbreviation directly to a drug name. Techniques for taking advantage of this feature differ among the various databank implementations of *EM-*

BASE. Proximity operators are usually employed, such as WITH or (L): e.g., *perindopril with ct.de.* on DataStar or *select perindopril(L)ct* on Dialog.

In *BIOSIS Previews* and *SciSearch*, no special indexing feature has been consistently used to identify clinical trials, so a series of synonyms will be required to locate relevant bibliography. A sample strategy on Dialog would be

> s ((open or controlled or randomized or multicenter or clinical)(1w)(trial? or study
> or studies or evaluation?) or phase(w)(1 or 2 or 3 or I or II or III) or placebo? or
> double(w)blind)/ti,de,id

This search statement specifies that the words in the first parenthesized group (open, controlled, etc.) be searched within one word of any terms in the second group. Another alternative is the word *phase* searched adjacent to either Arabic or Roman forms of stage numbers. In addition, *placebo* (truncated) implies a clinical study, as does *double-blind*. All of these alternative terms are qualified to occurrence in the title, descriptor, or identifier fields in an attempt to achieve higher precision in results. Results of the search statement would be combined (ANDed) with a drug name set to retrieve references to clinical study results.

Since *BIOSIS* and *SciSearch* are clearly more difficult to search when clinical trials are needed, why are they included in the list of recommended databases? *BIOSIS* is the only one of these major biomedical indexes to cover conference papers published in primary sources other than journals.[5, 6] Both *MEDLINE* and *EMBASE* limit their scope to journal literature, thereby missing an important form of scientific communication: the spoken word. Results of clinical trials are often first reported at meetings. Although some conference papers or meeting abstracts appear in biomedical journals, many are documented only in separate proceedings publications, which *BIOSIS* systematically collects and indexes. Therefore, searches in *BIOSIS* can, literally, preview what may later find its way into peer-reviewed journals. Results frequently uncover research in progress not cited elsewhere.

SciSearch usually contributes unique data to clinical bibliographies because of two important characteristics mentioned earlier in this chapter, but worth repeating. Produced by the publishers of *Current Contents*, *SciSearch* is known for its short lag time. It often adds references within one to two weeks of publication in primary sources (compared to an average of two to three months for *MEDLINE*). Furthermore, all of the 5,600 journals included on the *SciSearch* source list are indexed cover to cover (excluding ephemera, such as advertising), thus filling in gaps sometimes encountered in more selective subject indexing of many of the same titles by other biomedical databases.

Other good sources of references to current clinical trial results are *ADIS In-Pharma*, *LMS Drug Alerts*, the *IDIS Drug File*, and the *Federal Research in Progress (FEDRIP)* database. The *Derwent Drug File* flags clinical trial records with the section heading 64. If a question involves a cancer drug or research into

AIDS therapy, *CANCERLIT* and *AIDSLINE* are obvious choices. *International Pharmaceutical Abstracts* will also provide access to a selection of clinical trials in retrospective searches, but is less timely in its indexing of more recently published literature than other sources cited in this section.

14.23 *Evidence-Based Medicine Reviews.* New York: Ovid Technologies, 1991–. Updated quarterly. Available on Ovid.

Introduced in 1998, *Evidence-Based Medicine Reviews* (*EBM Reviews*) draws its data from the *Cochrane Database of Systematic Reviews*, the American College of Physicians (ACP) *Journal Club*, and the journal *Evidence-Based Medicine.* Ovid has implemented links from the *EBM Reviews* database to *MEDLINE*, enabling searchers to use an *EBM* limit to restrict results to articles that meet evidence-based criteria. Reciprocal links are also available from references in Ovid's version of *MEDLINE* back to *EBM Reviews.* The latter also hotlinks its bibliographic references to full-text selections, when available, in Ovid's impressive journal collection.

14.24 *The Cochrane Library.* Oxford, England: Update Software, 1995–. Updated quarterly. Available on CD-ROM and the Internet.

The full *Cochrane Library* includes not only the *Cochrane Database of Systematic Reviews* (*CDSR*) covered in Ovid's *EBM Reviews* file, but also the *Database of Abstracts of Reviews of Effectiveness* (*DARE*), the *Cochrane Controlled Trials Register* (*CCTR*), and the *Cochrane Review Methodology Database.* The latter is a bibliography of articles and books on the science of research systems. Available on the Internet and in CD-ROM format (both for a fee), *The Cochrane Library* also offers a glossary of methodological terms and a handbook on the science of reviewing and critically appraising clinical research. The core *CDSR* currently includes 1,014 full-text entries.

Abstracts of the entire set of Cochrane reviews can be searched and viewed free of charge at http://www.update-software.com/ccweb/cochrane/cdsr.htm. The full *DARE* database is also searchable without fee at http://nhscrd.york.ac.uk.

14.25 *MetaMaps.* Philadelphia: Institute for Scientific Information, 1998–. Available on CD-ROM.

MetaMaps is a CD-ROM series of relational databases that compile clinical data extracted from primary sources and arrange them in tables. The resulting hierarchical tabular display is based on a systematic review and critical appraisal of key clinical trial literature related to a particular drug or therapeutic area. Tables enable users to access clinical trial information by study type, patient criteria, treatment options, efficacy outcomes, and safety data. Results of meta-analysis often uncover significant variability in study design and competitive drug performance. The first *MetaMaps* title offered for sale was *Alzheimer's Dementia*, closely followed by an *Asthma MetaMap.* Selected cancers are planned as future topics, and release of a Web-based product is expected in 1999.

Free Internet coverage of clinical trials is, for the most part, dedicated to protocol locator services. Designed for the purpose of patient recruitment, they outline study objectives, parameters for patient participation, and key contacts. Some better known examples include *CenterWatch Clinical Trials Listing Service* (http://www.centerwatch.com) and *HIV Clinical Trials in the United States* (http://hivinsite.ucsf.edu/bin/keywords). A new Web-based initiative introduced late in 1998, *Current Controlled Trials*, promises to be a welcome addition. The site currently features a *meta Register of Controlled Trials* (*mRCT*) that compiles a minimum set of data elements for each ongoing and completed trial listed. Database records provide hotlinks to more detailed information, where available, from external registries participating in the collaborative service. A separate *Controlled Trials Links Register* is still under construction, but aims to facilitate access to the multitude of other registers on the Internet. The URL is http://www.controlled-trials.com.

When results of trials are needed, users generally will have to await publication in the peer-reviewed primary literature and access will rarely be free. The broad based abstracting and indexing services highlighted thus far in this chapter will be the most efficient route to results released in journals and presented at scientific conferences. However, as notes on *The Cochrane Library* have shown, small subsets of data are offered without fee at a few Web sites. See Chapter Fifteen's discussion of probing the Internet for health economics and outcomes research for additional relevant URLs.

When Subject Population Is Important

When a specific age group or gender is an important delimiter in measuring search success, *MEDLINE* and *EMBASE* step to the head of the class. Both routinely identify factors such as age groups in humans and gender of the subject population in sources cited. *MEDLINE* accomplishes this through "check tags." Options include:

infant, newborn	(up to one month old)
infant	(1–23 months)
child, preschool	(2–5 years)
child	(6–12 years)
adolescence	(13–18 years)
adult	(19–44 years)
middle age	(45–64 years)
aged	(65 years old and above)
aged, 80 and over	(80 years old and above)

female
male
pregnancy

Gender and pregnancy tags are used in indexing references to either humans or animals, but age terms apply only to humans in *MEDLINE*. To take advantage of the human-only policy, single word age tags should be qualified to limit retrieval to indexer-added segments of records (e.g., DE or MH fields). Otherwise, on some search systems, output will include references where the terms occur in the title or abstract and may, therefore, include citations to animals or other unintended populations (e.g., *adult* Wistar rats, children *aged* five to ten).

MEDLINE has the added advantage of age pre-explosions. This rather peculiar jargon refers to the fact that all citations tagged with any of the five terms referring to children (0–18 years old) can be retrieved with just one search entry, and those with any of the four other age terms can be searched using another shortcut entry. On the MEDLARS search system, entries would be *child (px)* or *adults (px)*. On Dialog, pre-explosions are indicated with an exclamation mark: *select child!* or *s adult!*

Special subject population indexing options in *EMBASE* include:

embryo	
fetus	
newborn	
infant	
preschool child	male
school child	female
adolescent	pregnancy
child	
adult	
aged	

All of these index terms are applied to both human and animal references in *EMBASE*, so if bibliography on humans only is needed, add the special Human qualifier supplied by the databank being searched. This usually requires a special entry format, which varies among vendors.

Other life science literature files do not make it as easy to specify age or gender in studied populations. For example, the *Derwent Drug File* uses section code 67 to represent both children and elderly populations. In *International Pharmaceutical Abstracts*, all discussions of drug use that indicate significance related to age are indexed with the subject terms pediatrics (anyone younger than an adult) or geriatrics. Natural language (multisynonym) strategies will be needed to augment or refine *Derwent*, *IPA*, and other database retrieval of age groups: e.g., *infant or neonate or newborn, teenage or adolescent, adult or men or women*, etc.

Retrieving Routes of Administration

Because of its extensive coverage of the pharmaceutical literature, *EMBASE* identifies most routes of drug administration through use of one or more of the following terms.

inhalational
intraarterial
intraarticular
intracardiac
intracerebral
intracerebroventricular
intradermal
intragastric
intralymphatic
intramuscular
intranasal
intraperitoneal
intrathecal
intratumoral
intravaginal
intravenous
oral
rectal
regional perfusion
subcutaneous
sublingual
topical
transdermal

Routes of drug administration identified in *MEDLINE*'s indexing vocabulary are listed in Figure 14.4. In a quick search for representative bibliography comparing routes of administration in either database, drug generic name entries can be qualified with the subheading AD (administration and dosage), then "ANDed" with the descriptor *comparative study* in *MEDLINE* or *drug comparison* in *EMBASE*. Suppose, for example, you were asked to find references comparing clonidine administered in transdermal patches versus the oral route. An initial, step-by-step strategy in *MEDLINE* would be to search

1. clonidine linked with AD
2. administration, cutaneous AND administration, oral
3. comparative study
4. AND together results of steps 1–3

Figure 14.4   MEDLINE Descriptors for Routes of Drug Administration

Drug Administration Routes
    Administration, inhalation
    Administration, intranasal
    Administration, oral
        Administration, buccal
        Administration, sublingual
    Administration, rectal
    Administration, topical
        Administration, buccal
        Administration, cutaneous
        Administration, intranasal
        Administration, intravaginal
        Administration, intravesical
        Administration, rectal
    Infusions, parenteral
        Infusions, intraarterial
        Infusions, intraosseous
        Infusions, intravenous
    Injections
        Injections, intraarterial
        Injections, intraarticular
        Injections, intralesional
        Injections, intralymphatic
        Injections, intramuscular
        Injections, intraperitoneal
        Injections, intravenous
        Injections, intraventricular
        Injections, spinal
            Injections, epidural
                Blood patch, epidural
        Injections, subcutaneous
            Injections, intradermal
            Injections, jet
        Microinjections
    Instillation, drug
    Iontophoresis
    Perfusion, regional
    Phonophoresis

In *EMBASE*, a comparable strategy would substitute the terms *transdermal* and *oral* in step 2, and the descriptive phrase *drug comparison* in step 3.

    International Pharmaceutical Abstracts, as might be expected from its subject specialty orientation, is another excellent source for compiling references when route of administration is a key factor. *IPA* systematically identifies the route by which a drug is administered to the patient in the first paragraph of abstracts. Controlled terms include:

buccal
intraperitoneal
nasal
ophthalmic
oral
oral inhalation
otic
parenteral
rectal
sublingual
topical
transdermal
urogenital (urethral)
vaginal

If route of administration is actually studied and compared, the phrase *drug administration routes* is added to *IPA* records.

The *IDIS Drug File* (14.13) is another good choice for quick retrieval of bibliography related to drug administration routes, offering controlled descriptors for twelve types of administration, including portable pump. Consult *IDIS* user aids for additional options.

Brand Name Comparisons

International Pharmaceutical Abstracts and *EMBASE* are the best sources of bibliography on drug brand name products. Both add trade names to indexing if the author refers to proprietary preparations in the full text of the original article, even if the title and abstract reproduced in database records do not identify brands. *EMBASE* goes one step further by identifying manufacturers, as well, when cited by primary source authors. In 1998, *EMBASE* extended its brand name and company indexing policy to include medical devices.

IPA also frequently rewrites abstracts to ensure that important details are immediately accessible. Compare, for example, the *IPA* reference shown in Figure 14.5 with its counterpart from *MEDLINE* reproduced in Figure 14.6. The original author's abstract, as found in *MEDLINE*, provides fewer user access points for brand name comparison strategies.

EMBASE indexing for the same citation includes only one of the brand names mentioned in the original article and identified in the *IPA* record (*Valisone*), but

Figure 14.5   Sample IPA Record Showing Indexing/Abstract of a Brand Name Comparison

DIALOG(R)File 74:Int.Pharm.Abs.
© 1995 Amer.Soc.of Hosp.Pharmacists Inc. All rts. reserv.

00187900 28-08836
DOUBLE-BLIND CONTROLLED COMPARISON OF GENERIC AND TRADE-
NAME TOPICAL STEROIDS USING THE VASOCONSTRICTION ASSAY
Olsen, E. A.
Box 3294, Duke Univ. Med. Ctr., Durham, NC 27710, USA
Archives of Dermatology (USA), V127, (Feb), p197–201, 1991
CODEN: ARDEAC ISSN: 0003-987X LANGUAGE: English RECORD TYPE: Abstract

A double-blind, placebo-controlled comparison study evaluating the bioequivalency, based upon vasoconstriction following administration, of 6 generic preparations of 5 topical steroids with their trade name counterparts was conducted in 96 volunteer subjects, aged 18–65 yr, who received either 50 mg of the steroid or placebo applied to the forearm and maintained for 16 h; the steroids evaluated were: 0.1% betamethasone valerate (Valisone) cream and ointment, 0.01% fluocinolone acetonide (Synalar) cream, 0.025% fluocinolone acetonide (Synalar) cream, and 0.05% betamethasone dipropionate (Diprosone; Diprolene) cream.

Vasoconstriction seem with Valisone cream was significantly greater than with the generic preparation. There was no significant difference in vasoconstriction between the 2 ointment preparations of betamethasone. Within a given concentration of fluocinolone cream, there was no difference between preparations, but both generic and trade name preparations of 0.025% fluocinolone cream produced significantly greater vasoconstriction than the 0.01% cream. Vasoconstriction with Diprosone cream was greater than with one generic preparation and equivalent to a second generic preparation. However, the vasoconstriction seen with Diprosone was greater than that seen with Diprolene.

It was concluded that differences in the vehicle of a given topical steroid may lead to relative differences in vasoconstriction that may not mirror clinical potency. (21 references)

CAS REGISTRY NUMBERS: 2152-44 (Betamethasone valerate); 67-73-2 (Fluocinolone acetonide); 5593-20-4 (Betamethasone dipropionate)
CHEMICAL/BRAND NAMES: Valisone; Synalar; Diprosone; Diprolene
DESCRIPTORS: Steroids, cortico—betamethasone valerate, generic equivalency, topical preparations; Steroids, cortico—fluocinolone acetonide, generic equivalency, topical preparations; Steroids, cortico—betamethasone dipropionate, generic equivalency, topical preparations; Equivalency, generic—betamethasone valerate, topical preparations; Equivalency, generic—fluocinolone acetonide, topical preparations; Equivalency, generic—betamethasone dipropionate, topical preparations; Topical preparations—betamethasone valerate, generic equivalency; Topical preparations—fluocinolone acetonide, generic equivalency; Topical preparations—betamethasone dipropionate, generic equivalency; Creams—betamethasone valerate, generic equivalency; Ointments—betamethasone valerate, generic equivalency; Creams—fluocinolone acetonide, generic equivalency; Creams—betamethasone dipropionate, generic equivalency; Methodology—steroids, cortico, topical, generic equivalency
SECTION HEADINGS: Biopharmaceutics (08); Methodology (18)
THERAPEUTIC CLASS: 68.04 (Steroids, cortico-); 84.00 (Topical preparations); 84.24 (Creams)

Figure 14.6   Sample MEDLINE Reference on DIALOG

DIALOG(R)File 154:MEDLINE(R)
© format only 1995 Knight-Ridder Info. All rts. reserv.

07600434 91119434
A double-blind controlled comparison of generic and trade-name topical steroids using the vasoconstriction assay.
Olsen EA
Department of Medicine, Duke University Medical Center, Durham, NC 27710.
Arch Dermatol (UNITED STATES) Feb 1991, 127 (2) p197–201, ISSN
0003-987X Journal Code: 6WU
Languages: ENGLISH
Document type: JOURNAL ARTICLE
JOURNAL ANNOUNCEMENT: 9105
Subfile: AIM; INDEX MEDICUS
Six generic formulations of five topical steroids were compared for bioequivalence with their trade-name counterparts using an in vivo vasoconstriction assay. Two of six generic formulations were found to show significantly less vasoconstriction than the respective trade-name topical steroids. The issue of generic equivalence of topical steroids is discussed, with particular emphasis on the vagaries of the vasoconstriction assay.
Tags: Comparative Study; Human; Support, U.S. Gov't, Non-P.H.S.
Descriptors: *Betamethasone—Analogs and Derivatives—AA; *Betamethasone—Pharmacokinetics—PK; *Fluocinolone Acetonide—Pharmacokinetics—PK; *Glucocorticoids, Topical—Pharmacokinetics—PK; Adult; Betamethasone—Administration and Dosage—AD; Double-Blind Method; Fluocinolone Acetonide—Administration and Dosage—AD; Glucocorticoids, Topical—Administration and Dosage—AD; Middle Age; Therapeutic Equivalency; Vasoconstriction
CAS Registry No.: 0 (Glucocorticoids, Topical); 378–44–9 (Betamethasone); 5593–20–4 (betamethasone-17,21-dipropionate); 67–73–2 (Fluocinolone Acetonide)

---

adds value by transcribing manufacturer names of both generic and proprietary brands used in the cited comparison, as shown in the following extract.

> TRADE NAME/MANUFACTURER NAME: valisone/USA schering; USA fougera; USA pharmacderm; USA syntex pharmaceuticals; USA thames; USA lemmon

Does this mean that other bibliographic databases should be ignored when searching for brand name comparisons? The answer is no, but bear in mind that in sources such as *MEDLINE*, recall is dependent on whether authors have included proprietary designations in their titles or abstracts reproduced online. Also, be prepared to supplement initial strategies with additional search terms. For example, simply "ANDing" together brand names in biomedical files does not ensure that results will include comparative data. Articles retrieved may cite both products because they are used to treat the same condition, but fail to offer any assessment of their relative efficacy.

Additional qualifying terms are usually needed to focus a strategy involving two or more proprietary names. As mentioned previously, *MEDLINE* assigns the phrase *comparative study* and *EMBASE* offers *drug comparison* to assist in fine tuning searches. A sample cross-file strategy to locate comparisons of the two brand name pulmonary surfactants Exosurf and Survanta would be to search: *exosurf and survanta and (comparative study or drug comparison)*. If databases other than *MEDLINE* and *EMBASE* were accessed, the entry would need more synonyms to retrieve the comparison concept, e.g., *exosurf and survanta and (assess? or evaluat? or compar? or versus or bioequivalen? or equivalen?)*.

Far more difficult to answer are questions involving comparisons of brand name products with their generic counterparts (drugs marketed under nonproprietary names). For example, how would you answer the question: Are there any articles comparing Tegretol with generic brands of carbamazepine? Since generic names are universally preferred as index terms in bibliographic databases, how can the searcher distinguish between the name used as a marketing term rather than as part of routine indexing? Strategies to retrieve references of this type start with the brand name "ANDed" to keywords that imply comparisons.

1. Tegretol
2. compar? or assess? or evaluat? or versus
3. commercial? or trade? or brand? or proprietary or nonproprietary or generic? or bioequivalen? or bioinequivalen? or equivalen? or formula? or excipient? or switch? or substitut?
4. AND together results of steps 1–3

Initial review of output from step 4 would show that separate brand and manufacturer name indexing in *EMBASE* facilitates searching for this type of comparison. Combining a generic name and manufacturer can retrieve additional citations from *EMBASE* where brand names are omitted. For example,

5. carbamazepine AND Ciba adjacent to Geigy
6. step 5 NOT step 4

Drug Category Searching

Another typical type of inquiry requires searching for bibliography related to an entire category of drugs. For example, how does the half-life of diclofenac compare to that of other nonsteroidal anti-inflammatory agents? What other differences among NSAIDs affect their potential to interact with antihypertensives in patients with arthritis who are also being treated for high blood pressure? Pharmacological action and therapeutic use are an essential part of these questions.

To avoid having to identify and key in alternative names for individual drugs in order to retrieve relevant bibliography, experienced researchers turn to databases that systematically classify references to specific compounds under their appropriate "action" or "application" terms. Three major biomedical literature files facilitate comprehensive retrieval of categories of drugs: *MEDLINE, EMBASE,* and *International Pharmaceutical Abstracts.* Each does so by providing a hierarchical thesaurus of controlled descriptors.

Figure 14.7   Extracts from *Medical Subject Headings—Annotated Alphabetic List*

Diclofenac
D2.241.223.601.210

a cyclooxygenase inhib & non-steroidal anti-inflamm agent

• **Anti-Inflammatory Agents, Non-Steroidal**
 D16.850.14.40.50   D17.25.30 +
 D17.50.30 +

Figure 14.7 reproduces extracts from *MEDLINE*'s hardcopy user aid, *Medical Subject Headings—Annotated Alphabetic List.* By consulting the alphabetical index of descriptors, preferred drug functional class terms and their corresponding Tree codes can be identified.

Diclofenac, for example, is classified as both a cyclooxygenase inhibitor (action) and a non-steroidal anti-inflammatory (use). *MeSH* entries for broad drug categories, such as NSAIDs, give code cross references to the *Tree Structures* user aid. As extracts reproduced in Figure 14.8 illustrate, subsequent look-up by code shows the drug category in its logical context within functional groups. For example, the Tree code D17.50.30 places NSAIDs side by side with other antirheumatic drug classes, while D16.850.14.40.50 indents NSAIDs under non-narcotic analgesics. The *Tree Structures* resemble an outline, designed to reflect broader and narrower relationships among concepts that an alphabetical list cannot express (their name is a metaphor for the "branches" of medicine that the hierarchical arrangement graphically depicts).

Still another metaphorical term is used to describe a related, extremely powerful feature built into the *MEDLINE* database: explode. When a user explodes a Tree, the computer software quickly locates references indexed under either the broad Tree category term or any of its branches (specific headings indented under it). For example, to retrieve bibliography on any of the five types of antirheumatic agents listed in Figure 14.8, the user simply enters the broad term with either a special prefix or a special suffix. For example: *antirheumatic agents (px)* on MEDLARS, or *antirheumatic-agents#* on DataStar.

MEDLINE's explode feature is also useful when searching for references to broad categories of adverse effects, such as bone marrow disorders or skin dis-

Figure 14.8 Extracts from *Medical Subject Headings—Tree Structures*

Analgesics, Non-Narcotic	D16.850.14.40
Anti-inflammatory Agents, Non-Steroidal	D16.850.14.40.50
Anti-Inflammatory Agents	D17.25
Anti-Inflammatory Agents, Non-Steroidal	D17.25.30
Anti-Inflammatory Agents, Steroidal	D17.25.50
Glucocorticoids, Topical	D17.25.50.180
Antirheumatic Agents	D17.50
Anti-inflammatory Agents, Non-Steroidal	D17.50.30
Anti-Inflammatory Agents, Steroidal	D17.50.40
Antirheumatic Agents, Gold	D17.50.50
Gout Suppressants	D17.50.337
Uricosuric Agents	D17.50.337.900

eases. Exploding the Tree for bone marrow diseases precludes the need to enter a multiplicity of specific effect terms, such as acute erythroblastic leukemia or thrombocytosis or myelofibrosis or hemoglobinuria.

EMBASE offers a similar hierarchical approach in its *EMTREE* thesaurus (see Figure 14.9). Although keyword phrases used may differ from *MEDLINE* (nonsteroid antiinflammatory agent versus anti-inflammatory agents, non-steroidal, dipeptidyl carboxypeptidase inhibitor versus angiotensin-converting enzyme inhibitors), the underlying indexing concept and retrieval capabilities are identical. EMTREEs can be exploded on Ovid, for example, by entering preferred terms with a special prefix: *ex nonsteroid antiinflammatory agent*.

As noted in Chapter Two, *International Pharmaceutical Abstracts* has adopted

Figure 14.9 Extract from EMBASE Classification Scheme (EMTREE)

Analgesic, Antiinflammatory, Antirheumatic and Antigout agents	D14
Analgesic agent	D14.10
Antipyretic analgesic agent	D14.10.10
Narcotic analgesic agent	D14.10.50
Fentanyl derivative	D14.10.50.300
Antigout agent	D14.20
Uricosuric agent	D14.20.70
Antiinflammatory agent	D14.30
Antirheumatic agent	D14.30.40
Nonsteroid antiinflammatory agent	D14.30.500
Ocular antiinflammatory agent	D14.30.650
Central Nervous system agents	D15

the drug classification scheme developed for the *American Hospital Formulary Service* (6.4). An extract is shown in Figure 14.10. Users of this database in machine-readable form can take advantage of its hierarchical indexing of drug classes by entering *AHFS* codes, which are "pre-exploded" or "cascaded" (no need to use a special command prefix or truncate to retrieve indented terms). For example, searching the therapeutic code 28.08 locates literature related to any of the four broad classes of analgesics and antipyretics.

Derwent Drug File (14.10) section headings classify drugs into more than thirty-five action or application categories (e.g., section 12 = antidiabetics, 33 = respiratory). *BIOSIS Previews* offers some category searching capabilities through drug modifier or affiliation indexing. However, drug affiliations are assigned as descriptors only when the primary source being indexed discusses therapeutic use of a drug. Thus, if adverse effects of a category of drugs are the topic under investigation, drug modifier terms may miss relevant items.

Figure 14.10   Extract from AHFS Pharmacological-Therapeutic Classification Scheme

28.00	**Central Nervous System Agents**
28.04	General Anesthetics
28.08	Analgesics and Antipyretics
28.08.04	Nonsteroidal Anti-Inflammatory Agents
28.08.08	Opiate Agonists
28.08.12	Opiate Partial Agonists
28.08.92	Miscellaneous Analgesics and Antipyretics
28.10	Opiate Antagonists
28.12	Anticonvulsants
28.12.04	Barbiturates
28.12.08	Benzodiazepines
28.12.12	Hydantoins
28.12.16	Oxazolidinediones
28.12.20	Succinimides
28.12.92	Miscellaneous Anticonvulsants

Indexing of Author Affiliation or Address

Tracking down research conducted at a given institution or corporation is another common search problem.[7] In most bibliographic databases, the address of the first author listed for each citation is transcribed from the original source and is directly searchable. This feature can help narrow down strategies to retrieve references to clinical trials, when a location is known (e.g., drug + indication + address). "ANDing" in address keywords can also reduce ambiguity in author searches when the surname is common and only initials of first and middle names are indexed.

Both search and display of author affiliation are used in identifying candidates to serve as clinical investigators. One technique for approaching this type of inquiry is to search for individuals publishing the most in the area of specialization (clinical indication) to be targeted in a trial. After the subject set of citations is isolated, a country of origin can be specified by searching the author address segment of records (e.g., *s cs = usa* on Dialog, *usa.in.* on Ovid, *s usa/cs* on STN). Then, in computer systems that offer a ranking capability, the next step would be to RANK AU in order to analyze results by author name occurrence. Subsequent review of output could, therefore, be confined to works by individuals whose names appear at the top of the ranked list.

Another useful analysis to gauge the status of prospective investigators in the scientific community can be conducted in *SciSearch*, where a set of references related to the subject specialty can be ranked not only by author name, but also by cited author name. The resulting list identifies individuals whose work is most frequently referred to by others writing about the topic in question.

People preparing for job interviews or sales calls at specific departments can use the author address field to locate recent publications produced by department members to be visited. Results of searches for certain terms (e.g., epidemiology, pharmacoeconomics) as part of department or institution names in addresses can also be used to supplement bibliography retrieved by accessing segments of online records more traditionally associated with subject content, such as titles or abstracts.

Corporate affiliation indexing can sometimes also supply a vital piece in drug identification puzzles. Suppose, for example, you're given a drug name, use, and company as starting points. A search on the drug name yields zero results (it will later be found to have been misspelled). A strategy that combines drug indication or action keywords with the company name may lead to the sound-alike (correctly spelled) substance name. In *EMBASE*, the company name should be searched in both the author address and manufacturer name fields for maximum effect.

Corporate source indexing can also play a role in collection development or subscription justification decisions.[8] When shrinking budgets dictate journal subscription cancellations, costly errors can be avoided by first determining where resident staff publish. Rather than attempting to key in all known author names, users can simply create a set of citations where their company, institution, or department name is listed as part of the reprint address in online records. The set can then be analyzed numerically by ranking journal names. Sources high on this list would obviously not be good candidates for cancellation.

Another factor to consider in subscription "rationalization" is: What sources do staff authors most frequently cite (and therefore use)? Only *SciSearch* facilitates this type of analysis, which is easily accomplished in two steps: 1) using the author address field, isolate publications by company-affiliated staff, then 2) rank cited work(s). Using online sources to compile statistical data on journal usage provides a solid basis for title retention, cancellation, or subscription subsidy allocation decisions.

A comparable approach could be used for collection building to meet anticipated needs. Perhaps a new department or academic degree program is planned, or a corporation is branching out into a new area of research. Strategies could build around known core authors or competing companies (the latter, again, searched as author affiliations) already working in the field. Where do they publish most often, what sources do they cite, and where do authors citing them typically publish?

As these examples illustrate, author address or corporate affiliation can become a key element in information problem solving. When a query calls for address searching, *EMBASE* and *SciSearch* are better choices than *MEDLINE*. *EMBASE* has indexed the first author's address in all of its records online since 1974. *SciSearch* coverage also dates from the same year and has the added advantage of making all author affiliations accessible, not just that of the first or senior author. *BIOSIS Previews* has added author affiliation to *Biological Abstracts* records from January 1978 forward, and, in the *BA/RRM* subfile, author addresses are present from January 1980 to date.

MEDLINE, on the other hand, includes author address only in those citations indexed from "Priority 1 or 2" journals (approximately 1,500 out of 3,600 titles covered in the database). Furthermore, search capabilities for accessing author addresses in *MEDLINE* vary dramatically from vendor to vendor. For example, in the MEDLARS (NLM) system, author address is searchable in only the latest month of *MEDLINE* (known as *SDILINE*). In contrast, most commercial search systems offer several years of retrospective access to addresses, but starting dates differ.

Retrieval methodologies are also vendor- and database-dependent. Different mnemonics (field or paragraph labels) are often used. Addresses may be single-word-indexed (rather than phrase-accessible), necessitating use of proximity operators. Search systems also differ in their requirements for pre- or post-qualification of search terms (e.g., *merck.in.* or *cs = merck* or *merck/cs*). Consult vendor documentation for precise entry guidelines.

However, one general tip transcends system differences in entry protocols. Beware of abbreviations and variations in spacing, spelling, or language. Words such as university, college, hospital, institute, laboratory, clinical, clinic, pharmacy, medicine, and surgery are often abbreviated, as are state and other regional names. Imaginative (and careful) use of truncation is advisable. Address components are transcribed in online records exactly as listed in the original document, including variations such as *Wien* for *Vienna*. Company names are not standardized, so strategies should anticipate variations such as Du Pont or DuPont, Smith-Kline or Smith Kline, etc.

Publication Types

Discussion and search examples included in previous sections illustrate several key features that can influence database selection, such as age group and gender indexing or consistent identification of routes of drug administration. Database annotations have also touched on major differences in publication type indexing. Figure 14.11 lists publication type options that can tip the scales toward *MEDLINE* in answer to many search requests.

Because meta-analysis and practice guidelines are both hot topics in medicine of the 1990s, it's important to note that *MEDLINE* provides separate indexing for these sometimes elusive categories of documents. When searching for *MEDLINE* references to standards of care, use not only *practice guideline*, but also *guideline* and *consensus development conference* headings.

The National Institutes of Health home page on the Internet makes the full text of NIH clinical practice guidelines, consensus statements, and technology assessment statements available for immediate display at http://www.nih.gov/health. Bear in mind, however, that online searches in commercial databases can also uncover official recommendations from other sources important to clinicians (e.g., those of professional societies).

Databases to Answer Adverse Effects and Interactions Questions

Virtually any biomedical bibliographic source will assist users in compiling information on drug adverse effects, overdose or poisoning, toxicity, and interac-

Figure 14.11   Selected Publication/Document Types Identified in MEDLINE Indexing

Bibliography	(1991–)
Clinical Conference	(1991–)
Consensus Development Conference	(1991–)
Consensus Development Conference, NIH	(1991–)
Directory	(1991–)
Editorial	(1991–)
Guideline	(1991–)
Letter	(1991–)
Meta-Analysis	(1993–)
Practice Guideline	(1992–)
Review	(1991–)
Review of Reported Cases	(1991–)
Review, Academic	(1991–)
Review, Multicase	(1991–)
Review, Tutorial	(1991–)
Twin Study	(1995–)

tions. The primary factor that influences database selection for bibliography in this subject area is not subject scope, but, rather, indexing and retrieval capabilities. Both *MEDLINE* and *EMBASE* offer the refinement of subheadings to fine-tune adverse effect searches. (See Figures 14.1 and 14.2.) In both files, appropriate qualifying terms can be linked directly to a drug name. To reinforce the cause-effect relationship when an association between a given disease or condition (e.g., somnolence, drowsiness, psychomotor performance) and administration of an agent is the topic under investigation, CI (chemically induced) or DE (drug effects) can be linked with disease or condition terms in *MEDLINE*. SI (side effect) is the counterpart link term in *EMBASE*. For example,

In MEDLINE: *terfenadine with (ae or po or to or ct) AND psychomotor disorders with (ci or de)*

In EMBASE: *terfenadine with (ae or to) AND psychomotor disorder with si*

In databases where direct coordination of drug names and adverse effect concept terms is not an option, strategies are likely to retrieve a disconcerting mixture of relevant and irrelevant citations. Consider, for example, the lack of precision when an analgesic is ANDed with phrases such as *adverse effect* or *adverse reaction*. Bibliography may well include references to the therapeutic use of the analgesic to treat the adverse effects of another drug. Co-occurrence of terms in the same database record, or even in the same field or paragraph of records, is a poor quality filter compared to direct linkage within the same descriptor offered in *MEDLINE* and *EMBASE*.

Searching for drug interactions data presents special challenges.[9] As with brand name comparisons, it is easy to be lured into the trap of assuming that merely ANDing together drug names of agents suspected of interacting with one another will be sufficient to retrieve pertinent references. Unfortunately, names can co-occur in records without the concept of interaction being discussed. *EMBASE* offers the option, once again, of linking the additional qualifying term directly to drug name descriptors; for example, *(theophylline and cimetidine) with IT*. *IPA* allows for direct coordination, as well: *phenytoin with interactions*. Both of these files, in consequence, provide the best capabilities for searching the topic of interactions.

In *MEDLINE*, drug terms can be ANDed with the *MeSH* descriptor *drug interactions*. In the *Derwent Drug File*, the section code 66 (drug interactions) can be ANDed with descriptors for suspected agents. A comparable strategy would seem to be possible in *BIOSIS Previews*, where the controlled keyword phrase drug-drug interaction has been in use since 1985. However, it will be important to realize that *BIOSIS* uses its interaction terms to index citations to both intentional, as well as undesired, effects. To limit *BIOSIS* retrieval to undesirable interactions, the major concept term toxicology should be included in the strategy.

Tips on technique for retrieving bibliography related to two other types of interactions, incompatibilities and drug-lab test interferences, have been the topic of previous installments in the "Caduceus" series of columns for online searchers.[10, 11] Two Internet sources of specialized adverse effects data, the *Cutaneous Drug Reactions Database* and *MotherRisk*, were singled out in Figure 7.1.

ADIS Press produces an outstanding subject specialty database dedicated to monitoring the current literature on adverse drug experiences, including reports of overdose, abuse, and drug dependency. *Reactions* is among baseline sources checked by the World Health Organization as an indicator of whether a drug adverse event reported to them is already known or should be the subject of a signal alert to national pharmacovigilance agencies.[12]

14.26 *ADIS Reactions Database.* Auckland, NZ: ADIS International, 1993–. Updated daily. Available on DataStar, Dialog, and SilverPlatter; also on CD-ROM.

This database is the machine-readable counterpart of *Reactions* (7.5), a printed newsletter from the same publisher, with the advantage of daily (versus weekly) prepublication updates and enhanced bibliographic screening capabilities available to the online, versus hardcopy, user. Particularly helpful is the ability to isolate first reports of adverse drug effects (search *first* adjacent to *report* in titles). Another useful refinement is the addition by ADIS of the keyword *serious* to titles of pertinent references. Records flagged in this way report reactions meeting FDA criteria for serious effects: those that result in death, severe or permanent disability, or hospitalization. The *Reactions Database* also includes drug interactions in its scope, identifying reports of adverse clinical experience with patients, evaluating their significance, and emphasizing clinical management strategies. "Views and Reviews," a recurring section, tracks trends in adverse drug use experience, citing epidemiology and incidence studies, as well as analyses identifying determinants of reactions.

14.27 *TOXLINE.* Bethesda, MD: U.S. National Library of Medicine, 1965–. Updated monthly. Available on DataStar, Dialog, MEDLARS, Silver-Platter, and STN; also on CD-ROM.

TOXLINE is a collection of bibliographic references to published material and research in progress, focusing on the adverse effects of chemicals, drugs, and physical agents on living systems. Topics covered include air pollution, animal venoms, antidotes, carcinogenesis, chemically induced diseases, food contamination, occupational hazards, radiation effects, waste disposal, and water treatment. This database also covers drug toxicity evaluation, analysis, or screening studies. To achieve this broad scope, information from several different agencies or publishers has been compiled (see Figure 14.12). Sixteen separate sources provide nineteen subfiles, not all of which are available in all vendor implementations of this database. For example, DataStar's version of *TOXLINE* omits references supplied by *BIOSIS* and *IPA*.

Figure 14.12   TOXLINE Subfiles

ANEUPL—Aneuploidy
   A special collection of references prepared by the Environmental Mutagen Information Center of the Oak Ridge National Laboratory (Tennessee) on the subject of numerical chromosomal abnormalities in humans and experimental systems. Includes population and screening studies. 1969 + . No abstracts.

BIOSIS
   A Toxicological Aspects of Environmental Pollutants subfile derived from *BIOSIS Previews*, this segment of *TOXLINE* covers the effects of environmental chemicals, other than medicinals, on health (1985 +). 1970–1984 material from *BIOSIS* is available in HEEP (Health Effects of Environmental Pollutants). *MeSH* terms have been added since August 1985 (Trees searchable, but not displayable), and CAS registry numbers from 1970 forward (assigned by machine). Abstracts found in comparable records in *BIOSIS Previews* are sometimes omitted in *TOXLINE* counterparts.

CIS—International Labour Office (ILO) Abstracts
   The CIS subfile, starting in 1981, contains toxicology-related material selected from the International Occupational Safety and Health Information Centre's database, *CIS Abstracts*, produced by the ILO, a United Nations organization in Geneva.

CRISP—Toxicology Research Projects (RPROJ)
   The RPROJ/CRISP subfile contains descriptions of toxicology and epidemiology research projects selected from the CRISP (Computer Retrieval of Information on Scientific Projects) database by the U.S. National Institutes of Health. Included are projects either supported through the various research grants and contracts programs of the U.S. Public Health Service or conducted intramurally by NIH and the National Institute of Mental Health. Older references are routinely removed.

DART—Developmental and Reproductive Toxicology
   The DART subfile provides a continuation of ETIC and covers literature on birth defects and other aspects of reproductive and developmental toxicology since 1989. DART is funded by the U.S. National Institute of Environmental Health Sciences, the EPA, and the Agency for Toxic Substances and Disease Registry. Approximately 60% of DART documents are derived from *MEDLINE*.

EMIC—Environmental Mutagen Information Center File
   Prepared by the Environmental Mutagen Information Center of Oak Ridge National Laboratory, this subfile covers environmental mutation literature from 1965 forward, with some earlier citations also present. No abstracts, but CAS RNs are included in indexing.

EPIDEM—Epidemiology Information System (EIS) File
   The EIS subfile, developed and maintained for the FDA by the Toxicology Information Response Center at Oak Ridge National Laboratory, was added to *TOXLINE* in July 1987. It contains citations to published and unpublished literature on the distribution and health effects of food contaminants, issued from 1940 to the present.

ETIC—Environmental Teratology Information Center File
   Another product of the Oak Ridge National Laboratory, ETIC covers literature published from 1950 through 1989, when it was superseded by DART. Includes CAS RN indexing, but no abstracts.

FEDRIP—Federal Research in Progress (RPROJ)
  The RPROJ/FEDRIP subfile contains information on projects in toxicology and related
  areas supported by various U.S. government agencies. Abstracts are available, but no
  CAS RN indexing. Added to *TOXLINE* in October 1991.

HAPAB—Health Aspects of Pesticides Abstract Bulletin
  See PESTAB.

HEEP—Health Effects of Environmental Pollutants
  See BIOSIS subfile.

HMTC—Hazardous Materials Technical Center File
  The *HMTC Abstract Bulletin* is a publication of the U.S. Department of the Army's
  Hazardous Material Technical Center in Rockville, Maryland. It cites scientific and
  technical literature on hazardous materials, including safety, handling, storage, and dis-
  posal of hazardous wastes. Material dates from 1981 and includes abstracts, plus CAS
  RN indexing.

IPA—International Pharmaceutical Abstracts subfile
  All of *International Pharmaceutical Abstracts*, from 1970 forward, was included in
  TOXLINE until 1982, when NLM began omitting references derived from *IPA*'s "Phar-
  macy Practice Track" sections. Includes CAS RN indexing.

KEMI—RISKLINE
  Created by the Swedish National Chemicals Inspectorate (KEMI), RISKLINE compiles citations dating back to 1983. Sources include IARC monographs, WHO publications, and numerous non-English-language publications. These are made more accessible via lengthy abstracts in English provided by KEMI.

NTIS—Toxicology Document and Data Depository (TD3)
  TD3 is obtained from the U.S. National Technical Information Service (NTIS) and contains citations from the *Government Reports Announcements and Index* related to toxicology (October 1979 +). Records include abstracts, in which CAS RNs are sometimes
  embedded in unhyphenated format (no separate RN field).

PESTAB—Pesticides Abstracts (formerly HAPAB)
  PESTAB was a monthly publication from the EPA, containing reports on the epidemiological effects of pesticides (1967–1981). From 1967 through 1973, it was known as
  Health Aspects of Pesticides Abstracts Bulletin (HAPAB). Records include abstracts
  and, sometimes, CAS RN indexing. Publication terminated in 1981.

PPBIB—Poisonous Plants Bibliography
  The Poisonous Plants Bibliography was created for NLM by Dr. Jesse Wagstaff and
  added to *TOXLINE* in September 1987. PPBIB contains 2,508 citations to English-
  language literature, most of which was published prior to 1976. Abstracts and CAS RN
  indexing included. PPBIB is no longer updated in *TOXLINE*, but has been continued
  on the Internet as PLANTOX.

TOXBIB—Toxicity Bibliography
  Currently the largest subfile of *TOXLINE* (approximately 50%), TOXBIB is derived
  from the *MEDLINE* database (1967 +). References selected cover adverse effects, poisoning, and toxicity of drugs and other chemicals; drug interactions; environmental
  pollution; occupational diseases; radiation disorders; and substance use disorders.
  MeSH index terms are included in records, as are author abstracts (1975 +) and CAS
  RN indexing (1980 +).

TSCATS—Toxic Substances Control Act Test Submissions File
This subfile, generated by the EPA, was added to *TOXLINE* in April 1988. TSCATS is a unique and extensive collection of unpublished, industry-generated and -sponsored information on chemical testing results mandated by TSCA legislation. Records include abstracts and CAS RN indexing.

More than half of *TOXLINE* is derived from *MEDLINE*, delivered in a segment labeled TOXBIB. *BIOSIS Previews* contributes 26% of *TOXLINE* references, and 10% of citations come from *IPA*. The Toxicology Document and Data Depository is derived from the *NTIS* database. FEDRIP references are drawn from the larger *Federal Research in Progress* database. In point of fact, only about 12% of *TOXLINE* records represent unique references unlikely to be found elsewhere.

Why search a database with so little exclusive material? Bibliography derived from other sources is often accessible in different ways than would be available in their original "home" file. For example, *TOXLINE* records originating in *BIOSIS Previews* have been augmented with CAS registry numbers (assigned using a computer algorithm, 1970–) and with *MeSH* terms added since August 1985.

On the other hand, it can be difficult to exploit the undoubted advantages of this subject specialty database due to its inconsistencies in record content and indexing. These inconsistencies can be attributed to the incredible diversity of contributing agency subsets. For example, not all *TOXLINE* references routinely identify language of source documents (EPIDEM, FEDRIP, NTIS, PPBIB, and TSCATS subfiles omit language indexing). Registry numbers are searchable in some subfiles of *TOXLINE*, but not others. If the searcher avoids these pitfalls, there remains the challenge of anticipating different indexing terms likely to be assigned in this collection of minidatabases. Clearly, multiple synonyms should be used in searches for references to chemical substances, as well as other subject concepts.[13]

Another set of databases potentially relevant to the pharmaceutical searcher are toxic substances directories. *RTECS*, already discussed briefly in Chapter Eight, is by far the largest directory in this family of resources, covering more than 140,000 substances.

14.28 *Registry of Toxic Effects of Chemical Substances (RTECS)*. Cincinnati, OH: U.S. National Institute for Occupational Safety and Health, 1971–. Updated quarterly. Available on DataStar, Dialog, MEDLARS, SilverPlatter, and STN; also on CD-ROM.

14.29 *Hazardous Substances Data Bank (HSDB)*. Bethesda, MD: U.S. National Library of Medicine. Current information, updated quarterly. Available on DataStar, MEDLARS, SilverPlatter, and STN.

14.30 *CHEMTOX Online*. Brentwood, TN: Resource Consultants. Current information, updated quarterly. Available on DataStar and Dialog.

14.31 *MSDS-OHS.* San Leandro, CA: MDL Information Systems. Current information, updated quarterly. Available on Dialog and STN; also on CD-ROM.

14.32 *MSDS-CCOHS.* Hamilton, Ontario: Canadian Centre for Occupational Health and Safety. Current information, updated quarterly. Available on SilverPlatter and STN; also on CD-ROM.

The *Hazardous Substances Data Bank (HSDB)* is a scientifically peer reviewed database of factual material compiled from a core set of standard texts and monographs, many of which were discussed in Chapters Seven and Eight. Additional data have been extracted from government documents, technical reports, and the primary journal literature. Each of the 4,500 monographs dedicated to single chemical compounds presents information in nine broad topical categories, including toxicity or biomedical effects, safety and handling, pharmacology, environmental fate or exposure potential, exposure standards and regulations, and monitoring or analysis.

Like *HSDB, CHEMTOX Online* is not limited to coverage of drug substances. It includes more than 10,300 monographs dedicated to compounds regulated or governed by legislation, because they raise environment, health, or safety issues. Each lengthy record collects information from one or more manufacturers' Material Safety Data Sheets, together with government-agency-derived reference data and other material from journals, books, and technical reports.

MSDS-OHS is comparable in content, dedicated to providing identification, handling, and hazard disclosure information for more than 56,300 substances that require documentation by chemical manufacturers under the Hazard Communication and Labeling Standard of OSHA (see Chapter Four). The MDL collection (originally begun by Occupational Health Services—hence *OHS*) has the advantage of providing more regulatory data from foreign government sources than would be found in *CHEMTOX Online.*

MSDS-CCOHS covers more than 118,000 substances, with 140,890 Material Safety Data Sheets for brand-named Canadian and U.S. products from 660 producers or distributors. The CCOHS database is also available by subscription on the Web-based interface *CCINFOWeb*, where it is updated monthly at http://www.ccohs.ca.

The U.S. Pharmacopeial Convention produces Material Safety Data Sheets for pharmaceutical substances covered by *USP* (11.8) reference standards. The small collection of approximately 1,000 MSDS can be licensed in machine-readable form with quarterly updates. A free sample data diskette and ordering information are featured in the product catalog on the USP's Web site at http://www.usp.org.

Complementary Hazardous Chemical Data Sources on the Internet

Hotlinks to manufacturer-produced MSDS and other repositories maintained at various academic institutions worldwide have been assembled at a site entitled

Where to Find Material Safety Data Sheets on the Internet (http://www. ilpi.com/msds/index.html) and at *MSDS-SEARCH* (http://www.msdssearch. com). In addition, three free Internet sites are noteworthy complements to commercially available databases cited in this section: the *Environmental Chemicals Data and Information Network* (*ECDIN*), *HAZDAT*, and *OPPT Chemical Summaries*. Other Web sources annotated below could be helpful in answering questions from consumers. The *CERCLA Priority List* is included in anticipation of regulatory status requests. For Web-based repositories of botanical toxicity data, refer to Figure 8.2.

Environmental Chemical Data and Information Network (ECDIN)
  ⇨ http://ecdin.etomep.net

The *Environmental Chemicals Data and Information Network* (*ECDIN*) is an outgrowth of research programs of the Commission of European Communities. It closely resembles the *Hazardous Substances Data Bank* (14.29) in its content and quality. The file can be searched by generic substance name and synonyms, CAS RN, or molecular formula. Lengthy monographs can be selectively displayed, enabling users to carve out sections devoted to, for example, identification, physical-chemical properties, uses, legislation and regulations, human health effects, occupational exposure limits, experimental toxicity, or detection methods. Textual summaries for each of the 120,000 substances covered in *ECDIN* are thoroughly referenced and conclude with lengthy bibliographies. Exposure limits cited (TLV, PEL, etc.) typically encompass standards established in many nations, each of which is identified.

HAZDAT
  ⇨ http://atsdrl.atsdr.cdc.gov:8080/hazdat.html

Much more limited in scope than *ECDIN*, the *HAZDAT* database focuses on Superfund site data assessments, augmented by toxicological profiles for about 150 substances. Queries in this resource can zero in on any of the 1,300 geographic sites targeted by the EPA or simply search by contaminant keywords. Site searches (location or company name) identify contaminants found and an overall hazards rating. Records for each substance include, at minimum, CAS RN, substance class, and regulatory status under various U.S. government programs. Some entries provide a hypertext link to a consumer oriented *ToxFAQ* sheet. Additional data may include health effects by route and duration of exposure, metabolites, interactions, susceptible populations, and biomarkers of exposure. *HAZDAT* is produced by the Agency for Toxic Substances and Disease Registry (ATSDR).

ToxFAQs
  ⇨ http://atsdrl.atsdr.cdc.gov:8080/toxfaq.html

Another product of the Agency for Toxic Substances and Disease Registry, *ToxFAQs* is a series of individual summaries, each focusing on a given hazardous substance. Chemicals covered are those found at hazardous waste sites. ATSDR offers two routes to the collection 1) a browsable alphabetic list by substance name or 2) a keyword search to delve into textual content, such as requesting all *ToxFAQs* mentioning "burn." Each consumer oriented data sheet includes a CAS RN, empirical formula, and answers to questions such as What is substance X? What happens when it enters the environment? How might I be exposed to it? How could it affect my health? How likely is it to cause cancer? Is there a medical test to determine if I've been exposed? Where can I find more information?

CERCLA Priority List of Hazardous Substances
  ➪ http://atsdr1.atsdr.cdc.gov:8080/97list.html

Every two years, ATSDR prepares a *Priority List of Hazardous Substances* identified under the Superfund and Comprehensive Environmental Response, Compensation, Liability Act (CERCLA) programs. Factors affecting priority ranking include frequency of occurrence, toxicity, and potential for human exposure. The *List* is presented as a simple table by priority rank number, cross referenced to chemical name, ranking on the previous biennial list, and CAS number. A new list is due to be released in 1999.

Chemicals in the Environment: OPPT Chemical Fact Sheets
  ➪ http://www.epa.gov/opptintr/chemfact

The Office of Pollution Prevention and Toxics (OPPT) of the U.S. Environmental Protection Agency publishes both consumer oriented *Fact Sheets* and professionally oriented *Chemical Summaries*. The latter compile information from secondary sources to provide basic chemical identification and physical/chemical property data, as well as summaries of production and use, environmental fate, and health effects. Each lengthy *OPPT Chemical Summary* concludes with a bibliography of cited references.

Drug Information for the Consumer or Patient

Most biomedical databases singled out for discussion thus far index publications intended for practitioners and trained scientific researchers. The vocabulary employed and the selection of topics reported assume a common ground of highly specialized education and experience. Nonetheless, a great deal of time and effort has been spent in the past ten years on building user-friendly interfaces to these sources, with the objective of making them more readily accessible to all.

Simplifying software will not solve patient information problems. Making *MEDLINE*, for example, easily searchable by the general public cannot change the fundamental barriers to understanding posed by the primary professional literature. What's needed, instead, are databases that tap into the medical consumer press.

14.33 *IAC Health & Wellness Database*. Foster City, CA: Information Access Company, 1976–. Updated weekly. Available on DataStar, Dialog, and Ovid; also on CD-ROM.

The best online source of general (not just medication related) consumer health information is the *IAC Health & Wellness Database* (*HWD*), formerly entitled *Health Periodicals Database*. *HWD* not only indexes and abstracts relevant literature, but also provides the option for immediate full-text display of many primary sources, including numerous high quality newsletters and more than 550 information pamphlets published by patient support groups such as the American Diabetes Association or the American Lupus Society. All titles in the *Consumer Health & Nutrition Index* are also monitored in *HWD*. Full-text coverage includes *USP DI Volume 2—Advice for the Patient* (9.1); *Consumer Health Information Source Book* (9.21); *The People's Book of Medical Tests*; *Mosby's Medical, Nursing, and Allied Health Dictionary*; and the *Columbia University College of Physicians and Surgeons Complete Home Medical Guide*.

The *IAC Health & Wellness Database* also features more than 1,800 topical overviews of a wide range of diseases, medical conditions, symptoms, treatment alternatives, and preventive measures, written for the lay researcher. Referral information for consumer hotlines and support groups is provided in *HWD* by *The Complete Directory for People with Chronic Illness*. In addition to health periodicals published for the layman, *IAC Health & Wellness* indexes more than 120 journals intended for a professional medical audience, including the *Archives of Internal Medicine, British Medical Journal, JAMA, Lancet, RN*, and the *Western Journal of Medicine*. Consumer summaries accompany citations to these sources, which can provide excellent patient education material for practitioners seeking ways to improve physician-patient communication.[14]

The *IAC Magazine Database* (formerly *Magazine Index*), another frequently cited source to help locate medical literature appropriate for laypeople, is one of several IAC "feeder files" contributing to *HWD*. Most health related materials found in the *Magazine Database* are also included in the *Health & Wellness Database*, which offers the added advantage of more subject-specific and detailed topical indexing than found in the *IAC Magazine* file.

14.34 *MDX Health Digest*. Merlin, OR: Medical Data Exchange, 1988–. Updated monthly. Available on Ovid and SilverPlatter; also on CD-ROM.

MDX Health Digest draws from a list of 200 publications in providing access to patient-oriented medical information. Sources include professional journals, popular health magazines and newsletters, general interest magazines (e.g., *Family Circle, Good Housekeeping, Redbook*), newspapers, and medical school publications. Medical Data Exchange indexes and creates substantive abstracts for articles from these sources.[15] Selected records are also derived from *MEDLINE*.

Although it includes no full-text items and covers fewer publications than the *IAC Health & Wellness Database*, *MDX Health Digest* is handy for quick-reference access to a selection of material appropriate for answering consumer inquiries.

14.35 *Physician Data Query Patient Information File.* Bethesda, MD: U.S. National Cancer Institute. Current information, updated monthly. Available on MEDLARS and Ovid; also on CD-ROM.

14.36 *Physician Data Query Directory File.* Bethesda, MD: U.S. National Cancer Institute. Current information, updated monthly. Available on MEDLARS and Ovid; also on CD-ROM.

For succinct, consumer oriented cancer information, the *Physician Data Query (PDQ) Patient* file offers menu-assisted access to prognostic statements and explanations of cancer stages and treatment options. The *PDQ* family of databases (see also 14.22) includes a referral *Directory*, enabling patients to locate specialists by region and by type of cancer therapy, and offering an organization or institution locator.

Remember, also, the *Allied and Alternative Medicine* database (14.15) is expressly devoted to indexing the literature of alternative medicine. *AMED* screens both popular and professional publications for citations pertinent to hot, but often hard to find, topics such as acupuncture, homeopathy, diet therapies, and herbalism. *MANTIS* (formerly *CHIROLARS*, see Appendix B), with its emphasis on preventive medicine (not limited to chiropractic), also includes acupuncture, biofeedback, naturopathy, and herbal therapy in its scope. Like *AMED*, it blends both popular and professional bibliography in references cited.

The *FDA Home Page* on the Internet, to be discussed later in the context of regulatory information (see Chapter Sixteen), includes much material appropriate for patients. For example, under the human drugs icon, *Consumer Drug Information Sheets* cover a selection of drugs approved from January 1998 to the present. Under the foods icon, an opening menu offers a hotlink to consumer advice and material for educators. Other menu options that can provide answers in everyday language address the topics of food additives and food labeling. Choosing the latter leads to a well organized list of information modules about using food labels to cope with diabetes, lose weight, prevent heart disease, or monitor sodium and other nutrients important to high blood pressure. Items available for immediate display free of charge include a list of publications consumers can order and the complete text of a special food labeling issue from the *FDA Consumer*. Clicking on "Food Additives" from the menu links to a set of questions and answers that convey a wealth of easily understood background information on why additives are used and related safety issues.

Content assembled under the cosmetics icon on the *FDA Home Page* is almost wholly dedicated to the general public, presenting succinct answers to anticipated inquiries about, for example, testing in animals, cosmeceuticals, over-the-counter drugs versus cosmetics, shelf-life and expiration dating, aromatherapy, or tattooing. Hair loss, weight loss, hypoallergenic, and suntan products are also featured. The *FDA Home Page* is located at http://www.fda.gov on the Internet.

Another Web site offering quality filtered consumer oriented materials is the *Centers for Disease Control and Prevention Home Page* at http:www.cdc.gov. Its "Health Information" option links users to substantive modules on specific diseases, injuries and disabilities, and immunizations. The Travelers' Health icon leads to both patient and professional selections, including the full text of the latest edition of CDC's *"Yellow Book"* (6.45). Many other consumer oriented Internet sites are discussed in Chapter Nine.

Pharmaceutics and Pharmaceutical Technology Sources

For searching pharmaceutics and pharmaceutical technology topics, *International Pharmaceutical Abstracts* is the database of choice. In addition to separate section headings devoted to these two broad subject areas, *IPA* also compiles relevant material under "drug analysis" and "drug stability" (see Figure 14.3). Rigorous indexing of dosage forms, when relevant, is especially helpful in answering requests for bibliography on biopharmaceutics topics (i.e., the effects of formulation on drug action within the body). The policy regarding dosage form identification in *IPA* records is comparable to that applied to route of administration indexing, discussed earlier in this chapter. "Form" keywords are always included in the first paragraph of abstracts. Many specific descriptors are also available in the *IPA Thesaurus* (14.9) for concepts such as dissolution rates, hydrogen ion concentration, surface active agents, coatings, microencapsulation, and the like.

EMBASE (14.4) introduced a link term for pharmaceutics (PR) in 1988, enabling direct coordination of this concept with specific drug descriptors. The *Derwent Drug File* (14.10) includes a section heading (SH code 29) to isolate references to pharmaceutics. Given the close relationship of pharmaceutics techniques with chemistry, it's not surprising that CAS and Royal Society of Chemistry databases are additional sources for background bibliography.

14.37 *CA SEARCH.* Columbus, OH: Chemical Abstracts Service, 1967–. Updated biweekly. Available on DataStar, Dialog, QUESTEL-ORBIT, and Ovid.

14.38 *CA File.* Columbus, OH: Chemical Abstracts Service, 1967–. Updated biweekly. Available on STN.

14.39 *Analytical Abstracts.* Cambridge, U.K.: The Royal Society of Chemistry, 1980–. Updated monthly. Available on DataStar, Dialog, QUESTEL-ORBIT, SilverPlatter, and STN; also on CD-ROM.

CA SEARCH indexes more than 14,000 journal titles annually, plus conference and symposia proceedings, dissertations, books, government and technical reports, and patents. It includes references to literature published in any of 130 countries and forty-seven languages; 62% of citations are to English-language sources. Patents records constitute 30% of online coverage, surveying applications filed with any of twenty-eight nations and other authorities. *CA SEARCH* includes all bibliography published in the hardcopy counterpart *Chemical Abstracts*, but excludes the abstracts. The publisher makes summaries available online only in the *CA File* on STN. The *Analytical Abstracts* database provides author summaries in every record. Narrower in subject scope, this Royal Society of Chemistry database indexes approximately 1,300 journal titles each year, along with conference papers, books, standards, and technical reports.

Both *CA SEARCH/CA File* and *Analytical Abstracts* are of primary interest as secondary literature sources in pharmaceutics. Neither is clinically oriented. *CA SEARCH/CA File* does cover early drug development studies, such as synthesis/isolation, chemical/physical characterization, initial screening, and toxicity testing in animals. However, factors such as subject population identification (e.g., animal species), age groups, gender, routes of administration, and organ systems or parts of the body affected are not consistently included in CAS indexing. The emphasis is on chemistry, rather than biomedicine, as is reflected in the selection of section headings listed below.

Air Pollution and Industrial Hygiene
Alkaloids
Biochemical Methods
Enzymes
Essential Oils and Cosmetics
Food and Feed Chemistry
Immunochemistry
Mammalian Biochemistry
Mammalian Pathological Biochemistry
Organic Analytical Chemistry
Pharmaceutical Analysis
Pharmaceuticals
Steroids
Toxicology

Specific compounds should be searched by CAS registry numbers, including current, alternate, or replaced RNs. This is the only database where these codes take precedence over all other forms of drug nomenclature. Strategies that omit them will result in woefully incomplete bibliographies. Simplified generic names and brand names are sometimes included in online indexing. Such terms, if present, are derived from the source author's own words; hence, locants and isomeric designations tend to be omitted. For example, *2,6-dichloropyridine* would appear simply as *dichloropyridine*. Individual compounds or substituents in chemical names are usually searchable as separate segments: e.g., *dichloropyridine* is also indexed as *di chloro pyridine*. Element names (iron, lead), rather than atomic symbols (Fe, Pb), are preferred. Enzyme Commission numbers are cited only when used by the author in the original source.

Retrieving bibliography on groups of pharmacologically- or therapeutically-related compounds is somewhat difficult in *CA SEARCH* or *CA File*. Broad category keywords, such as antiinflammatory agents or nitroso compounds, are generally added to online records only when the primary source mentions three or more substances of a given class or category, or if the source author emphasizes such a category in discussion. Thus, it is easy to miss references to individual substances belonging to a drug class, but not identified as such.

14.40 *MethodsFinder*. Philadelphia, PA: BIOSIS, 1998–. Updated weekly. Available on the World Wide Web at http://www.methodsfinder.org.
14.41 *ISI Reaction Center*. Philadelphia, PA: Institute for Scientific Information, 1985–. Updated monthly. See http://www.isinet.com.

Two fee-based Internet databases designed to support laboratory research needs were introduced in 1998. *MethodsFinder* focuses on references to hard-to-find scientific protocols for conducting laboratory experiments. Sources scanned include journals, books, meeting papers, and technical literature published by commercial biological suppliers. In its initial release, *MethodsFinder* contained more than 25,000 records, relaying either bibliographic references with abstracts or hypertext links to the full text of protocols found elsewhere on the Web.

ISI's *Reaction Center* compiles citations to synthetic methods reported in the primary journal and patent literature. The interface accommodates searching by structure, reaction conditions (e.g., pressure, temperature), catalyst or solvent names, and biological activity of reactants or their products.

Pharmacognosy

International Pharmaceutical Abstracts (14.8) and *BIOSIS Previews* (14.6) both offer excellent coverage of the literature of pharmacognosy (drugs derived from nature). *IPA* designates pertinent references under the section heading Pharmacognosy, and *BIOSIS* has implemented the word as a major concept term. The *Allied and Alternative Medicine* database (14.16) will also contribute unique material, as will the *CAB Health* collection (14.17), which includes the *Review of Aromatic and Medicinal Plants* among its printed counterparts.

14.42 *Natural Products Alert (NAPRALERT)*. Chicago: College of Pharmacy, University of Illinois at Chicago, 1975–. Updated monthly. Available on STN.

An outgrowth of the Program for Collaborative Research in the Pharmaceutical Sciences at the University of Illinois, the *Natural Products Alert* database contains more than 141,000 citations to articles and books on the chemical constituents, pharmacology, and ethnomedicinal uses of 121,000 compounds and 135,000 plant, microbial, and animal (primarily marine) organisms. Sources include a small collection of 200 scientific journals, augmented by scans of *Chemical Abstracts, Biological Abstracts, Index Medicus, Current Contents-Life Sciences, Medicinal and Aromatic Plant Abstracts,* and *Current Indian Titles.* Although half of the file is derived from literature published from 1975 to date, this database also contains records for sources dating from as early as the year 1650.

NAPRALERT includes information on the chemistry and pharmacology of secondary metabolites found to be present in, or isolated from, natural sources. Special profile records compile basic nomenclature and other data. For example, ethnomedical profiles for plants include Latin binomials, common names, and notes on traditional (folk) medicinal uses. Pharmacological profiles include genus-species, taxonomic family, organism part, habitat, type of pharmacological test, extract used, route of administration, dose, and identification of the test species and gender. Results are characterized as active (weak or strong), equivocal activity, or inactive.

Searchers can look forward to the release of *AltMedDex* in 1999. The supplier, Micromedex, has announced plans to publish fifty evidence-based monographs on herbals, vitamins, and other dietary supplements. Remember, also, that the *USP* (11.8) has begun issuing monographs for a small selection of phytomedicinal compounds. The Internet offers several intriguing sites of potential interest to pharmacognosy searchers. Professionally oriented sources are discussed in Chapter Twelve and consumer resources are identified in Chapter Nine.

Drug Identification and Nomenclature Sources

A thorough search for drug related literature should take into account changes in author terminology when referring to compounds at different stages in their life cycle (laboratory to launch). For example, references to studies conducted early in the R&D pipeline, such as synthesis/analysis or toxicity, often cite laboratory codes, rather than generic names (see Figure 2.1). Locating alternative names and codes under which a compound may appear in the literature is an important part of search preparation for thorough retrospective surveys.

Any online system intended to serve pharmaceutical literature searchers must provide adequate drug identification and nomenclature support. A baseline requirement is access to the full Chemical Abstracts Service registry file. Available under different names on various vendors, this CAS database offers access to alternative names, current and replaced or alternate RNs, and structural data for every substance cited in *Chemical Abstracts* from 1967 forward.

14.43 *CAS Registry File.* Columbus, OH: Chemical Abstracts Service, 1957–. Updated weekly. Available on STN.
14.44 *Chemical Registry Nomenclature (CNAM).* Columbus, OH: Chemical Abstracts Service, 1957–. Updated monthly. Available on DataStar.
14.45 *CHEMSEARCH.* Cary, NC: Dialog and CAS, 1957–. Updated monthly. Available on Dialog.

Each of the three sources cited here represents the full CAS database, with records for more than 16 million substances. In addition to differences in update frequency, these files differ in the pointers they provide to other online databases. STN adds information about the availability of literature references in several other databases within the system. Dialog tallies the number of citations in *CA SEARCH* as part of *CHEMSEARCH* records, but relies on its cross-system-*DIALINDEX* to help users locate additional bibliographies.

Identification of chemical compounds by their structural attributes is rarely needed in clinical information settings, but is an extremely useful tool for scientists in industry who are engaged in drug discovery. Graphical structure searching software is available as an interface to the CAS registry file through STN Express and on the QUESTEL-ORBIT online system.

14.46 *CHEMLINE.* Bethesda, MD: U.S. National Library of Medicine. Current information, updated bimonthly. Available on MEDLARS.

CHEMLINE compiles identification and nomenclature information on a relatively limited selection of chemicals (one million substances, compared to the more than 16 million registered). It includes entries for compounds identified by CAS RNs in other MEDLARS databases, such as *TOXLINE, TOXLIT, RTECS, MEDLINE, HSDB, CCIS, CANCERLIT,* as well as the *TSCA* (Toxic Substances Control Act) *Inventory* maintained by the U.S. Environmental Protection Agency. Because registry number indexing has not been added to all pertinent citations in each of these databases, not all substances cited in NLM files have nomenclature records in *CHEMLINE.*

Replaced or alternate registry numbers (useful in retrospective searching) are usually absent in *CHEMLINE* records. Offsetting this omission are references to related registry numbers (RR) for many (but not all) salts. Because *MEDLINE* assigns parent compound RNs to salts and stereoisomers, this RR indexing, updated annually, is a helpful user aid. Synonyms listed in *CHEMLINE* records are derived from a variety of sources, including the *USP Dictionary* (3.1) and the *CTFA Cosmetic Ingredient Dictionary* (11.29). Ambiguous names are flagged, and designations with official status are identified (e.g., USAN, BAN, INN, DCF). Most useful of all are cross references to drug or chemical classification for each substance. With each annual regeneration, locator information is also added to *CHEMLINE* records to assist users in locating other MEDLARS databases where references to each substance are available.

Other good sources of drug nomenclature online are databases equivalent to hardcopy publications discussed earlier in this *Guide*, such as *Drug Information Fulltext* (14.18), *USP Dictionary of USAN and International Drug Names* (available on Dialog and STN), *The Merck Index Online* (Dialog, QUESTEL-ORBIT, STN), and *Martindale Online* (DataStar). Computer-assisted, versus manual, consultation of such resources is particularly advantageous when the vendor system where they reside offers automatic extraction of RNs and synonyms listed in substance records, formulation into logical search entries, and easy capabilities for cross-file carryover without pausing to rekey terms.[16]

Another valuable, but sometimes overlooked, source of new drug names is the growing family of files designed for competitive intelligence, discussed in Chapter Fifteen. Drugs-in-development directories such as *Pharmaprojects*, *ADIS R&D Insight*, and *IMSworld R&D Focus* can often help identify products not found elsewhere, or provide more alternative names than the CAS registry databases for use in searching literature files.

Statistics from a study conducted in April 1992 illustrate the value of these pipeline directories as drug identification tools.[17] Using all new molecular entities approved by the FDA in 1991 as a starting point, generic names for thirty NMEs were searched across nomenclature sources to compile a list of brand names and research codes associated with each product (191 names in all). The cumulative list was then used to gauge the identification capabilities of several databases. The number of proprietary names from the test list that could be found in each file, expressed as a percentage of the total available, is an indicator of their relative utility as pharmaceutical nomenclature sources when preparing to search for bibliography on new products.

Pharmaprojects	94%
Merck Index Online	52%
CHEMSEARCH	30%
Martindale Online	23%

Data from a comparable study conducted in 1996, presented in Chapter Fifteen, paint a similar picture. A key distinction to bear in mind is the difference between product and chemical compound identification. CAS registry files and *The Merck Index Online* provide access to individual compounds. On the other hand, drugs-in-development directories such as *Pharmaprojects* focus on products, which consist not only of active chemical constituents, but also formulation agents (excipients). Identification information in these product-, versus compound-oriented, research tools also takes into account dosage form and strength as part of the unique formulation that constitutes a drug administered to patients. Furthermore, by focusing on competitive intelligence about research in progress, pipeline directories offer far more timely access to proprietary product news, as examples will illustrate in the next chapter.

References

1. Frisse ME, Florance V. A library for internists IX: Recommendations from the American College of Physicians. *Ann Intern Med* 1997 May 15;126:836–846.

2. Snow B. SciSearch changes: Abstracts and added indexing. *Online* 1991 Sep;15:102–106.

3. Snow B. Tapping into the invisible college: Online cited reference searching. *Online* 1986 Mar;10:83–88.

4. Snow B. Online database coverage of pharmaceutical journals. *Database* 1984 Feb;7:12–26.

5. Snow B. Online puzzles: Conference papers and proceedings. *Database* 1988 Aug;11:94–103.

6. Van Camp AJ. Searching the published conference literature: A Caduceus update. *Database* 1990 Aug;13(4):100–102.

7. Snow B. Author addresses or corporate affiliations. *Database* 1985 Dec;8:58–61.

8. Snow B. RANK: A new tool for analyzing search results on DIALOG. *Database* 1993 Jun;16:111–118.

9. Snow B. Searching for drug interactions data. *Database* 1986 Feb;9:69–74.

10. Snow B. Parenteral incompatibilities. *Database* 1986 Apr;9:75–83.

11. Snow B. Laboratory test modifications. *Database* 1986 Jun;9:81–85.

12. Fucik H, Edwards IR. Impact and credibility of the WHO adverse reaction signals. *Drug Inf J* 1996;30:461–464.

13. Snow B. TOXLINE search tips. *Database* 1991 Aug;14:100–105.

14. Snow B. Health Periodicals Database: A closer look. *Database* 1991 Feb;14:84–89.

15. Wehmeyer JM. MDX Health Digest: A consumer health database. *Med Ref Serv Q* 1995;14(2):53–60.

16. Snow B. MAPping in medicine: An update on options for automatic search-saves of drug names. *Online* 1993 Jan;17:93–100.

17. Snow B. Trade names in medicine: Searching for brand name comparisons and new product news. *Database* 1992 Jun;15:99–105.

Additional Sources of Information

Armstrong CJ, Large JA, eds. *Manual of online search strategies.* 2nd ed. Aldershot, Hants, England: Ashgate, 1992.

Barber J et al. Case studies of the indexing and retrieval of pharmacology papers. *Infor Process Manage* 1988;24(2):141–150.

Branch K. Computerized sources of AIDS information. *Med Ref Serv Q* 1988;7(4):1–18.

Bronson RJ. Alcohol information for clinicians and educators database. *Med Ref Serv Q* 1989;8(2):65–76.

Bruce NG, Farren AL. Searching BIOSIS Previews in the health care setting. *Med Ref Serv Q* 1987;6(2):17–37.

Buntrock RE. Gold (CASRN equals 7440–57–5) is where you find it, or caveats on finding chemical substances using CASRN. *Database* 1995 Jun;18(3):50–55.

Cassidy SL, Kostrewski BJ. An evaluation of information sources in household product poisoning. *J Info Sci* 1986;12(4):143–151.

Cosmides GJ. Electronic surveillance of the pharmacology-toxicology literature—the need for controlled vocabularies and registry systems. *Regul Toxicol Pharmacol* 1995 Apr;21(2):208–210.

Funk ME, Reid CA. Indexing consistency in MEDLINE. *Bull Med Libr Assoc* 1983 Apr;71(2):176–183.

Harbourt AM, Knecht LS, Humphreys BL. Structured abstracts in MEDLINE, 1989–1991. *Bull Med Libr Assoc* 1995 Apr;83(2):190–195.

Haynes RB et al. Developing optimal search strategies for detecting clinically sound studies in MEDLINE. *J Am Med Inform Assoc* 1994 Nov;1(6): 447–458.

Haynes RB et al. Performances of 27 MEDLINE systems tested by searches with clinical questions. *J Am Med Inform Assoc* 1994 May;1(3):285–295.

Hewison NS. Current Contents Search. *Med Ref Serv Q* 1988;7(4):57–66.

Johnson ED, McKinin EJ, Sievert ME. The application of quality filters in searching the clinical literature: some possible heuristics. *Med Ref Serv Q* 1992;11(4):39–59.

Judkins DZ. Searching hints: a chronic disease hedge for use on MEDLINE. *Med Ref Serv Q* 1984;3(2):72–73.

McCain KW. Biotechnology in context—A database-filtering approach to identifying core and productive non-core journals supporting multidisciplinary research-and-development. *J Am Soc Info Sci* 1995 May;46(4):306–317.

McKibbon KA, Dilks CW. Panning for applied clinical research gold. *Online* 1993 Jul;17:105–108.

Morisseau AL. Online databases: Information sources for the pharmacist. *Consult Pharm* 1986 Nov/Dec:261–272.

O'Leary M. *The online 100*. Wilton, CT: Pemberton Press Books, 1995.

Perry CA. Online information retrieval in pharmacy and related fields. *Am J Hosp Pharm* 1986;43(6):1509–1524.

Pratt GF. Searching the gene symbol field in MEDLINE. *Database* 1991 Dec;14(6):39–43.

Sayers M, Joice J, Bawden D. Retrieval of biomedical reviews—A comparative evaluation of online databases for reviews of drug therapy. *J Info Sci* 1990;16(5):321–325.

Schwarzwalder R. The brave new world of biotechnology online. *Database* 1994 Aug;17(4):103–105.

Self DA. Searching the literature of veterinary medicine. *Med Ref Serv Q* 1985/86;4(4):17–28.

Sievert ME, Verbeck A. The indexing of the literature of online searching: A comparison of ERIC and LISA. *Online Rev* 1987;11(2):95–104.

Snow B. Creating customized search shortcuts: The SET feature on DIALOG. *Online* 1992 May;16:97–102.

Snow B. Database selection in the life sciences. *Database* 1985 Aug;8:15–44.

Snow B. Differences in CANCERLIT on MEDLARS and DIALOG. *Online* 1986 Nov;10:118–123.

Snow B. EMBASE update for the pharmaceutical searcher. *Database* 1991 Dec;14:93–96.

Snow B. Online searching for alternatives to animal testing. *Online* 1990 Jul;14:94–97.

Snow B. Online sources for alternative medicine. *Database* 1998 Jun;21:19–29.

Snow B. People in medicine: searching names online. *Online* 1986 Sep;10:122–127.

Snow B. Review articles in MEDLINE: past and present. *Online* 1989 Mar;13:101–105.

Snow B. Searching online for articles about online: Where to find references to biomedical databases. Part 1. *Online* 1993 Nov;17:101–105. Part 2. *Database* Dec;16;100–104.

Snow B. TARGET for the biomedical searcher. *Online* 1994 Nov;18:58–65.

Snow B. What jargon is really necessary when teaching (and learning) online skills? *Online* 1986 Jul;10:100–107.

Sodha RJ, Vanamelsvoort T. Multi-database searches in biomedicine—Citation duplication and novelty assessment using carbamazepine as an example. *J Info Sci* 1994;20(2):139–141.

Tousignaut D, Spigai F. Searching "pharmacy" databases: nomenclature problems and inconsistencies. *Database* 1982 Feb;5:23–29.

Van Buskirk NE. The review article in MEDLINE: Ambiguity of definition and implications for online searchers. *Bull Med Libr Assoc* 1984 Oct;72(4):349–352.

Van Camp AJ. DIRLINE—An online directory of health information and resources. *Online* 1990 Nov;14(6):109–111.

Van Camp AJ. Fast-track databases for drug and biomedical searchers. *Online* 1993 Sep;17(5):113–115.

Van Camp AJ. The many faces of PDQ, the cancer therapy databases. *Database* 1992 Apr;15(2):95–98.

Van Camp AJ. Material safety data sheets: Online and CD/ROM sources. *Online* 1990 Mar;14(2):97–100.

Van Camp AJ. Online sources for alternative medicine information. *Database* 1993 Oct;16(5):100–103.

Van Camp AJ. Starsearch for the health-sciences. *Database* 1991 Oct;14(5):99–101.

Van Camp AJ. Strategies and codes for searching cancer information online. *Database* 1990 Oct;14(5):114–117.

Van Camp AJ. Subject code searching in biomedical databases. *Online* 1990 Jan;14(1):90–94.

Wexler P. HSDB and material safety data sheets. *NLM Tech Bull* 1987;219:10–13.

Wexler P, Goshorn J. Searching RTECS on TOXNET. *NLM Tech Bull* 1987;224:1,5–8.

Wilczynski NL, Walker CJ, McKibbon KA, Haynes RB. Quantitative comparison of pre-explosions and subheadings with methodologic search terms in MEDLINE. *J Am Med Inform Assoc* 1994 Sep;1(5):905–909.

Willis J, Powell T, Passarelli P, Johnston D, Van Lenten B. New MeSH and indexing policy change for 1996 MeSH chemical and pharmacological action headings and Trees. *NLM Tech Bull* 1995;286;9–16.

Wood MS, Horak EB, Snow B, eds. *End user searching in the health sciences.* New York: Haworth Press, 1986.

Yerkey N, Glogowski M. Scattering of library and information science topics among bibliographic databases. *J Am Soc Info Sci* 1990;41(4):245–253.

15

Market Research and
Competitive Intelligence Online

Competitive intelligence means many things to many people. To the uninitiated, the phrase may conjure up cloak and dagger images of industrial espionage or, at the very least, unethical information-gathering activities. While it is true that stealth and wealth are both involved, much of the spying takes place at the desktop computer. Competitive intelligence professionals today rely heavily on commercial databases to conduct their investigations, substituting online surveillance skills for backstreet vigilance. With potential sales from new molecular entities providing a powerful inducement to use, the high stakes healthcare marketplace has spurred the development of many specialized directories, news sources, and syndicated research reports designed to serve the business research needs of pharmaceutical corporations and industry watchers.

Drugs-in-Development Directories

What is company X currently working on? Who will be launching new cardiovascular drugs in France three years hence? Is anyone testing the application of this mechanism of action to treat condition Y? Do the number and types of compounds corporation Z currently has in clinical trials support their long-term sales predictions? How do they compare with multinational A? If we dedicate more of our resources to this therapeutic area, how long will it be before we can expect a return on our investment? Are there drug delivery technologies we could license to leverage growth in this product line? What new antineoplastic antibiotics have reached phase III? What impact will compounds currently under development have on therapeutic areas our company is targeting? How will these agents, if approved, affect the commercial viability of products we're currently working on?

447

Answers to questions such as these require resources designed for R&D pipeline assessment. A very distinctive type of online database is needed. It must provide access by company names (both originators and licensees), drug categories (therapeutic or pharmacological), country names (targeted markets), stages of development (lab to launch), and coordinate any or all of these factors with one another. Ideally, it would provide historical timeline data, recording dates of significant milestones such as transition from preclinical to clinical investigations, passage through trial phases, and filing of documents necessary for approval with government authorities. Pointers to the primary scientific literature on specific compounds would be helpful, both a few starter references and sufficient nomenclature to retrieve others. The source should also offer leads to patent applications, enabling follow-up investigations into claims, intellectual property protection, and expected expiration.

Most important of all, it should maintain constant and timely surveillance of current pharmaceutical research activities worldwide, updating information on individual compounds as soon as it is available. That one such paragon among competitive intelligence resources could exist would be welcome news. That an entire family of such files is, in fact, readily accessible online today is definitely a cause for rejoicing. The impressive collection includes: *Pharmaprojects*, *IMSworld R&D Focus Drug Updates*, *ADIS R&D Insight*, *NME Express*, *Drug Data Report*, *Drugs of the Future*, *Investigational Drugs Database* (*IDdb*), and *NDA Pipeline*.

15.1 *Pharmaprojects*. Richmond, Surrey, England: PJB Online Services, 1980–. Updated weekly. Available on DataStar, Dialog, Ovid, and STN; also on CD-ROM.

The oldest, in terms of online availability, of these drugs-in-development directories is *Pharmaprojects*, a database compiling records for products in active development since 1980. Produced by the publishers of the respected newsletters *Scrip* and *Clinica*, *Pharmaprojects* reports on the progress of drugs from early preclinical studies through each phase of clinical trials, on to preregistration with government authorities in various countries, approval (registration), and final launch. Subsequent investigations into new uses and important changes in formulation affecting therapeutic applications are also monitored. Discontinued, withdrawn, or suspended development, whether for commercial or toxicological reasons, is documented. Out of a total of more than 27,700 records, approximately 6,400 represent products actively in development, but not yet on the market anywhere in the world. Pharmaprojects monitors progress toward introduction in any of twenty-eight countries generally considered to be major world markets.

Every one of the access points identified above as desirable attributes of a competitive pipeline assessment research tool is included in this database (see Figure 15.1). Individual records list originating company, licensees, pharmacological action, therapeutic applications under investigation, and stage of development

Figure 15.1   Sample Pharmaprojects Record Online

DIALOG(R)File 128:PHARMAPROJECTS
© 1999 PJB Publications,Ltd. All rts. reserv.

0020009
DRUG NAME: cytarabine, DepoFoam
ORIGINATOR: DepoTech (USA) [Pre-registration]
LICENSEE: Chiron [Pre-registration]
              Pharmacia & Upjohn [Pre-registration]
SYNONYMS: ara-C, DepoTech
              cytarabine, DepoTech
              DepoCyt
              DTC-101
              Savedar
CHEM NAME: 2(1H)-Pyrimidone, 4-amino-1-beta-D-arabino furanosyl- (CAS)
CAS REG NO: 147–94–4

TEXT: DepoTech is developing a sustained-release formulation of cytarabine (DepoCyt), using its DepoFoam encapsulation technology (qv), for intra-CSF therapy of leptomeningeal metastases (Scrip, 1994, 1904, 26 and 1995, 1991, 16; Company communication, DepoTech, Feb 1995).

Marketing

Chiron has exclusive marketing rights in the US (Scrip, 1994, 1915, 10). Pharmacia and Upjohn (PandU) has exclusive marketing and distribution rights outside the US in return for an initial upfront cash payment and regulatory milestones totalling up to US$19 million and a share of net product sales. DepoTech retains manufacturing rights and remains responsible for clinical development and US registration. PandU will be responsible for regulatory filings outside the US (Scrip, 1997, 2249, 11; Press release, DepoTech, Jul 1997). DepoTech and Chiron filed a US NDA for the treatment of neoplastic meningitis (NM) arising from solid tumours, leukaemia and lymphoma, but the FDA declined to recommend approval (Press releases, Chiron, Apr and Dec 1997; Scrip, 1997, 2249, 11). The FDA then agreed to accept data from the one pivotal Phase III trial and from a 30-patient Phase IV trial in solid tumours, but subsequently declined approval again due to inadequate information (Scrip, 1998, 2317, 13; Press release, Chiron, May 1998). A subsequently filed US NDA has been recommended for accelerated approval for intrathecal treatment of lymphomatous meningitis, a subtype of NM (Press release, DepoTech, Nov 1998). An approval application has been filed in Canada for the treatment of NM arising from solid tumours. Orphan drug status has been awarded for NM (Scrip, 1994, 1904, 26; 1997, 2267, 22 and 1998, 2317, 13; Company communications, DepoTech, Nov 1994 and Aug 1995; Company pipeline, PandU, Nov 1997). A centralized EU application has been withdrawn (Scrip, 1998, 2381, 10).

Clinical

A 40 patient, non-controlled Phase IV trial in solid tumours treated with 2x 50mg q 2wk is ongoing (Scrip, 1998, 2317, 13). A trial is also being conducted in Europe (Scrip, 1996, 2144, 19). In Phase III trials in Canada and the US for the treatment of NM arising from solid tumours, DepoCyt showed an increased response rate and extended survival cf standard therapy (36% of 25 evaluable patients treated with DepoCyt had CRs cf 17% of 29 evaluable patients with methotrexate) (Company communications, Chiron and Depo-Tech, Aug 1995; Scrip, 1996, 2144, 19; Press releases, Chiron, Jun 1996 and DepoTech, Nov 1996). Additional analysis of these Phase III results demonstrated a median survival of 168 days for DepoCyt-treated patients cf 87 days for methotrexate-treated patients, and a mean time to progression of 108 days and 48 days, respectively (Scrip, 1996, 2178, 26). A response rate of 47% was seen in 15 patients receiving DepoCyt cf 6% for those on methotrexate, and the mean survival time was 227 days (cf 68 days for methotrexate) (Company communication, Chiron, Aug 1995). In 12 patients with leptomeningeal metastases, ventricular and lumbar CSF cytarabine concentrations were maintained for 3.6 and 14 days, respectively, following intrathecal lumbar administration of DepoCyt (29th ASCO (Orlando), 1993, Abs 505). DepoCyt is in Phase I trials in paediatric patients with advanced meningeal malignancies (Scrip, 1997, 2213, 27). Updated by WM on 24/11/1998.

STATUS:	World	Pre-registration
	Austria	Phase III Clinical Trial
	Belgium	Phase III Clinical Trial
	Canada	Pre-registration
	Denmark	Phase III Clinical Trial
	France	Phase III Clinical Trial
	Greece	Phase III Clinical Trial
	Ireland	Phase III Clinical Trial
	Italy	Phase III Clinical Trial
	The Netherlands	Phase III Clinical Trial
	Portugal	Phase III Clinical Trial
	Spain	Phase III Clinical Trial
	Sweden	Phase III Clinical Trial
	UK	Phase III Clinical Trial
	USA	Pre-registration
	Germany	Phase III Clinical Trial

THER. CLASS:	F1K	(Formulation, anticancer)
	K1C	(Anticancer, antimetabolite)
ORIGIN:	CH-SY	(Chemical synthesis, synthetic)
RTE OF ADMIN:	P-SP	(Parenteral, intraspinal)
INDICATIONS:	Cancer, brain; Meningitis	
PHARM. CODE:	DNA-SYN-AN, Physiological, Biochemical, DNA synthesis inhibitor, Antimicrobial e.g. quinolones, Antineoplastic e.g. cytarabine, cy-	

tosine arabinoside, Antineoplastic e.g. dactinomycin, Antimicrobial
e.g. aciclovir, P-B-DNA-SYN-AN

	Therapy	Pharmacology	Status
LINKING:	F1K	NA	Pre-registration
	K1C	DNA-SYN-AN	Pre-registration

RATING:	NOVELTY: 1 (New formulation of established compound)
	DEVELOPMENT SPEED: 1 (Slower than average development speed for therapy)
	MARKET SIZE: 2 (Therapeutic category market $501–2000 million worldwide)
	TOTAL RATING: 4 (Overall rating of novelty + market size + speed)
UPDATED:	19930528 New Product
	19930528 Licensing Opportunity (Worldwide)
	19940415 Status changed (Phase III Clinical Trial)
	19940506 New Licensee (Chiron)
	19961220 Registration submission (The US)
	19970131 Registration submission (The US)
	19970516 Change in Licensee Status (Chiron, Pre-registration)
	19970704 Licensing Opportunity (Additionally worldwide except the US)
	19970725 New Licensee (Pharmacia and Upjohn)
	19971003 Change in Licensee Status (Pharmacia and Upjohn, Pre-registration)
REVISED:	19981127; 1998

reached in each country targeted as a potential market. Beginning in 1999, indication keywords, routes of administration, and terms identifying the origin of each compound (e.g., natural products, chemical synthesis, biologicals) were added to *Pharmaprojects* records. Clinical trial summaries, supported by bibliographic references, highlight results of studies conducted and usually cite at least one reference to the primary scientific literature, such as a conference paper. Many *Pharmaprojects* records also include patent application numbers, countries, and dates. As information is updated on a given compound, historical milestones are meticulously noted (e.g., year and month of entry into Phase III, dates of subsequent development stage changes). Stages recorded include

preclinical
phase I clinical trial
phase II clinical trial
phase III clinical trial
clinical trial

pre-registration
registration
launched
discontinued
suspended
withdrawn

"Clinical trial" is used when studies in humans are known to be under way, but the precise phase is unknown. Each stage descriptor can be precisely coordinated with a country, with a company, with a therapeutic class, or with a pharmacological descriptor code. Country of origin (headquarters of originating company) is also searchable, as are various types of drug names (chemical, generic, brand, or lab codes). CAS registry numbers have been assigned to 45% of *Pharmaprojects* records. More than 18,100 parent companies and other organizations (laboratories, clinics, universities, government agencies) are indexed.

Drug therapeutic categories are based on the European Pharmaceutical Market Research Association (EPhMRA) anatomic/application classification, which *Pharmaprojects* has adapted and refined to reflect projected uses of agents currently under investigation. For example, PJB has added codes for various types of formulations and drug delivery systems (category F) not identified in the original EPhMRA scheme. Other supplements to EPhMRA include separate classification of immunological products (I), anticancer compounds (K), and biotechnology products (T). With a structure reminiscent of the Trees in *MEDLINE* and *EMBASE*, therapeutic codes assist retrieval of related categories of products. An extract from a portion of this hierarchical scheme devoted to cardiovascular products (C) will illustrate its potential.

C1D	Coronary therapy
C1D1	Coronary vasodilators
C1D3	Antiangina agents
C2	Antihypertensives
C2B1	Antihypertensives, adrenergic
C2B2	Antihypertensives, renin system

Introduction of codes, versus keywords, into strategies to retrieve therapeutic classes of drugs will serve to bring together records for products with related uses without resort to keying in alternative phrases. For example, by truncating C1D, products classified either as coronary vasodilators or antiangina agents can be isolated. Entry of C alone retrieves records for all cardiovascular products (single letter codes are automatically "cascaded or "exploded" in *Pharmaprojects*).

The database is unique among the drugs-in-development directories in having introduced a separate hierarchical classification scheme to index each product's mechanism of action, thus enabling searches on classes of drugs with similar pharmacological profiles. Using this feature, it is possible to identify and quantify the different approaches under study to achieve the same therapeutic outcome. Furthermore, comparing results of pharmacology codes linked with different stages of development will show which modes of action appear to be leading to marketable drugs. With a given drug activity as a starting point, you can also survey the range of potential therapeutic indications and perhaps identify an opportunity for expanding the scope of clinical investigations. This could, in turn, lead to new sources of revenue for compounds already in the pipeline.

15.2 *IMSworld R&D Focus Drug Updates.* London: IMS Global Services, 1977–. Updated weekly. Available on DataStar, Dialog, and STN; also on CD-ROM.

Known for sixteen years as *Drug License Opportunities, R&D Focus* was renamed in 1992 when it was made available for the first time for searching on an ad hoc basis. Prior to that time, this database was marketed only through subscription to a private online service. *R&D Focus* is well known for its timely and detailed reporting on new pharmaceutical products. Its geographic scope is more extensive than *Pharmaprojects*, monitoring progress through the pipeline in more than forty countries. This directory contains more than 18,800 drug entries, with at least 7,700 documenting active investigations of products not yet launched.

Although records assemble all items on the wishlist that began this section, *R&D Focus* differs from *Pharmaprojects* in several ways. More company information is provided by IMSworld, which routinely identifies both parent and subsidiary names of originators and licensees (parent companies only in *Pharmaprojects*). More than 14,270 companies and organization names are indexed. *R&D Focus* patent data are generally more extensive than found in the PJB file and often include not only application numbers, countries, and dates, but also a summary of their implications from a commercial standpoint. As a drug draws nearer to launch, *R&D Focus* tends to provide more discussion of its market potential, rather than focusing solely on reporting scientific findings. Another enhancement introduced in 1997 is bibliographic references drawn from *EMBASE* to support IMS scientific summaries.

CAS registry numbers have been assigned to 36% of records. Stage keywords differ in *R&D Focus* compared to *Pharmaprojects* in subtle ways that are important to the searcher of both files.

Stage keywords in IMSworld R&D Focus	**Counterparts in Pharmaprojects**
preclinical	preclinical
phase I	phase I clinical trial
phase II	phase II clinical trial
phase III	phase III clinical trial
clinicals	clinical trial
pre-registration	pre-registration

registration	registration
marketed	launched
discontinued	discontinued
suspended	suspended
withdrawn	

Note that "clinicals" is used when the specific phase is unknown, and that the word "clinical" does not accompany each phase indicator. This distinction means that while the *Pharmaprojects* user can retrieve all drugs in clinical trials, regardless of phase, simply by entering *clinical*, a comparable strategy in *R&D Focus* requires *phase OR clinicals*. Note, also, that the word *marketed* is preferred in the IMSworld file, rather than *launched*.

EPhMRA categories are, once again, the basis of drug classification. Users should not assume, however, that options available are identical from file to file, as is illustrated when the extract below is compared with codes used in *Pharmaprojects*.

EPhMRA codes in IMSworld

R&D Focus		**Codes in Pharmaprojects**	
C1D	Coronary therapy	C1D	Coronary therapy
C1E	Nitrates and nitrites	C1D1	Coronary vasodilators
C1F	Positive inotropic agents	C1D3	Antiangina agents
C2	Antihypertensives	C2	Antihypertensives
C3	Diuretics	C2B1	Antihypertensives, adrenergic
		C2B2	Antihypertensives, renin system

Although C1D represents products intended for coronary therapy in both databases, the separate codes for vasodilators and antiangina agents seen in *Pharmaprojects* are omitted in *R&D Focus*. On the other hand, *R&D Focus* offers codes for nitrates and nitrites and for positive inotropic agents, while *Pharmaprojects* does not. The entire category of cardiovascular products is searchable with the same single letter (C) in both databases, but must be truncated in *R&D Focus* to "cascade" or "explode" (i.e., retrieve related entries). Why has *Pharmaprojects* modified the EPhMRA scheme as shown in these extracts? Major changes were made in 1994, when *Pharmaprojects* introduced its separate mechanism of action classification scheme. At that time, EPhMRA codes that expressed pharmacological concepts were eliminated as redundant (e.g., positive inotropic agents, diuretics, beta blockers).

In contrast, *R&D Focus* searchers intent on surveying possible therapeutic applications for compounds with a given pharmacological profile will find that better known action-indication combinations are already coordinated within the drug category coding scheme (e.g., diuretics-cardiovascular use, as shown above). Those not precoordinated can be searched as keywords in the Action segment of records. Because words, rather than codes, are used to identify pharmacological concepts in *R&D Focus*, synonyms may be needed to retrieve records for drugs with similar modes of action described in different ways (e.g., agonist OR stimulant, antagonist OR inhibitor OR blocker).

Just as significant is a difference in the way the two directories coordinate access points. In *R&D Focus*, stage keywords can be directly linked with countries, as shown in Figure 15.2. Other factors, such as company name, therapeutic class, or pharmacological action, can be brought into no closer relationship than the Boolean AND expresses (i.e., in the same record). In contrast, *Pharmaprojects* offers direct and detailed linkage capabilities between company and stage indicators and between stage indicators and specific therapeutic or pharmacological hierarchical classification codes (with their built-in explode capability). This type of precision may not be needed in all competitive intelligence queries, but enhanced coordination capabilities are important to bear in mind when answering certain types of information requests.

15.3 *ADIS R&D Insight*. Auckland, NZ: ADIS International, 1992–. Updated weekly. Available on DataStar, Dialog, Ovid, and STN; also on CD-ROM.

ADIS R&D Insight is a newer pipeline directory, launched online in January 1996. With more than 5,900 out 14,100 total records documenting products actively under development, this database is comparable in size and scope to *Pharmaprojects* and *IMSworld R&D Focus Drug Updates* (when the latter are limited to research in progress, versus launched or discontinued projects). However, several features set the ADIS file apart from its competitors. One extra is that *R&D Insight* uses the World Health Organization's therapeutic classification scheme, in addition to EPhMRA code indexing. Another bonus is that a thesaurus of controlled keywords has been developed to provide consistent and predictable descriptors for two other important product attributes: indications and mechanism of action. (Both keyword lists are available for immediate full-text display free of charge on the DataStar search system.)

Furthermore, *ADIS R&D Insight* offers direct linkage between stage of development, indication, and target markets (see Figure 15.3). In addition, each record in *R&D Insight* includes a commercial summary from Lehman Brothers, who forecast eventual value with an estimated sales figure (in U.S. dollars). As a product nears the end of the pipeline, a launch date will appear in this section of *R&D Insight* records, as well as a patent expiration date.

A portion of *R&D Insight* records especially attractive to end users is the concluding bibliography of references to primary sources. Instead of only a few citations embedded in textual discussion, as found in directories described thus far, ADIS entries typically list many more journal articles, giving full bibliographic details (author, title, source, volume, pagination, date) for easy follow-up. These starter references save time and provide needed back-up documentation for ex-

Figure 15.2   Sample Record from IMSworld R&D Focus Drug Updates

---

DIALOG(R)File 445:IMSWorld R&D Focus
(c) 1999 IMSWorld Publ. Ltd. All rts. reserv.

02000901
Drug Name: cytarabine ocfosfate; phosteabine sodium
Brand Name: STARASID
R&D Focus— February 02, 1998 (980202)

COMPANY INFORMATION:
   Originator: Yamasa Shoyu; (Japan); NA; licensor; NA
   Licensee/Licensor: Nippon Kayaku; (Japan); NA; licensee; Japan
                          ASTA Medica Kayaku; (Germany); ASTA Medica :
                          Nippon Kayaku; licensee; Europe
   Patent Assignee: Nippon Kayaku
                          Yamasa Shoyu

DRUG INFORMATION:
   CAS Registry Number: 73532–83–9, cytarabine ocfosfate; 65093–40–5, mono-
                          sodium salt; 116459–64–4, monosodium salt monohy-
                          drate
   Laboratory Code: YNK 01; C18PCA
   Pharmacological Action: antimetabolite; nucleoside analogue
   Therapeutic Class Code: L1B (Antimetabolites)
   Clinical Indications: cancer
   Chemical Name: 4-amino-1-|5-O-|hydroxy(octadecyloxy)phosphinyl-beta-
                          D-arabinofur anosyl 2(1H)-pyrimidinone

LATEST INFORMATION:
   In a phase I study of cytarabine ocfosfate (YNK 01), conducted by ASTA Medica in
Germany, 2 of 23 patients with acute myelogenous leukemia (AML) showed complete
responses, 4 partial, and 3 stable disease. Of 20 patients with non-hodgkins lymphoma, 2
showed partial responses, and 6 stable disease. Diarrhea grade 3–4 was seen in 2 patients
with AML at 1200 mg.

CURRENT DEVELOPMENT STATUS:
   Highest Phase: Marketed (80)
   Development Phase/
   Country/Indication: Marketed, Japan
                          Phase II, Europe

DEVELOPMENT HISTORY:
   JAN 1993: Marketed, Japan. Phase II, Europe.
   SEP 1991: Pre-registration, Japan. Phase I, Europe.
   FEB 1990: Phase III, Japan.
   FEB 1988: Phase II, Japan.
   1986: Product patent priority appln Japan

ABSTRACT:

Records selected from EMBASE, copyright, and used with permission of Elsevier Science B.V., Amsterdam. AUTHORS: KOGA K.;IIZUKA E.;SATO A.; EKIMOTO H.;OKADA M. AUTHOR'S ADDRESS: PHARMACEUTICALS GROUP, ANTICANCER DRUGS DEPARTMENT, NIPPON KAYAKU CO. LTD., 3–31–12 SHIMO, KITA-KU, TOKYO 115 TITLE: CHARACTERISTIC ANTITUMOR ACTIVITY OF CYTARABINE OCFOSFATE AGAINST HUMAN COLORECTAL ADENOCARCINOMA XENOGRAFTS IN NUDE MICE JOURNAL: CANCER CHEMOTHER. PHARMACOL. 1995 36/6 (459–462) EMBASE NUMBER: 95291463

AUTHORS: UEHARA T. AUTHOR'S ADDRESS: DEPARTMENT OF INTERNAL MEDICINE, TOKYO MEDICAL COLLEGE, TOKYO TITLE: APPROPRIATE DOSES OF CYTOSINE ARABINOSIDE (ARA-C) AND CYTARABINE OCFOSFATE (SPAC) IN HIGH DOSE ARA-C THERAPY AND ORAL SPAC THERAPY FOR HEMATOLOGICAL MALIGNANCIES JOURNAL: J. TOKYO MED. COLL. 1995 53/4 (523–530) EMBASE NUMBER: 95284151

Single copies of the full text of the above records are generally available from EMDOCS. To place an order, call +1–800–282–2720 or +1–212–301–4003, fax +1–212–301–4060, or email dds@work4u.artx.com

COMMERCIAL SUMMARY:

The antimetabolite anticancer drug, cytarabine ocfosfate, is marketed in Japan by Nippon Kayaku under license from Yamasa Shoyu, and is indicated for the treatment of hematological malignancies resulting from osteomyelodysplasia. The joint venture company, ASTA Medica Kayaku, which was set up in 1991 between Nippon Kayaku and ASTA Medica, is conducting phase I/II trials with this agent in Europe and will eventually apply for product registration in Europe. Phase II studies are also planned in Europe with cytarabine ocfosfate as maintenance therapy in elderly patients with AML in first remission and for a further six weeks with interferon alpha2b in patients with newly diagnosed CML. Clinical studies are planned in the USA (IMS, SEP 1997). Cytarabine ocfosfate is a prodrug of cytosine arabinoside.

SCIENTIFIC SUMMARY:

Cytarabine ocfosfate is a cytosine arabinoside derivative and is the first orally active drug of this chemical series. In vivo mouse xenograft studies suggest it may be useful for induction and/or post-operative chemotherapy against colorectal adenocarcinomas (Koga, K. et al, EMBASE: 95291463). In a phase I study cytarabine ocfosfate shows one compartment pharmacokinetics and a mean half life of 32 h. This compares with a half life of 2.4 h for a conventional dose of cytarabine. Further pharmacokinetics data suggest cytarabine ocfosfate should be given in doses of 200–300 mg/day (Uehara, T., EMBASE: 95284151). In patients with acute or myelogenous leukemia, MDS or non-Hodgkin's lymphoma cytarabine ocfosfate is well tolerated up to a dose of 1200 mg, with a bioavailability of around 16%. Mild toxicity is seen at dose levels of 900 mg daily over 14 days and the dose-limiting toxicity is diarrhea. For hematological malignancies, a suggested oral dose is 200–300 mg/day (Uehara, T. et al, EMBASE: 95284151). Responses have been seen in patients with AML, low-grade NHL and MDS, as well as patients with CML who received combination therapy with interferon. In patients with AML (n = 23), 9% show complete responses, 17% partial, and 13% stable disease. In patients with NHL (n = 20), 10% show partial responses, and 30% stable disease. Diarrhea grade 3–4 is seen in patients with AML at 1200 mg (39th ASH, abs 1473, DEC 1997).

PATENT SUMMARY:
   Product: EP 239015 B 1991, priority JP 63963 1986, designating 8 states.
   Equivalents identified in 6 countries.

---

tensive summaries of preclinical and clinical studies, adverse events, pharmacokinetics, and pharmacodynamics included in preceding sections of each record. Particularly user-friendly is numbered cross referencing from statements in the text to specific cited works.

Longer (nine-digit) numbers following selected citations in each bibliography indicate the availability of more complete and structured study summaries in the *ADIS LMS Drug Alerts Online* (14.12) database. All of these cross references are compiled at the end of each record in the XR paragraph to facilitate rapid carryover into *LMS* by use of "mapping" (an automatic strategy formulation, saving, and execution function built into DataStar and Dialog software). When a user maps XRs from *R&D Insight*, there is no need to conduct a subject keyword or author/title search to locate companion records in *LMS Drug Alerts*. This exploitation of the synergy between two databases supplied by the same publisher is an innovative response to requests for more information that inevitably arise after pipeline directory consultation.

15.4 *NME Express*. Barcelona, Spain: J.R. Prous, 1993–. Updated biweekly.
      Available on DataStar and Dialog.

NME Express from Prous focuses on identifying new molecular entities just entering the R&D pipeline. Compounds represented are novel, biologically active molecules revealed for the first time in current journal literature (1,500 titles scanned per year), congresses (more than 150 meetings attended annually), and company communications. As soon as these drug prospects are cited by lab code number or chemical name, they are added to *NME Express*. Because coverage is restricted to new molecular entities, this drugs-in-development directory is much smaller in size than others discussed thus far (approximately 1,500 records). One company name (usually the originator, rather than a licensee) is provided in each entry and only one drug classification is assigned (see Figure 15.4). Prous has developed its own set of codes and keywords to facilitate drug category searching, a combination of therapeutic and pharmacological descriptors. For example,

           29000   antiarrhythmic agents
           30000   antianginal agents, antihypertensive agents

Figure 15.3   Sample Online Record from ADIS R&D Insight

---

1 ADRD [DataStar]

AN 00001191 960726.
TI Pramipexole.
SO Adis R&D Insight.
SY Generic name: Pramipexole
Synonyms: SND 919, SND 919Y
Chemical name: (S)-2-Amino-4,5,6,7-tetrahydro-6-(propylamino)-benzo-thiazole.
RN 104632–26–0.
MF C10 H17 N3 S.
CC N4A (Anti-Parkinson Drugs), N5A (Neuroleptics), N6A (Anti-Depressants/Thymo-analeptics).
AC N04B-C (Dopamine agonists), N05A-X (Other antipsychotics), N06A-X (Other anti-depressants).
ME Dopamine D2 receptor agonists, Dopamine receptor agonists.
CO Originator:
Boehringer Ingelheim (Germany).
Licensee(s):
Pharmacia & Upjohn.
PA Boehringer Ingelheim.
OT Nonindustrial source.

PH

Phase	Country	Indication
Preregistration	USA	Parkinson's disease.
Phase III	Germany	Affective disorders.
Phase III	USA	Affective disorders.
Phase III	Europe—unknown countries	Parkinson's disease.
Phase III	Europe—unknown countries	Schizophrenia.
Phase II	USA	Schizophrenia.
Clinical (Phase Unknown)	Japan	Affective disorders.
Clinical (Phase Unknown)	Japan	Parkinson's disease.
Clinical (Phase Unknown)	Japan	Schizophrenia.

HP Preregistration.
HI 22-Jul-96: Phase-III for Affective disorders in USA (Unknown route)
12-Jun-96: A preclinical study has been added to the Affective Disorders pharmaco-dynamics field (445479)
23-May-96: A study in patients with Parkinson's disease has been added to the therapeutic use field (437521)
16-Feb-96: Phase-III for Affective disorders in Germany (Unknown route)
30-Jan-96: Preregistration for Parkinson's disease in USA (Unknown route)
27-Oct-95: A study in patients with Parkinson's disease has been added to the therapeutic trials and side effects fields (389147)
22-Aug-95: Clinical-Phase-Unknown for Parkinson's disease in Japan (Unknown route)
22-Aug-95: Clinical-Phase-Unknown for Affective disorders in Japan (Unknown route)
22-Aug-95: Clinical-Phase-Unknown for Schizophrenia in Japan (Unknown route)

22-Aug-95: Phase-II for Schizophrenia in USA (Unknown route)

22-Aug-95: Phase-II for Affective disorders in USA (Unknown route)

22-Aug-95: Phase-III for Parkinson's disease in USA (Unknown route)

20-Jul-95: Phase-II for Affective disorders in Europe—unknown countries (Unknown route)

20-Jul-95: Phase-III for Parkinson's disease in Europe—unknown countries (Unknown route)

20-Jul-95: Phase-III for Schizophrenia in Europe—unknown countries (Unknown route).

CS Parkinsons/dopamine agonist

Company	Major Markets	Launch Date	Commercial Value	Patent Expiry
B Ingelheim	Wrld	95	$50–100m sup (p)	

Footnote description

p–product sales total

SU Pharmacodynamics:

Antipsychotic activity; potential antiparkinsonian and antidepressant activity

Mechanism of action:

Dopamine D2 receptor agonists

Dopamine receptor agonists.

IT Introduction:

Pramipexole (SND 919, SND 919Y) is a dopamine D sub(2) autoreceptor agonist structurally related to talipexole (BHT 920). Pramipexole may also possess D sub(1) and D sub(3) agonist activity. Pramipexole is currently in phase II/III clinical trials with Boehringer Ingelheim in Germany as a potential antipsychotic agent. It is also undergoing phase II/III trials for Parkinson's disease and phase II/III trials for depression. Clinical trials in the treatment of Parkinson's disease have been conducted in the USA in association with Pharmacia & Upjohn, and an NDA for this indication has recently been submitted. Fukuoka University is also conducting clinical trials in Japan.

AE Adverse Events:

In a trial involving patients with acute exacerbation of schizophrenia, pramipexole was associated with fewer and less severe extrapyramidal adverse events/1/.

In 28 parkinsonian patients treated with pramipexole for 9 weeks, reported adverse events included asymptomatic hypotension (n = 28), dizziness (12), headache (9), nausea (6), insomnia (6), hallucinations (4), abnormal vision (3) and dry mouth (3). Nine patients experienced dose-limiting adverse events in the titration phase of the trial. ECG changes in pramipexole recipients included prolonged PR intervals (n = 1) and an asymptomatic increase in premature ventricular beats (1). No clinically significant abnormalities in laboratory parameters were observed/2/. In a trial involving 360 Parkinson's disease patients, the rate of treatment discontinuation was similar in pramipexole and placebo recipients. An increase in hallucinations and dyskinesias was reported/3/.

PC   Pharmacodynamics (Affective Disorders):
Low doses of pramipexole produced locomotor hypoactivity in rats; this was anta-gonised by spiperone. At higher doses, the compound caused hyperactivity which was antagonised by haloperidol, sulpiride and clozapine, but not SCH 23390. Repeat-edly administered pramipexole potentiated D-amphetamine- and quinpirole-induced locomotor hyperactivity. Pramipexole antagonised reserpine + alpha-methyl-p-tyro-sine-induced akinesia. It potentiated the hyperkinetic activity of L-DOPA in both naive and monoamine-depleted rats. When administered alone, pramipexole de-creased immobility time in the forced swimming test. Combined administration with imipramine or amitriptyline produced a greater effect than any of the compounds alone. The compound had no effects at alpha sub(1) or alpha sub(2) adrenoceptors or at serotonin sub(2) receptors/4/.
Pharmacodynamics (Psychotic Disorders):
Preclinical studies: SC injection of pramipexole 25–500 mug/kg (and talipexole) in rats produced yawning responses (inhibited by D sub(2) antagonists such as spiper-one) and reduced both basal and stimulated prolactin levels.
[portion of text omitted here]

TR   Parkinson's Disease and Movement Disorders:
In a double-blind study, 55 patients with early Parkinson's disease, who were not receiving levodopa therapy, were randomised to pramipexole 0.30–4.5 mg/day or placebo for 9 weeks. Activities of Daily Living scores on the Unified Parkinson's Disease Rating Scale (UPDRS) were significantly improved in pramipexole recipi-ents compared with placebo. A trend in favour of pramipexole was also observed for the motor examination scores of the UPDRS/8/. A placebo-controlled, multicentre, randomised study which enrolled 360 patients evaluated the efficacy of pramipexole in levodopa-treated PD patients with motor fluctuations. After a > 6-month treatment with pramipexole less than or equal to 4.5 mg/day, there were significant (p less than or equal to 0.01 vs placebo) improvements in the UPDRS part II on (18 vs 1%), part II off (24 vs 5%) and part III (25 vs 12%), as well as significant (p less than or equal to 0.01 vs placebo) reductions in levodopa dosage (25 vs 6%), mean time off (31 vs 8%) and severity of time off (17 vs 8%)/3/.
Psychotic Disorders:
Comparative studies: In a dose-ranging study, the efficacies of 3 dosages of prami-pexole (0.3, 0.75 and 3 mg/day for 6 weeks) were compared with that of haloperidol 15 mg/day. Haloperidol was more effective than pramipexole (at any of the 3 dos-ages). Efficacy was assessed using changes in the Brief Psychiatric Rating Scale, Schedule for Assessment of Positive Symptoms, Schedule for Assessment of Nega-tive Symptoms and Clinical Global Impressions scores/1/.

CR   1. Lecrubier Y. A dose response study of SND 919 vs haloperidol in the treatment of schizophrenia. Neuropsychopharmacology. 10 (Suppl. Part 1): 124, May 1994. (English)
2. Davis TL, Roznoski M, et al. Acute effects of COMT inhibition on L-DOPA phar-macokinetics in patients treated with carbidopa and selegiline. Clinical Neurophar-macology. 18: 333–337, Aug 1995. (English). 800389146
3. Lieberman A, Pramipexole Advanced PD Study Group. Efficacy and safety of pramipexole in advanced Parkinson's disease patients with the wearing-off phenome-non. Neurology. 46 (Suppl.): 475, Feb 1996. (English). 800437521

4. Maj J, Rogoz Z, et al. Pramipexole, a selective dopamine receptor agonist with potential antidepressant activity. European Neuropsychopharmacology. 6 (Suppl.1): 11– 12, Apr 1996. (English). 800445479

5. Carter AJ, Muller RE. Pramipexole, a dopamine D2 autoreceptor agonist, decreases the extracellular concentration of dopamine in vivo. European Journal of Pharmacology. 200: 65–72, 23 Jul 1991. (English).

6. Brooks DP, Weinstock J. The pharmacology of pramipexole in the spontaneously hypertensive rat. European Journal of Pharmacology. 200: 339–341, 6 Aug 1991. (English). 800096336

7. Schilling JC, Adamus WS, et al. Neuroendocrine and side effect profile of pramipexole, a new dopamine receptor agonist, in humans. Clinical Pharmacology and Therapeutics. 51: 541–548, May 1992. (English).

8. Hubble JP, Koller WC, et al. Pramipexole in patients with early Parkinson's disease. Clinical Neuropharmacology. 18: 338–347, Aug 1995. (English).800389147.
XR 800389146 800437521 800445479 800096336 800389147.
ED 960722.

Figure 15.4   Sample Record from NME Express

DIALOG(R)File 456:NME Express
© 1996 J.R. Prous, S.A. All rts. reserv.

0002614 238010
DRUG NAME: MDL-101628
PROUS LIST NUMBER: 9615
COMPANY: Hoechst Marion Roussel
LANGUAGE: English
TEXT: MDL-101628, from Hoechst Marion Roussel, is a potent inhibitor of neutral endopeptidase with potential as a treatment for hypertension [Warshawsky, A. M. et al., 25th Natl Med Chem Symp (June 18–22, Ann Arbor) 1996: Abst 87]. The compound is described in patent literature (US 5430145).
CLASSIFICATION: 34620 (Neutral Endopeptidase Inhibitor)
CHEMICAL NAME:
   7(S)-[2(R)-Sulfanyl-3-phenylpropanamido]-6-oxo-1,2,3,4,6,7,8,12b(R)-
   octahydropyrido[2,1-a]-2-benzazepine-4(S)-carboxylic acid

31250	beta-adrenergic blocker
31260	alpha-adrenergic blocker
31270	alpha- and beta-adrenergic blocker
31300	vasodilator

No attempt is made in *NME Express* to record subsequent changes in developmental status or to relate basic drug discovery data with its commercial implications, such as countries where the prospective product might eventually be marketed or licenses pending or granted. The text of each record briefly summarizes the drug's action and potential application in therapy. As in *Pharmaprojects* and *IMSworld R&D Focus*, at least one lead into the primary scientific literature is usually provided, in the form of a bibliographic citation, a patent application number, or both. No CAS registry numbers are offered as access points.

Yet, despite its comparatively lean and mean appearance as a competitive awareness research tool, *NME Express* complements coverage offered in other directories by conveying results of systematic screening of the patent literature. It can often provide early warning of significant new discoveries not yet documented in other directories.

15.5 *Drug Data Report*. Barcelona, Spain: J.R. Prous, 1988–. Updated monthly. Available on DataStar and Dialog; also on CD-ROM.

Literally hundreds of patent applications dealing with potential new drugs are published each month, and thousands of compounds are covered within the scope of these patents. In *Drug Data Report* (*DDR*), Prous identifies as "preferred" compounds those with specific pharmacological properties actively under investigation. Prous also constructs briefer secondary records for other chemical entities cited in patents. *DDR* includes references to more than 20,000 patents obtained from scans of applications to eleven authorities: Belgium, Canada, France, Germany, Great Britain, Japan, Spain, Switzerland, the United States, the World Patent Office, and the European Patent Office. The resulting database contains more than 92,300 directory entries, of which 1,700 show active investigation underway. Scientific meetings, company communications, and a collection of more than 1,500 journal titles also contribute to material summarized in *Drug Data Report*, which compiles more than 100,000 references to the primary (nonpatent) literature. A sample record is reproduced in Figure 15.5.

The bare bones approach of *NME Express* is here fleshed out to include a molecular formula, chemical name, lab code, and generic name, when available, as well as the latest (highest) phase of development reached. The originating company, licensees (if any), and all applicable descriptors for the drug's action and potential uses under investigation (not just one, as was found in *NME Express*) are also identified in *DDR*. CAS registry numbers have been assigned to 4% of records. Graphic formulas (displayable, but not searchable) enhance approximately 98% of the Prous drug monographs.

The textual portion of *DDR* entries tends to be briefer than that provided in *Pharmaprojects* or *IMSworld R&D Focus*, consisting of a concise description of biological activity deduced from reports of investigations published thus far. Development status information is also comparatively sparse, in that only the latest (highest) stage achieved is documented, with no retention of historical detail about when previous milestones were reached. Some consolation can be derived

Figure 15.5   Sample Record from Drug Data Report Online

DIALOG(R)File 452:Drug Data Report
© 1999 J.R. Prous S.A. All rts. reserv.

00153878
ENTRY NUMBER: 153878
COMPOUND TYPE: Preferred
DRUG NAME: C18PCA
                  YNK01
GENERIC NAME   Cytarabine ocfosfate
                  Fosteabine sodium hydrate
BRAND NAME: Starasid (Nippon Kayaku, JP)
CHEM NAME: 1-beta-D-Arabinofuranosylcytosine 5'-stearyl phosphate mono
                  sodium salt monohydrate
FORMULA: C27H49N3NAO8P.H2O
CAS REG. NO.:   65093–40–5 (anhydrous)
                  116459–64–4
                  73532–83–9 (anhydrous, free acid)

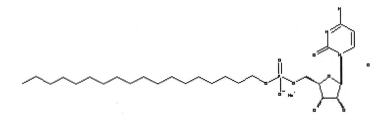

DEVEL. PHASE: Launched (1992)
ORIGINATOR: Nippon Kayaku
LICENSEE: Asta Medica
                  Yamasa Shoyu
CLASS: 75000 (Oncolytic Drugs (Miscellaneous))
                  75100 (Antimetabolites)
RELATED ENTRY: 103983 (non-specific)
PREV. PUB. IN: Drugs of the Future, Vol. 14, No. 11, p. 1056, 1989

PATENTS:

MEDICINAL COMPOSITION FOR INHIBITING CANCER METASTASIS TO LIVER
AND MEDICINAL COMPOSITION FOR CURING HEPATOMA
AUTHOR(s):   Ekimoto, H., Kobayashi, F., Kusano, S., Okamoto, K., Sasaki, H.,
                  Satoh, A.

APPLICANT(s):   Nippon Kayaku

FAMILY:	654269	[EP 654269]	European Patent Office, May 24, 1995
	6–107548	[JP 6107548]	Japan, April 19, 1994
	WO94–03183	[WO 9403183]	W.I.P.O., February 17, 1994
PRIORITY:	4–232699	[JP 92232699]	Japan, August 10, 1992
	5–170850	[JP 93170850]	Japan, June 18, 1993

REFERENCES:

Sato, T., Morozumi, M., Kodama, K., Kuninaka, A., Yoshino, H., "Sensitive radioimmunoassay for cytarabine and uracil arabinoside in plasma," Cancer Treat Rep 1984,68: 1357–66

Nakagawa, Y., Yamashita, K., Watanabe, K., Koga, R., Asakawa, N., Takayama, H., Kodama, K., Saito, K., Watanabe,Y., "Metabolism of YNK01," Xenobiotic Metabolism and Disposition 1987,2: 420

Kodama, K., Morozumi, M., Saitoh, K., Kuninaka, A., Yoshino, H., Saneyoshi, M., "Antitumor activity and pharmacology of 1-beta-D- arabinofuranosylcytosine 5'-stearylphosphate: An orally active derivative of 1-beta-D-arabinofuranosylcytosine," Jpn J Cancer Res 1989,80(7): 679–85

Yamada, K., Fukuoka, M., Masaoka, T., Kimura, I., Kimura, K., "Phase I and early phase II study of 1-beta-D-arabino- franosylcytosine-5'-stearyl phosphate (YNK01)," 16th Int Cong Chemother (June 11–16, Jerusalem) 1989, 52.

[62 additional references omitted in this example]

Braess, J. et al., "Phase I study of oral cytarabine-ocphosphate (YNK01) in AML and NHL—Pharmacokinetics and clinical results," Blood 1997,90(10, Suppl. 1, Part 1): Abst 1473

Blanco, M.D., Trigo, R.M., Garcia, O., Teijon, J.M., "Controlled release of cytarabine from poly(2-hydroxyethyl methacrylate-co-N-vinyl-2-pyrrolidone) hydrogels," J Biomater Sci-Polym Ed 1997,8(9): 709

---

from the fact that *DDR* is the only one of these directories identifying compounds in "biological testing," a stage in drug development even earlier than preclinical.

Perhaps as a result, the other end of the pipeline receives less attention. Target markets are completely ignored, precluding linkage of development stage with individual countries to assess future competition at the national level. Information on licensing companies is sometimes omitted, even when available in other directories.

But, what follows the basic nomenclature, identification, and summary information that researchers have come to expect in such a directory is the real bonus:

information on the patent family protecting the discovery, presented in an easy-to-read tabular format, and, in many records, a list of bibliographic references. As a drug proceeds through the pipeline, the length of bibliographies provided can be extended to as many as sixty core citations to respected journals. Although a patent family and bibliography are included only in Prous records for preferred compounds, the prospect of their availability prompts many competitive intelligence researchers to pull *DDR* records for drugs already identified elsewhere. Furthermore, cross-file surveys inevitably reveal that *Drug Data Report* also includes products not identified in other databases.

15.6 *Drugs of the Future.* Barcelona, Spain: J.R. Prous, 1990–. Updated
     monthly. Available on DataStar and Dialog; also on CD-ROM.

A third pipeline directory from Prous, *Drugs of the Future*, limits its scope to compounds judged to be the most promising new therapies. More than 1,600 records similar to that shown in Figure 15.6 make prospective products accessible by the various types of nomenclature expected in such files, as well as by highest (latest) development stage reached worldwide, originating company, and therapeutic/pharmacological classification codes and keywords. Once again, specific phases linked with target markets are conspicuously absent. The emphasis seen in other Prous files on chemistry, versus commercial development, is exemplified here.

Monographs in *Drugs of the Future* include detailed summaries of synthesis, cross referenced to structural illustrations of schemes of synthesis available for separate display. For compounds recently launched or in the final stages of clinical research, links to "Context Table" records are also included. These unique entries graphically illustrate structure/activity relationships within a given product class, lining up structures of compounds with comparable actions and applications to assist in quick comparisons. For example, the Context Table for antiplatelet therapy begins with three formulas for cyclooxygenase inhibitors, four for thromboxane A2 antagonists, two for thromboxane synthase inhibitors, and so on.

Records in *Drugs of the Future* summarize clinical and preclinical study data in the same detail shown in *Adis R&D Insight*. Textual statements are meticulously cross referenced to numbered citations in bibliographies concluding each monograph. Basic patent information is typically included among references cited, enabling follow-up, if desired.

15.7 *Investigational Drugs Database (IDdb).* London: Current Drugs Ltd,
     1995–. Updated weekly. Available on the Internet at http://www.
     current-drugs.com.

The *Investigational Drugs Database* takes a different approach to compiling pipeline data. Information is presented in the form of tabular reports targeting either drug classes, individual companies, or patent families. Elements in each

Figure 15.6   Sample Record from Drugs of the Future Online

DIALOG(R)File 869:Drugs of the Future
© 1997 J.R. Prous S.A. All rts. reserv.

00203961
ENTRY NUMBER: 203961 (Actively Investigated)
DRUG NAME: BMS-180291 sodium salt
   BMS-180291–02
GENERIC NAME   Ifetroban sodium (recommended INNM; USAN)
CHEM NAME: (+)-(1(S)-(1alpha,2alpha,3alpha,4alpha))-3-(2-(3-(4-(N-Pentyl-carbamoyl)oxazol-2-yl)-7-oxabicyclo(2.2.1)hept-2-ylmethyl) phenyl)propanoic acid monosodium salt
   (+)-(1S-(exo,exo))-2-((3-(4-((n-Pentylamino)carbonyl)-2-oxazolyl)-7-oxabicyclo(2.2.1)hept-2-yl)methyl)benzenepropanoic acid monosodium salt
FORMULA: C25H31N2NAO5
CAS REG. NO.:   143443–90–7 (free acid)
   156715–37–6

DEVEL. PHASE: Phase II
ORIGINATOR: Bristol-Myers Squibb
CLASS: 37200 (Platelet Antiaggregatory)
   37231 (Thromboxane Antagonist)
SYNTHESIS: 236186
CONTEXT TABLE: 37200C (Antiplatelet Therapy)

Synthesis

BMS-180291 sodium salt was prepared from optically active 7-oxabicyclo(2.2.1)heptane lactol (I) as shown in Scheme 1. The interphenylene side chain was introduced by deprotonation of (I) with ethylmagnesium bromide (0.95 eq.) followed by treatment with excess aryl Grignard (II) to afford crystalline diol (III). The extraneous benzylic hydroxyl group in (III) was removed by reduction with hydrogen in the presence of Pearlman's catalyst to give alcohol (IV).

Transformation of the alpha-side chain silyloxy carbinol to a carboxy methyl ester was accomplished by initial protection of the omega-side chain alcohol as the acetate (Ac2O/py) followed by oxidation under Jones conditions and then exposure of the resulting crude acetate-acid to methanolic hydrogen chloride to afford crystalline alcohol-ester (V). Oxidation of (V) under Jones conditions furnished acid-ester (VI).

The oxazole side chain was introduced into (VI) via serine-derived amino alcohol (VII). Standard coupling of acid (VI) with (VII) mediated by water-soluble carbodiimide (EDAC) gave amide (VIII). Acyclic side chain intermediate (VIII) was converted into oxazole (X) in three steps by mesylation followed by treatment with triethylamine to furnish cyclized oxazoline (IX). Dehydrogenation of (IX) employing a novel oxidative protocol (1) involving treatment with a mixture of copper (II) bromide and 1,8-diazabicyclo(5.4.0)undec-7-ene (DBU) in chloroform/ethyl acetate solvent yielded oxazole (X). Saponification of (X) followed by acidification afforded (XI) (BMS-180291) as a white solid which could be purified by recrystallization from acetonitrile.

The water-soluble sodium salt was available as a precipitate from (XI) by treatment with sodium methoxide/methanol in acetone.

Description

Free acid: white solid, m.p. 148–50 C (CH3CN).

Sodium salt: white solid, m.p. 248–50 C (CH3OH/acetone).

Introduction

Thromboxane A2 (TxA2) and prostaglandin endoperoxides (PGH2) are potent, short-lived arachidonic acid metabolites which induce platelet aggregation and smooth muscle contraction via activation of TxA2/PGH2 (TP) receptors (2). These and other agonists at TP receptors have been implicated in the pathogenesis of cardiovascular, renal and pulmonary diseases. Preclinical studies have indicated that TP receptor antagonists with pharmacokinetic and pharmacodynamic properties suitable for chronic administration may serve as useful therapeutic agents in these areas. However, the clinical efficacy of this class of agents has yet to be demonstrated, in part due to limitations of potency, specificity and/or pharmacokinetics of the examples that have previously been advanced to clinical trials (3, 4).

BMS-180291 is the result of over a decade of synthetic, pharmacological and metabolism studies focused on substituted 7-oxabicycloheptanes. Pioneering work in this area led to the identification of oxabicycloheptanes SQ-28,668, SQ-29,548 and SQ-30,741, all of which are selective, short-acting agents with lesser TP receptor-antagonistic potency. Structural modification of the alpha-side chain to suppress rapid metabolic deactivation via beta-oxidation and the introduction of a novel 4-amido oxazole into the omega-side chain has resulted in compounds with increased antagonistic potency and, importantly, a long duration of action (5). We describe from this series BMS-180291 as an orally active, potent, selective and long-acting TP receptor antagonist with a pharmacological profile suitable for evaluating the clinical efficacy of this class of agents (6).

Pharmacological Actions

BMS-180291 is a potent and highly selective antagonist of TP receptors in vascular and airways smooth muscles and in platelets (6).

BMS-180291 inhibited TP receptor-dependent platelet aggregation in an insurmountable manner, but it inhibited TP receptor-dependent platelet shape change competitively. Although BMS-180291 blocked platelet activation in response to arachidonic acid and the TP receptor agonists, U-46,619 and I-BOP, it did not inhibit ADP- or the primary wave of collagen-induced platelet aggregation, which is consistent with its being a selective TP receptor antagonist. (3H)-BMS-180291 bound with high affinity (kd i 3 nM) in a slowly, but completely reversible manner to a single class of specific binding sites in washed human platelets. This is different from GR-32,191, which recognizes two classes of platelet binding sites, from which its binding to one is not readily reversible.

[portion of text omitted here]

Pharmacokinetics and Metabolism

In rats, BMS-180291 showed 25% oral bioavailability at a dose of 3 mg/kg, with the maximal plasma concentration of about 600 nM being reached very early, approximately 5 min post-dose. Following the distribution phase, plasma concentrations declined with a terminal half-life of 7.7 h. Since intestinal absorption was at least 86%, a significant first-pass elimination appeared to be operating. The Vdss value of 3 l/kg is consistent with extensive distribution of BMS-180291 into tissues. More than 90% of the radioactivity was recovered in feces following intravenous dosing of (3H)-BMS-180291, indicating primarily biliary elimination. Less than 3% of the radioactivity was recovered in urine. Essentially the same percentages of biliary and urinary excretion of radioactivity were seen with dogs.

[portion of text omitted here]

Manufacturer

Bristol-Myers Squibb (USA).

In a double-blind, randomized, placebo-controlled study in 63 healthy male volunteers given BMS-180291 (10–1000 mg p.o.), pharmacokinetic results indicated rapid absorption, a long half-life consistent with once-daily dosing and enterohepatic recirculation. Therapy was well tolerated, with no severe side effects over the dose range studied. (17)

In a double-blind, placebo-controlled study in 45 healthy male volunteers, ifetroban sodium (10–500 mg once daily for 9 days) was well tolerated, with dose-proportional pharmacokinetics, a long half-life (about 17 h) and no accumulation. Marked, dose-dependent ex vivo antiplatelet effects without excessive prolongation of bleeding time were reported. (20)

[portion of text omitted here]

PREV. PUB. IN: Drugs of the Future, Vol. 19, No. 2, p. 107, 1994

REFERENCES:

1. Barrish, J.C.; Singh, J.; Spergel, S.H.; Han, W.-C.; Kissick, T.P.; Kronenthal, D.R.; Mueller, R.H., "Cupric bromide mediated oxidation of 4-carboxyoxazolines to the corresponding oxazoles," J Org Chem 1993, 58: 4494–6.

2. Hamberg, M.; Svensson, J.; Samuelsson, B., "Thromboxanes: A new group of biologically active compounds derived from prostaglandin endoperoxides," Proc Natl Acad Sci USA 1975, 72: 2994–8.

[remaining references omitted in this example]

41. Liao, W.; Manning, J.; Panting, L.; Delaney, C.; Norton, J.; Williams, S.; Ogletree, M.; Hammett, J.; Swanson, B.; Uderman, H., "The ex-vivo anti-platelet potency of ifetroban and aspirin," Pharmacology 97 (March 7–11, San Diego) 1997, Abst 47.

42. Misra, R.N.; White, R.E.; Ogletree, M.L., "Ifetroban Sodium," Drugs of the Future, Vol. 19, No. 2, p. 107, 1994 (Synthesis Scheme available. SEE 236186).

table are hotlinked to supportive references, including literature evaluations, discovery research commentaries, and current opinions prepared by Current Drugs staff, as well as hypertext links to pertinent *MEDLINE* records. The database covers more than 13,600 investigational drugs, including at least 640 launched products and 2,570 compounds where development has been discontinued.

IDdb incorporates a structural search capability. It also integrates a diverse range of optional current awareness services, such as a daily Internet news bulletin, weekly updates from scientific meetings, and new additions each week to the *Investigational Drug Patents Fast-Alert* file profiled in Chapter Sixteen (16.6). *EMBASE Alert* is another choice offered to *IDdb* subscribers.

15.8 *NDA Pipeline.* Chevy Chase, MD: FDC Reports, 1991–. Updated monthly. Available on DataStar and Dialog.

NDA Pipeline in hardcopy format was discussed in Chapter Four (4.20). The online database has the advantage of monthly, rather than annual, updates and more ways to access information than are possible in the printed publication. FDC monitors the progress of all drugs and biologic products undergoing clinical development with a goal of marketing in the United States. *NDA Pipeline* also includes products already approved since its online launch in January 1991. This database includes more than 15,800 records, of which approximately 11,000 document active investigations.

NDA Pipeline is compiled from original data collected by investigative reporters on the staff of FDC Reports (also responsible for the timely, in-depth coverage offered in *The Pink Sheet*). FDC journalists regularly attend meetings of FDA drug evaluation panels and briefings by financial analysts, as well as conduct interviews of company representatives. Other published sources from which *NDA Pipeline* data are derived include company reports, Securities and Exchange Commission (SEC) filings, press releases, research findings published in major scientific journals, and official new drug listings issued by the FDA.

Although much more limited in scope than worldwide drugs-in-development tracking sources, *NDA Pipeline* cites specific milestones within the U.S. regulatory process that other directories do not. For example, more information is included on Abbreviated New Drug Applications, such as date of suitability petition filing for ANDA and date of FDA response. Entries for products designated as orphan drugs can easily be isolated, with date of orphan designation and date of marketing approval, if granted.

Other access points include drug names (lab codes, generic names, brands), company names (originators or licensees, parents or subsidiaries, dependent on the likely NDA applicant), current status (phase or stage), and drug category terms. Vocabulary for the latter is based on *U.S. Pharmacopeia* (11.8) keywords, expressing either pharmacological action or therapeutic use.

Rather than compiling all information on a given compound into one record, *NDA Pipeline* typically divides status and indication data into separate entries when a drug is under investigation for multiple therapeutic applications. Thus, for the product featured in Figure 15.7, there were additional records showing different phase indicators for other indications (e.g., Phase III-antischizophrenic, Phase II-antidepressant).

Another difference is that text paragraphs in *NDA Pipeline* focus on commercial, rather than scientific, details, such as joint development or marketing agreements, expected NDA filing dates, or current regulatory status abroad. Cross ref-

Figure 15.7   Sample Online Record from NDA Pipeline

DIALOG(R)File 189:NDA Pipeline: New Drugs
© 1996 F-D-C Reports Inc. All rts. reserv.

00005435   F-D-C Accession Number   14N05435
The NDA Pipeline.   F-D-C Reports, Inc.
July 19, 1996

DRUG NAME: pramipexole dihydrochloride
GENERIC DRUG NAME: pramipexole dihydrochloride
DESCRIPTORS: treatment for Parkinson disease

COMPANY: Boehringer Ingelheim Corporation; Boehringer Ingelheim Pharmaceuticals, Inc.
CAS REGISTRY NUMBER: 104632–26–0
SUBFILE: DIR (Drug in Research)
STATUS: NDA filed 12/95 –ACTIVE
THERAPEUTIC CATEGORY: Nervous system—antiparkinsonian

LICENSING INFORMATION: Licensed to Pharmacia & Upjohn for co-development and worldwide marketing.
CROSS REFERENCE: "The Pink Sheet" 11/23/92 page 1

erences to *The Pink Sheet* (4.49, 15.10) are frequently included for a head start on competitive trade and industry follow-up investigations, but citations to the scientific literature are rarely offered. Patent information is sometimes, but not always, provided in *NDA Pipeline* entries online.

A complementary resource on the Internet is a *New Medicines in Development Database* offered free of charge at the Pharmaceutical Research and Manufacturers of America (PhRMA) Web site (http://www.phrma.org/webdb). Searchable by disease, indication, or drug name, it provides access to basic information about products in the pipeline in the United States. Each entry identifies the factors itemized here as searchable elements, as well as developing company and U.S. status (e.g., phase II). Entries are also dated, to help users gauge the accuracy of stage or phase data. Given its limited geographic scope and minimal information provided, the primary audience for PhRMA's database is the consumer or casual investigator. It would be a good place to gain an overview of pipeline trends, but could not be relied upon for in-depth business intelligence.

Summary of Key Differences in Pipeline Directories

Annotations in this section have emphasized distinguishing factors among these databases: 1) overall size (number of records), 2) geographic scope, and 3) record content and access points. Pricing will also, undoubtedly, influence source selection, but cannot easily be summarized here, because it is dependent on hardcopy subscriber status, search system accessed, user affiliation with academia or industry, and on what portions of records are displayed. However, content and searchability can, and should, be compared with a view to maximizing search efficiency. (Note: *IDdb* was not available for hands-on evaluation and has, therefore, been excluded from the following discussion.)

Because the ability to search for large categories of drugs is critical to competitive assessments, all pipeline directories offer some form of drug classification (use, target disease, or action). Although *Pharmaprojects*, *IMSworld R&D Focus Drug Updates*, and *ADIS R&D Insight* all base their "use" indexing on the same anatomic/therapeutic scheme originally developed by the European Pharmaceutical Market Research Association (EPhMRA), each file has introduced variations. It's important to remember that EPhMRA codes are not necessarily equivalent in each source.

Prous databases use their own classification system, a mixture of therapeutic and pharmacological terminology, but Prous generally applies codes less rigorously. For example, only one category is assigned per record in *NME Express*, and codes should definitely be augmented with keywords in strategies. Recall from codes in *Drug Data Report* and *Drugs of the Future* can also be considerably enhanced by using synonyms. Least accessible of all by drug category, *NDA Pipeline* demands creative lists of terms to anticipate numerous variations found in product records.

When drug action, as well as application, is needed, *Pharmaprojects* offers the most detailed hierarchical indexing. *ADIS R&D Insight* also provides controlled and consistent mechanism-of-action access, but lacks hierarchical (explode) capabilities. Still another type of product categorization that may be requested is indication, which requires isolation of functional subsets from more broadly defined therapeutic groups by focusing on specific diseases or conditions to be treated (e.g., thrombosis, leukemia, angina). The best directories for this type of search are *IMSworld R&D Focus* and *ADIS R&D Insight*, because both consistently assign vocabulary drawn from a published and predictable list. (Note: each uses its own, separately published thesaurus.)

Ideally, a drugs-in-development database will cross-tabulate or precoordinate target market(s) with stage of development and indications or actions. Information on these factors influences decisions regarding where, when, and for what use(s) a competing product should plan submissions. *ADIS R&D Insight* provides the most precise search and display capabilities in this respect, coordinating country with status for each indication under investigation. Next, in order of accessibility, is *Pharmaprojects*, which links phase with both mechanism of action and therapeutic use, but segregates target market and stage indicators into a separate portion of records. *Drug Data Report* and *Drugs of the Future* identify just the highest phase reached, with no linkage to indications and no mention of potential market. Remember, however, that *DDR* focuses on notices of first entries into the pipeline and is the only directory with a stage indicator for biological testing. Confined to U.S. product candidates, *NDA Pipeline* cannot be meaningfully compared to other directories with regard to status indexing. *NME Express* is similarly disqualified from evaluation on this point, because it does not index either status or market at all.

Assessment of commercial potential is another obvious difference among these directory databases. In general, *IMSworld R&D Focus* devotes more space and effort to this area of competitive intelligence, routinely summarizing licensing and other collaborative agreements, as well as projecting launch dates and sales data as a product proceeds through the pipeline. *ADIS R&D Insight* presents comparable data unaccompanied by textual discussion. In contrast, such information is totally absent from Prous files, but is included in *Pharmaprojects* records when a drug nears launch.

Accessibility ratings related to patent protection data shift the spotlight to *Drug Data Report*, with its inclusion of full patent citations and families in the majority of preferred compound records. Next in line comes *IMSworld R&D Focus*, which may include only one or two patent numbers (not full citations), but often complements its coverage with notes on possible intellectual property issues. Third choices would be *Drugs of the Future*, *Pharmaprojects* and *NME Express*, each of which often (but not always) cites at least one patent number and priority. *ADIS R&D Insight* offers no patent information.

Knowing how each file handles company name indexing is critical to search success. *IMSworld R&D Focus* is the easiest to use in this respect, because it consistently identifies both parent companies and subsidiaries (when applicable) for both originators and licensees. *Pharmaprojects* requires more advance home-work (and supplies user aids to support it), because it consistently prefers parent company names in indexing either originators or licensees. *ADIS R&D Insight* generally includes the parent company for originators, but not for licensees. *Drug Data Report* usually lists parents, along with subsidiaries, for originating organizations (does not distinguish which name is which), but is less thorough in its identification of licensees. *Drugs of the Future* is similar in this respect. *NME Express* is somewhat inconsistent in company name indexing, but usually confines itself to identification of parent originating companies; licensees are rarely cited. *NDA Pipeline* uses "applicant name" for entries, which equates to a diverse and fairly unpredictable company name field.

User wishlists in pharmaceutical intelligence always ask for development history and record updating information. Cumulative analysis of timeline data can assist in educated guesses about competitor launches, which can prompt reevaluations of project priorities and reallocation of internal resources to support them. *Pharmaprojects* fulfills both of these requirements by providing thorough recaps of development stage transitions and always disclosing when each record was last updated. *ADIS R&D Insight*, having a shorter publication history, shows fewer retrospective historical milestones, but does include latest record update and precisely delineates what changes to look for in newly enhanced entries. *IMSworld R&D Focus* offers comparatively limited milestone data (although depth varies among entries), but consistently dates records. Neither Prous files nor *NDA Pipeline* include development history. *Drug Data Report* also omits a record update field.

Product name accessibility facilitates both rapid record location and follow-up searches in other online sources. Highest honors in this category go to *Pharmaprojects*, with *ADIS R&D Insight* a close second. Both compile a wealth of alternative nomenclature, making initial product identification easier and providing more synonyms for effective segue into biomedical literature databases. A good test of name accessibility uses all new chemical entities approved for marketing in a given year. Starting with generic nomenclature for thirty-eight NCEs registered in 1995 in any of eleven countries worldwide, a total of 179 proprietary names could be located in April 1996, using a variety of online sources discussed in these pages. When the comparative contributions of each database were measured against this gold standard cumulative list, their relative performance (number of names accessible, expressed as a percentage of the total) was:

Pharmaprojects	75%
ADIS R&D Insight	74%
Drug Data Report	72%
IMSworld R&D Focus	65%

Drugs of the Future had yet to be launched at the time of this comparison. *NDA Pipeline* was omitted, due to its relatively limited (geographic) scope. However, it's interesting to note that when the same test was applied to the CAS registry file (*CHEMSEARCH*), only 38% of names were found. *Merck Index Online* contributed just 16% of names available for 1995 NMEs.

These data have implications not just for ease of follow-up in literature files, but also for search sequencing among pipeline directories. Standard operating procedure is, after all, not to limit competitive intelligence searches to just one directory, but rather to create composite reports based on information drawn from (and carefully cross checked among) multiple files. Starting a search in sources richer in nomenclature will assist users in locating complementary records in less readily accessible databases.

If composite data analysis and report preparation are typical sequelae to directory consultation, so, too, are searches for back-up bibliography. Decision makers need to know more about types of trials conducted and study findings, as these may disclose strengths and vulnerabilities that could be usefully addressed in competing product research. Can, for example, adjustments in patient population or dosage form and regimen carve out a profitable niche in the potential market? It is "not enough to identify critical competitors and their stage of developments. Often key attributes . . . advantages and disadvantages may be identified which prove very beneficial in differentiating one's own product. Designs of pivotal trials can be modified *a priori* in order to attempt to obtain slightly different labeling from regulatory agencies. . . ."[1] *ADIS R&D Insight*, *Drug Data Report*, and *Drugs of the Future* all provide excellent starter lists of references from which to work, growing in extent as a drug progresses through the pipeline. ADIS records also include much more detailed discussion of investigations, providing summaries of adverse events, pharmacokinetics, and pharmacodynamic data and results of preclinical and clinical studies. Moreover, when cross references to *ADIS LMS Drug Alerts Online* are pursued, further details about study design are immediately available for analysis.

Taken together, the drugs-in-development directories are a formidable set of research tools for competitive intelligence in the pharmaceutical industry. One company, BizInt Solutions, was quick to recognize the value of pooling results from individual pipeline databases and offering users the ability to construct tables for detailed analysis. *BizInt Smart Charts* provides an interface to searching three online directories with the objective of creating, sorting, and formatting various types of tabular reports. The highly sophisticated, but user-friendly software currently works with *Pharmaprojects*, *IMSworld R&D Focus*, and *Adis R&D Insight*, with Current Drugs' *IDdb* file soon to be added to the list of compatible resources. Data from another IMS publication online, *New Product Launches* (15.18), can also be incorporated into *Smart Charts* reports, as can information extracted from the *Incidence & Prevalence Database* (15.39).

By integrating results of cross-file queries in these complementary resources, users can prepare composite reports on individual compounds, analyze research in progress in an entire therapeutic category, survey a single company's R&D pipeline and compare it with that of others, uncover potential new applications for compounds with a given pharmacological activity, or identify methods that could cut development time from lab to launch. Indeed, applications for information found in these files are as diverse as the new chemical entities and treatment modalities they are designed to monitor.

Tracking Pharmaceutical News Online

Keeping up-to-date on business developments is just as challenging as current awareness monitoring of the scientific literature. Fortunately, when the business is health care, there are several outstanding sources specifically created to convey important news rapidly and in a convenient format.

15.9 *Pharmaceutical and Healthcare Industry News Database (PHIND)*. Richmond, Surrey, England: PJB Online Services, 1980–. Updated daily. Available on DataStar, Dialog, Ovid, and STN.

By far the best known newsletter in the pharmaceutical industry is a publication called *Scrip*. Its title is a highly appropriate *double-entendre*; "scrip" is a synonym both for "prescription" and for paper currency (i.e., money). This neatly expresses the subject matter: drug business news that will affect revenue. Issued twice a week in paper copy format since 1972, *Scrip* entries first appear online in the *Pharmaceutical and Healthcare Industry News Database (PHIND)*. Daily updates to *PHIND* enable users to preview full *Scrip* contents days before printed copies may reach their desks. This has ensured a large audience of dedicated online readers. The full text of all articles is available for immediate display, and each keyword is separately searchable. This feature enables prescreening of newsletter contents for items of interest that may not be uncovered in perusal of article titles alone. It also assists quick location of relevant items in *Scrip* back issues, incorporated into *PHIND* from January 1982 forward.

The *PHIND* online database also contains the full text of *Clinica World Medical Device and Diagnostic News*, *Animal Pharm World Animal Health and Nutrition News*, *BioVenture View*, and the European Pharma Law Centre publication *ERA News* (4.58). As with *Scrip*, online access to the contents of these sources predates paper copy publication by days (or weeks). Pharmaceutical companies typically license the rights to download and redistribute the contents of *Scrip* to interested personnel through internal electronic mail. Similar subscription agreements are common in the medical device industry, where *Clinica* is an essential current awareness source.

Why are these PJB newsletters so popular, as eagerly awaited each morning as the daily newspaper? The answer lies in their scope and timeliness. *Scrip* and

Clinica report on a broad spectrum of scientific, political, regulatory, and financial news of vital interest to their respective drug and device industry audiences. Coverage includes informed commentary, critical evaluation of current events, and trend analysis. *BioVenture View* focuses on news events in the biotechnology industry. *ERA News* (formerly *EPLC Update*) highlights developments in European regulatory affairs likely to affect the human and animal drug or device markets.

15.10 *F-D-C Reports*. Chevy Chase, MD: FDC Reports, 1987–. Updated weekly. Available on DataStar, Dialog, and Ovid.

In addition to *Scrip*, pharmaceutical business personnel generally regard *The Pink Sheet* (4.49) as compulsory reading to remain *au fait*.[2] Discussed in the context of regulatory affairs in Chapter Four, this newsletter's formal title is: *Prescription Pharmaceuticals and Biotechnology*. Its publisher, FDC Reports, is the source of a widely read series of current awareness newsletters, each published on colored paper. Titles include *Medical Devices, Diagnostics, and Instrumentation* (*The Gray Sheet*, 4.45); *Toiletries, Fragrances, and Skin Care* (*The Rose Sheet*, 4.53); *Health Policy and Biomedical Research* (*The Blue Sheet*, formerly *Drug Research Reports*, 4.56); and *Nonprescription Pharmaceuticals and Nutritionals* (*The Tan Sheet*, 4.52). The full text of each of these publications is available online in the *F-D-C Reports* database, which also includes *Pharmaceutical Approvals Monthly* (4.21) from September 1995 forward.

All of these specialty titles provide up-to-date information on companies, products, markets, personnel, regulatory and legislative activities, financial performance, and scientific or legal developments of importance to businesses involved in health care in the United States. FDC's reporting on FDA activities, U.S. professional and trade association news, and managed care organization issues is particularly thorough, filling in gaps left by *Scrip* and *Clinica*, which have a more Eurocentric slant.

15.11 *Health News Daily*. Chevy Chase, MD: FDC Reports, 1989–. Updated daily. Available on DataStar and Dialog.

Health News Daily (*HND*, 4.55), another respected publication of FDC Reports, offers more timely coverage of topics that will often also be covered later (in greater depth) in one of the other newsletters contained in the *F-D-C Reports* database online. Regular "departments" in each *HND* issue are retained in the machine-readable version of the newsletter, making browsing online as easy as in the paper copy. Recurring sections include product news, people, litigation, legislative news, industry news, research, regulatory news, financing, reimbursement, and public health. A section devoted to Washington This Week lists scheduled Congressional hearings, U.S. government agency meetings, and industry conferences immediately forthcoming in the District of Columbia area. The Calendar section compiles notices of forthcoming meetings, conferences, and seminars slated throughout the United States during the coming months. "Legislative Roundup" tracks Congressional bills, committee activities, and votes on health-care legislation.

Due to the time sensitive nature of much of the material, pharmaceutical and device companies usually contract for daily feeds of *HND* and weekly electronic delivery from the *F-D-C Reports* database, thus licensing downloading, controlled redistribution, and limited archiving rights to needed data without violation of copyright.

15.12 *IMSworld R&D Focus Drug News*. London: IMS Global Services, 1991–. Updated weekly. Available on DataStar, Dialog, and STN.

R&D Focus Drug News is comparable to *Scrip* in its subject scope, but has the added advantage, from the online searcher's perspective, of controlled indexing. The unvarnished truth about full-text sources online is that they are wonderful for systematic current awareness, combining convenient document delivery with redistribution capabilities (subject to copyright observance), but they can also be quite difficult to search. When background on a specific fact, event, or issue is needed, users must construct strategies that take into account all the quirks and quiddities of the English language. Ambiguity is rife, acronyms and abbreviations are the Scylla and Charybdis of the full-text database user, and unsuspected synonyms set further snares for the unwary. It is easy to miss pertinent material hidden under alternative terminology not included in a full-text strategy, and it is equally easy to retrieve totally irrelevant items due to unpredictable double meanings, metaphors, and keyword occurrence outside the context desired. These characteristics of full-text files are widely acknowledged, leading to frequent requests from users for value-added controlled indexing.

In *R&D Focus Drug News*, IMS has responded by systematically identifying company names, therapeutic categories of drugs cited, and typical events in descriptors ending each record. These enhancements mean that results of subject searches in the database are usually more precise than would be possible in many other full-text news files. Regular newsletter sections cover drug approvals and launches, pipeline news, conference news, company news (acquisitions, collaborations), biotechnology, and a listing of newly reported drugs entering the *R&D Focus Drug Updates* (15.2) database.

15.13 *Drug News & Perspectives*. Barcelona, Spain: J.R. Prous, 1988–. Updated monthly. Available on DataStar and Dialog.

Prous, the providers of *NME Express* (15.4) and *Drug Data Report* (15.5), also publish a monthly news journal entitled *Drug News and Perspectives*. The online database of the same name, launched in 1995, is not a direct full-text counterpart of the hardcopy journal. It is both more selective and more inclusive. The online version of *Drug News & Perspectives* (*DNP*) omits feature articles published in each printed issue, and focuses, instead, on archiving material drawn from recurring sections or columns in the journal. In doing so, *DNP* has also drawn from its internal archives, and includes many previously unpublished records omitted in print due to space limitations or because they represent items awaiting publication in a forthcoming issue. More than 72% of *Drug News & Perspectives* records online have not, or will not, appear in the hardcopy counterpart.

DNP subject sections online include Licensing Line (January 1995–), Line Extensions (July 1993–), New Product Introductions (January 1995–), NMEs This Month (current), People on the Move (January 1992–), R&D Briefs (January 1992–), and The Year's New Drugs (January 1988–). The latter are lengthy review articles, published on an annual basis, that offer an historical and evaluative perspective on new product introductions worldwide.

15.14 *PharmacoEconomics & Outcomes News*. Auckland, NZ: ADIS International, 1994–. Updated daily. Available on DataStar and Dialog.

Although not yet required for drug approval, pharmacoeconomics data submissions are already mandated for reimbursement applications under government-subsidized health delivery systems in Australia and Canada. Cost-efficacy and cost-benefit comparisons also play a major role in marketing to managed care organizations in the United States. Knowing what types of studies have been completed by competitors or outside agencies and what validation measures are being used by developers and accepted by prospective purchasers has become increasingly important to ensure commercial success of products still in the pipeline. Integrating pharmacoeconomic evaluations earlier in the development cycle is a rising trend that has, in turn, escalated demands for resources that focus on providing early intelligence and detailed data analysis.

ADIS was the first publisher to produce a full journal entirely devoted to the subject of pharmacoeconomics. More recently, they have begun publishing a weekly newsletter offering rapid access to summaries of important news regarding this very hot current topic. Launched in full-text format online in August 1995, *PharmacoEconomics & Outcomes News* (*PEO News*) offers prepublication previews of items that will later appear in the weekly printed newsletter, as well as retrospective coverage of its contents (and that of its biweekly predecessor *PharmacoResources*), dating from 1994.

A rough simile to characterize *PEO News* content would be "an economic *InPharma*." As does *InPharma* (14.11), *PEO News* provides extremely timely, original, evaluative summaries of papers presented at major international meetings and symposia and of articles published in biomedical journals (more than 2,300 are scanned). But in this case, the focus of such reporting is on cost-efficacy data. Records report on pharmacoeconomic studies of a particular drug or class of drugs, identify regulatory developments pertinent to the issue, and provide critical commentary on the clinical relevance of studies or the implications of government activities. Descriptors added to each record are drawn from the same *ADIS Drugs and Disease Thesaurus* used to index the *InPharma*, *ADIS Reactions* (14.26), and *LMS Drug Alerts Online* (14.12) databases.

15.15 *IAC Newsletter Database.* Foster City, CA: Information Access Company, 1988–. Updated daily. Available on DataStar, Dialog, and STN.

Approximately eighty of the more than 600 newsletters cited in the *IAC Newsletter Database* are devoted to biomedical or pharmaceutical news, and all are accessible cover to cover (excluding graphic data and images). At least thirty-nine of these healthcare titles are not available elsewhere online. Many of them are hidden treasures: specialty newsletters easily overlooked because of their limited hardcopy distribution, but tailor-made for focused current awareness or for background searches on topics such as biotechnology transfer, venture capital financing, medical economics and pharmacoeconomics, or new biomaterials. Notes on selected titles are included in Appendix C. Timeliness, breadth of coverage, and a source selection policy that blends science with business have earned the *IAC Newsletter Database* high marks among most competitive intelligence searchers.

15.16 *ESPICOM Pharmaceutical & Medical Device News.* Chester, England: ESPICOM Business Intelligence, 1995–. Updated daily. Available on DataStar and Dialog.

ESPICOM is the new name of a publisher formerly known as MDIS. Their *News* database is the full-text online counterpart of four hardcopy sources: *MDCA News* (weekly medical device companies analysis), *PCA News* (monthly pharmaceutical companies analysis), *MediStat News* (monthly healthcare market and epidemiological statistics), and *Cancer Drug News* (monthly). Daily updating online provides much earlier access to articles slated for later publication in printed form. This collection is a particularly good source for market intelligence related to healthcare technologies. Other strengths are coverage of emerging markets, such as Eastern Europe or Southeast Asia, novel companies, strategic alliances within the industry, and discussion of market trends. Company financial results, R&D funding, and product developments are regularly featured. Approximately 40% of database records focus on news from Europe, 40% for the USA, and 20% for the rest of the world.

15.17 *Pharmaceutical News Index.* Louisville, KY: UMI Company, 1974–. Updated weekly. Available on Dialog and Ovid.

Pharmaceutical News Index (*PNI*), once a premier source for current awareness, has been overshadowed in recent years by more convenient full-text access offered through other databases discussed in this section of the *Guide*. However, it's important to remember that *PNI* is a source of systematic (cover-to-cover) indexing for a collection of key industry newsletters, including two titles from

FDC not yet incorporated into the *F-D-C Reports* database: *Quality Control Reports-The Gold Sheet* (4.54) and *Weekly Pharmacy Reports—The Green Sheet* (4.57). *Pharmaceutical News Index* provides bibliographic citations (no abstracts) and natural language indexing for these publications from December 1977 to date.

Figure 15.8 identifies other newswatch databases of potential interest to the pharmaceutical market researcher and competitive intelligence professional. The distinction between *IAC PROMT* and the *IAC Newsletter Database* is sometimes confusing. Searchers often assume that, because both are full-text business files produced by the same company, one is merely a subset of the other. While it is true that many of the same titles are found in both databases, the depth of coverage offered can vary considerably. If a title is on the *Newsletter Database*'s source list, cover-to-cover access is usually provided, while *PROMT* may include only selected articles.[3] Another resource that causes some confusion is *Marketletter* (formerly *IMS Marketletter*). This popular publication is available both as a separate file or as one of many titles covered in *IAC PROMT* and the *IAC Newsletter Database*.

Because it is best known for indexing FDA regulatory documents (discussed in Chapter Sixteen), *Diogenes* (16.1) is often undervalued as a source of business oriented news. Yet, part of this "file with the funny name" is a collection of newsletters produced by Washington Business Information, including *Washington Drug Letter*, *The GMP Letter*, *Washington Health Costs Letter*, *The Food & Drug Letter*, *Devices & Diagnostics Letter*, *The Drug GMP Report*, and *European Drug & Device Reports*.

Once discovered, *Business Dateline* is usually also a much favored resource, because of the unique perspective it can provide into local business conditions in many U.S. and Canadian metropolitan areas. Regional business publications included in *Business Dateline* can help uncover investment opportunities, activities of state supported programs such as small business development networks or biotechnology centers, marketing and advertising leads, and even important details about multinational corporations not reported elsewhere.

Probing the Internet for Health Economics and Outcomes Research

To complement coverage offered in *PharmacoEconomics & Outcomes News* and other specialty titles cited in the previous section, users will find that six Internet subject hubs can serve as useful pathfinders to related material on the World Wide Web.

HealthEconomics.Com
⇨ http://www.exit109.com/~zaweb/pjp

Figure 15.8   Pharmaceutical and Health Technology Industry News Sources Online

Database	Availability	Notes
ADIS Reactions Database	1993 to date, updated daily DataStar, Dialog, SilverPlatter	Clinical literature monitoring service focusing on timely identification of adverse effects, interactions, overdose, abuse, and dependency case reports.
Aerzte Zeitung Online	1984 to date, updated weekly DataStar	Full text of the daily medical newspaper *Aerzte Zeitung* and the biweekly journal *Arzneimittel Zeitung*, both in German. Covers new therapies, national and international health policy, company news, and market data.
BioBusiness	1985 to date, updated weekly DataStar, Dialog, Ovid, STN	Bibliographic citations and brief abstracts for references from more than 600 sources, including selective indexing of U.S. patents.
BioCommerce Abstracts and Directory	1981 to date, updated twice monthly DataStar, Dialog, STN	Bibliographic database for monitoring new business applications of biotechnology worldwide. Citations are derived from 100 English-language specialty journals and popular media sources, primarily U.S. and U.K.
BNA Daily News from Washington	1990 to date, updated daily Dialog	Full-text Bureau of National Affairs newsletters focus on government activities. Newsletters online include: *Chemical Regulation Daily*, *Health Care Daily*, *Product Liability Daily*, *Toxics Law Update*, and *Washington Insider*.
Business & Industry	1994 to date, updated daily DataStar, Dialog, SilverPlatter	Mixture of bibliographic records with abstracts and full-text source records, both with value-added controlled indexing. See Appendix C for sample titles.
Business Dateline	1985 to date, updated weekly Dialog	Full text of articles from regional business publications originating in the United States and Canada.
Chemical Business NewsBase	1984 to date, updated weekly DataStar, Dialog, STN	Bibliographic references to market, product, legal and regulatory, and company news.
Chemical Industry Notes	1974 to date, updated weekly DataStar, Dialog, QUESTEL-ORBIT, STN	Bibliographic citations accompanied by brief extracts from business-oriented publications dealing with recent events in the chemical industry.
Diogenes	1981 to date, updated weekly DataStar, Dialog, SilverPlatter	In addition to its coverage of FDA regulatory documents, *Diogenes* provides the full text of newsletters from Washington Business Information and the FDA. Titles include: *Washington Drug Letter*, *The GMP Letter*, *Washington Health Costs Letter*, *The Food & Drug Letter*, *Devices & Diagnostics Letter*, *The Drug GMP Letter*, *European Drug & Device Report*, the FDA *Drug Bulletin* and *Radiological Health Bulletin*.
Drug News & Perspectives	1988 to date, updated monthly DataStar, Dialog	Full text of recurring columns or sections of the J.R. Prous publication of the same name, plus additional items never before published. Licensing, line extensions, new product introductions, NMEs, R&D briefs are regularly featured.

ESPICOM Pharmaceutical & Medical Device News	1995 to date, updated daily DataStar, Dialog	Full text of *MDCA News* (medical device companies analysis), *PCA News* (pharmaceutical companies analysis), *MediStat News* (healthcare market and epidemiological statistics), and *Cancer Drug News.*
European Chemical News	1984 to date, updated weekly DataStar	Full-text online source for monitoring market trends, new technology, company news. Selective coverage of the pharmaceutical and biotechnology industries.
F-D-C Reports	1987 to date, updated weekly DataStar, Dialog, Ovid	Full-text of the key industry newsletters: *The Pink Sheet* (pharmaceuticals), *The Gray* Sheet (medical devices), *The Rose Sheet* (cosmetics and toiletries), *The Tan Sheet* (nonprescription drugs and nutritional products), *The Blue Sheet* (biomedical research news and health policy), and *Pharmaceutical Approvals Monthly.*
Health News Daily	March 1989 to date, updated daily DataStar, Dialog, Ovid	Full-text news items are timely precursors to coverage later offered in *F-D-C Reports.*
IAC Newsletter Database	1988 to date, updated daily DataStar, Dialog, STN	Full text of more than 130 specialized industry newsletters, including biotechnology, pharmaceutical, and healthcare titles. (See Appendix C for sample selections.)
IAC PROMT	1981 to date, updated daily DataStar, Dialog, QUESTEL-ORBIT, STN	Includes a mixture of full-text and bibliographic records with abstracts and provides consistent indexing by SIC code, event, and geographic, product, or company names. Ecumenical in scope, covering more than 2,000 sources. (See sample titles in Appendix C.)
IAC Trade & Industry Database	1983 to date, updated weekly DataStar, Dialog	Full text from more than 200 trade journals, enhanced with company, SIC, and controlled subject term indexing. Additional records provide citations and abstracts for an expanded list of sources.
IMSworld R&D Focus Drug News	1991 to date, updated weekly DataStar, Dialog, STN	Full-text newsletter for monitoring new developments around the world. Value-added indexing includes company names, therapeutic classification, and event keywords.
InPharma	1983 to date, updated daily DataStar, Dialog, SilverPlatter	Full-text, prepublication access to the weekly newsletter of the same title. Reports on clinical developments and new product introductions worldwide.
Marketletter	1985 to date, updated daily DataStar	Full-text file focusing on financial and other commercial news from the pharmaceutical and biotechnology industries (formerly an IMS publication). (*Marketletter* is also available in *IAC PROMT* and *IAC Newsletter Database*.)
PharmaBiomed	1990 to date, updated weekly DataStar	Full text of approximately 30 trade journals from the pharmaceutical, biotechnology, and healthcare industries. A subset of *IAC PROMT.*
Pharmaceutical and Healthcare Industry News Database (PHIND)	1980 to date, updated daily DataStar, Dialog, Ovid, STN	Full-text, prepublication and archival access to the major industry newsletters: *Scrip, Clinica, Animal Pharm, BioVenture View,* and *ERA News.*

| Pharmaceutical News Index | 1974 to date, updated weekly Dialog, Ovid | Bibliographic citations (no abstracts) and natural language indexing for more than 20 industry publications, including *Biomedical Safety & Standards, Biomedical Technology Information Service, Clinical Lab Letter, Pharma Japan, Quality Control Reports—The Gold Sheet, Radiology & Imaging Letter*, and *Weekly Pharmacy Reports—The Green Sheet*. |
| PharmacoEconomics & Outcomes News | 1994 to date, updated daily DataStar, Dialog | Full-text, prepublication and archival access to the weekly newsletter of the same name. |

HealthEconomics.Com, formerly *Patti Peeples' Health Economics Resource Page*, is a good place to start, because it adds informative annotations to each hotlinked entry in separate indexes to databases, associations, consulting companies, journal/news sources, questionnaires and performance assessment instruments, government sites, education, and pharm/biotech companies. This hub has also added a search engine for targeted keyword access. The scope encompasses pharmacoeconomics, outcomes research, managed care, quality of life, and value in medicine.

Health Economics—Places to Go
⇨ http://www.medecon.de/healthec.htm

A narrower, and somewhat sharper, focus characterizes *Health Economics— Places to Go*. Maintained by Ansgar Hebborn of the University of Bayreuth, this home page provides pointers to associations, books, databases, education and training, institutions, journals, mailing lists, people, resource collections, and software. Entries are assembled under main menu selections that include economic evaluation, health economics, health policy, managed care, evidence-based medicine, pharma market, public health, and jobs. A bonus at this site is a library of full-text articles that Hebborn has bookmarked after searching the primary literature and gathered under the heading "Topics" in each category.

Outcomes
⇨ http://www.sph.uth.tmc.edu/www/res/outcomes/outcomes.htm

Outcomes is an attractively organized index to handouts, bibliographies, and external hotlinks used by the author, Carl Slater, MD, in courses at the University of Texas School of Public Health. It provides an overview of outcomes research and a menu of research topics, including tools for outcomes measurement and risk adjustment, as well as data sources. The combined bibliography and URLography identifies examples and actual applications of this specialized type of investigation.

Quality of Life Assessment in Medicine
⇨ http://www.glamm.com/ql/url.htm

Stater recommends this site as "one of the richest sources of links to topics in outcomes research, although the title would indicate otherwise." The list compiled by Ello Tamburini and published by Glamm Interactive, an Italian software development company, is a lengthy directory of assessment instruments, major associations and research groups, methodology sources, bibliographies, top quality of life journals, and specialty focused URLs for specific diseases, symptoms, and population subsets.

Pharmacy, Medicine and Managed Care
⇨ http://members.aol.com/_ht_a/bertrx/phamedmc.htm

The self-styled "Hypertext Guide" to *Pharmacy, Medicine and Managed Care* is maintained by Carl T. Bertram. It compiles a selection of links to insurance companies, associations, and their outcomes research or health economics publications.

The Health Economics Website
⇨ http://metz.une.edu.au/~mkortt

Michael Kortt, author of *The Health Economics Website*, is a doctoral student at the University of New England in New South Wales, Australia. His subject hub organizes links to university departments, research organizations, government agencies, and health associations under the flags of Australia, Canada, Sweden, the United Kingdom, and the United States. Two other icons lead to collections of journal sites and other literature and data sources.

Each of these pathfinders identifies sources not found in the others, reflecting its author's different view of a subject area new enough to lack clearly defined boundaries. Accordingly, inquiries are likely to demand an interdisciplinary approach that can only be achieved by consulting more than one guide. Other resources of potential interest are small databases hosted by universities in the United Kingdom.

Outcomes Literature Database
⇨ http://www.leeds.ac.uk/nuffield/infoservices/UKCH/chld.html

This is one of a trio of electronic files offered by the U.K. Clearinghouse on Health Outcomes. It is intended to provide details of published and gray literature (internal reports, papers) related to the study and development of methods for assessing changes in health status that may result from health or social interventions. U.K., U.S., European, and Australasian documents are among those cited. Other searchable files at the same site include an *Outcomes Activities Database* and an *Outcomes Database of Structured Abstracts*. Titles of studies, aims, setting, and measures used are analyzed and recorded in brief records.

NHS Economic Evaluation Database
⇨ http://nhscrd.york.ac.uk

The University of York houses the NHS Centre for Reviews and Dissemination (CRD), which has developed the *Economic Evaluation Database* of structured abstracts. References have been culled since January 1994 from a variety of sources through searches of *Current Contents-Clinical Medicine, MEDLINE, EMBASE, EconLit,* and *CINAHL.* They are subsequently assessed by CRD staff using standardized quality criteria. The focus of this file is on identifying cost-benefit, cost-effectiveness, or cost-utility analyses. The same URL provides access to two additional online bibliographic collections: a *Database of Abstracts of Reviews of Effectiveness (DARE)* and a *Health Technology Assessment Database.*

A complementary, and presumably more comprehensive, source on the same general theme is the *Health Economics Evaluations Database (HEED)* on CD-ROM. Available by paid subscription, it is described on the home page of the Association of the British Pharmaceutical Industry (http://www.abpi.org.uk) as a joint project of ABPI and the International Federation of Pharmaceutical Manufacturers Associations (IFPMA).

The U.S. Department of Defense Pharmacoeconomic Center
⇨ http://www.pec.ha.osd.mil

The U.S. Department of Defense (DOD) would seem to be an unexpected companion to other Web collections found in this section. However, the military is as interested in cost-effective and rational drug prescribing as other organizations. It publishes its basic core formulary at this site, as well as a preferred drug list. Both are searchable by generic and brand names and *American Hospital Formulary Service (AHFS)* classification. Nonmilitary visitors could benefit from DOD disease state reviews, available for downloading in PDF format. Each is a pharmacoeconomic analysis of a disease state commonly encountered within the military health system and includes treatment guidelines, drug usage evaluation criteria, and preferred drugs. Reviews have been published for helicobacter pylori eradication, gastrointestinal reflux diseases, benign prostatic hyperplasia, obesity, vulvovaginal candidiasis, asthma, and typhoid vaccines.

Exploring Licensing Opportunities

Alliances between companies have steadily increased since 1989, as pressures have mounted to improve productivity in research and development operations and reduce overlap in marketing and sales force activities. The cradle to grave approach to product development, whereby new drug introductions are dependent on the solo efforts of individual firms, is rapidly disappearing. "Licensing in" drug delivery or production technologies can jumpstart products stalled in the pipeline, just as marketing alliances can energize flagging distribution channels. Broadening product portfolios or accelerating portfolio turnover are additional motivations for licensing agreements in an industry where an innovation deficit has been forecast.[4]

All of the databases discussed thus far in this chapter can be used to monitor licensing opportunities. Three of the drugs-in-development directories make isolating relevant information especially easy. *IMSworld R&D Focus Drug Updates* (15.2) tags records for each new product as "available" when the originating company announces its intention or willingness to seek joint marketing or research agreements. At the same time, contact information is added to records for quick follow-up. *ADIS R&D Insight* (15.3) notes licensing availability in the Introduction segment of pertinent product records.

Pharmaprojects (15.1) identifies licensing opportunities in two different locations in online records: the country/status field and the update field. To monitor newly announced licensing opportunities, search the update segment of records on a regular basis. If agreements for rights in specific geographic areas are a further requirement, add country/status delimiters to the update search statement. For example,

On Dialog: *s 9507?(s)licensing(w)opportunity/up and japan(s)licensing/st*
On DataStar: *9507$ with licensing adj opportunity.dt. and japan with licensing.cn.*

Consult vendor documentation for help in translating these strategies to other search systems. For follow-up company contact information, *Pharmaprojects* searchers can turn to *Pharmacontacts* (15.23).

Another technique for surveying licensing opportunities is to examine, on a periodic basis, pipeline directory records for products where the status listed is *suspended* or *discontinued*. Although developing companies may not yet have announced that these compounds are available for joint development agreements, suspended status is an early indicator that pipeline reassessment may be under way. Sometimes, even promising candidates for development are judged not to be a good fit with a company's overall strategic direction or marketing capabilities. Alternatively, other research projects may have required reallocation of resources away from the candidate compound. In either case, originators may respond favorably to licensing inquiries.

The ADIS *Drug News & Perspectives* (15.13) database devotes an entire section to licensing opportunities in each monthly update. Announcements include availability notices for technology transfer of government funded products, as well as those offered by for-profit organizations. Material is organized under titles characterizing the type of opportunity: e.g., dermatologic drugs, diagnostic agents, drug delivery, pharmacological tools.

Several sources accessible in the *IAC Newsletter Database* (15.15) monitor licensing offers (see Appendix C). *Biotech Patent News, Pharmaceutical Business News, Healthcare Technology & Business Opportunities, Antiviral Agents Bulle-*

tin, and *Life Sciences & Biotechnology Update* frequently cite pertinent inventions and their applications of potential interest to the industry.

A good source for tracking licensable government owned inventions is *NTIS*. This online resource from the U.S. National Technical Information Service systematically cites patent applications filed in the United States and includes brief summaries of technology available for transfer to the private, for-profit sector. *The Blue Sheet* (4.56), available in full-text format as part of the *F-D-C Reports* database (15.10), also includes announcements of patents available for licensing from the National Institutes of Health (NIH). Once applicants are accepted, notices of intent to license to individual firms are published in the *Federal Register* (4.24). Some information professionals monitor the latter on a regular basis for early intelligence of competing companies' augmentation of their patent portfolios courtesy of NIH.

The Biotechnology Information Institute, publisher of *Antiviral Agents Bulletin*, has developed a database wholly dedicated to monitoring federal patents available for licensing, as well as Collaborative Research and Development Agreements (CRADAs). The *Federal Bio-Technology Transfer Directory*, updated quarterly, can be searched by paid subscription on the Internet or purchased for loading on company in-house computers. See http://www.bioinfo.com/biotech/ for a complete description of its features.

Investigating Line Extensions

Line extensions, in the context of pharmaceutical products, refer to new indications, new combinations, or other changes in formulation, packaging, and presentation, such as dosage form alternatives or additional strengths. New indications for established products are generally considered sufficiently newsworthy to warrant mention in sources such as *Scrip* or *The Pink Sheet*, accessible in *PHIND* (15.9) and *F-D-C Reports* (15.10), respectively. Work in progress toward gaining approval for new indications is also documented in *Pharmaprojects* (15.1), *R&D Focus Drug Updates* (15.2), and *ADIS R&D Insight* (15.3). However, no special indexing feature alerts users of these pipeline files that line extension investigations are commencing. This is one reason why searchers conduct periodic surveys of a competitor's product records in these directories, even after launch, to maintain a watching brief for such developments.

ADIS *Drug News & Perspectives* (15.13) also announces a selection of line extensions in each monthly update. This section of the database accounts for 13% of records, 56% of which have not also been announced in the hardcopy counterpart. Three types of line extensions are noted: new uses, new combinations, and new formulations. As mentioned previously, Prous maintains constant vigilance of the patent literature. Hence, *Drug News & Perspectives* often provides very early warning of possible extensions based on patent claims.

Because changes in dosage form or strength are usually considered less exciting news, these two types of line extensions are less meticulously documented in the literature and notoriously more difficult to verify. However, any such change made to a prescription drug marketed in the United States must, by law, be subject to prior approval by the FDA in the form of a supplemental NDA. Both *Diogenes* (16.1) and the *FDA Home Page* routinely index U.S. drug approvals of all types, whether original, abbreviated, or supplemental NDAs (see Chapter Sixteen).

News of line extensions for nonprescription products or for Rx or OTC drugs marketed abroad can prove to be much more elusive. Fortunately, two IMS databases are specifically designed to track such events.[5]

15.18 *IMSworld New Product Launches.* London: IMS Global Services, 1982–. Updated monthly. Available on DataStar, Dialog, and STN; also on CD-ROM.

15.19 *IMSworld Product Monographs.* London: IMS Global Services, 1965–. Updated quarterly. Available on DataStar, Dialog, and STN.

IMSworld New Product Launches documents initial drug product introductions in individual countries worldwide (fifty nations are currently covered). First launches of new chemical entities (NCEs) and of products produced by biotechnology are flagged by IMS for quick retrieval. All records include company name (parent and subsidiary), nonproprietary drug name, brand name, launch date, country, therapeutic class, composition (active ingredients and strength), packaging (e.g., "Tabl 28"), price in local currency, and indications. Since September 1995, excipients have been added to composition data, when supplied by manufacturers. Unbranded generic drug product launch information is another recent enhancement. *IMSworld Product Monographs* compile comparable, detailed information for all line extensions (new packs or presentations), although pricing data in these records are accessible only to subscribers.

The global venue of *IMSworld New Product Launches* is reflected in portions of records derived from labeling. Description of dosage form is typically transcribed in native vernacular as found on packaging, as is indications information. Languages used include English, Spanish, German, French, Portuguese, Danish, Italian, and Swedish. Therefore, strategies to retrieve specific dosage forms may require use of alternative, non-English terms. For example, *kap? or cap?* (truncated) would be needed to locate *kapsel, kapseln, kapslar, kapsler, capsule,* or *capsula.* For ointments, *salbe or unguento,* and abbreviations thereof, are likely alternatives; for vials, use *vial? or fial?*—and so on.

When searching indications keywords, liberal use of truncation will break down some language barriers, since the word root of a Latin- or Greek-derived medical term is identical in many languages. Internal spelling differences can be accommodated with embedded variable character search entry shortcuts available in most online systems; e.g., *select h?pert?n?* retrieves hipertension, hypertonie, or hypertension on Dialog. Choice of proximity operators should take into account inverted noun-adjective phrases common in many languages (e.g., *bronchites chroniques*), and it's a good idea to aim for the same sentence, rather than specifying direct word adjacency. Frequent searchers of the *New Product Launches* database may find it helpful to consult references cited in Chapter Ten's section on multilingual guides.

Both *IMSworld New Product Launches* and *Product Monographs* databases provide worldwide marketing information not replicated elsewhere. They can help answer such questions as: What's the competitive picture for ACE inhibitors in Canada? What types of drugs were launched in Colombia during the latter half of 1997? By whom? Has anyone tried introducing this kind of product in suppository form? Who would our competitors be in this therapeutic area in these countries? Would our product portfolio benefit from launching this line in extended-release capsules?

Company and Product Directories

As general business information specialists are well aware, there are far too many company directories available online today to contemplate discussing here. However, company files specifically devoted to coverage of the pharmaceutical and medical device industries should certainly be cited.

15.20 *IMSworld Pharmaceutical Company Profiles.* London: IMS Global Services. Current information, updated monthly. Available on DataStar and Dialog; also on CD-ROM.

IMSworld Company Profiles are full-text, in-depth reports on more than 110 public and private pharmaceutical firms headquartered in any of more than twenty countries. Each profile includes sections related to finance, research and development, historical milestones, and mergers or acquisitions. Principle sources include interviews with executives at profiled companies, reports from independent financial analysts, press conferences, investor meetings, newswires, and the trade press. All company profiles are completely revised each year. Monthly additions to the online database include updates to specific sections of individual company reports. Only portions of text or selected tables, rather than full company profiles, need be displayed, if desired.

15.21 *ESPICOM Pharmaceutical and Medical Company Profiles.* Chester, UK: ESPICOM Business Intelligence. Current information, updated monthly. Available on DataStar and Dialog.

The *ESPICOM* (formerly *MDIS*) *Pharmaceutical and Medical Company Profiles* database corresponds to two hardcopy publications, *Pharmaceutical Companies Analysis* and *Medical Device Companies Analysis*. The latter contributes the majority of records, making this online resource an excellent complement to the collection of company profiles maintained by IMSworld. Coverage currently includes lengthy reports on more than 110 device companies and 50 drug firms. Each *ESPICOM* profile provides a five-year financial analysis; corporate history and strategy sections; an overview of company products; a summary of agreements, alliances, and international activities; performance ranking within the industry; and an evaluation of R&D efforts. Separate segments present sales, profit, capital expenditures, and assets data by business area and geographic area. Selected portions of these reports, rather than full company profiles, can be singled out for searching and display.

15.22 *IMSworld Company Directory.* London: IMS Global Services. Current information, updated monthly. Available on DataStar and Dialog; also on CD-ROM.

Equivalent to the hardcopy *World Drug Market Manual—Companies*, the *IMSworld Company Directory* database online includes information on more than 4,000 firms, including subsidiaries of multinational corporations, located in any of more than eighty countries. *Directory* entries vary in length. Some offer only basic address data, as found in *Pharmacontacts* (15.23). Many others, however, provide full summaries of local operations, including manufacturing, importing, and distribution details, corporate ownership, key executives, number of medical representatives or detailers (i.e., size of local sales force), and year of establishment. Provision of these types of data for company operations at the local (country or state) level is what sets this IMSworld database apart. Company records include annual sales in U.S. dollars (again, sales are specific to the locale cited), top five branded products, top selling therapeutic categories, and the percent contribution to total sales that each therapeutic category delivers.

In addition to approaching this database on a company by company basis, another way to compile data is to search by country. For example, when the competitive environment in Taiwan is the subject of inquiry, entry of "Taiwan" might yield 110 company records. These entries could then be sorted (rearranged) by annual sales in descending order (highest to lowest) and only the top ten company records be displayed for a quick snapshot of leading competitors in that market. Other typical questions this database can answer are: Who are the leading companies in sales of (therapeutic category) X? Which brand name products are best sellers? Where has this type of product ranked highest in sales? What these examples illustrate is the potential range of useful information provided in the *IMSworld Company Directory*. Data compiled on local company operations are a veritable gold mine for the market researcher.

15.23 *Pharmacontacts.* Richmond, Surrey, England: PJB Online Services. Current information, updated monthly. Available on DataStar, Dialog, and Ovid.

Pharmacontacts contains the names and addresses of more than 12,700 pharmaceutical companies in Europe and the Americas, 5,500 chemical firms, and 5,500 service suppliers to the industry. This database was enhanced in 1996 with sources produced by PJB in conjunction with KYM publishers, including *The International Directory of Pharmaceutical Personnel*, *The International Directory of Pharmaceutical Companies*, and *The International Directory of Chemical Companies* (a good source for bulk drug ingredient producers).

Standardized record format facilitates use of *Pharmacontacts* for generation of mailing lists, in addition to individual company look-ups. Indexing of position titles has also been conveniently rotated (i.e., permuted), so that it is not necessary to anticipate all possible variations before compiling contact lists of individuals with specific responsibilities. For example, regulatory affairs personnel bear titles beginning with terms such as Director, Manager, Chief, Head, Vice President, Executive, Officer, etc. However, a search on keywords such as *regulatory* or *registration* in the position title index of *Pharmacontacts* will quickly locate relevant entries, regardless of precise title.

15.24 *Medical Device Register*. Montvale, NJ: Medical Economics. Current information, updated annually. Available on Dialog.

The *Medical Device Register* online corresponds to the multivolume *Medical Device Register* (13.8) for U.S. companies and the *International Medical Device Register* published by Medical Economics in hardcopy format. Taken together, these directories provide a detailed census of companies worldwide producing medical devices. The database incorporates entries for more than 11,600 domestic firms producing 65,000 products, plus 7,500 companies located outside the United States, listing 30,000 additional devices. Records for individual companies can be searched by sales level, FDA standardized product nomenclature, brand name, and geographic delimiters (country, city, state). Other searchable data elements include CE Mark status and ISO certification or registration. Federal procurement eligibility and contract types are also indicated in online records, when applicable. For example, female- or minority-owned businesses can be isolated, as can entries for companies granted General Services Administration (GSA) or Veterans Administration (VA) contracts.

15.25 *Health Devices Sourcebook*. Plymouth Meeting, PA: ECRI. Current information, updated annually. Available on Dialog; also on CD-ROM.

The *Health Devices Sourcebook* (*HDS*) database provides current address and marketing information for more than 6,000 North American manufacturers, distributors, and service companies associated with any of more than 4,000 classes of products. Listings include sources for diagnostic and therapeutic devices and materials, including laboratory equipment and reagents, systems and instruments used to monitor and test equipment, and selected hospital furniture or supplies. Product records in *HDS* (49% of entries) list devices by generic name. When available, a typical industry price range for the product is included, as well as a cross reference to a brand name product comparison conducted by ECRI. Formerly known as the Emergency Care Research Institute, ECRI is an independent nonprofit agency that evaluates healthcare technology.

Another type of listing in the *Health Devices Sourcebook* is manufacturer records (44% of *HDS* entries). Each manufacturer record includes name, address, telephone number, generic and brand names of the company's products, and chief executive officer, financial officer, and marketing officer. Service company entries (6% of *HDS*) show category of service (e.g., repairs, leases), geographical areas covered, and contact information.

Because brand names are included for a broad range of devices, *HDS* can be valuable in answering product identification questions. The *Sourcebook* database also includes records for many smaller private companies difficult to locate in other directories. Inclusion of price data for selected products is a bonus, as well. Citations to brand comparisons and evaluations, when available, make *Health Devices Sourcebook* an unusual combination of business directory and bibliographic reference tool for prospective device purchasers and competitive intelligence researchers.[6]

15.26 *Healthcare Organizations Database.* Montvale, NJ: Medical Economics. Current information, updated annually. Available on Dialog.

It's no secret that group purchasing agents now exercise considerable control over the U.S. healthcare market, negotiating over 65% of all medical products purchased by hospitals. The *Healthcare Organizations Database*, by including the full text of Medical Economics' *Directory of Healthcare Purchasing Organizations*, can provide background information on more than 500 such groups. Entries include address and telephone contact data, names of officials, standard requirements for vendor proposals, product categories negotiated, and types of contracts awarded.

A second full-text component of this database is the *HMO/PPO Directory* from the same publisher. Like its hardcopy counterpart, this source provides information about nearly 2,000 U.S. Health Maintenance and Preferred Provider organizations. In addition to basic address and phone data, entries typically list key administrative and purchasing contacts, year founded, current enrollment, geographic area served, number of affiliated physicians and hospitals, monthly subscriber fees and co-payments, and nonprofit or for-profit status.

A third subfile in the *Healthcare Organizations Database* is the *Directory of Hospital Personnel* issued each year by Medical Economics. Its coverage encompasses nearly 7,000 hospitals located in the United States. Name of administrators, numbers of interns, nursing students, employees, and licensed and actual beds, as well as insurance plans accepted, are all data elements included in online records from this source.

Information on chemical producers is also likely to be needed. From a business intelligence perspective, predetermination of the availability of bulk chemical suppliers at the local level can be a predictor of speed in brand name sales erosion to be expected following a product's patent expiration in a given geographic market. Would-be generic manufacturers will need to find a convenient source of supply that meets quality specifications, is compatible with manufacturing methods, and is sufficiently economical to support formulations for introduction at a competitive price, once approved by government authorities.

15.27 *Chem Sources Chemical Directory (CSCHEM)*. Clemson, SC: Chemical Sources International. Current, updated annually. Available on DataStar and STN; also on CD-ROM.

15.28 *Chem Sources Company Directory (CSCORP)*. Clemson, SC: Chemical Sources International. Current, updated annually. Available on DataStar and STN; also on CD-ROM.

Since its inception in 1958, *Chem Sources* in hardcopy has become the standard reference tool for finding out who makes what. Information published in both *Chem Sources U.S.A.* (13.6) and *Chem Sources-International* (13.7) is available online in a pair of directory databases. The *Chemical Directory (CSCHEM)* file lists suppliers for each of its 200,000 generic (simplified) chemical name entries and indicates, when known, whether products are sold as "high purity" or "bulk commercial quantity." More than 60% of records are accessible by CAS registry number.

The companion *Company Directory* database (*CSCORP*) compiles information on more than 7,400 suppliers of the chemicals indexed in *CSCHEM*. Company entries include main and branch office addresses in any of 120 countries, functions (sales, shipping, or manufacturing), telephone numbers, and categories of chemicals available (e.g., additives, food). Brand names, when relevant, are also listed. Because of this feature, the *Chem Sources Company Directory* can be added to the list of possible sources for product identification, especially when standard drug directories fail to yield results. More commonly, these *Chem Sources* directories will be used to locate local suppliers of raw materials for drug formulation and manufacture. Such inquiries can begin with either a specific substance name in the *Chemical Directory* or a category term in the *Company Directory*.

15.29 *Directory of Chemical Producers—Products*. Menlo Park, CA: SRI Consulting. Current information, updated annually. Available on Dialog.

15.30 *Directory of Chemical Producers—Companies*. Menlo Park, CA: SRI Consulting. Current information, updated annually. Available on Dialog.

SRI Consulting (formerly known as the Stanford Research Institute) is responsible for another set of companion files dedicated to assembling information on chemical producers and their products. First published in 1961, the *Directory of Chemical Producers* (*DCP*) originally limited its scope to U.S. manufacturers. *DCP-Europe* followed in 1978, *DCP-Canada* in 1988, and *DCP-East Asia* in 1989. Today, more than fifty-five countries are covered in nine regional directories for: Canada, China, East Asia, Europe, India, Mexico, the Middle East, South America, and the United States. The online *Directory of Chemical Producers* databases include the entire contents from more than 6,000 pages published in these hardcopy directories. The result is ready-reference access to information on more than 13,300 companies operating 19,000 plants and manufacturing 37,000 commercial chemical products.

The *Products* directory enables quick location of chemicals through extensive cross referencing of alternate names. Functional group indexing facilitates surveys for classes of related products, such as enzymes, plasticizers, or surface-active agents. Producers and plant locations are listed for each product, as well as plant-by-plant production capacity data for selected chemicals. The *Companies* database is analogous to the manufacturer section available in each hardcopy *DCP* edition, but has the advantage of multiregion searchability. Entries provide corporate and divisional headquarters address and telephone data, individual plant locations, and complete listings of products manufactured at each facility. Ownership and subsidiary or affiliates are routinely identified.

15.31 *Chemicals and Companies.* Cambridge, England: The Royal Society of Chemistry. Current information, updated quarterly. Available on CD-ROM.

The *Chemicals and Companies* (short title for *Chemicals, Formulated Products and Their Company Sources*) CD-ROM database is available by subscription directly from the Royal Society of Chemistry. Its coverage includes 35,000 company sites in the United States, Europe, India, and Japan. Substance entries for 61,000 formulated products and 15,000 chemicals include graphic structural formulas (displayable, but not searchable) and physical/chemical property information, such as molecular weight, melting and boiling point, and specific gravity. Hazard information is also provided.

Another fee-based source of comparable information is offered to subscribers as part of *ChemWeb* on the Internet: *ACD—The Available Chemicals Directory*. Compiled by MDL Information Systems, *ACD* enhances accessibility by enabling structure and substructure searching. Entries can also be retrieved using chemical names, synonyms, name fragments, molecular formulas, or CAS registry numbers as starting points. Information on 240,000 compounds and 600,000 products from 300 suppliers is updated twice a year. Listings provide details of suppliers, distributors, and their agents, as well as package size, grade, purity, and price data. *ACD* records are also cross-linked to the *OHS Material Safety Data Sheets* (14.31) in their *ChemWeb* implementation (see http://chemweb.com).

The American Chemical Society offers a free *CHEMCYCLOPEDIA* on its ACS publications Web site at http://pubs.acs.org/chemcy. This resource is the online equivalent of an annual supplement to *Chemical & Engineering News*. Suppliers listed have been asked to provide brand names, packaging information, special shipping requirements, keywords for potential applications, chemical names, and CAS RNs. Remember, also, that the Cosmetic, Toiletry, and Fragrance Association's Internet site provides an electronic edition of the *CTFA International Buyers' Guide* (13.15).

Statistical Sources: Market Share, Sales, and Epidemiological Data

Tracking down market share and sales statistics for pharmaceutical companies and products is much easier today than it was twenty years ago, due to the advent of interactive online systems and widespread use of microcomputers to collate and manipulate data at the desktop. Data gathering, storage, transmission, and communication have all been simplified, the result being an impressive collection of business resources readily accessible to the public. Determining where and how to locate the precise statistics needed is, nonetheless, difficult. This section of the *Guide* can scarcely do more than highlight some of the major resources where data needed are more likely to be found.

15.32 *IMS World Drug Markets*. London: IMS Global Services. Current, updated quarterly. Available on Dialog and DataStar; also on CD-ROM.

IMS World Drug Markets corresponds to the hardcopy *World Drug Market Manual—Countries*, a source which offers authoritative overviews of the pharmaceutical industry and healthcare provision in seventy-six nations. Lengthy entries for each country summarize government regulations affecting drugs, including registration (premarket approval) procedures, price controls, packaging and labeling guidelines, and rules regarding laboratory and clinical research, manufacturing, distribution, dispensing, promotion, post-marketing surveillance, and product liability. Patent and trademark laws are always reviewed in country monographs.

All of this information is augmented with healthcare statistics. Both general demographic and economic health indicators data are provided, with an assessment of primary and outpatient facilities, number and type of hospital beds, and numbers and types of healthcare personnel. The quantity and quality of these data vary from country to country, as might be expected, being dependent on the level of sophistication in statistics collection activities of local governments. Information is obtained from 250 statistical yearbooks and other government publications, as well as the journal literature and local contacts or IMS offices in countries covered.

What does not vary is the level of detail found in sections devoted to analysis of the pharmaceutical market in each locale. Total market estimates and sales data are systematically presented and evaluated. Users can expect to find sales statistics broken down by the ten leading therapeutic classes in a given country, with top-selling brand names in each class itemized. Another lengthy section in each country's profile compiles sales data for the ten leading companies and each of their leading products. Commentary identifies historical shifts in market share and presents growth rate calculations. Data are derived from the IMS MIDAS database, a massive repository of international market data from which customized reports and subsets can be commissioned, for a fee. Individual sections of each country's profile are easily identified online and can be separately displayed.

15.33 *ESPICOM Country Healthcare Database.* Chester, England: ESPICOM Business Intelligence. Current information, updated monthly. Available on DataStar and Dialog.

ESPICOM supplies a good complement (and competitor) to the *IMS World Drug Markets* database. Corresponding to the hardcopy *Medistat World Medical Market Analysis*, *ESPICOM Country Healthcare* online assembles in-depth reports for seventy-two nations. Each report includes extensive statistical data on population and health status indicators, health expenditures, and imports and exports of specific product categories. Where ESPICOM market research differentiates itself from IMS is in the level of detailed data available for medical devices and equipment, versus pharmaceuticals. In addition to impressive compilations of trade statistics, each country report also presents directories of hospitals, healthcare organizations, and device manufacturers, distributors, and their agents. Online implementations of this database on DataStar and Dialog make it easy to isolate needed sections of a given country's report for targeted searching and separate display.

Searching the Trade Literature

Digging out statistical data buried in trade and business publications can be quite difficult. One obstacle is that titles of individual articles are often poor indicators of textual content: e.g., "The Consumer Connection," "Rx for Success." Another barrier is that indexing added by database producers often fails to identify the presence of tables or graphs in primary sources cited. Moreover, in many online databases where these sources are transcibed in full-text format, illustrative material is often omitted or abridged. This is a common problem in traditional ASCII files. In contrast, PDF documents, now ubiquitous on the Internet, can replicate original publications with tables intact. The drawback is that their content (individual keywords and numbers) is not directly searchable using Web search engines. Recognizing the need for better access to tabular data, a company called Responsive Database Services (RDS) launched *TableBase* early in 1998.

15.34 *TableBase*. Beachwood, OH: Responsive Database Services, June 1977–. Updated weekly. Available on DataStar and Dialog; also on CD-ROM.

RDS extracts tables from more than 900 business magazines, as well as from separate publications issued by more than 100 trade associations and 200 research organizations. Each table is presented as an individual record and indexed in depth by industry name, Standard Industrial Classification (SIC) code, company, and concept. Geographic terms are also added to each record to indicate the scope of data included. Approximately 60% of *TableBase* documents address conditions in the United States, 20% in Europe, and 14% in the Pacific Rim.

Among more than 90 industries covered, searchable industry names include pharmaceutical, medical devices and diagnostics, personal care products, healthcare delivery, and chemical. Data are available on market share, production and consumption, imports and exports, usage and capacity, and number of outlets or users. Company and brand rankings, industry and product forecasts, and trade and general demographics can all be found in *TableBase*.

In addition to terms added to each record by RDS indexers, searchable keywords in this database include table title and textwords, original story title, and journal name. Titles of tables have been enhanced with one-sentence descriptions of content to ensure precise retrieval. Displaying the full text of articles from which tables have been extracted is also an option in about 80% of records. Growing at a rate of 25,000 citations per year, *TableBase* is updated weekly online and quarterly on CD-ROM. Online implementations include not only DataStar and Dialog, but also pay-per-view and flat rate subscription access through a Web-based interface at http://www.rdsic.com.

Industry newsletters discussed earlier in this chapter, such as *Scrip*, *Clinica* (both in *PHIND* online, 15.9), and F-D-C Reports' publications (*The Pink Sheet*, *The Gray Sheet*, 15.10) are also good sources of business statistics. Bear in mind, however, the exigencies of full-text searching when unassisted by controlled indexing; second guessing synonyms under which relevant items will be found demands creativity and flexibility. For example, suppose someone asks for market share data for cough and cold preparations. Although "cough" within one word of "cold" can certainly be searched, adding alternative keywords such as antitussives, expectorants, or decongestants would be a good idea. Not everyone writing about a category of drugs will use the same terms, and an answer to such an inquiry may need to be culled from isolated sources and coordinated after the fact.

For that matter, references to the concept of "market share" can be challenging to find in full-text sources. A strategy needs to take into account different word order and degrees of proximity. The concept can be expressed as "share of the—market" or "share of the total—market" (where — may be a drug class term, such as analgesic or cardiovascular). Because the words *of* and *the* are stop words not directly searchable in most online systems, perhaps the best way to retrieve references to market share is to search for *market* within four to five words of *share*, or simply in the same sentence, and specify that drug category keywords appear in the same paragraph of text. Similar guidelines would apply to strategies seeking *market size*.

15.35 *IAC PROMT*. Foster City, CA: Information Access Company, 1972–. Updated daily. Available on DataStar, Dialog, QUESTEL-ORBIT, and STN; also on CD-ROM.

15.36 *IAC Trade & Industry Database*. Foster City, CA: Information Access Company, 1981–. Updated daily. Available on DataStar and Dialog; also on CD-ROM.

Other online sources of market share, size, and sales data are not devoted exclusively to the pharmaceutical industry, so even more effort may be required to uncover statistics. For example, answers to many questions are likely to be found in the business journal literature and trade press. Databases such as *IAC PROMT* and *Trade & Industry Database* cover relevant sources and add controlled indexing to assist in isolating facts needed. Both are accessible by Standard Industrial Classification (SIC) codes and their successor, NAICS (North American Industry Classification System) codes, which can be located through database user aids.

Another type of indexing used in *IAC PROMT* is event codes. Consultation of the *PROMT* user manual prior to going online will help in selecting pertinent codes, covering such diverse areas as

43	capital expenditures
45	research & development outlays
48	use of services
51	population
60	market data
62	production information
65	sales & consumption
69	goods & services distribution
74	commodity & service prices
83	sales, profits, & dividends
87	financial assets

By coordinating SIC/NAICS indexing with event codes and further restricting results to subject keywords (e.g., nebulizers), experienced searchers can quickly isolate pertinent bibliography. In addition, the keywords *survey* or *statistic?* (truncated), when ANDed with specific subject terms in *IAC PROMT*, often yield references containing numeric data.

Useful controlled descriptors in *IAC Trade & Industry Database* include "Pharmaceutical Industry—Statistics" and "Market Share." Limiting recall from a subject keyword strategy to records where the word *table* appears in the "special feature" field or paragraph is another reliable approach to obtaining numeric data in the *Trade & Industry* file. Results often include the full-text of articles from specialty journals such as *American Druggist, Cosmetics & Toiletries,* and *Drug Topics. IAC PROMT* offers cover-to-cover full-text access to *Bio-Pharm, Chemist & Druggist, Community Pharmacy* (UK), *Drug & Cosmetic Industry, Drug Store News, Manufacturing Chemist, Pharmaceutical Executive,* and *Pharmaceutical Manufacturing Review.*

15.37 *Business & Industry.* Beachwood, OH: Responsive Database Services, 1994–. Updated daily. Available on DataStar, Dialog, and SilverPlatter; also on CD-ROM.

The *Business & Industry* database offers several types of controlled indexing to assist market researchers. Concept terms include market size, market share, sales, and consumption. Results of a search on any of these terms can be combined with SIC/NAICS codes, industry names (e.g., pharmaceuticals), or company, country, and product names. Retrieval can, once again, also be limited to records that contain tables. This database offers access to more than 600 trade publications, at least half of which are available for immediate full-text display online. Sample industry specialty titles offered in full-text format include *Gene Therapy Weekly, Pharma Japan, PharmaBusiness, Pharmaceutical Industry Weekly, Supermarket Pharmacy,* and *Pharmacy Today.*

Syndicated Market Research & Investment Analyst Reports

Syndicated market research and investment analyst reports are another rich source of business statistical data. Publishers who provide syndicated market research, also referred to as "off-the-shelf" research, gather data through extensive interviews with key industry leaders, specially commissioned consumer panels, and surveys. Suppliers of this type of business intelligence develop expertise in particular areas and often sell their reports to customers as publication series. The same organizations usually also conduct customized market research under contract to private clients (companies), tailored to their specific needs, but not widely disseminated.

Both public and privately issued reports add value to statistical data compiled by including analyses in which trends are identified and forecasts explained. They include discussion of external factors affecting an industry (government regulation, customer or consumer behavior), comparisons of key players in a market segment, and informed insight into competitive dynamics. For staff (including information professionals) newly assigned to a given segment, such reports can fulfill a mentoring function. Review of one or two of these focused overviews will quickly enable them to gain familiarity with the technological and trade environment, current issues, and insiders' vocabulary.

Databases such as *FIND/SVP Market Research, Frost & Sullivan Market Intelligence, Datamonitor Market Research,* and others listed in Figure 15.9 offer the option of searching and displaying selected segments of in-depth studies and industry analyses from expensive research publications that would otherwise have to be purchased in their entirety. What kinds of data are available? A *FIND/SVP* report entitled "Generic Drugs Market," issued in October 1995, included tables showing annual U.S. sales by company, domestic generics market share of new prescriptions over a seven-year period, top thirty prescribed drugs, and sales forecasts through the year 2000 broken down by therapeutic category.

Online strategies in market research report databases can zoom in on pages likely to contain statistical data on the topic desired simply by ANDing in the keywords *table* or *figure*. In the same way, *Investext* opens windows into financial analysts' reports, enabling users to track down valuable statistical data embedded in lengthy documents.

15.38 *Investext*. Boston: Thomson Financial Networks, 1982–. Updated daily or weekly on DataStar, Dialog, and STN; also on CD-ROM.

This database contains the full text of company, industry, geographic, and topical reports by analysts affiliated with any of more than 270 of the world's leading investment banks, brokerage firms, consulting companies, and other business research organizations. It covers more than 21,000 public and private companies and fifty-three industry categories, including biotechnology, health care, medical supplies, personal care products, and pharmaceuticals. Report segments are consistently indexed by business subject (e.g., competition, market share, sales and earnings estimates), product, SIC/NAICS code, company name or industry category, geographic name, and report type (industry, company, topical, or geographic). By combining two or more of these factors, pertinent material can easily be located. A further search restriction that almost guarantees numbers will be provided is to confine output to portions of reports with tables. *Investext* strategies can be limited to any of forty-seven business subjects, where choices include

Competition. Defined as tabular or textual information about companies or products vying for greater market share or profits.

Customer Base. Explains who the market is for a product or service, covering demographics, customer statistics and analyses, target markets, consumer profiles.

Government Relations/Regulations. Discussion of a company's or an industry's interaction with government regulatory agencies.

Industry Overview. Discussion of factors or conditions affecting the current market for goods.

Industry Statistics. Tabular statistical information about an industry.

Figure 15.9   A Selection of Market Research Report Databases Online

Database	Availability	Notes
Asian Business Intelligence Reports	Current, updated monthly Dialog	Detailed local reports focusing on developing markets, industries, and products in Australia, China, Hong Kong, Indonesia, Malaysia, New Zealand, the Philippines, Singapore, South Korea, Taiwan, Thailand, and Vietnam.
BCC Market Research	1990–, updated monthly Dialog	Business Communications Company (BCC) reports address industry structure, market segmentation, production and consumption statistics, new technologies, as well as providing company profiles. Subject coverage includes biotechnology, healthcare materials, and medical technology. Geographic scope: 80% of coverage devoted to U.S. market, 20% to world markets.
Datamonitor Market Research	1992–, updated bimonthly DataStar and Dialog	Syndicated research, drawing from commissioned Gallup surveys and consumer panels. Points addressed include market share, pricing, competitive environment. OTC products and Rx pharmaceuticals are among subjects covered. Published in the United Kingdom, reports cover developments in France, Italy, Germany, Spain, Europe, the U.K., and USA.
Decision Resources Pharmaceutical Industry Reports	1996–, updated monthly Dialog	The *DR Link* series of reports from Decision Resources analyzes and interprets advances and emerging trends in the healthcare industry. The *Pharmacor* series examines the commercial outlook for drugs in development to treat cardiovascular, CNS, or immune system diseases, cancer, and bacterial or viral infections.
Euromonitor Market Research	1992–, updated bimonthly DataStar and Dialog	Reports focus on consumer goods and services, including consumer healthcare and cosmetics and toiletries, in France, Germany, Italy, Spain, the United Kingdom, and the USA. Publications include items from the *Market Directions* series, *Euromonitor Emerging Markets*, and *Strategic Management Overviews*.
FIND®/SVP Market Research	1993–, updated monthly Dialog	FIND/SVP's *Packaged Facts* and other market studies are based on extensive executive interviews and secondary literature research. Data compilations address size and growth of market, trend assessment, forecasts, and profiles of influential competitors. Subject coverage includes biotechnology, drugs, healthcare products and services, with a geographic scope encompassing both the USA and international markets.
Freedonia Market Research	1990–, updated monthly DataStar and Dialog	Freedonia produces analyses of industries and products and profiles major players. Detailed historical and forecast data are often presented in tabular format. Healthcare and medical products industry coverage, with 80% of data devoted to USA, 10% USA and Canada, and 10% world data, by country.
Frost & Sullivan Market Intelligence	1994–, updated monthly DataStar and Dialog	In-depth analyses and forecasts of technical market trends, including market share, sales, and vendor profiles. Industries covered include biotechnology, medical devices, pharmaceuticals, and veterinary medicine. European, U.S., and worldwide reports are included.

Snapshots International Markets Research	Current, updated annually Dialog	More than 1,000 concise reports on market segments for consumer, business-to-business, and industrial goods, with market size, growth, and share figures included. Geographic scope includes the USA, United Kingdom, and Europe.

Market Share. Textual or tabular information about a company's percentage of total market volume.

New Products. Discussion of previously unavailable products or services.

Research and Development. News of what's in the pipeline.

As this selection of subject term options indicates, *Investext* content is by no means limited to financial data, in the narrowly defined sense of sales and earnings reports and forecasts. Market share and size projections involve investigation of political, legal, and demographic factors. For example, investment analysts routinely investigate a company's patent portfolio as part of their overall assessment of its long-term health and wealth. A surprising amount of epidemiological data is also compiled in *Investext* reports.[7]

Several free Internet sources of drug sales and utilization data, such as Miller Freeman's *dotpharmacy* site and the National Association of Chain Drug Stores home page, are discussed in Chapter Thirteen. Although much more limited in scope than fee-based services described in this section, sites such as these can often supply quick answers to casual inquiries, when time and money are limited.

Other Sources of Incidence, Prevalence, Patient Demographics, and Procedures Data

Disease demography is an important part of market research in the pharmaceutical industry. Prelaunch sales projections based on patient population assessments exercise a strong influence on research and development decisions. IND applications, in outlining proposed protocols for clinical testing, must define selection criteria for trial participants, showing the comparability of the population to be studied with the ultimate target population that the drug is intended to treat.

Once a drug is approved, still more statistical data will be needed to support marketing the product to managed care organizations. If a company hopes to compete with established drugs on factors other than pricing, material presented to formulary decision-makers must include data on quantifiable measures of effectiveness beyond per unit cost. Can the new product lower the number of hospital admissions or decrease length of stay? Does the course of therapy require fewer office visits to physicians, either by shortening recovery time or reducing side effects? How does the drug affect the cost of illness compared to other alternatives?

Although several of the bibliographic databases discussed in Chapter Fourteen cover sources that contain statistical data, their records do not always identify the presence of numeric tables embedded in the full text of primary sources cited. In many medical literature files, when "statistics" is used as an index term, citations retrieved tend to focus on statistical methodologies, rather than containing epidemiological data. In other words, their emphasis is on statistics as a subject, rather than as an attribute, of the bibliography. To overcome this barrier, elaborate strategies must often be constructed to separate the gold from the dross.[8, 9]

Full-text files in machine-readable form offer more opportunities for successful retrieval of medical and healthcare statistics, provided that extra indexing has been added to identify the presence of tables, charts, graphs or other illustrative material implying succinct, but substantive, presentation of numeric data. For example, the co-occurrence of terms such as asthma, child or pediatric, and mortality or death does not necessarily ensure relevance, but if a strategy can be further restricted to items containing tables or graphs, reliability of results increases. Unfortunately, few biomedical databases offer users this option. On the other hand, business and consumer oriented literature sources often do, as was illustrated in discussion of *Investext* and market research report databases.

Another example is the *IAC Health & Wellness Database* (14.33), which consistently notes the presence of illustrations in sources cited. The many full-text pamphlets and topical overviews of diseases and conditions reproduced in this database frequently provide a quicker route to epidemiological data than is afforded in *MEDLINE, EMBASE*, or other professional literature indexes. Patient education and support materials produced by organizations such as the American Diabetes Association, National Hemophilia Foundation, National Kidney Foundation, or the American Lupus Society often assemble authoritative numbers. The need for more readily accessible statistical and numeric data in medicine led to the introduction of a unique new online resource in 1995, the *Incidence and Prevalence Database* (*IPD*).

15.39 *Incidence and Prevalence Database.* Palo Alto, CA: Timely Data Resources, 1988–. Updated quarterly. Available on DataStar and Dialog; also on floppy disk.

IPD compiles information on epidemiology, incidence, prevalence, morbidity, mortality, risk factors, trends, and costs associated with diseases or surgical procedures. It monitors hospital, emergency room, physician's office, and inpatient/outpatient visits, extracting data from more than 3,000 scientific, business, and trade journals, investment reports, audits, and national and international surveys.

By consolidating and summarizing statistics from many different sources, the *Incidence and Prevalence Database* has become an important tool for assessing market opportunities and size, and assembling evidence for cost-of-illness analyses as part of pharmacoeconomics evaluations. Searchable by *ICD-9* codes, subject keywords, and country, *IPD* records generally consist of both narrative text and statistical breakdowns by year, gender, and age, when such data are pertinent and available. *IPD* is a good place to start when questions involve disease and treatment demographic data. For example, What risk factors are associated with hormone replacement therapy? What are the costs associated with back pain? In which diseases is compliance a problem?

Like *TableBase*, *IPD* has also been implemented as a pay-per-view service on the Web, available at http://www.tdrdata.com. There, it has many competitors offered free of charge. However, locating and extracting epidemiological and outcomes data from a succession of separate sites must be weighed against the convenience of ready-made, consistently indexed compilations offered by Timely Data Resources.

Healthcare Statistics on the Internet

Predictably, the Centers for Disease Control and Prevention's Internet site is a rich repository of communicable disease demographic data, including information gathered by the National Center for Health Statistics. NCHS sources cited in Chapter Thirteen (13.31–13.33 and 13.36) are available as downloadable full-text files. Answers in the "Frequently Asked Questions" section of the CDC home page anticipate ready-reference queries about average length of hospital stays, contraceptive practices, or physician visits. "Data from Death Investigations" leads to predefined tables correlating mortality with any of seventy-two causes. CDC Wonder, another menu option, facilitates retrieval from forty text-based and numeric databases, including *Morbidity and Mortality Weekly Reports*, *Surveillance Summaries*, and *MMWR Supplements*. Using this search engine, it is possible to find numbers and rates (incidence and prevalence) of specified diseases. The CDC's Internet address is http://www.cdc.gov.

The Federal Interagency Council on Statistical Policy *FEDSTATS* search engine enables keyword queries to locate statistical publications produced by any of twenty-eight U.S. government agencies. Its index is updated monthly, and the search form includes a selection of databases or agencies for limiting and focusing results (http://www.fedstats.gov/search.html). For a direct route to two other specialized Internet sources of epidemiological data, see Chapter Eight's discussion of reports from the *Drug Abuse Warning Network* (*DAWN*) and the *National Household Survey on Drug Abuse* (8.43–8.44).

The *WHO Statistical Information System* maintains a home page at http://www.who.int/whosis. The *Global Health-For-All* database is located here, as is the full text of the *Weekly Epidemiological Record*, along with instructions for establishing ongoing e-mail subscriptions.

Probably the best approach to building knowledge of healthcare statistics available on the World Wide Web is to start with some of the major subject hubs identified in Figure 15.10. Each uncovers unique sites not included in other pathfinders, so it's a good idea to set aside time to explore them all and begin constructing a personal bookmark list for quick reference in the future.

Figure 15.10   Subject Hubs to Locate Healthcare Statistics on the Internet

- *EpiVetNet* (Massey University, NZ)
  ⇨ http://epiweb.massey.ac.nz
- *Health Statistics—College & Research Libraries News* (Auditore & Stoklosa)
  ⇨ http://www.ala.acrl/resoct97.html
- *HealthLinks: International Health and Social Statistics* (University of Washington)
  ⇨ http://www.hslib.washington.edu/statistics
- *HealthWeb Public Health Statistics* (University of Michigan)
  ⇨ http://www.lib.umich/hw/public.health/health.stats.html
- *HSLS Health Statistics* (University of Pittsburgh)
  ⇨ http://www.hsls.pitt.edu/intres/guides/statcbw.html
- *MedNets Epidemiology & Public Health*
  ⇨ http://www.internets.com/epidemio.htm
- *Resources in Epidemiology* (University of Pittsburgh)
  ⇨ http://www.pitt.edu/~epidept/resource.html
- *The Wellcome Trust Centre for the Epidemiology of Infectious Disease*
  ⇨ http://www.ceid.ox.ac.uk/Links/sql.asp
- *World Wide Web Virtual Library: Epidemiology* (University of California, San Francisco)
  ⇨ http://www.epibiostat.ucsf.edu/epidem/epidem.html

Summary and Segue

Analysis of 6,729 online searches carried out in the information department at a major pharmaceutical company from 1989–1993 showed that marketing and sales departments submitted the most requests for information (14% and 42%, respectively, compared to 35% originating in R&D).[10] Three general topics topped marketing's list: finding new indications for established drugs, answering epidemiological questions related to potential new forms of therapy, and evaluating license opportunities. Because such inquiries are typical (and often troublesome), ways and means to solve these and similar information problems have been the primary focus of this chapter.

Monitoring U.S. Food and Drug Administration activities is yet another form of competitive intelligence. As the primary gatekeeper to the lucrative drug and medical technology marketplace, the FDA's decisions regarding new therapeutic product introductions or what constitutes acceptable industry practice (manufacturing, promotion, testing) affect an incredibly broad range of interrelated commercial enterprises, including not only competing companies, prospective investors, and insurers, but also advertising agencies, legal counsel, shipping companies, and packaging firms. Knowing why, when, and where to search for regulatory documents is the topic of Chapter Sixteen.

References

1. Krol TF, Coleman JC, Bryant PJ. Scientific competitive intelligence in r&d decision making. *Drug Inf J* 1996;30:252.

2. Snow B. Keeping up-to-date with full-text F-D-C Reports. *Online* 1990 May;14:94–97.

3. Snow B. Full-text healthcare business sources online. *Online* 1993 Mar;17:103–108.

4. Drews J, Ryser S. Innovation deficit in the pharmaceutical industry. *Drug Inf J* 1996;30:97–108.

5. Snow B. Global guides to launched drug products: IMSworld New Product Launch Letter and Product Monographs databases. Part 1. *Database* 1994 Aug;17:93–97. Part 2. *Database* 1994 Oct;17:107–110.

6. Snow B. A new medical device directory online: ECRI's Health Devices Sourcebook. *Online* 1989 May;13:103–107.

7. Snow B. Noneconomic healthcare information in Investext: epidemiologic data and background on legislation and regulation. *Database* 1994 Apr;17:96–99.

8. Snow B. Finding medical and health care statistics online. *Online* 1988 Jul;12:86–95.

9. Snow B. Health care statistics online: business, news, and government resources. *Online* 1988 Sep;12:102–109.

10. Thomas M, Gretz M. From serum cholesterol in elephants to morbidity in Nepal: An empirical analysis of 6,729 on-line searches at Boehringer Mannheim GmbH. *Drug Inf J* 1996;30:217–236.

Additional Sources of Information

Bootman JL, Townsend RJ, McGhan WF, eds. *Principles of pharmacoeconomics*. Cincinnati, OH: Harvey Whitney Books, 1996.

Bradley CA et al. Quality assessment of economic evaluations in selected pharmacy, medical, and health economics journals. *Ann Pharmacother* 1995 Jul;29:681–689.

Clement GP. *Science and technology on the Internet: an instructional guide*. Internet workshop series, no. 4. Berkeley, CA: Library Solutions Press, 1995.

Desai BH, Bawden D. Competitor intelligence in the pharmaceutical industry, the role of the information professional. *J Info Sci* 1993;19(5):327–338.

Drug outcomes sourcebook. A progress report and resource guide to pharmaceutical cost-effectiveness and outcomes research. New York: Faulkner & Gray, 1995.

Haas LM. Online ready reference searching for company and market share information. In: *Proceedings of the eleventh National Online Meeting*. Medford, NJ: Learned Information, 1990, 149–153.

Hancock L, ed. *Key guide to electronic resources: Health sciences*. Medford, NJ: Learned Information, 1995.

Nye JB, Brassil EC. Online searching in selected business databases for management aspects of health care. *Med Ref Serv Q* 1984 Spr;3:33–48.

Ojala M. The business of medicine. *Online* 1988 Nov;12(6):88–93.

Ojala M. Business searching for biotechnology. *Database* 1994 Aug:17(4):74–76.

Snow B. Creating tables of data from multiple records: The REPORT feature. *Online* 1992 Sep;16:97–102.

Snow B. General business statistics and r&d specifics—Pharmaprojects has the answers. *Database* 1990 Oct;13:111–115.

Snow B. They stood up and were counted: Health surveys and public opinion polls online. *Database* 1992 Feb;15:88–93.

Snow B. When corporate human resource departments look for healthcare information. *Online* 1989 Sep;13:112–118.

Snow B. When hospitals mean business: Online sources for health care marketing information. *Online* 1989 Nov;13:112–116.

16

Regulatory Sources Online

The need for drug and device regulatory information is not confined to an isolated group of legal staff within the pharmaceutical industry. A financial analyst might ask: What are the top five generic drug companies in terms of numbers of new products approved in the past twenty-four months? And what percentage of each company's total represents first-time approvals for off-patent drugs? Medical engineers might benefit from a survey of adverse experience reports for the purpose of identifying potential defects to avoid in designing new products of a similar type. Market researchers could use the same data to assess perhaps unavoidable hazards and consequent product liability costs. The director of pharmacy services to a chain of nursing homes may need a list of all approved formulations, generic and brand name, of an antiarthritic drug. Developers of a novel drug delivery system will want to review types of drugs already approved using competing technology. A bulk chemical supplier needs to monitor drug patent expirations to gauge potential markets for long-range planning. The list of possible applications could go on and on. Once their implications are understood, regulatory documents are rapidly transmuted from arcane to essential research tools.

For this startling metamorphosis to take place, it's necessary for prospective beneficiaries of regulatory data (and their information mediators) to know what's available and its potential significance. Background on drug and device law provided in Chapter Four, with particular reference to regulatory hot topics and frequently asked questions, is a prerequisite to effective use of documents that are the focus of discussion here. For example, knowing whether a 510k, a PMA, or a PMA supplement is the end point affects resource selection in answering medical device regulatory queries. This distinction also influences the strategy employed, timing of published notices, and the likelihood of success in locating relevant materials.

Finding Information on Product Approvals

Three online sources provide access to U.S. drug or device product approval information: the *FDA Home Page* on the Internet, *Diogenes*, and the *F-D-C Reports* database. Differences in scope, timeliness, and accessibility must be weighed each time a question calls for information about authorizations to market. Does the query involve recent approvals announced within the past one to two months? Or are retrospective data needed, e.g., all drugs approved for a given indication, or devices originating from a specified company? Is ongoing current awareness the objective, and for what types of approvals (original or supplemental NDAs, ANDAs, BLAs, etc.)? Are applicant company, ingredients, Rx versus OTC status, dosage form, strength, route of administration, or therapeutic use key elements in prescreening for answers? Factors such as these will sharply define source selection decisions, due to dramatic differences in how and when approvals are indexed by each database and which products are covered.

Drug Registrations

Announcements of new drug approvals are available for inspection free of charge on the FDA's World Wide Web site (http://www.fda.gov). Clicking on the human drugs icon will link users to the opening screen from the agency's Center for Drug Evaluation and Research (CDER). Choosing CDER's "Drug Info" option leads to a choice of 1) new and generic drug approvals, 2) FDA drug approvals list, September 1996 forward, or 3) FDA drug and device approval list legacy information from February 1991 through August 1996. The first option is an extremely timely listing of original, supplemental (both efficacy and labeling), abbreviated, and "approvable" human NDA authorizations, updated on a daily basis as information becomes available. Preliminary records for registrations typically appear within one week of FDA approval. These interim entries, sorted by brand name, provide generic names of active ingredients, dosage form and strength(s), applicant (company) name, application number, approval date, and Rx versus OTC status. Presented in tabular format, this list of newly approved products also adds hypertext links to the full text of the agency's approval letter and official labeling as soon as these materials are released after initial product postings.

The second CDER approvals option offers retrospective access to separate month by month listings, updated weekly, in which entries are organized in reverse chronological order by approval date and include the additional data elements of chemical type (NCE, etc.), therapeutic potential (FDA priority classification), and indications. An opening statement on the year/month selection page warns users that recent listings may not contain all approvals, referring to *Orange Book* (*Approved Drug Products with Therapeutic Equivalence Evaluations*, 4.42) monthly updates as a definitive source, instead. However, *Orange Book* supplements, another selection on CDER's drug information Web menu, are less than timely, lagging behind NDA authorizations by three to four months. For example, the latest update as of December 1998 was the August edition. Furthermore, *Orange Book* listings do not provide all of the data elements assembled in new drug registration records.

Under the "Legacy" information link, combined drug (human and animal), biologic, and device approval lists are available month by month from January 1995 through August 1996. Full year, downloadable WordPerfect files are the only option for viewing approvals from 1991 through 1994. Note, also, that since the combined approvals listing has been discontinued, it is necessary to look elsewhere on the FDA Web site for current registrations no longer included on CDER's menu. For example, coverage of biologic licenses (PLAs, ELAs, BLAs) disappeared from listings found under the human drugs icon in August 1996. Users are referred, instead, to the separate biologics section of the *FDA Home Page*. Similarly, NADAs are now segregated under the animal drugs icon, where an electronic database covers all veterinary pharmaceuticals approved for marketing in the United States, updated monthly.

Source selection within the FDA Web site will, then, be influenced by differences in types of approvals covered, timeliness, and retrospective availability. What is likely to prove even more important is searchability. Results of queries lead to, at minimum, full month displays, which must then be scanned for pertinent records. (The FIND function built into Web browser software can assist navigation to desired entries.) Only fee-based online services currently offer the ability to isolate, in advance, approval list subsets matching user-defined parameters such as company name, therapeutic class, active ingredients, and other combinations of data elements often specified in requests for registration information.

One such source is *F-D-C Reports Online* (15.10). It includes individual approval records for original NDAs, supplemental efficacy and supplemental labeling NDAs, biologics, approvable originals, abbreviated NDAs, and tentative approvals of ANDAs. From November 1987 through December 1995, indexing was included in *The Pink Sheet*. Since January 1996, registration announcements are accessible in the new F-D-C publication, *Pharmaceutical Approvals Monthly*. The *F-D-C Reports* database incorporates the full text of each of these newsletters. As the sample record reproduced in Figure 16.1 illustrates, searchable data elements include company name, active ingredients, dosage form, brand name, indication keywords, and date of approval. Results of user-defined queries lead to targeted displays of relevant records, with no necessity to scan full month listings. This quality filtered access to new U.S. drug approvals is available in *F-D-C Reports Online* within one month following registration.

The lag time for announcements of ANDA authorizations is shorter. Both tentative and final approvals are accessible in *F-D-C Reports* within one week of their release by the FDA. A sample record is reproduced in Figure 16.2. Search

Figure 16.1   Sample Drug Approval Notice in F-D-C Reports Online

DIALOG(R)File 187:F-D-C Reports
© 1997 F-D-C Reports Inc. All rts. reserv.

00174467 F-D-C Accession Number 06020020055
Pharmaceutical Approvals Monthly
February 1, 1997
Volume 2, Issue 2

FDA's DECEMBER-1996 PREPARED REPORT OF NDA APPROVALS

PRODUCT NAME: Zagam 20–677 (1 S)
APPLICANT: Rhone-Poulenc Rorer
ACTIVE INGREDIENTS: Sparfloxacin 200 mg, tab.
PRINCIPAL INDICATIONS: Fluoroquinolone antibiotic (community-acquired pneumonia, and acute bacterial exacerbations of chronic bronchitis)
DATE APPROVED: 12/19/96
TYPE OF APPROVAL: Original

capabilities enable users to isolate entries by active ingredients, company name, and dosage forms.

16.1 *Diogenes*. Rockville, MD: FOI Services, 1976–. Updated weekly. Available on DataStar, Dialog, and SilverPlatter.

Another source of information on U.S. drug approvals is *Diogenes*. Like its Greek philosopher namesake, *Diogenes* specializes in bringing things to light, specifically, FDA regulatory documents related to human drugs and medical devices, as well as full-text issues of six newsletters from Washington Business Information (see Figure 15.8). There are two publications searchable in *Diogenes* covering drug approval announcements. One is a monthly *Drug and Device Approvals List*. Unfortunately, coverage of this title in *Diogenes* is far less timely than registration announcements found on the FDA Web site. FOI Services generally takes three to four months to release its searchable list, while the FDA's issue of full, verified entries typically lags behind actual approval date by only two to three weeks. It should also be noted that *Diogenes* indexing of the monthly *Approvals List* omits supplemental labeling NDAs and veterinary drug approvals, both of which are included in FDA Web site coverage.

On the other hand, *Diogenes* offers powerful search and display capabilities and indexing of authorized NDAs and ANDAs retrospective to 1984. As sample records reproduced in Figure 16.3 illustrate, access points include brand name, generic name, company and location, approval date, dosage form, strength, and drug class. Retrieval can be further restricted by type of approval (original NDA,

Figure 16.2   Sample ANDA Approvals in F-D-C Reports Online

DIALOG(R)File 187:F-D-C Reports
© 1996 F-D-C Reports Inc. All rts. reserv.

00147967   F-D-C Accession Number   00580160042
The Pink Sheet
April 15, 1996
Volume 58, Issue 16

FDA's ANDA APPROVALS

TRADE/PRODUCT NAME: None 74–588
APPLICANT: Barre-National
ACTIVE INGREDIENTS: Minoxidil 2%, topical solution
DATE APPROVED (EFFECTIVE DATE)4/5/96
PRODUCT CATEGORY: ABBREVIATED NEW DRUG APPROVALS
    TRADE/PRODUCT NAME: None 74–589
APPLICANT: Lemmon
ACTIVE INGREDIENTS: Minoxidil 2%, topical solution
DATE APPROVED (EFFECTIVE DATE)4/5/96
PRODUCT CATEGORY: ABBREVIATED NEW DRUG APPROVALS
    TRADE/PRODUCT NAME: None 74–643
APPLICANT: Bausch & Lomb
ACTIVE INGREDIENTS: Minoxidil 2%, topical solution
DATE APPROVED (EFFECTIVE DATE)4/9/96
PRODUCT CATEGORY: ABBREVIATED NEW DRUG APPROVALS
    TRADE/PRODUCT NAME: None 74–216
APPLICANT: Biocraft
ACTIVE INGREDIENTS: Naproxen USP 250 mg, 375 mg, 500 mg, tab.
DATE APPROVED (EFFECTIVE DATE)4/11/96
PRODUCT CATEGORY: ABBREVIATED NEW DRUG APPROVALS
    TRADE/PRODUCT NAME: None 73–667
APPLICANT: Biocraft
ACTIVE INGREDIENTS: Nortriptyline HCl USP 10 mg, 25 mg, 50 mg, 75 mg, capsule
DATE APPROVED (EFFECTIVE DATE)4/11/96
PRODUCT CATEGORY: ABBREVIATED NEW DRUG APPROVALS

approvable original, ANDA, or supplemental NDA). When searching for the latter, users can also distinguish between new indications and new dosage regimens or designate, if desired, Rx to OTC switch. For original NDAs, FDA priority coding (e.g., 3S, 1P) is directly searchable. Among ANDA approvals, it is possible to single out those available for the first time generically.

Another bonus in *Diogenes* is access to additional retrospective approval data not fully searchable elsewhere online, through a cumulative *New Drug List*

Figure 16.3   Monthly Drug Approval Notices in Diogenes

DIALOG(R)File 158:Diogenes
© 1996 DIOGENES. All rts. reserv.
04423205   913750
ORIGINAL ABBREVIATED NDA (ANDA): DILTIAZEM HCL.
  DRUG BRAND NAME(S): DILTIAZEM HCL
  DRUG GENERIC NAME: DILTIAZEM HCL 5 MG/ML
  COMPANY NAME: BEDFORD BEDFORD, OHIO
  DRUG/DEVICE NO.: 74617
  SOURCE: FDA DRUG AND DEVICE PRODUCT APPROVALS FEBRUARY 1996.
  DOCUMENT TYPE: DRUG (DRG)
  PUBLICATION DATE: 960228
  IDENTIFIERS: CLASS: CALCIUM ION INFLUX INHIBITOR; FIRST TIME PROD-
UCT AVAILABLE GENERICALLY; DOSAGE FORM: INJECTABLE

DIALOG(R)File 158:Diogenes
© 1996 DIOGENES. All rts. reserv.
04423163   913708
ORIGINAL AND SUPPLEMENTAL NDA: ROGAINE.
  DRUG BRAND NAME(S): ROGAINE
  DRUG GENERIC NAME: MINOXIDIL 2%
  COMPANY NAME: UPJOHN KALAMAZOO, MICHIGAN
  DRUG/DEVICE NO.: 19501
  SOURCE: FDA DRUG AND DEVICE PRODUCT APPROVALS FEBRUARY 1996.
  DOCUMENT TYPE: DRUG (DRG)
  PUBLICATION DATE: 960209
  IDENTIFIERS: CLASS: RX TO OTC SWITCH; OTC; TYPE: SUPPLEMENT 12
DOSAGE FORM: SOLUTION

DIALOG(R)File 158:Diogenes
© 1996 DIOGENES. All rts. reserv.
03667779   912010
ORIGINAL AND SUPPLEMENTAL NDA: NEUTREXIN.
  DRUG BRAND NAME(S): NEUTREXIN
  DRUG GENERIC NAME: TRIMETREXATE GLUCURONATE EQ 25 MG BASE/
VIAL
  COMPANY NAME: US BIOSCIENCE WEST CONSHOHOCKEN, PENNSYL-
VANIA
  DRUG/DEVICE NO.: 20326
  SOURCE: FDA DRUG AND DEVICE PRODUCT APPROVALS DECEMBER 1993.
  DOCUMENT TYPE: DRUG (DRG)
  PUBLICATION DATE: 931217
  IDENTIFIERS: CLASS: FOLATE ANTAGONIST; PNEUMOCYSTIS CARINII
PNEUMONIA; TYPE: 1P, AA (PRIORITY CLASSIFICATION AIDS DRUG), V (DES-
IGNATED ORPHAN DRUG), E (DRUG FOR SEVERELY DEBILITATING/LIFE
THREATENING ILLNESS); DOSAGE FORM: INJECTABLE

(*NDL*). NDAs for all human drugs approved since the enactment of the current U.S. drug law in 1938 are listed in *NDL*, which is updated quarterly. A sample record is reproduced in Figure 16.4. Note that there are several differences, beyond retrospective coverage and update frequency, between quarterly *NDL* entries and monthly announcements of approvals. First, *NDL* records for original NDAs provide the U.S. patent number for a product, its patent expiration date, and date when patent and market exclusivity expires. When applicable, date of product discontinuation or withdrawal from the market can also be determined by consulting *NDL* records in *Diogenes*. In addition, route of administration is consistently identified in the quarterly *NDL* list, but can only be inferred from dosage form indicators in monthly new drug announcements (Figure 16.3). On the other hand, monthly NDA entries afford searchers opportunities for compiling lists of product approvals by drug class, whereas pharmacological or therapeutic keywords are omitted in quarterly *NDL* records. OTC (nonprescription) marketing status is indicated in monthly NDA approvals, but not in the retrospective *NDL* list. Figure 16.5 summarizes differences in sources of U.S. drug approvals in *Diogenes*.

For current awareness intended to track all new U.S. drug approvals, the *FDA Home Page* is probably the best choice. If timely coverage of generic product registrations is needed, *F-D-C Reports* supplies better search capabilities for prescreening. When a question calls for a thorough retrospective survey of approvals, *Diogenes* is currently the best option. Regardless of which database is used to locate U.S. drug approvals, beware of possible variations in company name

Figure 16.4 Sample Entry from the Quarterly New Drug List in Diogenes

DIALOG(R)File 158:Diogenes
© 1996 DIOGENES. All rts. reserv.

04420993   4027322
Original or Supplemental New Drug Application (NDA): ZOFRAN. ONDANSETRON HYDROCHLORIDE EQ 2MG BASE/ML. INJECTION; IV(INFUSION).
DRUG BRAND NAME(S): ZOFRAN
DRUG GENERIC NAME: ONDANSETRON HYDROCHLORIDE EQ 2MG BASE/
    ML. INJECTION; IV(INFUSION)
COMPANY NAME: Glaxo
DRUG/DEVICE NO.: 20007
SOURCE: FDA New Drug Application List (NDL). List Edition: FEBRUARY 1996.
DOCUMENT TYPE: DRUG (DRG).
PUBLICATION DATE: 910104
IDENTIFIERS: PATENT: 4695578 PATENT EXPIRATION: 200125 EXCLUSIVITY
    CODE: I-9
EXCLUSIVITY EXPIRATION: 960813

Figure 16.5   Differences in Sources of U.S. Drug Approval Information Online in Diogenes

Comparison Checklist	Monthly List	Quarterly New Drug List
Scope		
Original & Supplemental NDAs	√	√
Abbreviated NDAs ·	√	√
Supplemental Labeling NDAs	√	
Efficacy Supplements	√	
Record Content		
Therapeutic/Pharmacological class	√	
Dosage Form	√	√
Route of Administration		√
Applicant Company Location	√	
Patent/Market Exclusivity Data		√
Date of Discontinuation/Withdrawal		√
Indication of OTC Market Status	√	
FDA Priority Coding	√	

format and dosage form or drug category descriptive terms. For example, Johnson RW and R.W. Johnson have been used to designate the same company, just as Merrell-Dow or Marion Merrell Dow, Lilly or Eli Lilly, MSD or Merck Sharp Dohme have been used interchangeably. Some dosage forms are abbreviated (cap, tab, inj); others are spelled out in full (powder, solution, film, drops, aerosol, ointment, cream). Drug category terms are an unpredictable mixture of therapeutic and pharmacological terminology: e.g., antibacterial, decongestant, analgesic, calcium ion influx inhibitor, beta adrenergic blocker.

What about keeping up-to-date on launches worldwide? Two drugs-in-development directories discussed in the previous chapter are good sources for monitoring official registrations in other countries. In *Pharmaprojects* (15.1), the keyword *registration* can be coordinated with a country name or abbreviation in the update segment of records. Either first or additional registration can also be specified, along with year and month. A comparable current awareness strategy intended for *IMSworld R&D Focus Drug Updates* (15.2) would substitute *registered* as the approved status indicator. Selected product approvals are also announced in *Scrip* (15.9), *InPharma* (14.11), and *Drug News and Perspectives* (15.13).

Sources for Medical Device Approvals

Relative timeliness and searchability are also factors in distinguishing among sources for U.S. medical device premarket application (PMA) approvals. PMAs authorized from February 1991 through August 1996 are accessible on the Center for Drug Evaluation and Research (CDER) menu under the human drugs icon on the *FDA Home Page*, where they are mixed in with NDA approvals (as described in the previous section). A separate, PMA-only listing is linked to the main *FDA Home Page* under the medical devices/radiological health icon. From the Center for Devices and Radiological Health (CDRH) opening menu, click on "Program Areas" to locate the releasable PMAs option. Here, monthly PMA listings (originals and supplements) are available for immediate display from January 1995 forward.

In addition to month by month sequential displays, CDRH provides more targeted access through a PMA database search form, reproduced in Figure 16.6. Records can be isolated by applicant (company) name, brand name, product code, PMA number, date, and Advisory Committee Panel. What is unclear is whether the FDA's searchable database includes all PMAs (1976 forward) or only that portion of monthly listings offered elsewhere on the Web site (1995 forward under CDRH and 1991–1994 under CDER). What is clear is that the lag

Figure 16.6 PMA Database Search Form on the FDA Web Site

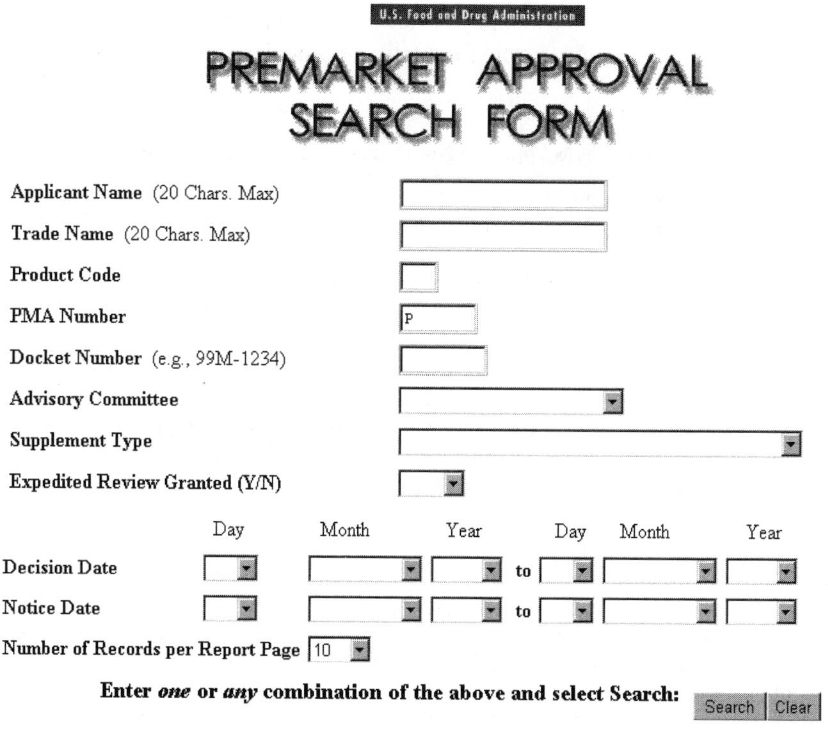
U.S. Food and Drug Administration

PREMARKET APPROVAL SEARCH FORM

Applicant Name (20 Chars. Max)

Trade Name (20 Chars. Max)

Product Code

PMA Number P

Docket Number (e.g., 99M-1234)

Advisory Committee

Supplement Type

Expedited Review Granted (Y/N)

	Day	Month	Year		Day	Month	Year
Decision Date				to			
Notice Date				to			

Number of Records per Report Page 10

Enter *one* or *any* combination of the above and select Search: Search Clear time between actual date of approval and announcement at the CDRH site is three to four weeks, on average.

If more timely access is needed, users will find that PMA approvals are usually indexed within one week of FDA announcement and converted to fully searchable format online in *The Gray Sheet*, part of the *F-D-C Reports* database (15.10, 1987–). As the sample record reproduced in Figure 16.7 illustrates, PMA entries are easily retrieved by approval date, applicant company name and location, brand name, and approval class.

PMA authorizations are also cited in the *Federal Register* and *Diogenes* (16.1). Full *Federal Register* notices contain information valuable in gauging timelines from submission to launch for selected types of products. For example, dates are given for the initial PMA submission to the FDA, agency referral to an advisory committee for review, and for the approval letter and any subsequent correspondence or other communications with the applicant company. Notices also fully describe the product and its use, as shown in Figure 16.8.

The drawbacks to monitoring new device approvals directly through the *Federal Register* are its limitations in scope and timeliness of PMA coverage. The *Federal Register* generally announces only original PMAs (omits supplements) and tends to lag behind both *F-D-C Reports* and the Center for Devices and Radiological Health Web site by at least three weeks.

Diogenes' posting of the monthly device premarket approvals list is even more dilatory.[1] However, as was seen in coverage of drug approvals, *Diogenes* offers

---

Figure 16.7   Sample PMA Approval Notice from F-D-C Reports Online

---

DIALOG(R)File 187:F-D-C Reports
© 1996 F-D-C Reports Inc. All rts. reserv.

00148029   F-D-C Accession Number   01220160061
The Gray Sheet
April 15, 1996
Volume 22, Issue 16

FDA's MARCH 1996 REPORT OF MEDICAL DEVICE APPROVALS

TRADE/PRODUCT NAME: Truquant BR RIA
SERIAL NUMBER: P950011
APPLICANT: Biomira Diagnostics, Inc., Rockville, MD
COMMENT: An in vitro diagnostic device for the quantitative determination of CA 27.29 antigen in serum or EDTA plasma of patients previously treated for stage II or III breast cancer.
APPROVAL CLASS: PREMARKET APPROVALS
APPROVAL DATE: 3/29/96

Figure 16.8 Sample PMA Approval Notice from the Federal Register

DIALOG(R)File 669:Federal Register
(c) 1996 Knight-Ridder Info. All rts. reserv.

00594078
Biomira Diagnostics, Inc.; Premarket Approval of TRUQUANT (R) BR(TM) RIA
Vol. 61, No. 142
61 FR 38206
Tuesday, July 23, 1996

AGENCY: DEPARTMENT OF HEALTH AND HUMAN SERVICES (HHS); Public Health Service (PHS); Food and Drug Administration (FDA)
DOC TYPE: Notices
NUMBER: Docket No. 96M-0216
DATES: Petitions for administrative review by August 22, 1996.
CONTACT: FOR FURTHER INFORMATION CONTACT: Peter E. Maxim, Center for Devices and Radiological Health (HFZ-440), Food and Drug Administration, 9200 Corporate Blvd., Rockville, MD 20850, 301-594-1293.
ADDRESSES: Written requests for copies of the summary of safety and effectiveness data and petitions for administrative review to the Dockets Management Branch (HFA-305), Food and Drug Administration, 12420 Parklawn Dr., rm. 1-23, Rockville, MD 20857.
ACTION: Notice.
SUMMARY: The Food and Drug Administration (FDA) is announcing its approval of the application submitted by Thomas Tsakeris, Devices and Diagnostics Consulting Group, Rockville, MD, U.S. Representative for Biomira Diagnostics Inc., 30 Meridian Rd., Rexdale, ON, Canada, for premarket approval, under the Federal Food, Drug, and Cosmetic Act (the act), of TRUQUANT (R) BR(TM) RIA. After reviewing the recommendation of the Immunology Devices Panel, FDA's Center for Devices and Radiological Health (CDRH) notified the applicant, by letter of March 29, 1996, of the approval of the application.

WORD COUNT: 684
TEXT:

SUPPLEMENTARY INFORMATION: On February 24, 1995, Thomas M. Tsakeris, Devices and Diagnostics Consulting Group, Rockville, MD, U.S. Representative for Biomira Diagnostics, Inc., Rexdale, ON, Canada, submitted to CDRH an application for premarket approval of TRUQUANT (R) BR(TM) RIA. The device is an in vitro diagnostic device indicated for quantitative determination of CA 27.29 antigen in serum or EDTA plasma of patients previously treated for Stage II or Stage III breast cancer. Serial testing for CA 27.29 antigen with TRUQUANT (R) BR(TM) RIA in patients who are clinically free of disease should be used in conjunction with other clinical methods used for the early detection of recurrence.
-On September 21, 1995, the Immunology Devices Panel of the Medical Devices Advisory Committee, an FDA advisory committee, reviewed and recommended approval of

the application. On March 29, 1996, CDRH approved the application by a letter to the applicant from the Director of the Office of Device Evaluation, CDRH.

-A summary of the safety and effectiveness data on which CDRH based its approval is on file in the Dockets Management Branch (address above) and is available from that office upon written request. Requests should be identified with the name of the device and the docket number found in brackets in the heading of this document.

-Opportunity for Administrative Review

-Section 515(d)(3) of the act (21 U.S.C. 360e(d)(3)) authorizes any interested person to petition, under section 515(g) of the act, for administrative review of CDRH's decision to approve this application. A petitioner may request . . . . [*text continues in the original, but is omitted here*]

Dated: June 21, 1996.

Joseph A. Levitt,

Deputy Director for Regulations Policy, Center for Devices and Radiological Health.
INTERNAL DATA: FR Doc. 96–18556; Filed 7–22–96; 8:45 am; BILLING CODE 4160–01-F

---

the advantage of full retrospective access online. All devices approved since the passage of the Medical Device Amendments in 1976 are documented in *Diogenes* through indexing of the FDA's quarterly *PMA List*. Company name, product name, and date are directly searchable, as well as the FDA advisory panel or committee with jurisdiction over each product. Using *Diogenes'* standardized panel abbreviations, searchers can locate approved devices by broad subject categories. For example, *DVCIRC*, the code for circulatory devices shown in the record reproduced in Figure 16.9, could be ANDed with *PMA* searched as a source to find all approved devices in that general category. FDA device classification codes offer a narrower approach to retrieving approvals in specified categories (e.g., *JOQ* in the sample record). Keywords can also be used to search categories of devices (such as *external* AND *pacemaker* as descriptors).

510ks

Technically, 510ks are not considered "approvals" by the FDA, merely "premarket notifications" (PMNs) mandated under Section 510(k) of the 1976 Medical Device Amendments. Nonetheless, requests for approvals of all medical devices manufactured or sponsored by a specified company will usually require finding 510ks, as well as PMAs. Both the CDRH menu accessible from the *FDA Home Page* on the Internet and *Diogenes* provide online access to 510ks retrospective to 1976. CDRH offers free month-by-month listings, organized in alphabetical order by company name, from November 1995 forward. CDRH also makes

Figure 16.9   Sample Diogenes Record from the FDA Quarterly PMA Listing

AN	03000736 9506. [DataStar]
OC	PARAGRAPH
	SO (1)
TI	MODEL 4553 DUAL CHAM. DDD TEMP.CARDIAC PACEMAKER: PMA Listing.
AU	Advisory committee : CIRCULATORY SYSTEMS DEVICE PANEL DEVICE PANEL (DVCIRC).
SO	FDA-PREMARKET-APPROVAL-LIST (PMA). LIST EDITION: MAY 1995.
YR	940310.
CO	Pace Medical.
NU	Drug/Device No.: P920032.
DE	(JOQ)-Generator,-Pulse,-Pacemaker,-External-Programmable. CLASS: 3. 870–.
PT	DEVICE (DEV).

zipped (compressed) files of approved 510ks available for the time periods 1976–1980, 1981–1985, 1986–1990, 1991–1995, and 1996 to date.

Manual or visual scanning of monthly or annual lists of 510ks is an impractical method for monitoring competitive developments or isolating entries in answer to specific queries. Fortunately, CDRH provides a search engine for accessing device premarket notifications. Users can limit recall to devices under the jurisdiction of a given FDA advisory panel and create subset listings by applicant (company) name, as shown in Figure 16.10. Searches can also focus on specific device names, product classification codes, or 510k numbers.

Diogenes also enables creation of customized device premarket notification listings. Queries can isolate subsets using any combination of date ranges, applicant name(s), advisory panel(s), and FDA device classification(s), as well as searches for specific K numbers or brand names (see Figure 16.11). FDA advisory panel codes are, again, one approach to retrieving broad categories of devices, while FDA device classification numbers or their keyword equivalents can be used to limit searches to more specific types of devices. When searching company names, remember to enter both subsidiaries and parents, when relevant (not all subsidiaries are also indexed under their parent company name). Variations in name format should also be anticipated.

Basis-of-Approval Documents

What was the basis for approval of product X? What data were submitted to substantiate bioequivalence of this product compared to drug Y? What kinds of stability studies and data analysis are generally submitted in NDAs for products of this type? Questions such as these require access to back-up documentation on file at the FDA.

Figure 16.10   510k Database Search Form on the FDA Web Site

U.S. Food and Drug Administration

RELEASABLE 510(k) SEARCH FORM

Panel	[▾]
Product Code	[ ]
510K Number	[K]
Applicant Name (20 Chars. Max.)	[allergan]
Device Name (20 Chars. Max.)	[ ]
Type	[▾]
Number of Records per Report Page	[10 ▾]

Center for Devices and Radiological Health — CDRH

Enter *one* or *any* combination of the above and select Search: Search | Clear

Figure 16.11   Sample 510k Record from Diogenes

AN	00771124 9405. [DataStar]
TI	JOBST ATHROMBIC PUMP –SYSTEM 2500 : 510(K) LISTING. FOI SUMMARY AVAILABLE FROM FOI SERVICES.
AU	Advisory committee : CIRCULATORY SYSTEMS DEVICE PANEL (DVCIRC).
SO	FDA-510-K-LIST (510K). LIST EDITION: APRIL 1994.
YR	940209.
CO	Jobst .
NU	Drug/Device No.: K934639 .
DE	(JOW)-Sleeve,-Compressible-Limb.-CLASS:-2. 870–5800. 870.5800.
PT	DEVICE (DEV).

Because of the volume of confidential business and patient information in an NDA or PMA, the full original document is not disclosable under Freedom of Information (FOI) provisions. Instead, summaries are prepared by the FDA and made available upon request, along with the approval letter, labeling, and reviewer commentary. For a drug, such documents are referred to as an SBA or SBOA (Summary Basis of Approval). In recent years, the agency has ceased preparation of SBAs, substituting, instead, relevant portions of written reviews (dubbed "SBA equivalents" by users). The counterpart document for a medical device premarket approval is known as an SS&E (Summary of Safety & Efficacy/Effectiveness) and for device premarket notifications, Substantially Equivalent (SE) 510k Summaries or Statements.

There are three routes to obtaining these basis-of-approval documents: 1) submission of a Freedom of Information Act request to the FDA, or a search of either 2) the *FDA Home Page* or 3) the *Diogenes* database. The first requires a formal letter following a carefully prescribed format; payment to the FDA for an archival search and review of documents by agency staff; public disclosure of requester name, affiliation, and the subject of each request; and patience. The other, more direct routes involve visual scans of free FDA document lists on the Web for requisite hypertext links or a quick, inexpensive ($3 to $4) online search—and no loss of requester confidentiality.

"Drug Approval Packages" are available for selected NDAs and ANDAs from 1997 forward on the Center for Drug Evaluation and Research Freedom of Information Office Web page (http://www.fda.gov/cder/foi/index.htm). Yearly lists of hyperlinks are sorted by brand name. Selected entries for drug products approved in 1996 and earlier are gradually being added to the FDA's Electronic Reading Room.

The path to SBA documents for NADAs is also smooth, thanks to the Center for Veterinary Medicine's (CVM) award winning site on the World Wide Web, found under the animal drugs icon on the *FDA Home Page*. There, the "On-Line Library" offers users access to FOI summaries through three browsable location aids, listing products by NADA number, generic name, or brand name. Links to newly released FOI summaries are singled out under a separate "What's New" icon on the opening screen of the CVM site. The search option on the opening menu enables users to enter keyword queries for streamlined access to all animal drug SBA document collections (1989–), regardless of their location within the CVM's databank. Searches lead to abbreviated entries showing product brand name, company sponsor, NADA number, generic name(s) of active ingredients, date of summary, and an informative abstract describing its content. A hotlink in each record retrieves the full text FOI summary submitted by the veterinary drug sponsor to support the NADA or ANADA approval. Note: Official product labeling is not necessarily included in these electronic FOIs.

References to medical device SS&Es offered for immediate display can be found in monthly PMA listings (January 1995–) located under the "Program Areas" option on the CDRH page of the FDA Web site. A highlighted PMA number within a given month's list indicates hypertext linkage to an approval letter and Summary of Safety and Effectiveness in PDF format. Listings of available Substantially Equivalent 510k summaries or statements are another option on the FDA Web site at http://www.fda.gov/cdrh/510khome.html. These documents, available from November 1995 forward, are generally released within one month of 510k posting online. Underlined 510k numbers in each month's list indicate when SE summaries have been hotlinked.

Sample SBA and SS&E records from *Diogenes* are illustrated in Figure 16.12. Although not all basis-of-approval documents are indexed in this database, those that are can be located by searching *FOI* in the source field or paragraph of re-

Figure 16.12   Sample Records for Basis-of-Approval Documents (SBA, SSE) in Diogenes

DIALOG(R)File 158:Diogenes
© 1996 DIOGENES. All rts. reserv.

03963380   117399
  LEVORA (SYNTEX): SBA EQV APRVD 12/13/93 (AL, PI, LBL, CH, B/E, DS)
PP:48.
  FDA NO.: F93–48753
  DRUG BRAND NAME(S): LEVORA
  DRUG GENERIC NAME: LEVONORGESTRELET
  DRUG/DEVICE NO.: 73592
  SOURCE: FOI SERVICES FULL TEXT (FT).
  DOCUMENT TYPE: DRUG (DRG). Freedom of Information Act Request

DIALOG(R)File 158:Diogenes
© 1996 DIOGENES. All rts. reserv.

03666909   117335
0060 SERIES ENDOTAK LEAD SYSTEM (CARDIAC PACEMAKERS) A/L, SSE PP: 25
  FDA NO.: F93–48451
  DEVICE CLASSIFICATION: CARDIAC LEAD
  COMPANY NAME: CARDIAC PACEMAKERS
  DRUG/DEVICE NO.: P910073
  SOURCE: FOI SERVICES
  DOCUMENT TYPE: DEVICE (DEV) Freedom of Information Act Request

cords, ANDed with the drug or device number previously published in the approval announcement record online. All documents with records in *Diogenes* that cite FOI as their source are available for immediate full-text hardcopy postal or fax delivery from the database supplier (for a modest fee). Immediate display of complete text online is also an option noted in many FOI records (see first example shown in Figure 16.12). The *Diogenes* collection of basis-of-approval documents provides retrospective access extending well beyond what is currently offered on the FDA Web site.

Sources for Product Recall Notices

Drug and device product recalls in the United States are announced in *FDA Enforcement Reports*. This weekly publication is indexed online in *Diogenes* (16.1, 1984–), *F-D-C Reports* (15.10, 1988–), *Health Devices Alerts* (16.2, 1982–), and the *IAC Newsletter Database* (15.15, 1992–). It is also displayable (and somewhat searchable) on the FDA's Web site. As might be expected, the agency's own *Home Page* offers the most timely access, posting recalls within one day of official announcement each week. Among nongovernment-subsidized sources, *Diogenes* is generally more up-to-date than other commercial files listed here, adding recall records within one week of issue by the FDA (closely followed by *F-D-C Reports*).

Issues of the *Enforcement Report* can be reached from several locations on the FDA Web site, but the most direct route to the *Enforcement Report* is clicking on the "What's New" icon on the opening screen. The latest issue is included under a link to "Other Press Releases, Talk Papers, and Other Publications." The full text includes food and cosmetic recalls, as well as those for drugs and devices. Archives are another selection on the same menu, where *Enforcement Reports* (all but the latest issue) can be searched back to February 21, 1990 using the FDA's implementation of the Verity search engine. Although Boolean and closer proximity combinations are possible, logical operators function at the whole issue (rather than individual recall notice) level. Thus, results of *FDA Home Page* archival document searches must still be followed up by time consuming visual surveys to pinpoint items needed (assisted by the FIND function built into browser software).

In contrast, commercial databases have created separate records for each product recall notice and implemented capabilities to search and view individual data elements (see Figure 16.13). Consequently, users can limit output to drug or device recalls only and isolate further subsets by factors such as company name, product name, and FDA classification of recalls by severity potential (I, II, or III, where Class I = highest risk of injury). Such features enable more selective scanning for current awareness purposes, as well as high precision retrospective research into recalls and product seizures (where date ranges can also be specified).

Among several commercial databases that index product recall notices, *Diogenes* alone offers access to additional background information from the FDA, when available. Under Freedom of Information Act provisions, the database supplier (FOI Services) has obtained and indexed documents that describe events leading to recalls in far more detail than is included in the *FDA Enforcement Report*. Although these documents are rarely offered for immediate full-text display, their availability for ordering from archives at FOI Services is always noted online. To check for the presence of background material on recalls, search *FOI* as the source, the word *recall* as a title keyword, and the company name associated with the product under scrutiny. Don't attempt to add date or product name as further restrictions. Many documents are undated and refer to products by recall number, rather than by name. Also, consider searching for warning letters regarding recalls to locate additional background information.

16.2 *Health Devices Alerts*. Plymouth Meeting, PA: ECRI, 1977–. Updated weekly. Available on Dialog; also on CD-ROM.

Figure 16.13   Sample Product Recall Notice in Diogenes

AN   00117363   9404. [DataStar]
TI   ALLSCRIPS PHARMACEUTICALS CLASS I RECALL 2/8/94: ALUPENT
     INHALATION AEROSOL COMPLETE.
SO   FDA-ENFORCEMENT-REPORT 3/30/94.
YR   940208.
CO   3M HEALTH CARE SPECIALTY. ST. PAUL, MINNESOTA. ALLSCRIPS
     PHARMACEUTICALS. VERNON HILLS, ILLINOIS.
PN   Trade name : ALUPENT INHALATION.
     Generic name : METAPROTERENOL SULFATE.
NU   FDA No.: D-218–4.
PT   REGULATORY ACTION (REG).
TX   1 OF 1.
     PRODUCT   Alupent Inhalation Aerosol Complete,
                              Metaproterenol Sulfate USP, 0.65 mg, 10 ml inhaler,
                              Rx bronchodilator for the relief of bronchospasm
                              in asthma patients and other patients with
                              respiratory ailments. Recall #D-218–4.
     CODE   Lot #3337026 EXP 7/95.
     MANUFACTURER   3M Health Care Specialty, St. Paul, Minnesota
                              (responsible firm).
     RECALLED BY   Allscrips Pharmaceuticals, Inc., Vernon Hills,
                              Illinois (relabeler), by letter February 8, 1994.
                              Firm-initiated recall ongoing.
     DISTRIBUTION   California, Washington state, Georgia.
     QUANTITY   50 canisters were distributed; firm estimates that
                              35% of the product remains on the market.
     REASON   Product does not meet particle size distribution
                              specifications.

Health Devices Alerts (*HDA*) focuses on medical device evaluations and problem reporting. Entries are derived from an extensive review of the medical, legal, and technical literature, government sources, and ECRI's own international problem reporting network. Coverage in this database complements that offered in ECRI's *Health Devices Sourcebook* (15.25). *HDA* can also supplement information on device recalls found in *Diogenes.*

Health Devices Alerts often provides details not readily available elsewhere online regarding FDA enforcement actions, such as specific follow-up recommendations to remedy or avoid further problems with cited devices. For example, when the FDA issues a safety alert in its weekly *Enforcement Reports*, the only background given is a relatively terse summary, such as "Reason—Blood cell separators could have spillage of blood undetected to users." However, the corresponding safety alert for the same product in *HDA* includes information provided by the manufacturer, as shown in Figure 16.14. In busy clinical settings, where printed safety bulletins may be overlooked or misplaced, *Health Devices Alerts* can be monitored for problems associated with equipment or supplies previously purchased.[2]

Checking a Device's Track Record of Adverse Experience Reports

Although increasingly stringent premarket clearance requirements generally ensure that benefits outweigh risks before medical devices reach the patient population, most diagnostic and therapeutic advances also represent potential hazards, given certain conditions of use. Recognizing this, the FDA instituted a mandatory medical device problem reporting system in 1984. Summaries of each adverse incident, submitted by device manufacturers, are published quarterly under the title *Medical Device Reports* (MDR). These documents are accessible on the FDA Web site under the devices and radiological health icon as an option on the CDRH "Program Areas" menu. Unfortunately, only MDRs submitted from 1992–1996 are keyword searchable in the government sponsored interface. Other MDRs are, as of the end of 1998, available only as full year downloadable compressed data files (1984–).

All *Medical Device Reports* are also indexed online in *Diogenes* and *Health Devices Alerts* (*Diogenes* offers more up-to-date coverage). Company names, FDA device categories (such as vascular graft prostheses, tracheal tubes), and product names are directly searchable access points to MDRs in both databases from 1984 forward. However, it's imperative to avoid over specification when searching product names. Model or catalog numbers are often omitted or truncated in MDR records online.

Searchers should also be aware that preliminary MDR entries sometimes include descriptions of events that are later corrected or clarified in a final MDR. Be sure to track down the final version, if reference in legal actions is contemplated. Because incidents are systematically flagged as "malfunction," "serious injury," or "death," output can also be restricted by severity of effects reported. For example, after designating *MDR* as the source in *Diogenes*, ANDed with a company name or FDA device category code, the keywords *death* or *serious* adjacent to *injury* can be searched in titles of records retrieved (see Figure 16.15). If references to specific effects are needed, synonyms should be used. How many mammary prosthesis recipients reported effects on breast feeding? To answer this question, terms such as lactation or breast milk would be necessary alternatives to breast feeding in the strategy.

As previously discussed in Chapter Four, monitoring the incidence of MDR citations to a given company, class of devices, or specific product can provide information important not only to legal investigators, but also to prospective purchasers, sellers, insurers, and industry analysts. Market researchers and product

Figure 16.14 Sample Action Item Record from Health Devices Alerts

DIALOG(R)File 198:Health Devices Alerts(R)
© 1995 ECRI-nonprft agncy. All rts. reserv.

00418543   AI-A2661   SUBFILE: AI
PRODUCT(s): 16–405   APHERESIS UNITS
COMMON DEVICE NAME: Blood Cell Separators: (1) Model CS -3000, (2) Model CS 3000 Plus
IDENTIFIER: All units manufactured since 1979, all serial numbers; approximately 2,576 units distributed in the U.S. and internationally

MANUFACTURER: Baxter Biotech {162923}, 1425 Lake Cook Rd (LC IV-2), Deerfield IL 60015

PROBLEM: Baxter Biotech Fenwal Division has become aware that, following unde-tected blood spills or leaks, blood may enter and collect in the interior of the pressure transducer assembly in the above units. Baxter Biotech issued a Safety Alert Letter dated August 15, 1994, informing customers of the issue and providing proper cleaning instructions for the units. The firm states that all transducer assemblies on the above units will be inspected by Fenwal field service representatives and replaced if blood is found in the transducer. Similar inspections will take place during routine preventive maintenance visits. FDA has designated this action Safety Alert Nos. N-001/002–5.
ACTION NEEDED: Verify that you have received the August 15, 1994, Safety Alert letter from Baxter Biotech. Complete and return the reply card provided to Baxter, indicating receipt of the letter. Ensure that all users are familiar with the following steps recom-mended by Baxter Biotech Fenwal to ensure that blood leaks or spills are detected: (1) Before the first procedure of each day and after each use of the unit, visually inspect and lightly wipe the 3 pressure transducers located on the monitor panel of the units with a tissue/cotton swab to identify if a blood leak has occurred. After removing the monitor assembly box from the unit, visually inspect and lightly wipe the surface of the 3 diaphragm assemblies with a tissue/cotton swab to identify if a blood leak has oc-curred. (2) If blood is found in either the monitor box diaphragm assembly area or in the transducers, discard any blood product, and do not use the unit. U.S. customers should contact Fenwal Post Market Quality Assurance (PMQA) at (800) 933–6925 to arrange for a service call to properly clean the transducer assembly. Customers outside the U.S. should contact their local Baxter Biotech Fenwal distributor. The manufacturer cautions that lightly wiping the transducer surface may remove lubricant. Customers should ensure that transducers are properly lubricated before use. Customers may con-tinue to use the units both before and after inspection by Fenwal field service represen-tatives provided that the above steps are followed and no blood is found. For further information, U.S. customers should contact Diane Mattucci, Baxter Biotech Fenwal, at the above number; customers outside the U.S. should contact their local Baxter Biotech Fenwal distributor.

SOURCE: "FDA Enforcement Rep" 1994 Nov 23; Manufacturer.
PUBLICATION DATE: 9412

Figure 16.15   Sample MDR Record from Diogenes

AN	01403764 9510. [DataStar]
TI	MDR REPORT—FINAL : EDWARDS CVS DIV. BAXTER HEALTHCARE CORP. CARPENTIER-EDWARDS BIOPROSTHESIS MODEL 2625 CATALOG NA SERIOUS INJURY.
AU	Advisory committee : CIRCULATORY SYSTEMS DEVICE PANEL (DVCIRC).
SO	FDA-MDR-LIST (MDR). LIST EDITION: JULY 1995.
YR	941014.
CO	EDWARDS CVS DIV. BAXTER HEALTHCARE CORP. (EDWACVS).
NU	FDA No.: M555686.
DE	(LWR)-Tissue,-Heart-Valve. CLASS: 3. CFR Cite Not Provided by FDA.
PT	DEVICE (DEV).
TX	1 OF 1.
	PT UNDERWENT REOPERATION FOR THE REPLACEMENT OF THE BIO-PROSTHESIS REPORTEDLY DUE TO STENOSIS, CALCIFICATION, CALCI-FIC 'DEGENERATION' AND CONGESTIVE HEART FAILURE. IMPLANT DATE: 9/30/86. IMPLANT DURATION: 7 YEARS, 10 MONTHS, 11 DAYS. PT'S SEX: MALE. PT'S AGE AT EVENT: 66 YEARS. DATE OF MFR: UNK. SEE DISCLAIMER STATEMENT.

developers survey MDRs to identify potential defects to avoid in designing new, competitive products and to assess liabilities in embarking on a new product line. Such surveys can include statistical analysis of MDRs, examining, perhaps, a given company's product line by ranked incidence of adverse experience reports or reviewing the track record of an entire category of medical devices. For example, it is possible to determine, among heart valve prostheses, which companies' products have been associated most often with death or serious injury due to stenosis, and what kinds of prostheses present the greatest hazard to patients (or liability to manufacturers).[3]

Establishment Inspection Reports and Form 483s

Failure to meet FDA standards can lead to delays in new product introductions or suspension of production. Any addition to approval lag time is costly. The longer it takes to commercialize a drug or device, the shorter its shelf life before patent expiry, thus decreasing its potential to offset research and development costs. Unsatisfactory FDA plant inspections can also have a devastating effect on products already well established in the marketplace. Correcting GMP (good manufacturing practice) violations could require expensive upgrades to equipment, necessitating higher prices. Market share losses in consequence could be further inflated by consumer migration to competing therapies, if inventories fail to sustain a temporary suspension in production. For generic manufacturers, delays imposed by GMP violations can be especially serious, because the availability of many alternatives may make re-entering the market far more difficult.

Inspections of clinical testing sites and Institutional Review Boards (IRBs) are also a cause for concern. Study sponsors (companies developing products) can be held liable for poor oversight of clinical and preclinical investigations. In worst case scenarios, unfavorable findings from FDA inspections can disqualify physician managers and invalidate study results pivotal to product approval, which not only wastes R&D investment, but also affects a company's good name.

Thus, planning for efficient product development and manufacture usually integrates proactive strategies to avoid failed establishment inspections. Prudent companies maintain a close watch on Form FD-483 filings, which are used by the FDA to record alleged violations that must be corrected. Their content can help identify areas of operations that could cause problems.

The *Diogenes* database (16.1) indexes Establishment Inspection Reports (EIRs) dating from 1976 forward, incorporating records for more than 14,000 EIRs and 7,300 Form 483s. Access points include both company name and location, as illustrated in Figure 16.16. Complete EIRs, once obtained, often provide a history of the company and outline the internal staff reporting structure (who reports to whom and their respective responsibilities). Because of its competitive value, such information is another reason why people request EIRs. Unfortunately, these regulatory documents are not available for immediate full-text display online, but they can be ordered through FOI's document delivery service. Expect copies liberally tattooed with blacked-out segments that have been "redacted" by the FDA Freedom of Information Office to avoid disclosure of confidential business or patient data. These reports are, nonetheless, hot commodities for industry watchers, due to the forewarnings they provide of standards expected and of company vulnerability.

Another point in drug or device development where checking Form 483s becomes critical is in the choice of investigators to oversee clinical trials. Before contracting with practitioners and hospitals to initiate human studies, drug and

Figure 16.16   Sample Establishment Inspection Report and Form 483 Record in Diogenes

AN	05127691 9510. [DataStar]
TI	CHESAPEAKE BIOLOGICAL, OWINGS MILLS, MD: EIR, 483 10/11–20/94 PP: 9.
SO	FOI-SERVICES.
CO	CHESAPEAKE. OWINGSMILLS, MARYLAND.
NU	FDA No.: F94–50248.
PT	INSPECTION REPORT (EIR).

device companies need to check for the existence of prior Form 483s. To find EIRs for a named individual, simply substitute a personal name for a company name in search strategies online.

Warning Letters as Competitive Intelligence Tools

Warning letters are the FDA's most used enforcement tool. They often spell out in detail violations somewhat cryptically noted on Form 483s. A close study of correspondence can fill in the blanks in official GMP guidelines, itemizing agency concerns and expectations on such diverse matters as validation of computerized process controls, wording on product labels, recommended employee training, and packaging standards to withstand shipping from offshore plants. In addition to clarifying regulatory requirements, the content of warning letters can signal shifts in enforcement initiatives that may affect future business. Moreover, because the FDA releases full copies of all warning letters, a company's reputation, stock value, and credit rating can be affected when customers, competitors, financial institutions, Wall Street, and the press learn that problems exist.

Known prior to May 1991 as "regulatory letters" or "notices of adverse findings," warning letters today carry more clout than previous types of correspondence, because they now almost invariably convey the threat of further enforcement action. The effect of such letters on the medical device industry has been especially profound. In the past, receipt of a warning letter automatically placed a device firm on the FDA's "Reference List," which meant that authorization of further product approvals could be blocked until alleged GMP deficiencies were corrected. After the controversial list began in April 1992, nearly 1,000 device approvals were delayed while their sponsors struggled toward compliance. Between 500 and 600 sites could be on the (unpublished) Reference List at any given time, thereby placing as many as 300 510ks in regulatory limbo. In April 1995, the FDA announced its intent to eliminate the Reference List. GMP violations related to a specific device are still grounds for delaying its approval, but premarket reviews of devices unrelated to alleged problems are no longer affected.

Post-marketing medical device tracking regulations, first implemented in August 1993, extend responsibility for monitoring and reporting adverse experiences with permanently implanted devices to the person or institution purchasing them. Physicians and hospitals are now considered final users or distributors and, in consequence, may find it advisable to check warning letters regarding standard operating procedures required for user surveillance and compliance.

This background on warning letters underscores their significance. The advantages of maintaining a close watch on these important documents are two-fold: 1) keeping up-to-date on the latest elaboration of guidelines, in order to be prepared when scrutiny shifts to your own company or to firms in which yours has a vested interest, and 2) identifying windows of opportunity in the marketplace while competitors cope with violations. The *FDA Home Page* began adding warning letters to its Freedom of Information Electronic Reading Room in 1996 (http://www.fda.gov/foi/warning.htm). Separate monthly files can be browsed for January 1995, selected months in 1996, and for every month from January 1997 forward. A warning letter search form (Figure 16.17) enables targeted searches of this collection by combinations of factors such as company name, subject line, date ranges, and issuing office (accessible from a pull-down menu).

There are two possible impediments to search success to be aware of when using this form. One is that subject keyword access is limited to the FDA correspondent's cryptic one line description. This tag tends to be distressingly uninformative (e.g., drug products, labeling, clinical studies). Lacking full-text search capabilities, this sole indicator of subject content makes it impossible to isolate letters on the FDA Web site dealing with specific topics of interest.

A second, less obvious barrier to search success is company name formatting. Entries on the search form are retrieved as literal character strings, making it easy to miss warning letters containing variations such as Bristol Myers (with a space) versus Bristol-Myers (with a hyphen). Fortunately, the FDA's interface also offers options to browse a list of letters arranged alphabetically by company name, where variant entries can be identified quickly. Lists arranged by issuing office, date, and subject line can also be viewed at the URL cited.

Diogenes (16.1) has assembled a larger retrospective collection of warning let-

Figure 16.17   Warning Letter Search Form on the FDA Web Site

FOIA WARNING LETTERS SEARCH

Warning Letters Search Form

Enter all or part of a search term in the text boxes below.

Company Name

Subject

Issuing Office

Date Issued   From: Month   Year

To: Month   Year

Search   Reset

ters, adding new records within one week of their release by the FDA. Of the more than 5,000 letters indexed in the database dating from 1984 forward, 98% are offered for immediate full-text display. The bonus in this commercial database's implementation of warning letters is that all keywords embedded in the complete text of these documents are searchable, not just company, product name, or cryptic subject lines. Thus, it is possible to find FDA policy statements regarding specific topics, such as Internet promotions, homeopathic drug labeling, or patient records, within the *Diogenes* collection of letters.

FDA Guidelines and Regulations

As was discussed earlier in Chapter Four, it's important to remember the distinction between regulations and documents resulting from their implementation. Most FDA related questions require hunting down records associated with implementation. In other words, answers will usually be found in sources featured thus far in this chapter. Occasionally, it will be difficult to determine whether the text of regulations is actually needed. Should this situation arise, the best solution is simply to start by searching Title 21 of the *Code of Federal Regulations* (*CFR*, 4.25).

Title 21 in hardcopy format is updated annually and poorly indexed. Online and CD-ROM versions are much easier to use and generally provide updates at least monthly, incorporating additions and corrections published in the *Federal Register* (4.24) since the last annual *CFR* edition. Check sources providing the full text of the *Federal Register* on a daily update schedule to complete a search for FDA regulations. It will only be necessary to scan daily issues of *FR* published since the last update to whatever version of Title 21 you are using as a starting point. When searching both of these regulatory sources, don't rely on keywords alone. Strategies should also include relevant *CFR* Section and Part codes to be comprehensive.

If you fail to find regulations related to the subject of inquiry, the next step is to look for an FDA guideline or guidance document. A guideline is a quasi-official publication, representing the agency's interpretation or elaboration of a formal legal requirement. It is one of a bewildering number of communication mechanisms used to define policy. For example, "guidance" documents, rather than guidelines, are often preferred by the FDA, because their development is not subject to stringent rules now applied to the latter (e.g., requiring dissemination of multiple drafts for public comment). Although not binding as legislative rules, both types of documents carry the weight of FDA sanctioned suggestions for handling a variety of situations. The broad spectrum of topics addressed includes test procedures, product standards, clinical protocols, record-keeping recommendations, and other criteria for performance or technical specifications. Note: Guidelines covering biologics are often called "points to consider."

Offices within the FDA with jurisdiction over human and animal drug products each issue guidelines and make them accessible on the Internet. However, navigating the home pages of separate FDA centers, all structured in widely different formats, to locate guidance documents is a daunting task. Fortunately, the FDA has added a convenient pathfinder under the "Special Information for Industry" icon on the opening screen of its Web site. Using this option, browsable lists of current proposed and final guidance collections compiled by each regulatory unit are only three mouse clicks away.

Diogenes also makes retrieval of guidelines easy by flagging pertinent references with the abbreviation GLS in the document or publication type field in online records. Both current and past guidance documents are indexed in this database from 1984 forward. The supplier, FOI Services, has also released its full-text collection on CD-ROM, searchable through SilverPlatter software. This annual compilation contains more than 1,200 FDA guidelines covering medical devices, human drugs, biologics, veterinary products, foods, and cosmetics.

Legally Permissible Additives

When a company is engaged in developing a new drug formulation, questions about permissible additives may arise. One way to avoid the lengthy and expensive testing that is required if entirely new (to regulatory authorities) drug excipients are selected is to survey additives already approved for use in foods or cosmetics.

16.3 *Foodline: Current Food Legislation (FOLE)*. Leatherhead, Surrey, England: Leatherhead Food Research Association. Current information, updated biweekly on DataStar and DIALOG.

A unique and authoritative source of additive standards in the worldwide food industry, *FOLE* is one of a family of databases produced by the Leatherhead Food Research Association (U.K.), an independent trade organization with more than 750 corporate members drawn from companies located in any of thirty-six countries. The file offers two types of full-text records, standards and additives. Standards documents provide information on composition and labeling requirements of foods in seven European Union countries and the United States. Entries include product definitions, permitted ingredients, and legal provisions regarding claims, quality, and quantity statements. Additives records give details on permitted uses, maximum levels, and labeling requirements for any of ninety countries.

Coordinating a country name with the word "introduction" searched as a descriptor is a good way to begin research in *FOLE*. Titles of records retrieved can then be scanned to survey what standards are available. For example, a search on *France* AND *vitamins*, when limited to *introduction* documents, locates a concise overview of regulations on dietary and dietetic products and recommendations on further search terms to use (e.g., essential amino acid product, fatty acid producer, exertion product). *FOLE* can also be used to investigate health food claims, such as what dietetic, nutrition, energy, or medicinal statements are permissible in labeling.

Complementary information on additives is also available under both the foods and the cosmetics icons on the *FDA Home Page*, discussed in more detail in the next section.

The FDA Home Page on the Internet

The *FDA Home Page* has already been discussed as an up-to-date source for product approvals, recall notices, and other frequently requested regulatory documents. Available free of charge on the Internet, this U.S. government subsidized service offers access to far more information than its menu-driven precursor, the FDA Bulletin Board Service (BBS).[4] It contains many items of potential interest not only to regulatory personnel, but also to healthcare practitioners, subject specialty industry watchers (Wall Street), and the general public.

The best way to gauge the utility of an Internet resource for answering questions in your own work setting is, of course, to use it. However, a detailed preview here may save time later, when information is needed quickly. This site is large and multilayered, so it's easy to become lost in the maze and miss professionally useful items mixed in with consumer offerings. At the same time, it must be recognized that this World Wide Web site is in a constant state of evolution, making it essential to review any of the segments described below for changes and additions in the future.

Human Drugs

The human drugs segment of the *FDA Home Page* is maintained by the Center for Drug Evaluation and Research (CDER) and is divided into four paths: About CDER, Drug Info, Regulatory Guidance, and What's Happening. The latter provides access to the full text of recent agency press releases and public health advisories, a calendar of advisory committee meetings and of conferences and workshops sponsored by CDER, links to the full text of *FDA Consumer* magazine and the *FDA Medical Bulletin,* descriptions of new program initiatives, and meeting presentations by CDER staff.

"Regulatory Guidance," as its name implies, is the place to look for guidance documents related to human drugs, a compilation of laws enforced by the agency, and forms required for compliance. Its resource menu includes an external link to the *Federal Register* in machine-readable form. A *Pharmacy Compounding Page* is a recent addition here. Created to assist users in monitoring documents associated with the implementation of FDA Modernization Act provisions affecting compounding, it includes a lists of products that have been withdrawn from the market (thereby excluded from permissible extemporaneous formulations) and a proposed list of bulk drug substances that may be used, as well.

"About CDER" contains the *Manual of Policies and Procedures* (MaPPs) written for FDA staff, various indexes to directories of agency personnel, Prescription Drug User Fee Act progress reports, and the latest CDER annual report. These reports are definitive sources for measures of FDA performance mandated under 1994's landmark legislation to reduce drug lag. Here, you will find median approval times, from submission of applications to final authorization, for each fiscal year from 1987 to date. Reports also list the number of submissions annually from 1983 forward, broken down by category, new drug applications (NDAs), product license and establishment license applications for vaccines and other biologics, efficacy supplements, manufacturing supplements, etc.

Other extremely useful documents replete with statistics are hidden behind the "About CDER" menu option labeled "Office and Subject Home Pages." A link to the FDA's Office of Compliance leads to annual reports for the past few years. Each describes the array of oversight activities for which the agency is responsible, many of which are not well documented elsewhere. Data compiled include number of inspections (and violations found) conducted at nonclinical animal labs, clinical investigator and sponsor monitor (drug trial) sites, hospital investigational review boards, bioequivalence determination facilities, and manufacturing plants. Enforcement tallies cover the number of product recalls, withdrawals, or discontinuations, and for what purpose (such as failure to meet standards for tamper-resistant packaging or for labeling).

Another link under "Office and Subject Home Pages" well worth bookmarking is the *Over-the-Counter Drugs Home Page.* Here, sources include indexes of significant OTC drug *Federal Register* publications from 1972 forward, a milestone list showing *FR* citations to all major OTC rulemakings, and the *OTC Drug Review Ingredient Status Report.* The latter's alphabetical list of active ingredients cumulates information released piecemeal over many years and often difficult to find elsewhere. CDER promises a searchable OTC active ingredient database in the near future. Meanwhile, the OTC drugs page, added in late July 1996, is a convenient way to tackle the task of answering questions related to nonprescription ingredient reviews still ongoing (background on which was provided in Chapter Four).

Figure 16.18 outlines a selection of particularly useful headings found under CDER's "Drug Info" option. The *Adverse Drug Reaction System* is a computerized database of reactions (ADRs) reported by health professionals since 1969. Downloadable data sets compile more than one million reports. The annual *Adverse Drug Experience Report* summarizes post-market ADRs evaluated by the FDA.

The *AIDS Clinical Trials Information Service (ACTIS)* offers simple search interfaces to the AIDSTRIALS and AIDSDRUGS databases also available through Internet Grateful Med. Their purpose is to provide quick and easy access

Figure 16.18   Useful FDA CDER Home Page "Drug Info" Options

☐ Adverse Drug Reaction System
☐ Adverse Drug Experience Report
☐ AIDS Clinical Trial Information Service (ACTIS)
☐ Approved Drug Products with Therapeutic Equivalence Evaluations (Orange Book)
☐ Consumer Drug Information Sheets (1998–)
☐ Drug Approvals
    √ New and Generic Drug Approvals
    √ FDA Drug Approvals List
    √ FDA Drug and Device Product Approval List: Legacy Information
    √ Drug Approval Packages
☐ Drug Master Files
☐ National Drug Code Directory
☐ Patent Term Extension and New Patents Docket
☐ SAS Drug Formulation Stability Program

to information on both federally and privately funded clinical trials for adults and children. Protocol descriptions include study locations, patient eligibility requirements and exclusion criteria, and names and telephone numbers of contact persons.

The Web implementation of the *The Orange Book* (*Approved Drug Products with Therapeutic Equivalence Evaluations,* 4.42), with its cumulative monthly supplement, has the advantage of an interactive query search form enabling quick retrieval of products by active ingredient, proprietary name, or applicant company. Results generated are far easier to read than tables found in the hardcopy counterpart.

Consumer Drug Information Sheets were introduced by the FDA in 1998, despite an earlier Congressional decision that patient package inserts should remain the province of industry and other nongovernment groups. Nonetheless, CDER staff pharmacists are now preparing attractive two-page summaries in lay language of basic package insert information. They describe what the featured medication is used for, who should not be treated with it, general precautions, administration instructions, concurrent medications or foods to avoid, and common side effects. Surprisingly, each *Sheet* concludes with a hypertext link to the full professional package insert. This policy seems to undermine the purpose of preparing a PPI or, at the very least, reflects some ambivalence about possible liabilities.

Distinctions among the three drug approval listings have already been discussed earlier in this chapter. *Drug Approval Packages,* launched on the FDA Web site late in 1997, provide digitally scanned documents as background to market authorizations, including chemistry, pharmacology, and toxicology reviews.

Drug Master Files (DMFs) are a series of directories listing companies registered with the FDA as manufacturing sites, as providers of drug substances or materials used in their preparation, or as packaging material suppliers. The Internet version of the *National Drug Code Directory* updates the 1995 hardcopy edition (10.9) with quarterly supplements. Used primarily for inventory purposes and reimbursement programs under Medicare, NDC data files classify products by brand name, drug class, and company code. Individual entries display brand, dose form, route, strength, active ingredients, and package size and types available.

The *Patent Term Extension and New Patents Docket* lists both new and cumulative drug patent extension and exclusivity term data. Arranged alphabetically by proprietary name, this compilation cites U.S. patent number, expiration date, reason for exclusivity, and extension expiration date for each product benefiting from Waxman-Hatch provisions.

The *SAS Drug Formulation Stability Program* is a downloadable PC software system designed to estimate expiration dating based on linear regression analysis. The statistical foundation for this program was established in a 1987 FDA guideline for submitting documentation for the stability of human drugs and biologics.

Medical Devices/Radiological Health

Clicking on the Center for Medical Devices and Radiological Health (CDRH) icon on the *FDA Home Page* leads to six choices, the most user-friendly being a topic index. All items cross referenced in this index are also offered at other points on this site's many menu screens, but accessing them through a single integrated alphabetic list saves time. The topic index is brief enough to browse and is generous in its document links, which are presented under both regulatory buzzwords or abbreviations and everyday language descriptive labels. Use this index to find recent safety alerts, public health advisories and notices, guidance memoranda (the Office of Device Evaluation's "Blue Book"), and new device approvals.

A valuable adjunct to searches for device approvals is the *Product Code Classification Database* found at http://www.fda.gov/cdrh/prodcode.html. Codes found here can assist retrieval of information on comparable—and competitive—products. The CDRH search interface to the FDA classification scheme enables users to locate relevant codes by entering broad medical specialty terms matching advisory committee jurisdictions (e.g., anesthesia, cardiovascular, orthopedic) or typing in more specific device keywords. For example, a search on *defibrillator* quickly compiles a list of device names containing this keyword, regardless of word order, such as:

atrial defibrillator
auxiliary power supply for low-energy DC-defibrillator
defibrillator, implantable, dual-chamber

tester, defibrillator
wearable, defibrillator, automatic, external

Each device name in the results list is hotlinked to an individual record showing advisory panel jurisdiction, product code, device class designation as 1, 2, or 3 (see Chapter Four), and *CFR* number. Product codes can then be used in the same database to locate additional devices of the same type or to form part of a query in the 510k or PMA databases on the FDA Web site or commercial vendors.

Animal Drugs

The icon for animal drugs leads to what is arguably one of the most sophisticated components of the *FDA Home Page.* In addition to the usual news announcements, staff directories, and pointers to recent *Federal Register* notices, the Center for Veterinary Medicine (CVM) site provides a fully searchable database (known as *The Green Book*) of all U.S. drugs approved for use in animals, updated monthly.

Through this Web site's "On-Line Library" link, users can also locate a complete collection of animal drug adverse experience reports, compiled annually from 1987 forward and arranged alphabetically by generic name. Summaries of adverse drug events note the total number of reports submitted for the category of drug, for specific species, and for given routes of administration. Structured records also identify the number of animals treated versus those exhibiting a drug-associated effect, clinical manifestations observed, and the number and percentage of total adverse experience reports citing specified signs and symptoms.

Another particularly welcome selection on the CVM library menu is *Freedom of Information Summaries*, which consist of safety and efficacy information submitted by drug sponsors to support the approval of their original or supplemental new animal drug applications (NADAs). See the section on basis-of-approval documents earlier in this chapter for a discussion of their organization and, more importantly, their significance.

Rounding out the CVM library of online resources is the copyright-free *FDA Veterinarian* magazine, published bimonthly. In addition, a link to information for consumers supplies answers to frequently asked questions about companion animal care and veterinary medical issues.

It should be noted that users of the CVM site will find complementary resources on the U.S. Department of Agriculture's *Veterinary Biologics Home Page* (http://www.aphis.usda.gov/vs/cvb/index.html). The USDA, rather than the FDA, is responsible for enforcement of the Virus-Serum-Toxic Act of 1913, amended in 1985. This means that the agency reviews license (i.e., approval) applications for biologic products intended for use in animals, applications for related production facilities, and applications for animal biologic drug imports. Accordingly, relevant guidance memoranda and *Federal Register* notices at the

Veterinary Biologics Internet site will supplement FDA Animal Drugs reference material.

Biologics

The *FDA Home Page* path to human biologics information is the least developed of the drug-related sections. Options found under publications and conferences/ meetings overlap, to a large extent, with links found elsewhere. Under "Inside CBER," users will find an organization chart and directory list for the Center for Biologics Evaluation and Research. Brief annual reports are also included in this section. "Product Info" assembles a menu of links to approvals and a cumulative directory of licensed establishments and products. The latter organizes data in four parts. Part I is an alphabetical list of establishments licensed for production of biologics, including their operating locations, mailing address, phone number, and primary contact person. Part II presents establishments by license number, cross referenced to products each is authorized to manufacture. Part III list biologic products alphabetically, coordinating them with the license number and name of approved manufacturers. Part IV organizes products by category.

Cosmetics

Content organized under the cosmetics icon is, for the most part, consumer oriented and distressingly brief. However, a ready-reference treasure for professionals is available under the menu choice "Cosmetic Information for Industry." Here, a *Cosmetic Handbook* contains separately displayable sections on regulatory requirements for marketing, good manufacturing practice guidelines, product related health hazard issues, and color additives. The latter includes two important lists: 1) dyes subject to FDA certification (requires submission and agency testing of each batch produced) and 2) color additives exempt from certification (both provisional and permanent categories). Either may be the subject of drug, as well as cosmetic, information inquiries.

Further down on the industry menu is a supplementary link, *Summary of Color Additives Listed for Use in the United States in Foods, Drugs, Cosmetics, and Medical Devices.* The table groups named additives according to their categories of use and cross references them to *CFR* citations.

Foods

Perhaps surprisingly, the foods icon on the *FDA Home Page* points the way to much of potential interest to readers of this book. For example, this Web location is a good place to find well written background material on the controversial (and confusing) Dietary Supplement Health and Education Act of 1994 and on health claims on foods. A food additive database is also available, covering more than

3,000 substances directly added to food, such as color additives and preservatives. These include many, but not all, GRAS (Generally Recognized as Safe) ingredients. The database, dubbed *EAFUS* (Everything Added to Food in the United States), lists substances alphabetically by generic name. CAS registry numbers are also cited, along with cross references to specific *CFR* section and part numbers where the chemical appears. Document type abbreviations indicate the status of toxicology information available for the chemical under the FDA's program of Priority-Based Assessment of Food Additives (PAFA). Because the entire database has been converted to HTML, users can invoke the FIND feature in their Web browser to locate specific substances by name or CAS RN. Abstracts of more than 7,000 toxicology studies related to EAFUS entries are available in *Food Additives: Toxicology, Regulation, and Properties* (11.25), published in CD-ROM format by CRC Press.

The complete text of a very useful reference resource, *Foodborne Pathogenic Microorganisms and Natural Toxins* (1992), popularly titled the "Bad Bug Book," is another option on the FDA Web site worth exploring. Its nickname notwithstanding, this publication includes mushrooms and shellfish in its scope, along with "bugs" such as viruses, parasitic protozoa, and pathogenic bacteria. Individual entries assemble basic facts such as characteristics, habitat and source, infectious or harmful dose, symptoms, and complications. In common with "bug" monographs, entries for toxic mushrooms include a history of recent outbreaks (accidental or other ingestions) and relative frequency of disease, treatment tables, and diagnostic guidelines. The Internet version of this book has the advantage of hypertext links to a glossary of useful definitions.

Another exceptionally well done section of the foods portion of the *FDA Home Page* is a subject directory to other sites, supported by hypertext links. Topics addressed include bioinformatics, botany, biodiversity, entomology, mycology, microbiology, toxicology, and biotechnology. The lengthy list also cites sources for relevant meetings calendars, course announcements, and full-text journals.

What's New

Tucked behind the "What's New" icon are not only the expected public calendar and summaries of recent *Federal Register* notices, but also the *Enforcement Report*, the *FDA Medical Bulletin*, and the full text of *FDA Consumer*. The main menu hides the latest issue of each under the general rubric "Other Press Releases, Talk Papers, and other Publications." An archives option leads to back issues of these titles dating from February 1990, January 1996, and April 1989, respectively. Other archived materials carried over from the former *FDA BBS* include:

Backgrounders (February 1990–)
Congressional testimony by FDA staff

Federal Register notice summaries (1995–, with selective coverage back to
   1991)
Major speeches (June 1988–)
Press releases (1992–)
Talk Papers (April 1990–)

Archived items (including the three FDA serial titles noted above) can be viewed
sequentially in reverse chronological order (heaven forbid) or, more sensibly,
searched by keyword(s). The search engine uses Verity protocols and permits restriction to one or more specific sources. *Diogenes* (16.1) also provides separate
records for search and full-text display of FDA press releases from 1982 forward,
Talk Papers and Backgrounders (1984–), Congressional testimony and speeches
(1979–), and Federal Register notices (1985–).

Other Options on the FDA Home Page

The FDA Electronic Reading Room found under the "Freedom of Information"
icon on the home page is rapidly evolving into a rich repository of long awaited
documents. For example, advisory committee agendas, minutes, and full tran-
scripts are gradually being released in this section. A directory of state officials
is available, as is the official list of disqualified or restricted clinical investigators.

   Contents compiled under the "International" icon have assumed increasing
importance in this era of global cooperation and mutual recognition agreements.
Items offered here encompass ICH documents, a directory of ministries of health
around the world, a hotlinked collection of international food and drug law resources, and another of international trade resources on the World Wide Web.

   Clicking on the "Year 2000" link leads to a database where the compliance
status of medical devices and scientific laboratory equipment can be checked.
Searchable by company name, records identify products with date-related problems that will affect their performance in the new millennium if they are not
corrected.

   Other FDA opening screen options currently include: children and tobacco,
MedWatch, toxicology research, FDA Modernization Act public feedback, FAQs,
dockets, and separate links to special information for consumers, industry, health
professionals, patients, state and local officials, women, and kids. Many of these
selections lead to sources that are offered elsewhere under other icons. Redundancy is rampant on the FDA Web site, but odd gaps in hypertext cross-linking
do occur. For example, consumer oriented information is scattered everywhere,
with no unifying index to assist in locating it. It's easy to overlook pertinent material of all types when browsing through lengthy menus, especially where the
rationale behind their order of presentation is undiscernible. Therefore, wise
users will reinforce visual scans of page headings with results of keyword

searches conducted through the site's search engine. Other recommended follow-up would be a thorough skim of the noteworthy FDA Web site index.

Summary

The *FDA Home Page* is an excellent and inexpensive source for many, but by no means all, answers to frequently asked questions about U.S. regulatory topics affecting the pharmaceutical and health technology industries. It's a good place to start when looking for statistics on agency activities accomplished during the previous year, such as number of NDA approvals, establishment inspections, or recalls. It's also the best bet for browsing recent *Federal Register* notice summaries, press releases, officially issued guidance documents, and talk papers or backgrounders on hot drug, cosmetic, or food topics. Staff directories and calendars of forthcoming advisory committee meetings are most readily accessible at this site. Furthermore, no other source online today comes close to providing the quantity and quality of veterinary drug information assembled under the animal drugs icon. Consumer oriented information on AIDS drug clinical trials certainly deserves a bookmark, as do menus of fast facts to answer inquiries from the general public regarding cosmetics and foods.

However, the old adage "you get what you pay for" springs to mind when comparing the capabilities of the *FDA Home Page* for answering product approval or recall queries with those of more powerful fee-based vendors. The *Home Page* is unrivaled for current awareness in these two important categories of documents, offering NDA, PMA, and 510k authorizations for public inspection sooner than any other source. But when retrospective searches on factors such as company name, ingredients, brands, and type of approval or recall are needed, answers can be uncovered more quickly and efficiently in commercial databases such as *Diogenes* or *F-D-C Reports*.

Specialty Fee-Based CD-ROM Services

The importance of regulatory documents is obvious in the number of specialized information services developed to make accessing them easier. Because online sources generally offer the largest collections of relevant data and greater flexibility in searching, they are the primary emphasis of this chapter. However, examples from five publishers will illustrate some of the exciting products in alternative formats on the market today.

IHS (Information Handling Services) has compiled several regulatory libraries on CD-ROM. *The Food and Drug Library* includes the full text of statutes and proposed legislation; relevant portions of Titles 9, 21, and 40 of the *Code of Federal Regulations*; DEA, FDA, and pertinent EPA and USDA notices from the *Federal Register*; manuals, guidelines, press releases, talk papers, and speeches from the FDA; court case decisions dating from 1938; *Enforcement Reports*; and warning letters (1991 forward). A *UK Pharmaceuticals Library* is also available.

The IHS *U.S. Medical Devices Library* transcribes *Medical Device Reports*, statutes, *Federal Register* notices, pertinent *CFR* extracts, FDA manuals and other publications, a partial list of guidance documents, warning letters, and establishment registration and product listings. It also includes an index of PMAs and 510ks. Complementary resources from IHS are a *European Union Medical Devices Library*, the *Japanese Pharma-Devices Update*, and a *Device Standards Library*. The latter offers full-text scanned images of industry documents from ISO, IEC (International Electrotechnical Commission), ASTM, and CEN/Cenelec (European Committees for Standardization). Each of these CD-ROM collections is updated monthly, with daily additions to the *Federal Register* accessible to subscribers through the IHS Internet site. Other regulatory collections from the same publisher focus on food and beverages, healthcare facilities, and Medicare/Medicaid. Descriptions of their content can be previewed at http://www.ihshealth.com. Most IHS libraries are now offered to paid subscribers through a Web-based interface, as well.

Another specialty publisher in the regulatory subject area is INCAD (*Computed-Automated-Digital Information*). In a joint venture with the Nonprescription Drug Manufacturers Association, an *OTC Electronic Library* was launched by this company in 1994. It consists of OTC monographs documenting the current status of every FDA-reviewed ingredient, sample labels, regulatory agency directories and phone books, and pertinent compliance policy guides. The CD-ROM set includes the full *Code of Federal Regulations*, historical *Federal Register* entries from the FDA dating back to DESI reviews, and the full text of major statutes.

A new collection from the same publisher is called the *Drugs-Biologics Regulatory Database* (formerly *Pharmaceutical Information Library* or *PhIL*). INCAD outlines its content at http://www.incadinc.com. Both CD-ROM products are updated quarterly, and late breaking news items, plus daily *Federal Register* extracts, are available to subscribers through a proprietary electronic bulletin board service on the Internet. The FolioViews interface permits full-text keyword and phrase queries, including truncation and ordered/unordered proximity searching, and field restrictions.

The European Pharma Law Centre, publishers of *ERA News* (4.58), markets an *EPLC EC Document Database* on either CD-ROM or ASCII diskette. The collection includes all directives, decisions, guidelines, proposals, amendments, and drafts issued by the European Commission, European Parliament, EMEA, and ICH that are relevant to the human or animal pharmaceutical and medical device industries. Clearly written abstracts summarize the contents of each of the more than 1,000 documents assembled by EPLC, and an automated cross reference system links related sources. The full text of all documents is directly searchable, as well. Annual subscriptions to the *EPLC EC Document Database* provide monthly updates.

IDRAC is another compact disc regulatory information service marketed by IMS. International in scope, the CD-ROM database is regenerated six times a year, with further updates made available to subscribers through the Internet at http://www.ims-int.com/idrac. Official explanatory documents and guidelines are the core of IDRAC, which covers publications of the European Union and national procedures of member states, in addition to FDA materials and mandates. A Central and Eastern European module was added in 1997, followed by one for Japan in 1998. A visit to IDRAC's Web site at http://www.ims-int.com/idrac will uncover further information about content and technical specifications of this huge regulatory resource collection. Other information offered to all visitors (not just subscribers) on the *IDRAC Home Page* is a Web guide with annotated hotlinks to pharmaceutical industry sites. This brief, but useful, directory also identifies government agencies and health authorities worldwide, as well as Internet locations for pertinent organizations and industry associations.

FOI Services has compiled a subset of the *Diogenes* database (16.1) entitled *DIOGENES-FDA Medical Devices*. Available on CD-ROM and through the SilverPlatter Internet service, this retrospective collection includes records for all PMA approval and 510k clearance announcements, as well as the full text of more than 70,000 archived MDRs. Annual subscriptions offer the option of receiving three to four updates per year.

Verifying Patent Numbers, Expirations, and Extensions

With passage of the Drug Price Competition and Patent Term Restoration Act (Waxman-Hatch legislation) in 1984 and GATT-enabling legislation in 1994, a new hot topic was added to an already daunting list of possible regulatory questions that has provided the impetus for this chapter of the *Guide*. Has company X applied for an extension on its patent for drug Y? In fact, whenever a query involves checking a patent expiration date, whether or not an extension has been mentioned, the possibility of supplementary protection must be considered.

Why do people ask about patent expirations? A generic drug manufacturer may use this information in long-term planning for me-too product introductions, in order to allocate resources needed to support abbreviated new drug applications and anticipate a timeline for additional revenues successful registrations may yield. A bulk chemical producer can use expiration dates to predict possible increases in demand for compounds essential to formulation of the products in question, which may require expansion of manufacturing facilities, enhancement of distribution channels, and stepped up marketing and sales programs. Competing companies in a therapeutic category where the patent expiration will occur must counter the threat of lower priced alternatives with strategically timed new product introductions of their own. Financial analysts and investors, in consequence, closely monitor probable moves by all players affected as patent expiration dates approach and attempt to analyze their impact on a given market, as well as on individual companies.

Before an expiration date can be determined, another question must be answered: What patent covers this product? This, in itself, is a typical inquiry to anticipate, and may owe its origin to preliminary investigations into joint ventures or licensing agreements. Although seemingly straightforward to the requester, it is a question that can be extremely difficult to answer. Drug information professionals will need to know some basic facts about patent law and publications resulting from its implementation in order to choose appropriate resources and use them effectively. When their job responsibilities involve service to legal staff, readers in industry settings are likely to require far more than the basic introduction provided in this section.

Amernick[5] offers a solid foundation on which to build knowledge of patent laws. Maynard and Peters[6] focus on understanding chemical patents. Simmons[7] augments an overview of legal issues with detailed discussion of online sources. The intent of this section of the *Guide* is to bring together background material sufficient to prepare readers for general reference service to regulatory personnel and market researchers in answer to typical patent inquiries. The emphasis here, as in other sections, will be on sources especially useful in the pharmaceutical subject area and on specialized vocabulary commonly encountered in this context. Additional information about databases mentioned in the course of discussion, but not singled out for separate annotations, is included in Appendix B.

Background on Patent Law

The purpose of patent laws is to encourage innovation by protecting the rights of inventors. Patents confer exclusive rights to inventors to make, use, or sell their discoveries by barring others from doing so for a specified period of time. At the same time, documents required to obtain such a monopoly guarantee survival of the scientific or technological advances that they protect by full disclosure of the inventions. Patent laws in most countries dictate that the "specification" portion of a patent application provide a written description sufficient to enable others working in the same field to make or use the discovery. Specifications must conclude with "claims," which precisely pinpoint the innovations to be regarded as inventions entitled to protection from commercialization by others. Thus, a patent application is a curious melding of technological and legal data, with equally important implications to business information seekers. It's important to recognize at the outset that indexing resources wholly devoted to patent publications vary in their potential utility, depending on which of these three applications (scientific, legal, or commercial) is facilitated.

Sources also differ in their geopolitical scope. Because patents offer protection of inventions only within the country where they have been granted, answers to questions about product patents and expiration dates may be linked to a given locale. Further complicating the issue is the fact that some countries do not allow claims for pharmaceutical products *per se*. (Examples include Spain, Greece, Portugal, and Argentina.) In such cases, legal protection may hinge, instead, on the process used to make the product, if it is sufficiently unique, or on a composition claim, if a novel formulation is the dominant factor. Method of use claims can also be proposed as a basis for monopoly, whereby the specific method for treating a disease would be protected from competition. Innovative dosage forms or ways of administering them may also be covered.

Reading between the lines in many inquiries means finding the "priority" patent. Priority generally refers to the date and country where the initial application was submitted and the serial number assigned to it at that time. Subsequent applications in other countries usually refer to these priority details, because they establish the petitioner's right to be considered the first inventor and set the twelve-month clock during which corresponding applications can be submitted in countries other than the first filing location (an acceptable interval agreed upon by participants in the Paris Convention of 1883). A group of patents claiming the same invention by the same applicant in different countries is referred to as a patent family, and its members are often called equivalents. The lineage they share in common is the priority filing.

Two international agreements have made multinational patent filings easier. The Patent Cooperation Treaty (PCT) of 1970, effective in 1978, permits filing of a single application as the first step in requesting protection in a group of eighty-five signatory countries. Any of these nations can be selected by an inventor as "designated states" where a commercial monopoly on the discovery will be sought within the next thirty months. One benefit of the PCT is time: additional time to determine, through ongoing preclinical and clinical studies, whether a compound will be commercially viable. Under its protection, decisions on whether to proceed with the application and where to file (not all nations initially designated need be pursued) can be delayed, as can expenses involved in follow-up at the national level (e.g., translation, hiring a local representative, government fees). If pursued, an application made under PCT provisions must still be examined for validity in individual countries before protection can be officially granted. (Validity depends on local patent laws, but centers on factors such as novelty, nonobviousness, and utility or applicability in industry.)

A second international agreement, the European Patent Convention of 1973, offers the additional benefit of a standardized examination process overriding national differences in validity determinations and allowable claims. A single filing with the European Patent Office (EPO) is examined by one authority and, if deemed valid, the resulting European Patent (EP) is enforceable in any designated states selected by the applicant from the list of eighteen participating countries.

Patent information sources should, ideally, offer users the capability to bring together families resulting from such agreements. A priority number is often a good starting point and, therefore, can be an acceptable answer to inquiries about a drug patent. However, many other numbers crop up in the course of such inquiries, such as (in each country where it is submitted) the number assigned to an application when filed, the number assigned to the published application, a separate number assigned to an examined or accepted application, and, finally, the number of the granted or issued patent. All of this can lead to a great deal of confusion and frustration, but it is best to be aware of the differences and to plan accordingly, assembling as much information as possible by checking multiple sources. It's particularly important to distinguish between published applications (referred to as "A" documents) versus granted patents ("B" publications) when reviewing online records.

In most countries, applications are published within eighteen months of filing. Prior to that time, do not expect to find substantive information about a new drug discovery. In general, publication describing an invention prior to patent filing automatically disqualifies the application's validity. Statutory protection, being predicated on novelty, will be denied. Laws governing the patent process in the United States are an exception to this rule, in that they permit a one year grace period between prior disclosure and application filing. However, because therapeutic innovations require a multinational monopoly to ensure return on investment, secrecy imposed by foreign filing rules prevails. "Prior art" searches, conducted by both applicants and patent examiners, must, in fact, show lack of precedents in order to demonstrate entitlement of claims to meet criteria of novelty and inventiveness ("nonobviousness"). Silence is, literally, golden in establishing rights to intellectual property protection and profitability, should the drug discovery ultimately be approved for marketing.

Linking Brand Name Products with Their Patents

By the time questions arise about what patent covers a product, statutory nondisclosure is unlikely to be the chief impediment to finding an answer. Instead, problems encountered will be inherent in the patent process. Claims are often deliberately written to encompass as broad a scope as possible (albeit subject to national legal restrictions), in order to gain protection for an invention that accommodates the fullest commercial exploitation. Where permitted, a group of compounds characterized by a generic structure will be reserved for exclusive use, with their applicability described in very general terms. In this way, specific therapeutic indications as yet undetermined will be covered. Descriptions in specifications are designed to block loopholes that could be used to defend infringements and, by intent, avoid potentially restrictive language.

This practice, while eminently sound from a legal point of view, makes patents frustratingly inaccessible to searchers accustomed to more precise clinical terminology and the straightforward writing style encountered in scientific publications. It is very difficult to determine, from examination of claims alone, what products currently, or soon to be, in commerce are actually covered by a patent. Needless to say, at the very early stage in drug development when patent protection is sought, simplified nonproprietary (generic) names or brand names have yet to be coined and, therefore, are not used to describe compounds to be covered. What's needed to answer product patent questions is not what are generally referred to as patent databases. Instead, sources that link lab codes, generic names, and brands to patent numbers are the best choice.

Diogenes (16.1) records derived from the FDA *New Drug List* (*NDL*, updated quarterly) include notes on intellectual property protection and U.S. market exclusivity, as was illustrated in Figure 16.4. This information is also released annually in hardcopy format under the title *Drugs Under Patent* (4.16). It is, in turn, based on *Orange Book* (4.42) listings of patent numbers and expiration dates for approved drug products in the United States. A new *Orange Book* query capability on the FDA Web site makes data far more accessible than in the hard-to-read printed version.

Don't assume, however, that patents cited in *The Orange Book* (or in *Diogenes* records derived from the same source) are definitive answers to product patent inquiries. The FDA currently exercises little oversight over intellectual property declarations submitted to the agency under Waxman-Hatch mandates. Sometimes the patent cited does not cover actual ingredients used or therapeutic uses approved. Companies have been known to substitute formulation patents granted after NDA approval, in order to delay generic introductions for a period beyond what original patents would ensure.[8]

16.4 *IMSworld Patents International*. London: IMS Global Services, 1987–. Updated monthly. Available on DataStar, Dialog, and QUESTEL-ORBIT.

The *IMSworld Patents International* database tracks pharmaceutical patent families through international registration and monitors expiration dates worldwide (fifty-six countries and other issuing authorities), not just in the United States. Unfortunately, only about 1,800 products have been selected for inclusion, based on IMS judgments regarding their commercial significance at Phase III (and beyond). Like *Diogenes*, *Patents International* accommodates searching by brand or generic drug names and by company. In addition, CAS registry numbers are searchable, as are therapeutic class (an exclusive feature), laboratory codes and alternative generic names (not just USAN, but also INN, BAN), and patent country.

Each record compiles information on a single product in a given country, citing patentee (assignee); parent company; patent type (product, process, composition, or method of use); numbers of both the national application and granted patent; dates of application filing and publication, patent issue, and expiration;

and priority details, such as country, number(s), and dates. Explanatory notes, when necessary, summarize important issues regarding a product's patent protection, including related applications by the same and competing companies (see Figure 16.19). A special tag enables searchers to isolate patents whose terms were amended by GATT implementation in the United States; search the phrase *term reset* to take advantage of this feature.

Other possible links to product patent data are drugs-in-development directories discussed in Chapter Fifteen. These publications, which monitor the pharmaceutical pipeline from the preclinical stage forward, often include patent numbers supplied by companies whose products are featured. Thus, patent numbers in *Pharmaprojects* (15.1) or *IMSworld R&D Focus Drug Updates* (15.2) records are likely to be those that will actually be relied upon for commercial protection when the products cited are launched. In contrast, patents cited in sources on which chemists depend, such as *The Merck Index* (3.5), *Beilstein*, or *Chapman & Hall Chemical Database* (formerly *Heilbron*), often represent the earliest publications describing the synthesis of targeted compounds and are not necessarily the much-sought-after "product" patents. To a certain extent, some of the same reservations apply to patent numbers provided in *NME Express* (15.4) or *Drug Data Report* (15.5), which may not turn out to be those finally claimed by companies for market exclusivity of finished products that will evolve. [Note: *The Merck Index* is, nonetheless, prized for its references to U.S. and foreign patents issued prior to 1950 (i.e., predating online indexing coverage). Also, *Merck* monographs newly added from the eleventh edition forward (1989–) have begun to cite, whenever possible, U.S. product patents.]

In answer to product related inquiries, any qualified lead into the patent literature is preferable to attempting a direct scan of data as they are presented in legally or technologically oriented databases such as *INPADOC* or *World Patents Index*. Although searches in these files can be confined to patents for specified companies (assignees) and countries, attempts to isolate records for specific therapeutic applications are often foiled by the unpredictability of language used in describing discoveries. In *INPADOC*, for example, cryptic titles offer little scope for effective free-text strategies and the alternative, International Patent Classification Codes, can be cumbersome to use and is inconsistently applied. *World Patents Index*, by providing natural language abstracts in place of verbatim claims transcription, affords greater opportunity for successful location of relevant records, but results can, nonetheless, be impractically lengthy to screen for answers to product patent questions.

Determining Expiration Dates and Tracking Down Term Extensions

Expiration inquiries cannot be easily answered by direct access to traditional patent literature files. Because terms of protection are subject to change, the original documents indexed in these databases do not include expiration dates. Status can

Figure 16.19 Sample Record from IMSworld Patents International

DIALOG(R)File 447:IMSworld Patents International
© 1996 IMSworld Publ. Ltd. All rts. reserv.

00016318
Drug Name: ondansetron
Patents International–May 28 1996 (19960528)

DRUG INFORMATION:
CAS Registry Number:	99614–02–5, ondansetron
	99614–12–7, maleate
	99614–51–4, citrate (2:1)
	99614–01–4, monohydrochloride
	99614–50–3, phosphate (1:1)
	103639–04–9, monohydrochloride, dihydrate
	110707–92–1, hydrochloride
	119884–17–2, monoHCl dihydrate, mixt with ranitidine monoHCl
	120180–61–2, monoHCl dihydrate, mixt with omeprazole
	128061–09–6, monoHCL monohydrate, mixt cont 116002– 70–1, (+,-)
	99614–60–5, (R)
	99614–74–1, (R),
	[R-(R*,R*)]-2,3-bis[(4-methylbenzoyl)oxy]butane dioate
	99614–61–6, (R), maleate
	99614–58–1, (S)
	99614–73–0, (S),
	[S-(R*,R*)]-2,3-bis[(4-methylbenzoyl)oxy]butane dioate
	99614–59–2, (S), maleate
	110204–46–1, replaced
Brand Name:	ZOFRAN ; ZOPHREN; ZOFRON
Laboratory Code:	GR 38032; GR 38032F; SN 307
Therapeutic Class Code:	A4 (Antiemetics and Antinauseants)
	N6D (Nootropics)
	L1 (Cytostatics)
Clinical Indications:	emesis
	cognitive defect
	cancer

PATENT INFORMATION:
Patentee:	Glaxo (UK)
Patent Type:	Product

Patent Country	Patent Number	Patent Date	Expiration Date
US (USA)	US 4695578	19870922	20050509

Priority Country	Priority Number	Priority Date
GB (UK)	GB 1888	19840125
GB (UK)	GB 25959	19841015

EXPIRATION COMMENTS:
Term reset;Extended

COUNTRY COMMENTS:
The normal expiry date of US 4695578 is 22 September 2004. The term was extended by 104 days under Waxman-Hatch provisions and this patent was set to expire on 3 January 2005. On 8 June 1995 the amendments to the US patent law under the General Agreement on Tariffs and Trade (GATT) came into force. Following a ruling on 4 April 1996, the Waxman-Hatch extension may be added to any GATT term reset if the patent (not including any Waxman-Hatch extension) was in force on 8 June 1995. As a result the estimated expiry date of US 4695578 has been reset to 9 May 2005. Glaxo has US 4753789, normal expiry 28 June 2005, term reset to 24 June 2006, claiming the use of ondansetron for the relief of nausea and vomiting, particularly when these conditions result from some form of anticancer therapy. Glaxo also has US 4929632, normal expiry 29 May 2007, term unaffected, claiming the use of ondansetron to promote gastric emptying in diagnostic radiological procedures. Both of these US patents are equivalent to Glaxo's European patent appln 226266, filed 24 June 1986. Beecham has a method of use patent in the USA for ondansetron. US 4783478, published 8 November 1988, normal expiry 8 November 2005, term reset to 12 March 2006, claims the treatment of emesis and/or irritable bowel syndrome, particularly when caused by cytotoxic agents. It is a divisional of US 4721720, published 26 January 1988, the claims of which were amended after grant to exclude ondansetron. Both of these US patents are equivalent to Beecham's European patent appln 201165, filed 10 March 1986.

be affected by nonpayment of maintenance fees, court decisions, and successful applications for term extension. Moreover, statutory terms of protection differ from country to country. For example, the clock may start at the date of application filing, of application publication, of final grant or issue, or of publication of the examined (accepted) specification. Term lengths, ranging from five to twenty years, also differ among nations and, even within a given country, can be dependent on legislation in force at the time of grant, rather than current law. This is one reason why databases such as *IMSworld Patents International* and *Diogenes* are highly valued as sources of expiry data, in addition to supplying direct links from product names to pertinent patent numbers. But, perhaps predictably, there are drawbacks to using them when questions specifically address patent term extensions, particularly when recently granted supplements to protection are a possibility.

The first announcement, in an official source, of an application for extension of U.S. patent exclusivity appears in the *Federal Register* (4.24). Several steps in the extension process have already been completed before such a notice appears: 1) the originating company submitted an application to the U.S. Patent and Trademark Office (PTO) within sixty days of product approval date, 2) the PTO sent a letter to the FDA requesting confirmation that the product underwent regulatory review, 3) the FDA affirmed eligibility, and 4) the PTO submitted a second formal request for FDA authorization of the company's claimed review period, the basis for patent term extension. Unless a company has previously issued a press release regarding its application, it is not possible to determine that an extension may be in the works until the FDA's response to the PTO is published in the *Federal Register*. A search for the phrase *patent extension* in the title of *FR* entries will isolate relevant notices, to which company or product brand name can be added to narrow down results.[9]

Federal Register notices of FDA determinations on patent term extensions include the exact dates of IND and NDA submissions and of subsequent approval, making them an accurate source on which to gauge estimations of length of time to market following completion of preclinical testing. An example is reproduced in Figure 16.20. Notices also state the number of days designated as the applicable regulatory review period for patent extension, a sum of the time period required for human testing and days elapsed in the preregistration phase. *Pharmaceutical Approvals Monthly* (4.21, 15.10), in its indexing of *FR* patent extension requests, adds value by identifying the issue date of the patent and calculating its expiration date with or without the restoration days petitioned (see Figure 16.21).

However, neither the original *Federal Register* announcement, nor its corresponding index entry in *Pharmaceutical Approvals Monthly*, should be regarded as proof of actual patent extension or as more than an estimation for an adjusted U.S. patent expiration. Both the FDA and the PTO sometimes adjust their calculations after further deliberation. Important questions that remain after a *Federal Register* notice is located are: Has legal protection subsequently been extended by the PTO and, if so, what is the adjusted expiration date?

To answer these questions, a search of patent databases is needed. Why consult the *Federal Register* or *Pharmaceutical Approvals Monthly* (in *F-D-C Reports Online*) first? As was previously noted, patent files generally do not cite proprietary names. Both the *Federal Register* and *F-D-C* provide a vital link between the approved product brand name and a patent number. With this number in hand, the quickest route to definitive U.S. patent term extension information is a search in the IFI/Plenum database *CLAIMS/Reassignment & Reexamination* (*CLAIMS/ RRX*), available on Dialog, QUESTEL-ORBIT, and STN. Term restorations resulting from the 1984 Waxman-Hatch legislation are first announced in the U.S. PTO *Official Gazette* and are added to *CLAIMS/RRX* records within one to two weeks (see Figure 16.22). Entry of a patent number will be sufficient to isolate data needed. The only task that remains is to calculate the precise expiration date, which involves adding the extension days to the statutory term. The statutory

Figure 16.20   Patent Extension Application Notice in the Federal Register Online

DIALOG(R)File 669:Federal Register
© 1996 Knight-Ridder Info. All rts. reserv.

00403223
Determination of Regulatory Review Period for Purposes of Patent Extension; Zofran (REG.)

Vol. 56, No. 87
56 FR 20622
Monday, May 6, 1991

AGENCY: DEPARTMENT OF HEALTH AND HUMAN SERVICES; Food and Drug
  Administration
DOC TYPE: Notices
NUMBER: Docket No. 91E-0109
CONTACT: Nancy E. Pirt, Office of Health Affairs (HFY-20), Food and Drug Administration, 5600 Fishers Lane, Rockville, MD 20857, 301-443-1382. Written comments and petitions should be directed to the Dockets Management Branch (HFA-305), Food and Drug Administration, rm. 4–62, 5600 Fishers Lane, Rockville, MD 20857.
Notice.
The Food and Drug Administration (FDA) has determined the regulatory review period for Zofran cumber and is publishing this notice of that determination as required by law. FDA has made the determination because of the submission of an application to the Commissioner of Patents and Trademarks, Department of Commerce, for the extension of a patent which claims that human drug product.
WORD COUNT: 990
TEXT:
SUPPLEMENTARY INFORMATION: The Drug Price Competition and Patent Term Restoration Act of 1984 (Pub. L. 98–417) and the Generic Animal Drug and Patent Term Restoration Act (Pub. L. 100–670) generally provide that a patent may be extended for a period of up to 5 years so long as the patented item (human drug product, animal drug product, medical device, food additive, or color additive) was subject to regulatory review by FDA before the item was marketed. Under these acts, a product's regulatory review period forms the basis for determining the amount of extension an applicant may receive.
   A regulatory review period consists of two periods of time: A testing phase and an approval phase. For human drug products, the testing phase begins when the exemption to permit the clinical investigations of the drug becomes effective and runs until the approval phase begins. The approval phase starts with the initial submission of an application to market the human drug product and continues until FDA grants permission to market the drug product. Although only a portion of a regulatory review period may count toward the actual amount of extension that the Commissioner of Patents and Trademarks may award (for example, half the testing phase must be subtracted as well as any time that may have occurred before the patent was issued), FDA's determination of the length of a regulatory review period for a human drug product will include all of the testing phase and approval phase as specified in 35 U.S.C. 156(g)(1)(B).
   FDA recently approved for marketing the human drug product Zofran sup (ondan-

setron hydrochloride). Injection is indicated for the prevention of nausea and vomiting associated with initial and repeat courses of emetogenic cancer chemotherapy, including high dose cisplatin. Subsequent to this approval, the Patent and Trademark Office received a patent term restoration application for Zofran sup (U.S. Patent No. 4,695,578) from Glaxo Group Ltd., and the Patent and Trademark Office requested FDA's assistance in determining this patent's eligibility for patent term restoration. FDA, in a letter dated April 2, 1991, advised the Patent and Trademark Office that this human drug product had undergone a regulatory review period and that the approval of Zofran sup represented the first commercial marketing of the product. Shortly thereafter, the Patent and Trademark Office requested that the FDA determine the product's regulatory review period. FDA has determined that the applicable regulatory review period for Zofran sup is 1,570 days. Of this time, 1,120 days occurred during the testing phase of the regulatory review period, while 450 days occurred during the approval phase. These periods of time were derived from the following dates:

1. The date an exemption under section 505(i) of the Federal Food, Drug, and Cosmetic Act became effective: September 19, 1986. FDA has verified the applicant's claim that the date the investigational new drug (IND) application became effective was September 19, 1986.

2. The date the application was initially submitted with respect to the human drug product under section 505(b) of the Federal Food, Drug, and Cosmetic Act: October 12, 1989. FDA has verified the applicant's claim that the new drug application (NDA20–007) was filed on October 12, 1989.

3. The date the application was approved: January 4, 1991. FDA has verified the applicant's claim that NDA 20–007 was approved on January 4, 1991.

This determination of the regulatory review period establishes the maximum potential length of a patent extension. However, the U.S. Patent and Trademark Office applies several statutory limitations in its calculations of the actual period for patent extension. In its application for patent extension, this applicant seeks 560 days of patent term extension.

Anyone with knowledge that any of the dates as published is incorrect may, on or before July 5, 1991, submit to the Dockets Management Branch (address above) written comments and ask for a redetermination. Furthermore, any interested person may petition FDA, on or before November 4, 1991, for a determination regarding whether the applicant for extension acted with due diligence during the regulatory review period. To meet its burden, the petition must contain sufficient facts to merit an FDA investigation. (See H. Rept. 857, part 1, 98th Cong., 2d Sess., pp. 41–42, 1984.) Petitions should be in the format specified in 21CFR 10.30. Comments and petitions should be submitted to the Dockets Management Branch (address above) in three copies (except that individuals may submit single copies) and identified with the docket number found in brackets in the heading of this document. Comments and petitions may be seen in the Dockets Management Branch between 9 a.m. and 4 p.m., Monday through Friday.

Dated: April 26, 1991.
Stuart L. Nightingale,
Associate Commissioner for Health Affairs.
INTERNAL DATA: FR Doc. 91–10591; Filed 5–3–91; 8:45 am; BILLING CODE 4160–01–M

Figure 16.21   Indexing of Patent Extension Requests in F-D-C Reports Online

```
        FDCR [DataStar]
AN     01M08364 9601.
TI     Patent Extension Requests: Zyrtec (cetirizine).
SO     Pharmaceutical Approvals Monthly, August 1, 1996, Page 42.
DT     960801.
TX     1 of 1
        Drug ................... Zyrtec (cetirizine)
        Number .............. 4,525,358
        Patentee(s) .......... Eugene Baltes, et al.
        Assignee .............. UCB Pharma (licensed to Pfizer)
        Issue Date ........... 6/25/85
        Exp Date ............. 6/25/2002
        Ext Request ......... 6/25/2007
        Footnote .............
```

Figure 16.22   Sample Record for a Patent Extension in CLAIMS/RRX

DIALOG(R)File 123:CLAIMS(R)/REASS.& REEXAM.
© 1996 IFI/Plenum Data Corp. All rts. reserv.

1798516
EXTENDED
Assignee: GLAXO GROUP LTD GB

	Patent Number	Issue Date	Extension Date	Recorded in OG
Patent:	US 4695578	870922	911230	920128
Extended for:			104 Days	

term for a U.S. patent is now twenty years from filing date; formerly, the term was seventeen years from issue date (see Chapter Four).

Because *Diogenes* and *IMSworld Patents International* cite exact U.S. expiration date, without requiring further calculation by the user, it is tempting to rely on their data. The problem in both of these files is that extensions granted within the last three months may not be reflected in record content. In addition to lag time, another drawback to *Diogenes* patent information is that extended expirations are not specifically identified (as they are in IMS), so that a searcher has no way of knowing if recent extensions have been incorporated. The same drawback applies to *Orange Book* expiration data. And, although *Diogenes* includes medical devices in its scope, patent data comparable to that compiled for drugs are not provided. The *Federal Register-CLAIMS/RRX* two-step approach described here will locate device and animal drug term extensions, as well as those granted for human medicinals.

The *Patent Term Extension and New Patents Docket* listed under the FDA's Center for Drug Evaluation and Research "Drug Info" option on the Internet is another source of term restoration data. When a cumulative retrospective list (excluding the last few months) is needed, users can download this PDF document. It compiles data by generic name of active ingredient, listing brand name, patent number, original expiration date, and extended exclusivity expiration date. Unfortunately, this Web site option is for display (and printing) only; there is no search engine that permits prescreening of the information it contains or isolation of list entries for given companies or brands.

Most (but not all) European Community countries have implemented a patent term extension program. The Supplementary Protection Certificate (SPC) is applicable to human, but not animal, drugs. Although the impetus for this EC initiative is encouragement of pioneer research by restoring part of patent life expended in testing and regulatory review, SPC terms are not actually determined by the length of time consumed in these two activities. This extension program also differs from Waxman-Hatch provisions in that multiple SPCs can be granted on the same patent when its claims cover more than one approved product. (Under the U.S. restoration law, only one NDA-approved drug product per patent can be used as a basis for term extension.) SPCs grant five years of continuing trade monopoly beyond a product's original patent expiration date, or a maximum of fifteen years of protection following the product's first marketing approval in any EC member state. A request for supplementary protection can be filed in a given country within six months of its official approval of a product. These requests are published in the national patent gazette of the member state recipient, as are announcements of SPCs granted.

Information regarding Supplementary Protection Certificates can be found in several sources. Derwent offers subscriptions to an SPC compilation for German pharmaceutical patents, as well as publications documenting Japanese and U.S. patent extensions, all in hardcopy format. The *IMSworld Patents International* database includes SPC data for major drug products. It is also a good source for determining extensions granted for foreign patents in Japan since January 1988. Applicable to both human and veterinary drugs, the Japanese term restoration program is predicated on time expended in regulatory review and permits a maximum extension of five years. Approval of additional indications can result in additional extensions.

When coverage of a product is not available in *IMSworld Patents International*, probably the best online source to answer questions about SPCs is *INPADOC*, produced by the European Patent Office and available on Dialog, QUESTEL-ORBIT, and STN. This database offers worldwide coverage of patents issued by at least one of sixty-four countries and other authorities, dating from 1968 to the present. With its expanded global scope, *INPADOC* will help verify expiry dates adjusted not only by Supplementary Protection Certificates (SPCs), but also extended protection authorized under French law prior to adoption of the EC program (Certificat Complémentaire de Protection, or CPC). *INPADOC*'s legal status information (available under the database title *LEGSTAT* on ORBIT) includes the actual length of extensions granted under any of these national patent term restoration programs, citing the serial number of the patent affected. However, neither original or adjusted expiration dates are included in *INPADOC/ LEGSTAT* records, leaving calculation tasks to the user.

It should be noted that, although *INPADOC* also documents U.S. patent extensions, *CLAIMS/RRX* is a far more timely source for verifying Waxman-Hatch restorations. *INPADOC*'s lag time in recording U.S. extensions varies, ranging from seven weeks to five months, while *CLAIMS/RRX* can be relied upon to add new data within one to two weeks of *Official Gazette* announcements. Other patent databases online may note that term extensions have been authorized, but do not provide further details. For example, some *CLAIMS/U.S. Patents Abstracts* records add the word "extended," but the length of the officially designated extension period is not specified.

Exploring Other Applications of Patent Data and Subject Specialty Sources

Because intellectual property issues exercise a profound influence on financial markets, several business databases discussed in Chapter Fifteen are other potential sources of patent information. Many reports in *Investext* (15.38), for example, provide useful tables correlating brand names with expiration dates. However, it is imperative that text accompanying tables be checked to ensure that post-GATT term adjustments and Waxman-Hatch extensions have been taken into account. *IMS World Drug Markets* (15.32) is a convenient place to check patent law provisions for any of the seventy-six countries covered. It can help answer questions about product versus process patent acceptability, statutory terms of protection and if extensions are permitted, and whether a country is a participant in the various international cooperative agreements cited previously. In addition, patent information supplied in *Investext*, *IMSworld* databases, and *Pharmaprojects* (15.1) is often augmented with useful licensing information. Background on licensing will, for example, help explain puzzling oddities that searches sometimes uncover, such as products from two different companies that both claim exclusivity from the same patent.

Patent databases afford excellent opportunities for trend analysis. Special software capabilities available on Dialog, QUESTEL-ORBIT, and STN permit ranked compilations of patent data when statistical comparisons are needed. For example, results of a subject search within a specific area of drug development can be analyzed to create a table showing companies and number of patents granted, in ranked order. An individual corporation's patent portfolio can be examined for subject shifts from year to year by requesting a ranked list of patent classification codes found in documents listing the company as an assignee and published in each year. Leading scientists can be identified with strategies that start with subject classification codes, then rank results by inventor name. Patents are, of course, an excellent way to monitor cutting edge technology. Some difficulties to anticipate in subject searching have already been mentioned. Strategies should never rely on subject keywords alone. The highly stylized language embodied in claims and specifications make it difficult to predict all possible descriptive terms that could be used in relevant documents. Furthermore, sentence structure and word order is somewhat peculiar, necessitating creative use of proximity operators, truncation, and many, many synonyms. Results of initial forays should be analyzed for high occurrence patent classification codes, which can then be incorporated into subject keyword strategies, both to eliminate ambiguity and to increase recall.

Several databases offer special advantages to pharmaceutical patent searchers. The most well known source is Derwent's *World Patents Index*, which adds descriptive titles to characterize document content and creates subject oriented abstracts that clarify the meaning of awkwardly worded claims. *CA Search* and *CA File*, although far more selective in coverage of the patent literature, add value with CAS registry number access and, on STN, descriptive abstracts. Structural search capabilities, such as *Markush DARC* on QUESTEL-ORBIT or *MARPAT* on STN, bring graphic retrieval options to accessing patent data. A new database from Derwent, *DGENE*, provides indexing of nucleic acid and protein sequences extracted from patent documents published in any of the forty countries and other authorities covered in *World Patents Index*, with the ability to display corresponding patent families derived from the latter, as well.

16.5 *Pharmsearch*. Paris: Institut National de la Propriété Industrielle, 1961–. Updated semimonthly. Available on QUESTEL-ORBIT.

Pharmsearch includes citations and abstracts for French, European (EPO), British, German, PCT, and U.S. pharmaceutical patents. French, EPO, and PCT documents are covered from 1985 to date, U.S., U.K., and German patents from 1992 to the present. Value-added index terms identify starting materials used in preparations, preparation processes, therapeutic effects, and mechanism of action of claimed substances. Images extracted from original documents accompany *Pharmsearch* records added since October 1993. Structural searches of this database can be conducted through *Markush DARC*.

16.6 *Investigational Drug Patents Fast-Alert*. London: Current Drugs Ltd, 1989–. Updated weekly. Available on DataStar and QUESTEL-ORBIT.

Updated weekly within ten days of patent application publication, *Investigational Drug Patents Fast-Alert* (formerly *Current Drugs Fast-Alert*) is designed for targeted current awareness in both the pharmaceutical and agrochemical sub-

ject areas. Coverage includes British, U.S., EPO, Japanese, and PCT applications
and granted patents in the following major therapeutic areas:

Anti-infectives
Arthritis
Biologicals & Immunologicals
Cardiovascular & Renal
Central & Peripheral Nervous Systems
Dermatological
Endocrine & Metabolic
Gastrointestinal
Oncologic
Pulmonary-Allergy

Database records provide key bibliographic details, such as priority, patent assignees, inventor names, and International Patent Classification, as shown in Figure 16.23. Each entry is also accompanied by an English-language abstract written by an expert in the specific subject area addressed by the discovery. Current
awareness scans can be limited to any of the broad drug categories listed above
or can focus on narrower topics identified by descriptors drawn from a controlled
vocabulary developed by Current Drugs. Descriptors assigned to each document
consist of three components: therapeutic category, mechanism of action, and
chemical classification. For example,

DE: Anxiolytic; 5HT2-antagonist; Ergoline derivative
DE: Antibacterial; Gyrase-inhibitor; Quinolone derivative

For patents dealing with a new chemical production process, the term "Process"
appears in the DE paragraph. Diagnostics are also consistently identified by indexers. The intent of this online resource is to characterize the "main embodi-
ment" of new pharmaceutical patents, at the same time enhancing accessibility
through systematic, clinically oriented indexing.

   Another specialized patent database is available free of charge on the Internet.
The Center for Networked Information Discovery and Retrieval (CNIDR), in collaboration with the U.S. Patent and Trademark Office and the National Science
Foundation, has created an international *AIDS Patents Database* for free public
access. The file is fully searchable by subject keywords, as well as by applicant
company and individual inventor name. Records consist of the full text and images of important patents relating to acquired immune deficiency syndrome, including applications for drugs, biologics, and diagnostic products. The Internet
URL is http://app.cnidr.org. Remember, also, another Internet source cited earlier, the *Biotechnology Law Web Server*, which offers a wealth of commentary
and analysis related to both U.S. and European patent news (see Chapter Four).

Figure 16.23   Sample Record from Investigational Drug Patents Fast-Alert

AN	BT15239 AC12645 950620. [DataStar]
TI	Method and composition for cancer therapy and for prognosticating responses to cancer therapy.
AB	Novelty: To determine/prognosticate the effectiveness of a therapeutic agent in the treatment of certain cancers the amount of expressed receptor-like oncogene is measured. Biology: Malignancy in some tumours is characterized by the expression or overexpression of at least the HER-2/neu oncogene. A ligand/antibody to this receptor-like protein induces terminal differentiation. Therefore an assay was developed to determine the induction of terminal differentiation. Cells of a biopsy sample are divided into two portions. One is treated with a specific ligand/antibody to the oncogene product, the other is cultured without this agent. After culturing, the percentage of cells that exhibit morphological evidence of terminal differentiation in both samples is compared. The method may be used with cells of a patient to choose a therapeutic drug combination tailored to the patient or, alternatively, the malignant cells are an established transformed cell line and the method is used as a general screening assay for selecting anti-cancer therapeutics. (pp28).
PA	Becton Dickinson & Co & et al.
IN	Bacus-S-S, Yarden-Y, Sela-M.
PN	EP-0656367-A.
DS	AT BE CH DE DK ES FR GB GR IE IT LI LU MC NL SE.
PD	950607.
PR	US-767042.
PY	910927.
FD	920821.
SC	Biotechnology (BT) Anti Cancer (AC).
DE	Neoplasm-Breast-tumour-Stomach-tumour; Receptor-Oncogene-Monoclonal-antibody; Enabling-technology.
IC	C07K-016–030 A61K-039–395 C07K-019–000.

The Importance of Regulatory Surveillance

The emphasis placed here on maintaining surveillance of regulatory documents may seem like paranoia rather than prudent professionalism. Yet, the industry press provides ample evidence to underline the wisdom of proactive vigilance. A "there-but-for-the-grace-of . . ." tone pervades when results of unsuccessful FDA inspections are reported in detail. Is this ghoulish relish over the misfortunes of others, or is there a sound reason for picking over the bones so meticulously?

Unusually thorough Form 483 post mortems arise from the fact that wording in written FDA guidelines is deliberately general, leaving ample room for inter-pretation in their practical implementation. A former associate chief counsel to the FDA has pointed out that a long-standing agency practice has been to set policy through speeches and warning letters, acknowledging that such piecemeal disclosure offers "little definitive guidance."[10] Specific criteria for compliance are often revealed only in enforcement documents. In this context, contents of warning letters cannot be viewed as isolated cautionary tales, but rather as test cases that will, in retrospect, define official policy. Another FDA employee has suggested that the agency could circulate lists of the most frequent violations found in Form 483s, to help the industry identify problems to avoid. "Companies need to learn about new and evolving requirements in time to implement changes before the next round of inspections."[11]

In the absence of FDA-initiated compilations of data from its own archives, the responsibility for gathering and analyzing living law revealed in many of the documents discussed in this chapter rests firmly on the shoulders of pharmaceutical information specialists and their clientele. In a sense, the entire subject focus of this book—preparation for effective literature research and reference service—could be called "practical paranoia." By whatever name, knowledge of issues, published sources, and search protocols in the pharmaceutical subject specialty area is a powerful tool to leverage scientific R&D, improve patient care, and maintain surveillance on competitive business developments.

References

1. Snow B. Finding information on new drug approvals. *Database* 1992 Oct;15: 83–87.

2. Snow B. Protecting patients and staff from medical equipment hazards: Health Devices Alerts online. *Database* 1990 Feb;13:87–90.

3. Snow B. Tracking down medical device regulatory data online. Part 1. *Database* 1995 Feb;18:93–96. Part 2. *Database* 1995 Apr;18:94–98. Part 3. *Database* 1995 Jun;18:98–103.

4. Snow B. The FDA electronic bulletin board service. *Database* 1993 Feb;16:80–85.

5. Amernick BA. *Patent law for the nonlawyer: a guide for the engineer, technologist, and manager.* 2nd ed. New York: Van Nostrand Reinhold, 1991.

6. Maynard J, Peters H. *Understanding chemical patents.* 2nd ed. Washington, DC: American Chemical Society, 1991.

7. Simmons ES. Patents. In: Armstrong CJ, Large JA, eds. *Manual of online search strategies.* 2nd ed. Aldershot, Hants, England: Ashgate, 1992: 51–127.

8. Glaxo bupropion patents are example of 'Orange Book' abuse—GPIA. *The Pink Sheet* 1998 Oct 26;60(43).

9. Snow B. Drug patent extension information online: Monitoring post-approval regulatory developments. *Online* 1994 Jul;18:95–100.

10. Ex-FDAer scores agency for ways it makes policy. *Drug GMP Rep* 1994 Sep;26:*Diogenes* accession no. 550166.

11. Former drug center topsider explains what works well at FDA. *Food Drug Letter* 1994 Jul 29;*Diogenes* accession no. 400763.

Additional Sources of Information

Berks AH. Patent information in biotechnology. *Trends in Biotechnology* 1994;12:352–364.

Cheeseman EN. Pharmaceutical patent alerting services—Patents Preview and Patent Fast-Alert. *Database* 1995 Aug;18(4);65–71.

Gotkis HK. Current Patents Fast Alert. *Database* 1992 Dec;15(6):58–67.

Simmons ES, Kaback SM. Patents (literature). In: *Kirk-Othmer encyclopedia of chemical technology*. 4th ed. v. 18. New York: John Wiley, 1996:102–156.

Snow B. Competitive intelligence in the health device industry. *Online* 1989 Jul;13:107–114.

Snow B. Diogenes sheds new light on FDA regulatory actions. *Database* 1988 Apr;11:72–80.

Snow B. Monitoring bioscience legal and regulatory news. *Online* 1988 Nov;12:107–117.

Snow B. Patents in non-patent databases: Bioscience specialty files. *Database* 1989 Oct;12:41–48.

Snow B. Searching the Federal Register. *Online* 1991 May;15:94–99.

Van Dulken S. *Introduction to patents information*. 2nd ed. London: The British Library Science and Information Service, 1992.

Practicum 5

This practicum exercise will help you evaluate your online database selection skills and review information presented in Chapters Fourteen through Sixteen. Questions posed can be answered without actually conducting an online search. Suggested answers are included in Appendix E.

Directions: Assume that you have available for your use all of the sources cited in previous chapters. Unless otherwise indicated, your response to each question should consist of:

a. a list of sources to be consulted, with order of priority indicated, and

b. a brief explanation of the rationale behind your selection of resources and sequence of consultation.

1. Find references to the effects of bromocriptine therapy in elderly patients with both Parkinson's disease and hypertension.
2. Document the medicinal uses of yarrow, a commonly cultivated flowering perennial.
3. What companies are investigating antibiotics for antineoplastic therapy? I'm particularly interested in topoisomerase inhibitors.
4. I need bibliography on the comparative efficacy of two brand name products with the same active ingredients.
5. Find references to EC 4.1.1.33.
6. Which pharmaceutical firms have FDA approval to produce generic equivalents of Zantac, and which have also launched equivalents abroad?
7. We've been asked to investigate a new group of anti-inflammatory compounds called "antedrugs." This isn't a *MeSH* or *EMTREE* descriptor, so where would be a good place to start?
8. Find toxicity data on Drug Z and on the class of compounds to which it belongs.
9. I'm planning a prescription audit for three long-term care institutions. Where can I find articles about conducting such a survey?
10. What is the product patent for Drug Y? When does it expire?

11. I've been asked to find literature references to an investigational immuno-suppressant called "gusperimus trihydrochloride." When I tried searching this name in *MEDLINE* and *EMBASE*, there were no records that cited this name, but I was able to find a few items that used the name "gusperimus" and gave a registry number. When I showed these to the requester, she said that the registry number is incorrect, so they can't be about the same compound. What should I do next?

12. What pharmaceutical companies have spent the most on research and development in the last three years? How did outlays compare with their total capital expenditures?

13. Are statistics available on noncompliance? For example, how many people don't bother to have their initial prescription filled? Have data been compiled correlating dose regimen with incorrect use? What about types of drugs? Do certain categories show more compliance problems than others? Can you find some numeric data related to this issue?

14. I'd like to assemble some consumer-oriented materials on the effects of herbal teas.

15. I need an up-to-date list of all bronchodilators approved by the FDA in the past six months.

16. On what date was labetalol hydrochloride approved for intravenous injection in the United States?

17. We're interested in pharmacoeconomic evaluations of prophylactic use of filgrastim and comparable drugs to reduce the incidence of cancer chemo-therapy-induced neutropenia.

18. I've been told that Company Z is investigating a new corticosteroid for asthma. I think it's called "ciclisonide," but I can't find any references to this name. What next? I need citations to clinical studies, if available.

19. We're looking for a drug delivery system we can license that will enable administration of our antitumor products in liquid form to form controlled-release solid biodegradable implants at the application site.

20. When was Drug Q recalled, and why? What tests were conducted to determine its safety and efficacy prior to its approval?

21. In what countries are nootropics best sellers? What brands rank highest in sales, and where?

22. I never know how far back to go when surveying the adverse effects literature on a given drug. Are there any general guidelines for establishing retrospective delimiters in this type of online search?

A

The Core Drug Information Collection

Choosing a core collection from the 495 hardcopy and CD-ROM publications discussed in the *Guide* is difficult. Accordingly, this Appendix includes two lists of recommended titles, one for hospitals and one for public libraries. Suggested follow-up to consultation of either list is review of resource annotations in the context of discussion in previous chapters, where their scope and organization can be compared to other options available. Reference numbers following each title will help you locate source descriptions quickly. Additional notes included here highlight important distinctions among resources and cite precedents for the bibliography selected. Following the two core lists is a section that suggests which titles to retain, where space permits, after newer editions are issued.

Basic (Minimum) Ready-Reference Bibliography for Hospitals

Notes	Title	Ref #	Price	Precedents
	AHFS Drug Information	6.4	$155	2,3,5,6,7,8,9,10
	American Drug Index	3.6	$55	5,7,8
	Basic and Clinical Pharmacology	6.57	$40	1,2
	Casarett & Doull's Toxicology: The Basic Science of Poisons	8.12	$75	1
	Catalog of Teratogenic Agents	8.23	$125	
	The Chemotherapy Source Book	6.22	$99	2
	Chemically Induced Birth Defects	8.24	$275	
A.	Drug Facts and Comparisons (monthly looseleaf subscription)	6.2	$330	1,2,3,4,5,7,8
	Drug Information Handbook	6.20	$393	
	Drug Interaction Facts	7.10	$100	3,5
	Drugs and Human Lactation	7.20	$310	2
	Drugs in Pregnancy and Lactation	7.19	$169	2,3
	Effects of Drugs on Clinical Laboratory Tests	7.29	$29	

567

Ellenhorn's Medical Toxicology	8.13	$106	1
Evaluations of Drug Interactions	7.9	$229	1
Geriatric Dosage Handbook	6.35	$42	3
Goldfrank's Toxicologic Emergencies	8.14	$180	1,2
Goodman and Gilman	6.51	$92	1,2,3,5,6,7,8
Handbook for Prescribing Medications During Pregnancy	6.24	$38	
Handbook of Basic Pharmacokinetics	6.56	$49	
Handbook of Cancer Chemotherapy	6.23	$38	2
Handbook of Clinical Drug Data	6.19	$60	6,7,8
B. Handbook of Nonprescription Drugs	6.6	$150	3,5,6,7,8
Handbook on Injectable Drugs	7.31	$150	3,5,6,7,8
Hansten and Horn's Drug Interactions	7.8	$63	1,3,5,6,7,8
The Harriet Lane Handbook	6.28	$35	1
Infectious Diseases Handbook	6.46	$41	3
Manual of Antibiotics and Infectious Diseases	6.47	$34	1,3
Manual of Pediatric Therapeutics	6.29	$36	1
Martindale: The Extra Pharmacopoeia	6.1	$299	3,5,6,7,8
Medication Teaching Manual	9.39	$81	
The Merck Index	3.5	$45	2,3,5,7,8
Meyler's Side Effects of Drugs	7.1	$344	3,5,7
Mosby's GenRx	6.3	$73	1,2
Mosby's Nursing Drug Reference	6.64	$30	
B. Nonprescription Products: Formulations and Features	6.7		
Nurses Drug Facts	6.62	$70	
Patient Drug Facts	9.40	$60	3
PDR Generics	6.8	$80	1
The Pediatric Drug Handbook	6.27	$35	1
Physicians' Desk Reference	6.10	$80	1,2,3
POISINDEX	8.10		7,8
Poisoning & Drug Overdose	8.1	$37	1
Poisoning & Toxicology Handbook	8.2	$90	3
C. Remington's Pharmaceutical Sciences	6.52	$125	5,6,7,8
Side Effects of Drugs Annual (companion to Meyler's)	7.2	$227	3,5
USP DI v. 1: Drug Information for the Health Care Professional	6.5	$130	1,4,5,7,8,9,10
USP DI v. 2: Advice for the Patient	9.1	$69	1
USP DI v. 3: Approved Drug Products and Legal Requirements	4.43,4.33	$115	1
USP Dictionary of USAN	3.1	$150	
C. USP/NF	11.8	$520	4,5,7,10
D. **Total estimated cost**		**$5,804**	

Notes on the Core Collection:

A. Brandon and Hill cite only the annual, bound edition of *Drug Facts and Comparisons*, but a subscription to the monthly looseleaf service is a better investment for up-to-date prescribing and product selection information.

B. The purchase price of APhA's *Handbook of Nonprescription Drugs* now includes the companion volume *Nonprescription Products: Formulations and Features*.

C. *Remington's* and *USP/NF* are recommended additions to the core collection for pharmacy departments (could be omitted in minimum hospital library drug information collections).

D. The total excludes the subscription cost of *POISINDEX*, which is dependent on the format implemented and is substantial enough to warrant shared budgeting across departments.

Comparisons with Other Reference Collection Standards

There are no universally recognized standards for drug information collections to support patient care. However, a title's presence on other published lists, indicated by numbered references, can, perhaps, be regarded as reinforcement of these selections. For example, the Brandon-Hill list[1] cites nineteen of the sources recommended here, but would add *Conn's Current Therapy* (6.15), the *Physicians' Desk Reference for Nonprescription Drugs* (6.9), and Griffith's *Instructions for Patients* (9.41). The Library for Internists IX,[2] compiled from recommendations by practitioners and endorsed by the American College of Physicians, concurs with twelve of the titles selected. Additional suggestions found on the Library list, but omitted here, are *Conn's Current Therapy* and the *PDR for Nonprescription Drugs* (in common with Brandon-Hill), as well as the *Essential Guide to Prescription Drugs* (9.14) and *DRUGDEX* (6.14).

Applied Drug Information,[3] a recently published guide to the literature annotated in Chapter Five (5.7), identifies thirty core texts in its bibliography of 107 sources. Twenty overlap with titles suggested in this core list, as well. Eight of the remaining ten references in James and Millares' list are discussed elsewhere in this book, but have not been singled out in the Appendix.

In *Goodman and Gilman*, Nies[4] endorses a short bibliography of ready-reference sources: *USP DI*, AMA *Drug Evaluations* (now deceased), *Drug Facts and Comparisons*, and *USP/NF* (at the same time acknowledging that the PDR is most often used instead). In a chapter dedicated to "Clinical Drug Literature" in *Remington's Pharmaceutical Sciences*, Amerson[5] cites as examples fifteen of the fifty-one titles suggested in this Appendix.

Results of three surveys of drug information centers (DICs) in the United States provide strong evidence of concurrence on the utility of several sources. Beaird, Coley, and Crea's assessment[6] of the current status of DICs draws on responses from 130 centers in 1990, 107 of which were hospital based. Eight titles were reported as present in at least 90% of the more than 117 collections. Rosenberg[7] pools results from 127 centers located in thirty-nine states, surveyed in 1986, and cites fifteen publications also included here. The national audit conducted by Dombrowski and Visconti in 1983[8] tabulated information supplied by 98 DICs, 85% of which were located in hospitals. Thirteen core collection titles were in use in centers surveyed and all but one (*POISINDEX*) present in at least 85%. Eight sources appear in results of all three national surveys, showing common use by subject specialists.

All three surveys of DICs also show the prevalence of the *PDR*. However, *Mosby's GenRx* and *PDR Generics* are far more comprehensive than the *Physicians' Desk Reference,* and thus are strongly recommended as necessary complements for the *PDR* (see Chapter Six for further discussion). By the same token, the APhA's *Handbook of Nonprescription Drugs* offers significant advantages when compared to the *PDR for Nonprescription Drugs.*

The Omnibus Budget Reconciliation Act (OBRA) of 1990[9] uses three sources as a basis for defining a medically accepted indication when establishing coverage for reimbursement purposes in state Medicaid prescription drug benefits programs: AMA's *Drug Evaluations Annual, USP DI Volume 1,* and *AHFS Drug Information.* The National Association of Boards of Pharmacy (NABP) minimum standard for "technical equipment and stock" in pharmacies[10] cites *USP/NF, USP DI,* and *AHFS.*

What about titles that lack the reinforcement of any of these precedents? Three selections address the critical area of medication use in pregnancy and lactation and possible teratogenic effects. Although other sources of pharmacotherapeutics and adverse reaction information will assist in answering questions related to these topics, the contributions of Shepard (8.23), Shardein (8.24), and Bennett (7.20) to the professional reference collection should not be underestimated. They are suggested here as valuable enhancements to libraries supporting patient care. *Effects of Drugs on Clinical Laboratory Tests* will augment the comparatively selective coverage of drug-lab test modifications offered in other sources.

For patient education beyond *USP DI Volume 2,* the *Medication Teaching Manual* from the American Society of Health-System Pharmacists and Patient *Drug Facts* are recommended here, instead of other consumer oriented publications cited in the Brandon-Hill and Library for Internists lists. Another extra title has been included in this core collection to expand coverage of pharmacokinetics, and two sources specifically address nursing considerations.

The *USP Dictionary of USAN* can scarcely require justification, considering the significance of U.S. Adopted Names in the indexing of other sources. Remember that this volume includes not only a cumulative list of USANs assigned since 1961, but also identifies International Nonproprietary Names established by the World Health Organization from the beginning of the INN program in 1953 to the present. Either or both types of nomenclature have been adopted as standards for nonproprietary drug identification by all reputable reference source publishers. Having this official publication on hand is essential for effective information service.

A Core Drug Information Collection for Public Libraries

A core drug information collection for public libraries must anticipate use by allied health personnel, legal researchers, and other professionals, as well as the lay public. The following bibliography has been selected to accommodate both groups. Hospital and medical libraries with an objective of expanding service to patients may also wish to review this list, along with additional selections annotated in Chapter Nine.

Professional Ready-Reference Bibliography

Notes	Title	Ref #	Price
	American Drug Index	3.6	$55
	Conn's Current Therapy	6.15	$59
	Drug Facts and Comparisons (annual hardbound edition)	6.2	$450
A.	Handbook of Nonprescription Drugs	6.6	$150
	Herbs of Choice	12.9	$30
	Medication Teaching Manual: The Guide to Patient Drug Information	9.39	$81
B.	Mosby's GenRx	6.3	$73
	Nonprescription Products: Formulations and Features	6.7	
	Patient Drug Facts	9.40	$60
	PDR for Herbal Medicines	12.11	$60
	Physicians' Desk Reference	6.10	$80
	USP DI Volume 1: Drug Information for the Health Care Professional	6.5	$130
	USP DI Volume 3: Approved Drug Products and Legal Requirements	4.43	$115
	Total estimated cost of professional bibliography		**$1,343**

Core Collection for Consumers

Notes	Title	Ref #	Price
C.	The American Druggist's Complete Family Guide to Prescriptions, Pills, and Drugs	9.7	$75
C.	AARP Pharmacy Service Prescription Drug Handbook	9.6	$30
C.	The AMA Guide to Prescription and Over-the-Counter Drugs	9.5	$25
	The American Pharmaceutical Association's Guide to Prescription Drugs	9.8	$7
	The American Pharmaceutical Association's Practical Guide to Natural Medicines	9.20	$25
	Complete Guide to Prescription and Nonprescription Drugs	9.13	$17
	Consumer Health Information Source Book	9.21	$60
	The Essential Guide to Prescription Drugs	9.14	$35
	The Essential Guide to Psychiatric Drugs	9.16	$17
	or		
	The Handbook of Psychiatric Drugs	9.18	$15
	The Honest Herbal	9.19	$20
	Parent's Guide to Childhood Medications	9.9	$14
	Taking Your Medications Safely	9.12	$20
D.	USP DI Volume 2: Advice for the Patient	9.1	$69
	What Do I Take? A Consumer's Guide to Nonprescription Drugs	9.10	$13
	Zimmerman's Complete Guide to Nonprescription Drugs	9.15	$60
	Total estimated cost of core collection for consumers		**$502**
	Combined total estimated cost of both collections		**$1,845**

Notes:

A. This title, along with the *Medication Teaching Manual* and *Patient Drug Facts*, would also be appropriate in a core collection for consumers. Its purchase price includes the companion volume *Nonprescription Products: Formulations and Features.*

B. *PDR Generics* (6.8) would be an acceptable alternative to *Mosby's GenRx* in a public library collection.

C. These three titles are currently out of print, but are of such high quality to justify retention. In other words, if your collection already includes these sources, don't discard them yet.

D. This edition is preferable to the bookstore version published by Consumer Reports (*The Complete Drug Reference*, 9.3) or the *USP Guide to Medicines* (9.4), both because it is more comprehensive in scope and because annual subscriptions include monthly updates.

Precedents

In the *Consumer Health Information Source Book* (9.21), Rees concurs with three titles (9.12, 9.14, and 9.16) singled out in the consumer collection here, but would add several other sources annotated in Chapter Nine. These include the *Handbook of Over-the-Counter Drugs and Pharmacy Products* (9.23), the *PDR Family Guide* series (9.24–9.26), *Worst Pills Best Pills* (9.28), *The Pill Book* (9.30), and *A Consumer's Guide to Medicines in Food* (9.34). In addition, the *Sourcebook* provides annotations for at least ten drug-related titles not selected for inclusion in this *Guide*. It is also interesting to find the *Physicians' Desk Reference for Non-Prescription Drugs* among Rees's listings for consumers, as well as the CDC's *Health Information for International Travel* (6.45) and the *Nutrition Drug Reference* (7.28).

References

1. Brandon AN, Hill DR. Selected list of books and journals for the small medical library. *Bull Med Libr Assoc* 1997 Apr;85(2):111–135.

2. Frisse ME, Florance V. A library for internists IX: Recommendations from the American College of Physicians. *Ann Intern Med* 1997 May 15;126:836–846.

3. James K, Millares M. Drug and medical information reference sources. Appendix 1 in: *Applied Drug Information.* Vancouver, WA: Applied Therapeutics, 1998: A1.1-A1.31.

4. Neis AS, Spielberg SP. Principles of therapeutics. In: Hardman JG, Gilman AG, Limbird LE, eds. *Goodman and Gilman's the pharmacological basis of therapeutics.* 9th ed. New York: McGraw-Hill, 1995: 77.

5. Amerson AB. Clinical drug literature. In: Gennaro AR, ed. *Remington's pharmaceutical sciences.* 19th ed. Easton, PA: Mack Publishing, 1995: 1838.

6. Beaird SL, Coley RMR, Crea KA. Current status of drug information centers. *Am J Hosp Pharm* 1992 Jun;49:103–106.

7. Rosenberg JM, Martino FP, Kirschenbaum HL, Robbins J. Pharmacist-operated drug information centers in the United States—1986. *Am J Hosp Pharm* 1987;44:337–344.

8. Dombrowski SR, Visconti JA. National audit of drug information centers. *Am J Hosp Pharm* 1985 Apr;42:819–826.

9. Omnibus Budget Reconciliation Act of 1990 (OBRA).

10. *Model state pharmacy Act and model rules of the National Association of Boards of Pharmacy* (4.29).

Baseline Historical Collection

Medical libraries have an understandable tendency to weed older editions of reference books when newer replacements are issued. However, where space permits in larger academic collections, it is helpful to retain (or acquire) older editions of many drug compendia. Questions often arise where accepted prescribing practices, known side effects, or products available (and their manufacturers) in previous years need to be investigated. Older editions of the following titles will help answer such inquiries.

American Drug Index, 1956– (3.6)

AMA Drug Evaluations Annual—formerly *AMA Drug Evaluations*, 1971–1995

Drug Facts and Comparisons, 1984– annual bound editions (6.3)

Martindale: The Extra Pharmacopoeia, 1883– (6.1)

Meyler's Side Effects of Drugs, 1957– (7.1)

Physicians' Desk Reference, 1947– (6.11)

Physicians' Generix, 1990–1992 (former title of *Physicians' GenRx*)

Physicians' GenRx, 1993–1997 (former title of *Mosby's GenRx*)

Mosby's GenRx, 1998– (6.3)

In addition to older editions of the titles listed above, don't turn down as gifts—or place in the circulating collection—the following resources. All of these publications qualify as reference classics still frequently cited today or are simply useful, in and of themselves. For example, the first twenty editions (1833–1960) of the *Dispensatory of the United States of America* offered encyclopedic coverage of botanicals, supported by background bibliography. Cases reported in Kingsbury's *Poisonous Plants of the United States and Canada* represent a baseline of human toxicity data that, in many cases, cannot be replicated.

Adverse Reactions to Drug Formulation Agents, 1989 (7.18)

The AMA Handbook of Poisonous and Injurious Plants, 1985 (8.49)

Birth Defects and Drugs in Pregnancy, 1977 (8.29)

Clinical Toxicology of Commercial Products: Acute Poisoning, 1984 (8.8)

Diet and Drug Interactions, 1989 (7.24)

Dispensatory of the United States of America, 1833–1960

Dispensing of Medication, 1984 (Additional Sources, Chapter Six)
Drug Effects in Hospitalized Patients, 1976 (7.7)
Drug-Nutrient Interactions, 1988 (7.25)
Drugs of Choice, 1958–
Handbook of Industrial Toxicology, 1987 (8.6)
Handbook of Poisoning: Prevention, Diagnosis and Treatment, 1987 (8.4)
Isolation and Identification of Drugs, 1969–1975 (8.18)
Kingsbury's Poisonous Plants of the United States and Canada, 1964 (8.48)
Modell's Drugs in Current Use and New Drugs, 1955–
Modern Drug Encyclopedia & Therapeutic Index, 1934–
Plant Contact Dermatitis, 1985 (8.50)
Poisoning: Toxicology, Symptoms, Treatments, 1986 (8.5)

B

Database Selection Aids and Additional Online Resource Annotations

Online Sources

Database selection aids included here are quick-reference guides to online sources in fifteen broad topical areas. Major resources for answering questions in each category are indicated with an asterisk (*). A total of 149 databases are cited, 86 of which are discussed in Chapters Fourteen through Sixteen. The subsequent directory of databases provides brief descriptions of 63 complementary files. A chart summarizing database availability follows the selection aids and directory.

Identification and Nomenclature

Adis R&D Insight (15.3)*
AIDSDRUGS
Beilstein Online
CAS Registry File (14.43)*
Chapman and Hall Chemical Database
Chem Sources Chemical Directory (15.27)
Chem Sources Company Directory (15.28)
Chemical Registry Nomenclature (14.44)*
Chemicals and Companies (15.31)
CHEMLINE (14.46)
CHEMSEARCH (14.45)*
CHEMTOX Online (14.30)
Derwent Drug Registry
Directory of Chemical Producers—
    Products (15.29)
Drug Data Report (15.5)

Health Devices Sourcebook (15.25)
IDdb (15.7)*
Imsmarq Pharmaceutical Trademarks In-Use
IMSworld R&D Focus Drug Updates
    (15.2)*
Kirk-Othmer
Markush Pharmsearch*
Martindale Online*
Medical Device Register (15.24)
Merck Index Online*
MSDS-CCOHS (14.32)
MSDS-OHS (14.31)
Natural Products Alert (14.42)
NDA Pipeline (15.8)
NME Express (15.4)
Pharmaprojects (15.1)*

Drug Information Fulltext (14.18)*
Drugs of the Future (15.6)
EMBASE (14.4)
Hazardous Substances Data Bank (14.29)

RTECS (14.28)
Unlisted Drugs
USAN*
USP DI Volume I (14.19)

Physical and Chemical Properties Information

Analytical Abstracts (14.39)
Beilstein Online*
CA File/CA Search (14.37–14.38)*
CASREACT
Chapman and Hall Chemical Database*
Chemical Engineering & Biotechnology
  Abstracts
CHEMTOX Online (14.30)*
Drug Information Fulltext (14.18)*
Hazardous Substances Data Bank (14.29)*

Kirk-Othmer*
KOSMET
Martindale Online*
Merck Index Online*
MSDS-CCOHS (14.32)
MSDS-OHS (14.31)
Natural Products Alert (14.42)
RTECS (14.28)
USP DI Volume I (14.19)*

Pharmaceutics and Pharmaceutical Technology

Analytical Abstracts (14.39)*
Beilstein Online
BIOSIS Previews (14.6)
CA File/CA Search (14.37–14.38)*
CASREACT*
Chemical Engineering and Biotechnology
  Abstracts
Current Contents Search
Derwent Drug File (14.10)*
EMBASE (14.4)*

IDIS Drug File (14.13)
International Pharmaceutical Abstracts
  (14.8)*
ISI Reaction Center (14.41)
Kirk-Othmer
KOSMET*
MEDLINE (14.1)
SciSearch (14.7)*
TOXLINE (14.27)

Coverage of Preclinical Studies

ADIS LMS Drug Alerts Online (14.12)
ADIS R&D Insight (15.3)*
AIDSLINE (14.14)
Allied and Alternative Medicine (14.15)
Analytical Abstracts (14.39)
BIOSIS Previews (14.6)*
CA File/CA Search (14.37–14.38)*
CANCERLIT (14.17)*
Conference Papers Index
Current Biotechnology Abstracts
Current Contents Search*
Derwent Drug File (14.10)*

IAC Newsletter Database (15.15)
IDdb (15.7)*
IDIS Drug File (14.13)
Immunoclones Database
IMSworld R&D Focus Drug Updates (15.2)*
InPharma (14.11)
Inside Conferences
International Pharmaceutical Abstracts
  (14.8)*
ISI Reaction Center (14.41)
KOSMET
Life Sciences Collection

Derwent Biotechnology Abstracts
Derwent Veterinary Drug File
Drug Data Report (15.5)*
Drug News & Perspectives (15.13)
Drugs of the Future (15.6)*
EMBASE (14.4)*
Federal Research in Progress

MEDLINE (14.1)*
MethodsFinder (14.40)
NME Express (15.4)
Pascal
Pharmaprojects (15.1)*
SciSearch (14.7)*
TOXLINE (14.27)*

Clinical Information

ADIS LMS Drug Alerts Online (14.12)*
ADIS R&D Insight (15.3)*
ADIS Reactions Database (14.26)*
AIDSDRUGS
AIDSLINE (14.14)*
AIDSTRIALS*
Alcohol and Alcohol Problems Science
    Database
Allied and Alternative Medicine (14.15)
AMA Journals Online
BIOSIS Previews (14.6)*
CAB Abstracts
CAB Health (14.16)
CANCERLIT (14.17)*
The Cochrane Library (14.24)*
Conference Papers Index
Current Biotechnology Abstracts
Current Contents Search*
Derwent Biotechnology Abstracts*
Derwent Drug File (14.10)*
Derwent Veterinary Drug File
Directory of Published Proceedings
Drug Data Report (15.5)*
Drug Information Fulltext (14.18)*
Drug News & Perspectives (15.13)*
Drugs of the Future (15.6)*
EMBASE (14.4)*
Evidence-Based Medicine Reviews
    (14.23)*
ExtraMED
F-D-C Reports (15.10)*
Federal Research in Progress
Health Devices Alerts (16.2)
Health News Daily (15.11)
IAC Health & Wellness Database (14.33)
IAC Newsletter Database (15.15)

IDdb (15.7)*
IDIS Drug File (14.13)*
IMSworld R&D Focus Drug News
    (15.12)*
IMSworld R&D Focus Drug Updates
    (15.2)*
Incidence and Prevalence Database
    (15.39)
InPharma (14.11)*
Inside Conferences
International Pharmaceutical Abstracts
    (14.8)*
Journal Watch
KOSMET
Lexi-Comp's Clinical Reference
    Collection (14.20)*
Life Sciences Collection
MANTIS
Martindale Online
MEDLINE (14.1)*
MetaMaps (14.25)
New England Journal of Medicine
NTIS
Online Journal of Current Clinical Trials
Pascal
Pharm-Line (14.21)
Pharmaceutical and Healthcare Industry
    News (15.9)*
PharmacoEconomics & Outcomes News
    (15.14)*
Pharmaprojects (15.1)*
Physician Data Query Protocol File
    (14.22)*
SciSearch (14.7)*
TOXLINE (14.27)
USP DI Volume I (14.19)*

Adverse Effects and Toxicity Resources Online

ADIS LMS Drug Alerts Online (14.12)
ADIS R&D Insight (15.3)
ADIS Reactions Database (14.26)*
AIDSLINE (14.14)
Alcohol and Alcohol Problems Science
    Database
Allied and Alternative Medicine (14.15)
AMA Journals Online
BIOSIS Previews (14.6)*
CA File/CA Search (14.37–14.38)*
CAB Abstracts
CAB Health (14.16)
CANCERLIT (14.17)*
Chapman and Hall Chemical Database
Chemical Safety NewsBase
CHEMTOX Online (14.30)*
Current Contents Search
Derwent Drug File (14.10)*
Derwent Veterinary Drug File
Drug Information Fulltext (14.18)*
Drugs of the Future (15.6)
EMBASE (14.4)*
Hazardous Substances Data Bank (14.29)*
Health Devices Alerts (16.2)*
HSELINE

IAC Health & Wellness Database (14.33)
IDdb (15.7)
IDIS Drug File (14.7)*
InPharma (14.11)
International Pharmaceutical Abstracts
    (14.8)*
KOSMET
Life Sciences Collection
MANTIS
Martindale Online*
MEDLINE (14.1)*
Merck Index Online
MSDS-CCOHS (14.32)*
MSDS-OHS (14.31)*
Natural Products Alert (14.42)
New England Journal of Medicine
NIOSHTIC*
Pascal
Pharm-Line (14.21)
RTECS (14.28)*
SciSearch (14.7)*
SEDBASE*
TOXLINE (14.27)*
USP DI Volume I (14.19)*

Coverage of Healthcare Biotechnology Research

ADIS R&D Insight (15.3)*
Biological & Agricultural Index
BIOSIS Previews (14.6)*
CAB Abstracts
Chemical Engineering and Biotechnology
    Abstracts*
Conference Papers Index
Current Biotechnology Abstracts*
Current Contents Search*
Derwent Biotechnology Abstracts*
Derwent Drug File (14.10)*
Directory of Published Proceedings
Drug Data Report (15.5)*
Drug News and Perspectives (15.13)
Drugs of the Future (15.6)
EMBASE (14.4)*
F-D-C Reports (15.10)*

IDdb (15.7)
Immunoclones Database*
IMSworld R&D Focus Drug News
    (15.12)*
IMSworld R&D Focus Drug Updates
    (15.2)*
InPharma (14.11)
Inside Conferences
International Pharmaceutical Abstracts
    (14.8)
Life Sciences Collection
McGraw-Hill Publications Online
MEDLINE (14.1)*
NME Express (15.4)
Pascal
Pharmaceutical and Healthcare Industry
    News (15.9)*

Health News Daily (15.11)
IAC Newsletter Database (15.15)*
IAC PROMT (15.35)*
IAC Trade & Industry Database (15.36)

Pharmaceutical News Index (15.17)
Pharmaprojects (15.1)*
SciSearch (14.7)*

Medical Device Information Sources

BioBusiness
BIOSIS Previews (14.6)*
Current Contents Search*
Diogenes (16.1)*
EI Compendex
EMBASE (14.4)*
F-D-C Reports (15.10)*
Health Devices Alerts (16.2)*
Health Devices Sourcebook (15.25)*
IAC Newsletter Database (15.15)

IAC PROMT (15.35)
IAC Trade & Industry Database (15.35)
INSPEC
International Pharmaceutical Abstracts
  (14.8)
Medical Device Register (15.24)*
MEDLINE (14.1)*
Pharmaceutical and Healthcare Industry
  News (15.9)*
SciSearch (14.7)*

Cosmetics and Toiletries Information

BIOSIS Previews (14.6)
CA File/CA Search (14.37–14.38)*
Current Contents Search
EMBASE (14.4)
F-D-C Reports (15.10)*
IAC Newsletter Database (15.15)*

IAC PROMT (15.35)
IAC Trade & Industry Database (15.36)
International Pharmaceutical Abstracts
  (14.8)*
KOSMET*
SciSearch (14.7)

Coverage of Veterinary Drugs

AGRICOLA*
AGRIS
BioBusiness
Biological & Agricultural Index
BIOSIS Previews (14.6)*
CAB Abstracts*
Current Contents Search
Derwent Veterinary Drug File*

Life Sciences Collection
Martindale Online
MEDLINE (14.1)
Merck Index Online
Pharmaceutical and Healthcare Industry
  News (15.9)*
SciSearch (14.7)

Pharmacy Practice Topics

ABI/Inform
BIOETHICSLINE
EMBASE (14.4)
HealthSTAR*
HSELINE

MEDLINE (14.1)
Pharm-Line (14.21)
Pharmaceutical News Index (15.17)
PharmacoEconomics & Outcomes News
  (15.14)

IAC PROMT (15.35)
IAC Trade & Industry Database (15.36)
International Pharmaceutical Abstracts
 (14.8)*

Social SciSearch
TOXLINE (14.27)

Pharmacognosy Topics

AGRICOLA
AGRIS
Allied and Alternative Medicine (14.15)*
Biological & Agricultural Index
BIOSIS Previews (14.6)*
CA File/CA Search (14.37–14.38)*
CAB Abstracts*
CAB Health (14.16)
Conference Papers Index
Current Contents Search*
Directory of Published Proceedings
EMBASE (14.4)*
ExtraMED

IAC Health & Wellness Database
 (14.33)
International Pharmaceutical Abstracts
 (14.8)*
Life Sciences Collection
MANTIS*
Martindale Online
MEDLINE (14.1)*
Natural Products Alert (14.42)*
Pascal
SciSearch (14.7)*
TOXLINE (14.27)
Unlisted Drugs

Marketing and Business Information

ABI/Inform*
ADIS R&D Insight (15.3)*
Aerzte Zeitung Online
Asian Business Intelligence Reports
BCC Market Research*
BioBusiness
BioCommerce Abstracts and Directory
Business & Industry (15.37)*
Business & Management Practices*
Business Dateline*
Chem Sources Chemical Directory (15.27)
Chem Sources Company Directory (15.28)
Chemical Business Newsbase
Chemical Industry Notes
Chemicals and Companies (15.31)
Datamonitor Market Research*
Decision Resources Pharmaceutical
 Industry Reports*
Diogenes (16.1)
Directory of Chemical Producers
 (15.29–15.30)
DIRLINE
Drug Data Report (15.5)*

IAC Newsletter Database (15.15)*
IAC PROMT (15.35)*
IAC Trade & Industry Database (15.36)
IMS World Drug Markets (15.32)*
Imsmarq Pharmaceutical Trademarks In-
 Use
IMSworld Company Directory (15.22)*
IMSworld New Product Launches (15.18)*
IMSworld Patents International (16.4)
IMSworld Pharmaceutical Company
 Profiles (15.20)*
IMSworld Product Monographs (15.19)*
IMSworld R&D Focus Drug News
 (15.12)*
IMSworld R&D Focus Drug Updates
 (15.2)*
IMSworld R&D Meetings Diary
Incidence and Prevalence Database
 (15.39)*
International Pharmaceutical Abstracts
 (14.8)
Investext (15.38)*
KOSMET

Drug News & Perspectives (15.13)*
Drugs of the Future (15.6)*
ESPICOM Country Healthcare Database (15.33)*
ESPICOM Pharma & Med Company Profiles (15.21)*
ESPICOM Pharmaceutical & Medical News (15.16)*
Euromonitor Market Research*
European Chemical News
EventLine
F-D-C Reports*
FIND/SVP Market Research*
Freedonia Market Research*
Frost & Sullivan Market Intelligence*
General Practitioner
Health Devices Sourcebook (15.25)
Health News Daily (15.11)
Health Organizations Database (15.26)
HealthSTAR

Marketletter*
MarketLine International*
McGraw-Hill Publications Online
Medical Device Register (15.24)
MediConf (Fairbase)
NDA Pipeline (15.8)*
NME Express (15.4)*
PharmaBiomed
Pharmaceutical and Healthcare Industry News (15.9)*
Pharmaceutical News Index (15.17)
PharmacoEconomics and Outcomes News (15.14)*
Pharmacontacts (15.23)
Pharmaprojects (15.1)*
Research Centers and Services Directory
Snapshots International Markets Research
Social SciSearch
TableBase (15.34)*

Legal or Regulatory Information

ADIS R&D Insight (15.3)*
BIOETHICSLINE
BNA Daily News from Washington*
Chemical Business Newsbase
Chemical Industry Notes
CHEMTOX Online (14.30)*
CLAIMS/RRX*
CLAIMS/U.S. Patents Abstracts*
Derwent Biotechnology Abstracts
Diogenes (16.1)*
Drug Data Report (15.5)*
F-D-C Reports (15.10)*
FOODLINE: Current Food Legislation (16.3)*
Hazardous Substances Data Bank (14.29)*
Health Devices Alerts (16.2)
Health News Daily (15.11)
HealthSTAR
IAC Newsletter Database (15.15)
IAC PROMT (15.35)
IAC Trade & Industry Database (15.36)
IMS World Drug Markets (15.32)
Imsmarq Pharmaceutical Trademarks In-Use

IMSworld Patents International (16.4)*
IMSworld R&D Focus Drug News (15.12)
IMSworld R&D Focus Drug Updates (15.2)*
INPADOC*
International Pharmaceutical Abstracts (14.8)
Investext (14.38)
Investigational Drug Patents Fast-Alert (16.6)
LEGSTAT*
Markush Pharmsearch
MSDS-CCOHS (14.32)*
MSDS-OHS (14.31)*
NDA Pipeline (15.8)*
NTIS
Pharmaceutical and Healthcare Industry News (15.9)*
Pharmaceutical News Index (15.17)
Pharmaprojects (15.1)*
Pharmsearch (16.5)
RTECS (14.28)*
World Patents Index*

Directory of Databases

ABI/Inform   Abstracted Business Information (ABI) compiled by UMI, with an emphasis on management. Healthcare and pharmacoeconomics are among topics covered in this bibliographic database, which includes citations, with abstracts, to 1,400 journals published from 1971 to date. The complete text of selected articles from 550 sources has also been included since 1991. Available on DataStar, Dialog, QUESTEL-ORBIT, Ovid, SilverPlatter, and STN, updated daily.

ADIS Drug News   Dialog database containing *InPharma, ADIS Reactions Database,* and *PharmacoEconomics & Outcomes News.*

ADIS LMS Drug Alerts Online   see 14.12.

ADIS R&D Insight   see 15.3.

ADIS Reactions Database   see 14.26.

Aerzte Zeitung Online   see Figure 15.8.

AGRICOLA   The USDA National Agricultural Library produces *AGRICOLA (Agric*ultural *OnL*ine *Access*), a bibliographic database containing citations to journal articles, books, theses, patents, audiovisuals, and technical reports. Subject coverage includes veterinary science, botany, and human and animal nutrition. References are drawn from more than 2,000 serial titles dating from 1970. Available on Dialog, Ovid, SilverPlatter, and STN, updated monthly.

AGRIS International   A bibliographic database covering worldwide agricultural literature, *AGRIS* corresponds, in part, to *AgrIndex,* a monthly publication from the United Nations Food and Agriculture Organization (FAO). Animal science and human nutrition are included in its scope. Available on Dialog and SilverPlatter, 1975 to date, updated monthly.

AIDSDRUGS   A directory prepared by the U.S. Centers for Disease Control of more than eighty drugs being tested for use against HIV and AIDS. Entries include generic and brand names, synonyms, CAS registry number, manufacturer, and information on physical and chemical properties, adverse reactions, contraindications, and pharmacology. References to clinical trials where these drugs are used can be found in *AIDSTRIALS.* Available on MEDLARS, updated monthly.

AIDSLINE   see 14.14.

AIDSTRIALS   A directory prepared by the U.S. Centers for Disease Control of more than 230 open, closed, and completed clinical trials of AIDS drugs. Entries list title and purpose of each trial, drug name, diseases under study, patient inclusion and exclusion criteria, trial sites, trial status, and telephone numbers for contacting the trial site or sponsor. Available on MEDLARS, updated biweekly.

Alcohol and Alcohol Problems Science Database   Produced by the U.S. National Institute on Alcohol Abuse and Alcoholism, this bibliographic database compiles citations, with abstracts, to the worldwide literature on alcoholism research. Sources include conference proceedings, reports, dissertations, and journals. Available 1972 to date on Ovid, updated monthly.

Allied and Alternative Medicine   see 14.15.

AMA Journals Online   Contains the complete text (minus illustrations) of ten medical journals published by the American Medical Association: *AJDC-American Journal of Diseases of Children, Archives of Dermatology, Archives of General Practice, Archives* *of Internal Medicine, Archives of Neurology, Archives of Ophthalmology, Archives of Otorhinolaryngology-Head and Neck Surgery, Archives of Pathology and Laboratory Medicine, Archives of Surgery,* and *JAMA,* 1982 to date. Available on Dialog, updated weekly.

AMED   see 14.15

Analytical Abstracts   see 14.39.

Asian Business Intelligence Reports   see Figure 15.9.

BCC Market Research   see Figure 15.9.

Beilstein Online   Contains data on carbon compounds from the *Beilstein Handbook of Organic Chemistry,* as well as citations to the primary literature. Each record provides available information on the structure, physical and chemical properties, natural occurrence and isolation, preparation and manufacture, and analytical methods for an organic compound, based on evaluative review of the literature published since 1830. Covers 3.4 million heterocyclic, isocyclic, and acyclic compounds. Available on Dialog and STN.

BioBusiness   see Figure 15.8.

BioCommerce Abstracts and Directory   see Figure 15.8.

BIOETHICSLINE   A bibliographic database from Georgetown University's Kennedy Institute of Ethics, with citations and abstracts for literature related to patients' rights, allocation of healthcare resources, human and animal experimentation, euthanasia, abortion, contraception, genetic intervention, reproductive technologies, organ transplantation, the practitioner-patient relationship, and comparable ethical issues. Available on DataStar, MEDLARS, Ovid, QUESTEL-ORBIT, and SilverPlatter, 1973 to date, updated bimonthly.

Biological & Agricultural Index   One of several bibliographic databases produced by H.W. Wilson, publishers of *The Reader's Guide to Periodical Literature. Biological & Agricultural Index* is broad in scope and easy to use, with its preference for familiar terms, rather than technical jargon. Biochemistry, botany, genetics, microbiology, neuroscience, nutrition, physiology, and veterinary medicine are among the many subject areas covered. Available on Dialog, Ovid, and SilverPlatter, 1983 to date, updated monthly; also on CD-ROM.

Biological Abstracts   see 14.6.

BIOSIS Previews   see 14.6.

BNA Daily News from Washington   see Figure 15.8.

Business & Industry   see 15.37.

Business & Management Practices   A database from Responsive Database Services that focuses on indexing literature dealing with practical processes, methods, and strategies for running a business, deriving data from more than 300 source publications. Available on Dialog and SilverPlatter, 1995 to date, updated weekly.

Business Dateline   see Figure 15.8.

CA File   see 14.38.

CA Search   see 14.37.

CAB Abstracts   A bibliographic database with extensive coverage of agricultural sciences and related fields, including veterinary medicine, as well as human nutrition. Archives online extend back to 1972, but coverage varies among vendors. Available on DataStar, Dialog, Ovid, SilverPlatter, and STN, updated monthly; also on CD-ROM.

CAB Health   see 14.16.

CANCERLIT   see 14.17.

CAS Registry File   see 14.43.

CASREACT   A bibliographic database compiled by Chemical Abstracts Service from the worldwide literature on chemical reactions. Entries include a reaction diagram; CAS RNs for all reactants, products, reagents, solvents, and catalysts; textual reaction notes; primary source citation; substance and subject indexing; and abstracts. Available on STN, 1985 to date, updated weekly.

CCOHS-MSDS   see 14.32.

Chapman and Hall Chemical Database   Contains the complete text of the *Dictionary of Organic Compounds; Dictionary of Antibiotics and Related Compounds; Carbohydrates, Amino Acids and Peptides;* and other sourcebooks from Chapman & Hall publishers. Entries provide identification information, physical and chemical properties data, and summarize uses and hazards. Graphic structures also accompany records. Former title: Heilbron. Available on Dialog, updated semiannually.

Chem Sources Chemical Directory   see 15.27.

Chem Sources Company Directory   see 15.28.

Chemical Abstracts   see 14.37.

Chemical Business NewsBase   see Figure 15.8.

Chemical Engineering and Biotechnology Abstracts   A bibliographic database prepared by the Royal Society of Chemistry covering literature on plant and process chemical engineering, plant and pilot-scale processing, laboratory research, safety and environmental matters, and commercial and technical information for the biotechnology industry. Current literature only, available on DataStar, Dialog, QUESTEL-ORBIT, and STN, updated monthly.

Chemical Industry Notes (CIN)   see Figure 15.8.

Chemical Registry Nomenclature   see 14.44.

Chemical Safety NewsBase   A bibliographic database provided by the Royal Society of Chemistry with a focus on occupational hazards in the chemical industry, biomedical and other types of laboratories, and hazards in the office environment. Citations, with abstracts, are drawn from 250 journal titles, as well as books and technical reports. Available on DataStar, Dialog, QUESTEL-ORBIT, and STN, 1981 to date, updated monthly.

Chemicals and Companies   see 15.31.

CHEMLINE   see 14.46.

CHEMSEARCH   see 14.45.

CHEMTOX Online   see 14.30.

CHIROLARS   see *MANTIS.*

CIN   see Figure 15.8.

CLAIMS/Reassignment & Reexamination (CLAIMS/RRX)   Compiles citations to patents for which ownership has been transferred (reassigned, 1980 to date) or for which the patentability has been reviewed and either rejected, reaffirmed, or extended by the U.S. Patent and Trademark Office. An IFI/Plenum Data Corporation database, available on Dialog, QUESTEL-ORBIT, and STN, updated weekly.

CLAIMS/U.S. Patents Abstracts   IFI/Plenum compilation of bibliographic data for granted U.S. patents, 1950 to date. Abstracts are included for chemical patents issued since 1950, as well as information on equivalent patents issued by Belgium, Germany, France, Great Britain, and the Netherlands. Abstracts also accompany records for electrical and mechanical patents issued since 1963, and design patents dating from 1976. Full-text claims and front-page information are provided in records from 1971 forward. Available on Dialog, QUESTEL-ORBIT, and STN, updated weekly.

Clinica   see 15.9.

CNAM   see 14.44.

The Cochrane Library   see 14.24.

COMPENDEX   see *EI COMPENDEX.*

Conference Papers Index   A bibliographic database provided by Cambridge Scientific Abstracts, with citations to individual conference papers presented 1973 to date. Entries include names and addresses of authors, conference title, location, and date, sponsors, and information required to order available proceedings. Available on Dialog and STN, updated bimonthly.

CSA Life Sciences Collection   see *Life Sciences Collection.*

CSCHEM   see 15.27.

CSCORP   see 15.28.

Current Biotechnology Abstracts   A bibliographic database from the Royal Society of Chemistry, with coverage of the literature from 1983 to date. Available on DataStar and Dialog, updated monthly.

Current Contents Search   A bibliographic database corresponding to seven hardcopy indexes from the Institute for Scientific Information. Coverage includes clinical medicine, life sciences, engineering, biology, and chemistry. Online access extends back to 1990, but varies from vendor to vendor. Available on DataStar, Dialog, and Ovid, updated weekly.

Current Drugs Fast-Alert   see 16.6.

Current Drugs IDdb   see 15.7.

Datamonitor Market Research   see Figure 15.9.

DCP   see *Directory of Chemical Producers.*

Decision Resources Pharmaceutical Industry Reports   see Figure 15.9.

Derwent Biotechnology Abstracts   A bibliographic database from Derwent, indexing journal and patent literature dealing with all aspects of biotechnology. Available on DataStar, Dialog, QUESTEL-ORBIT, SilverPlatter, and STN, 1982 to date, updated biweekly or monthly (check vendor documentation); also on CD-ROM.

Derwent Drug File   see 14.10.

Derwent Drug Registry   Also known as the *Standard Drug File,* this directory database includes records for the approximately 26,000 drugs indexed in the *Derwent Drug File* and the *Derwent Veterinary Drug File.* Entries include alternative nomenclature, CAS registry number, and information regarding activities and structure. Available on DataStar, Dialog, QUESTEL-ORBIT, and STN, updated semiannually.

Derwent Veterinary Drug File (VETDOC)   A bibliographic database, with abstracts, of the international journal literature on veterinary drugs, vaccines, growth promotants, toxicology, and hormonal control of breeding. Available on DataStar, QUESTEL-ORBIT, and STN, 1968 to date, updated monthly.

Derwent World Patents Index   see *World Patents Index.*

Dictionary of Organic Compounds   see *Chapman and Hall Chemical Database.*

DIF   see 14.18

Diogenes   see 16.1.

Directory of Chemical Producers—Products   see 15.29.

Directory of Chemical Producers—Companies   see 15.30.

Directory of Healthcare Purchasing Organizations   see 15.26.

Directory of Hospital Personnel   see 15.26.

Directory of Published Proceedings   Contains bibliographic and ordering information for published proceedings of more than 6,000 conferences, 1985 to date. Prepared by InterDok Corporation and available on DataStar, updated monthly.

DIRLINE   A directory database prepared by the U.S. National Library of Medicine, with information on more than 17,000 organizations that provide assistance in their areas of specialization. Available on MEDLARS, updated quarterly.

Drug Data Report   see 15.5.

Drug Information Fulltext   see 14.18.

Drug News & Perspectives   see 15.13.

Drugs of the Future   see 15.6.

EBM Reviews   see 14.23

EI COMPENDEX   An index to the engineering literature, including bioengineering and medical devices, prepared by Engineering Information, Inc. Citations, with abstracts, 1970 to date. Available on DataStar, Dialog, QUESTEL-ORBIT, Ovid, SilverPlatter, and STN, updated weekly. Also on CD-ROM.

EMBASE   see 14.4.

EMBASE Alert   A companion file to *EMBASE* (*Excerpta Medica* online), this bibliographic database is specifically designed for current awareness. Citations and abstracts, sans indexing, appear in *EMBASE Alert* within five days after Elsevier's receipt of primary sources. The same records, augmented with indexing, will appear later in *EMBASE*. Most recent eight weeks available on DataStar, Dialog, SilverPlatter, and STN, updated weekly.

ESPICOM Country Healthcare Database   see 15.33.

ESPICOM Pharmaceutical and Medical Company Profiles   see 15.21.

ESPICOM Pharmaceutical & Medical Device News   see 15.16.

Euromonitor Market Research   see Figure 15.9.

European Chemical News   see Figure 15.8.

EventLine   Lists forthcoming conferences, exhibits, trade fairs, and symposia scheduled worldwide through the year 2010. Emphasis is on events relevant to business, biomedicine, chemistry, and technology. Compiled by Elsevier Science Publishers and available on DataStar, Dialog, QUESTEL-ORBIT, and STN, updated monthly.

Evidence-Based Medicine Reviews   see 14.23

Excerpta Medica   see 14.4.

ExtraMED   The product of a World Health Organization initiative, *ExtraMED* was created to index journals published in countries with little or no *MEDLINE* coverage. WHO's selection includes 300 sources, only a few of which are scanned by other indexing services. Local journals in developing countries can provide unique information about communicable diseases once thought to have been eradicated, as well as AIDS, tropical biodiversity, and traditional medical practices. Available in Dialog, 1994 to date, updated 10 times per year.

Fairbase see *MediConf.*

F-D-C Reports see 15.10.

Federal Research in Progress (FEDRIP) A directory database prepared by the U.S. National Technical Information Service (NTIS), with descriptions of more than 138,000 projects in progress or recently completed under federal government sponsorship. Includes the CRISP subfile from NIH (also part of *TOXLINE,* see Figure 14.12), as well as NIOSH, Veterans Administration, EPA, and National Science Foundation projects. Available on Dialog, updated monthly.

FIND®/SVP Market Research see Figure 15.9.

FOLE see 16.3.

FOODLINE: Current Food Legislation see 16.3.

Freedonia Market Research see Figure 15.9.

Frost & Sullivan Market Intelligence see Figure 15.9.

General Practitioner A full-text file from Haymarket Medical publishers that includes three sources, including *MIMS Magazine,* a monthly newsletter covering pharmaceutical developments, prescription trends, therapeutics, detection and analysis of side effects, and reviews of drugs and other medical preparations. Available on DataStar, 1987 to date, updated monthly.

The Gray Sheet see 15.10.

Hazardous Substances Data Bank see 14.29.

Health & Wellness Database see 14.33.

Health Devices Alerts see 16.2.

Health Devices Sourcebook see 15.25.

Health News Daily see 15.11.

Health Periodicals Database see 14.33.

Health Planning & Administration see *HealthSTAR.*

Healthcare Organizations Database see 15.26.

HealthSTAR A bibliography co-produced by the U.S. National Library of Medicine and the American Hospital Association, with citations to the worldwide literature on healthcare delivery. Records are derived from *MEDLINE, CATLINE,* and the *Hospital and Health Administration Index* (formerly *Hospital Literature Index*). This file represents a 1996 merger of two databases: *Health Planning and Administration* and *HSTAR* (Health Services/Technology Assessment Research). Available on DataStar, Dialog, MEDLARS, Ovid, and SilverPlatter, 1975 to date, updated monthly; also on CD-ROM.

Heilbron see *Chapman and Hall Chemical Database.*

HMO/PPO Directory see 15.26.

HSDB see 14.29.

HSELINE A bibliographic database prepared by Great Britain Health and Safety Executive, with citations and abstracts for literature on occupational safety and health. Sources include journals, books, conference proceedings, technical reports, and legislation. Available on DataStar and QUESTEL-ORBIT, 1977 to date, updated monthly; also on CD-ROM.

HSTAR see *HealthSTAR.*

IAC Health & Wellness Database see 14.33.

IAC Newsletter Database see 15.15.

IAC PROMT see 15.35.

IAC Trade & Industry Database   see 15.36.

IDdb   see 15.7.

IDIS Drug File   see 14.13.

Immunoclones Database   A full-text, English-language directory originating from the Centre Européen de Recherches Documentaires sur les Immunoclones, that compiles immunological information on cells. Descriptions include cell types, immunogen, immunocyte donors, product, and reactivities. Sources include scientific literature, commercial catalogs of biotechnology firms, hybridoma collections from research laboratories, published patents and patent applications from the European Patent Office, and relevant articles from the *EMBASE, MEDLINE,* and *PASCAL* databases. Available on DataStar, 1986 to date, updated monthly.

IMS World Drug Markets   see 15.32.

Imsmarq Pharmaceutical Trademarks In-Use   A directory from Imsmarq AG, containing information on more than 300,000 pharmaceutical trademarks in use, whether registered or not, in more than fifty countries worldwide. Entries include the owner or distributor associated with each trademark, product launch date, recorded sales, and anatomical/therapeutic classification (EPhMRA). Current information only, available on DataStar, updated monthly.

IMSworld Company Directory   see 15.22.

IMSworld New Product Launches   see 15.18.

IMSworld Patents International   see 16.4.

IMSworld Pharmaceutical Company Profiles   see 15.20.

IMSworld Product Monographs   see 15.19.

IMSworld R&D Focus Drug News   see 15.12.

IMSworld R&D Focus Drug Updates   see 15.2.

IMSworld R&D Meetings Diary   A directory database from IMS Global Services, with information on forthcoming meetings worldwide of potential interest to the pharmaceutical industry. Available on DataStar, updated monthly.

Incidence and Prevalence Database   see 15.39.

INPADOC   Citations to more than twenty million patent documents issued by any of sixty-four countries and other patent-granting authorities, compiling patent family and legal status information (including extensions and Supplementary Protection Certificates) from 1968 to date, provided by the European Patent Office. Available on Dialog, QUESTEL-ORBIT, and STN, updated weekly.

InPharma   see 14.11.

Inside Conferences   A bibliographic database (*sans* abstracts) devoted to documenting papers presented at congresses, symposia, workshops, and other meetings for which proceedings are on file with the British Library Document Centre. Available on Dialog, 1993 to date, updated weekly.

INSPEC   A bibliographic database prepared by the Institution of Electrical Engineers (U.K.), with citations and abstracts for journal articles, conference papers, books, technical reports, and dissertations. Coverage includes information technology and topics relevant to bioengineering of medical devices. Available on DataStar, Dialog, QUESTEL-ORBIT, Ovid, SilverPlatter, and STN, 1969 to date, updated weekly; also on CD-ROM.

International Pharmaceutical Abstracts   see 14.8.

Investext   see 15.38.

Investigational Drug Patents Fast-Alert   see 16.6.

Investigational Drugs Database   see 15.7.

Iowa Drug Information Service   see 14.13.

IPA   see 14.8

ISI Reaction Center   14.41.

Journal Watch   Produced by the Massachusetts Medical Society (publishers of the *New England Journal of Medicine),* this bibliographic database is designed for current awareness. It contains citations, with abstracts, to clinical studies reported in twenty-five major medical journals. Available on Ovid, 1987 to date, updated twice weekly.

Kirk-Othmer Encyclopedia of Chemical Technology Online   Contains the complete text of the twenty volumes of the third edition of the *Encyclopedia,* published by John Wiley & Sons, as well as fourth edition volumes issued to date. Coverage includes drugs, cosmetics, and biomaterials, fermentation and enzyme technology. Available on DataStar and Dialog, 1978 to date, updated as new data become available; also on CD-ROM.

KOSMET   A bibliographic database prepared by the International Federation of the Societies of Cosmetic Chemists, covering literature on the manufacture of cosmetics, including raw materials, biological and chemical properties of active ingredients, formulations, quality control, safety, stability and packaging, clinical studies, and marketing. The emphasis is on indexing and abstracting scientific and technical research and studies. Available on DataStar and STN, 1968 to date, updated monthly.

LEGSTAT   A subfile of legal status information derived from *INPADOC,* available on QUESTEL-ORBIT (see also INPADOC).

Lexi-Comp's Clinical Reference Collection   see 14.20.

Life Sciences Collection   A bibliographic database compiled by Cambridge Scientific Abstracts, corresponding to nineteen abstracting journals from the same publisher, including: *Biotechnology Research Abstracts, Chemoreception Abstracts, Genetics Abstracts, Human Genome Abstracts, Immunology Abstracts, Toxicology Abstracts,* and *Biochemistry Abstracts.* Available on Dialog, SilverPlatter, and STN, 1978 to date, updated monthly.

LMS Drug Alerts Online   see 14.12.

MANTIS   A bibliographic database produced by Action Potential, *MANTIS* (Manual, Alternative and Natural Therapy) covers biomedical topics published in professional journals and the popular press, as well as conference proceedings. Known formerly as *CHIROLARS, MANTIS* was renamed in 1996 to reflect its expanded subject scope. This file focuses on several healthcare disciplines not significantly represented in major medical databases, such as *MEDLINE* and *EMBASE.* Particular emphasis is given to therapies for the relief of backache, muscle damage, nerve compression, and sports injuries (osteopathic, chiropractic, and physical therapy lierature). Other complementary or alternative medical treatments covered include acupuncture, herbal medicine, homeopathy, and traditional Chinese medicine. Citations, 70% with abstracts, are available on DataStar, Dialog, and Ovid, 1880 to date, updated monthly.

Marketletter   see Figure 15.8.

MarketLine International   Contains the full text of market research reports that provide more than 200 current analyses and forecasts for several market sectors, including cosmetics and toiletries. Available on DataStar, updated monthly.

Markush Pharmsearch Offers graphic representations of 65,000 generic (Markush) structures used in patents for new therapeutically active compounds with novel preparation processes or activities, and active ingredients of new drug compositions. Users can transfer graphic search results to *Pharmsearch* to facilitate retrieval of complete patent information. Coverage includes French, European, and U.S. patents since 1985, as well as patents from Great Britain and Germany dating from 1992. Available on QUESTEL-ORBIT, updated biweekly within four to eight weeks of patent publication date.

Martindale Online Corresponds to *Martindale: The Extra Pharmacopoeia* (6.1), enhanced with a hierarchical drug classification scheme and other precision indexing. Available on DataStar, updated annually; also on CD-ROM.

McGraw-Hill Publications Online Contains the complete text of thirteen business magazines and thirty-four newsletters published by McGraw-Hill, including *Biotechnology Newswatch* (1986 to date). Available on Dialog, updated weekly.

MDIS see ESPICOM.

MDX Health Digest see 14.34.

Medical Device Register see 15.24.

MediConf (Fairbase) A directory listing forthcoming medical and pharmaceutical conferences and exhibitions scheduled worldwide through the year 2000. Available on DataStar, Ovid, and STN, updated biweekly.

MEDLINE see 14.1.

Merck Index Online Corresponds to *The Merck Index* (3.5) in hardcopy, with additional monographs and revisions prepared since the latest printed edition. Available on Dialog, QUESTEL-ORBIT, and STN, updated semiannually.

MetaMaps see 14.25.

MethodsFinder see 14.40.

MSDS-CCOHS see 14.32.

MSDS-OHS see 14.31.

NAPRALERT see 14.42.

Natural Products Alert see 14.42.

NDA Pipeline see 15.8.

New England Journal of Medicine Full text, minus illustrations, of articles, letters to the editor, book reviews, and editorials from *NEJM,* 1983 to date. Available on Dialog and Ovid, updated weekly; also on CD-ROM.

New Product Launch Letter see New Product Launches.

New Product Launches see 15.18.

The Newsletter Database (IAC) see 15.15.

NIOSHTIC A bibliographic database maintained by the U.S. National Institute for Occupational Safety and Health, compiling citations, with abstracts, to journals, technical reports, and monographs dating from 1900. Available on Dialog and STN, updated quarterly; also on CD-ROM. Alternative title: *Occupational Safety and Health.*

NME Express see 15.4.

NTIS Compiled by the U.S. National Technical Information Service, NTIS is a bibliographic database with extensive coverage of worldwide government sponsored research. Citations, with abstracts, date from 1964 to the present, but the time period offered online varies from vendor to vendor. Available on DataStar, Dialog, Ovid, SilverPlatter, and STN, updated monthly.

Occupational Safety and Health   see *NIOSHTIC*.

OHS-MSDS   see 14.31.

Pascal   A bibliographic database, with abstracts, originating from the France Institut de l'Information Scientifique et Technique. Subject coverage encompasses both the biological sciences and medicine, and sources include books, theses, technical reports, conference proceedings, and journals. Index terms and titles are provided in French, English, German, and Spanish. Available on DataStar, Dialog, QUESTEL-ORBIT, and Silver-Platter, 1973 to date, updated monthly; also on CD-ROM.

Patents International (IMS)   see 16.4.

PDQ   see *Physician Data Query* databases.

Pharm-Line   see 14.21.

PharmaBiomed   see Figure 15.8.

Pharmaceutical and Healthcare Industry News Database   see 15.9.

Pharmaceutical News Index   see 15.17.

PharmacoEconomics & Outcomes News   see 15.14.

Pharmacontacts   see 15.23.

Pharmaprojects   see 15.1.

Pharmsearch   see 16.5.

PHIND   see 15.9.

Physician Data Query Directory File   see 14.36.

Physician Data Query Patient Information File   see 14.35.

Physician Data Query Protocol File   see 14.22.

The Pink Sheet   see 15.10.

PNI   see 15.17.

Product Monographs (IMS)   see 15.19.

PROMT   see 15.35.

R&D Focus   see 15.2.

R&D Focus Drug News   see 15.12.

R&D Insight   see 15.3.

Reactions Database   see 14.26.

Registry of Toxic Effects of Chemical Substances   see 14.28.

Research Centers and Services Directory   A Gale Research database compiling descriptions of 30,000 organizations conducting research in any of 145 countries, with entries for university based and other nonprofit facilities, government research units in the United States and Canada, and for-profit private sector firms. Available on Dialog and SilverPlatter, updated semiannually.

Ringdoc   see 14.11.

RTECS   see 14.28.

SciSearch   see 14.7.

Scrip   see 15.9.

SEDBASE   Corresponds to *Meyler's Side Effects of Drugs* (7.1) and *Side Effects of Drugs Annual* (7.2), enhanced with relevant *EMBASE* references and additional drug name indexing drawn from *Marler's Pharmacological and Chemical Synonyms* (3.12). Available on DataStar and Dialog, 1975–1995, when updates ceased. It is anticipated that this file will remain online for archival purposes. Also on CD-ROM.

Snapshots International Markets Research   see Figure 15.9.

Social SciSearch Similar in structure to *SciSearch* (14.8), *Social SciSearch* can be used to locate bibliographic citations, with abstracts, on pharmacy practice issues and health-care planning or administrative topics, including pharmacoeconomics. Produced by the Institute for Scientific Information and available on DataStar and Dialog, 1972 to date, updated weekly; also on CD-ROM.

Standard Drug File see *Derwent Drug Registry.*

TableBase see 15.34.

TOXLINE see 14.27.

TOXLIT A bibliographic database derived from *Chemical Abstracts,* focusing on references that cover interactions of chemical substances with biological systems *in vivo* and *in vitro.* Produced by Chemical Abstracts Service and available on MEDLARS, 1965 to date, updated monthly.

Trade & Industry Index see 15.36.

Unlisted Drugs Corresponds to *Unlisted Drugs* (3.8) in hardcopy, 1987 to date. Available on DataStar and Dialog, updated monthly.

USAN Corresponds to the *USP Dictionary of USAN and International Drug Names* (3.1). Available on Dialog and STN, updated annually.

USP DI Volume 1: Drug Information for the Health Care Professional see 14.19.

VETDOC see *Derwent Veterinary Drug File.*

World Drug Market Manual—Companies see 15.20.

World Drug Market Manual—Countries see 15.32.

World Patents Index A bibliographic database produced by Derwent Information, containing more than seven million citations, with abstracts, to patents issued by thirty-one major patent issuing authorities. Dating from 1992, selected chemical patent drawings (usually structures) accompany relevant citations. Available on Dialog, QUESTEL-ORBIT, and STN, 1963 to date, updated weekly.

Guide to Database Availability

	DataStar	Dialog	MEDLARS	Ovid	QUESTEL-ORBIT	Silver-Platter	STN
ABI/Inform	•	•		•	•	•	•
ADIS LMS Drug Alerts Online	•	•					•
ADIS R&D Insight	•	•		•			•
ADIS Reactions Database	•	•				•	
Aerzte Zeitung Online	•						
AGRICOLA		•		•		•	•
AGRIS International		•				•	
AIDSDRUGS			•				
AIDSLINE	•	•	•	•		•	•
AIDSTRIALS			•				
Alcohol & Alcohol Problems Science Database				•			
Allied and Alternative Medicine	•	•				•	
AMA Journals Online		•					
Analytical Abstracts	•	•			•	•	•
Asian Business Intelligence Reports		•					
BBC Market Research		•					

	DataStar	Dialog	MEDLARS	Ovid	QUESTEL-ORBIT	Silver-Platter	STN
Beilstein Online		•					•
BioBusiness	•	•		•			•
BioCommerce Abstracts and Directory	•	•					•
BIOETHICSLINE	•		•		•	•	
Biological & Agricultural Index		•		•		•	
BIOSIS Previews	•	•		•		•	•
BNA Daily News from Washington		•					
Business & Industry	•	•				•	
Business & Management Practices		•				•	
Business Dateline		•					
CA File							•
CA Search	•	•		•	•		
CAB Abstracts	•	•		•		•	•
CAB Health	•	•				•	
CANCERLIT	•	•	•	•		•	•
CAS Registry File							•
CASREACT							•
Chapman & Hall Chemical Database		•					
Chem Sources Chemical Directory	•						•
Chem Sources Company Directory	•						•
Chemical Business NewsBase	•	•					•
Chemical Engineering & Biotechnology Abstracts	•	•			•		•
Chemical Industry Notes	•	•			•		•
Chemical Registry Nomenclature	•						
Chemical Safety NewsBase	•	•			•		•
CHEMLINE			•				
CHEMSEARCH		•					
CHEMTOX Online	•	•					
CLAIMS/RRX		•			•		•
CLAIMS/U.S. Patents Abstracts		•			•		•
Conference Papers Index		•					•
Current Biotechnology Abstracts	•	•					
Current Contents Search	•	•		•			
Datamonitor Market Research	•	•					
Decision Resources Pharmaceutical Industry Reports		•					
Derwent Biotechnology Abstracts	•	•			•	•	•
Derwent Drug File	•	•			•		•
Derwent Drug Registry	•	•			•		•
Derwent Veterinary Drug File	•				•		•
Diogenes	•	•				•	
Directory of Chemical Producers—Products		•					
Directory of Chemical Producers—Companies		•					

	DataStar	Dialog	MEDLARS	Ovid	QUESTEL-ORBIT	Silver-Platter	STN
Directory of Published Proceedings	•						
DIRLINE			•				
Drug Data Report	•	•					
Drug Information Fulltext	•	•		•		•	
Drug News & Perspectives	•	•					
Drugs of the Future	•	•					
EI Compendex	•	•		•	•		•
EMBASE	•	•		•	•	•	•
EMBASE Alert	•	•				•	•
ESPICOM Country Healthcare Database	•	•					
ESPICOM Pharmaceutical and Medical Company Profiles	•	•					
ESPICOM Pharmaceutical & Medical Device News	•	•					
Euromonitor Market Research	•	•					
European Chemical News	•						
Eventline	•	•			•		•
Evidence-Based Medicine Reviews				•			
ExtraMED		•					
F-D-C Reports	•	•		•			
Federal Research in Progress		•					
FIND/SVP Market Research		•					
FOODLINE: Current Food Legislation	•	•					
Freedonia Market Research	•	•					
Frost & Sullivan Market Intelligence	•	•					
General Practitioner	•						
Hazardous Substances Data Bank	•		•			•	•
Health Devices Alerts		•					
Health Devices Sourcebook		•					
Health News Daily	•	•					
Healthcare Organizations Database		•					
HealthSTAR	•	•	•	•		•	
HSELINE	•				•		
IAC Health & Wellness Database	•	•		•			
IAC Newsletter Database	•	•					•
IAC PROMT	•	•			•		•
IAC Trade & Industry Database	•	•					
IDIS Drug File	•			•		•	
Immunoclones Database	•						
IMS World Drug Markets	•	•					
Imsmarq Pharmaceutical Trademarks In-Use	•						
IMSworld Company Directory	•	•					
IMSworld New Product Launches	•	•					•
IMSworld Patents International	•	•			•		
IMSworld Pharmaceutical Company Profiles	•	•					
IMSworld Product Monographs	•	•					•

	DataStar	Dialog	MEDLARS	Ovid	QUESTEL-ORBIT	Silver-Platter	STN
IMSworld R&D Focus Drug News	•	•					•
IMSworld R&D Focus Drug Updates	•	•					•
IMSworld R&D Meetings Diary	•						
Incidence & Prevalence Database	•	•					
INPADOC		•			•		•
InPharma	•	•				•	
Inside Conferences		•					
INSPEC	•	•		•	•	•	•
International Pharmaceutical Abstracts	•	•		•		•	•
Investext	•	•					•
Investigational Drug Patents Fast-Alert	•				•		
Journal Watch				•			
Kirk-Othmer	•	•					
KOSMET	•						•
LEGSTAT					•		
Lexi-Comp's Clinical Reference Collection						•	
Life Sciences Collection		•				•	•
MANTIS	•	•		•			
Marketletter	•						
MarketLine International	•						
Markush Pharmsearch					•		
Martindale Online	•						
McGraw-Hill Publications Online		•					
MDX Health Digest					•	•	
Medical Device Register		•					
MediConf	•			•			•
MEDLINE	•	•	•	•	•	•	•
Merck Index Online		•			•		•
MSDS-CCOHS						•	•
MSDS-OHS		•					•
Natural Products Alert							•
NDA Pipeline	•	•					
New England Journal of Medicine		•		•			
NIOSHTIC		•					•
NME Express	•	•					
NTIS	•	•		•		•	•
Pascal	•	•			•	•	
Pharm-Line	•	•					
PharmaBiomed	•						
Pharmaceutical and Healthcare Industry News	•	•		•			•
Pharmaceutical News Index		•		•			•
PharmacoEconomics & Outcomes News	•	•					
Pharmacontacts	•	•		•			
Pharmaprojects	•	•		•			•
Pharmsearch					•		

	DataStar	Dialog	MEDLARS	Ovid	QUESTEL-ORBIT	Silver-Platter	STN
Physician Data Query Directory File			•	•			
Physician Data Query Patient Information File			•	•			
Physician Data Query Protocol File			•	•			
Research Centers and Services Directory		•				•	
RTECS	•	•	•			•	•
SciSearch	•	•					•
SEDBASE	•	•					
Snapshots International Market Research		•					
Social SciSearch	•	•					
TableBase	•	•					
TOXLINE	•	•	•			•	•
TOXLIT			•				
Unlisted Drugs	•	•					
USAN		•					•
USP DI Volume 1		•					
World Patents Index		•			•		•
Number of featured databases from each provider	**103**	**120**	**16**	**36**	**29**	**36**	**61**

C

A Selection of Current Awareness Newsletters Available in Full-Text Format Online

AIDS Weekly Plus (formerly *CDC AIDS Weekly*) reports on clinical studies of AIDS-related drugs and testing or screening devices. Summaries of research are drawn from scientific journals and conference proceedings. Issued weekly by Charles W. Henderson (publisher). Complete coverage from January 1991 to date in the *IAC Newsletter Database* and *IAC Health & Wellness Database*; selected articles in *IAC PROMT* (1992–) and in *Business & Industry Database* (1995–).

Antiviral Agents Bulletin specializes in news and abstracts of AIDS and antiviral drug and vaccine R&D results, with selective coverage of relevant patents. Issued monthly by the Biotechnology Information Institute. Complete coverage from April 1988 to date in the *IAC Newsletter Database*; selected articles in *IAC PROMT* (December 1990–) and *Business & Industry Database* (February 1995–).

Applied Genetics News covers business and scientific developments in biotechnology, including applications in health care, food, waste treatment, and agriculture. Issued monthly by Business Communications Company, Inc. Complete coverage dates from September 1989 in the *IAC Newsletter Database*; selected articles in *IAC PROMT* (February 1990–).

BBI Newsletter (formerly *Biomedical Business International*) includes drug, diagnostics, and device product briefs for new approvals, market and technology updates, news of acquisitions and licensing agreements, and discussion of factors influencing the worldwide health technology marketplace. Issued monthly by American Health Consultants. Complete text online in the *IAC Newsletter Database* from January 1990.

Biomedical Market Newsletter monitors business, marketing, and regulatory issues with potential impact on biomedical equipment, device, diagnostic test, and supply industries. Issued monthly by Biomedical Market Newsletter, Inc. Complete coverage dates from September 1991 in the *IAC Newsletter Database*; selected articles in *IAC PROMT* (January 1992–).

Biomedical Materials focuses on research and development related to materials used in medicine, including ceramics, composites, metals, and polymers. Issued monthly by Elsevier Advanced Technology publications. Complete coverage from November 1992 to date in the *IAC Newsletter Database*.

Biotech Business provides detailed reporting on biotechnology products and companies, with growth forecasts and periodic financial assessments, as well as news of licensing opportunities. Issued monthly by Worldwide Videotex. Complete coverage dates from August 1988 in the *IAC Newsletter Database*.

Biotech Equipment Update relays news on laboratory equipment, drug delivery systems, test kits, and related technological developments and new product approvals. Issued monthly by Worldwide Videotex. Complete coverage from December 1993 to date in the *IAC Newsletter Database*; selected articles in *IAC PROMT* (December 1993–).

Biotech Financial Reports covers news of public offerings, venture capital financing, and other financial events and opportunities related to the biotechnology industry. Issued monthly by Worldwide Videotex. Complete coverage from July 1994 forward in *IAC Newsletter Database*; selected articles also in *IAC PROMT* (July 1994–).

Biotech Patent News reports on patenting, licensing, and related litigation, government actions, and special interest group activities. Issued monthly by Biotech Patent News. Complete coverage dates from January 1991 in the IAC Newsletter Database; selected articles also in *IAC PROMT* (January 1991–).

Biotechnology Business News (United Kingdom) focuses on the commercial implications of scientific developments and monitors government regulations and biotech companies' business performance. Issued 24 times/year by Financial Times Business Information. Complete coverage from January 1991 to date in the *IAC Newsletter Database*; selected articles in *IAC PROMT* (October 1991–) and *Business & Industry Database* (January 1995–).

Biotechnology Newswatch follows developments from the laboratory to the marketplace, featuring company profiles, regular review of patent filings, "JapanWatch," and news related to biotechnology applications in pharmaceuticals, agriculture, and bioremediation. Issued two times/month by McGraw-Hill, Inc. Complete coverage dates from September 1986 in *McGraw-Hill Publications Online*.

Blood Weekly monitors case reports and journal articles related to transplantation, transfusion, blood culture systems, and blood diseases, abstracting the current literature and reporting on industry news. Issued weekly by Charles W. Henderson (publisher). Complete coverage, August 1994 to date, in the *IAC Newsletter Database*; selected articles in *IAC PROMT* (August 1994–) and *Business & Industry Database* (January 1995–).

BT Catalyst covers biotechnology news, with special emphasis on university and industry programs. Issued 10 times/year by the North Carolina Biotechnology Center. Complete coverage from January 1991 to date in the *IAC Newsletter Database*.

Cancer Biotechnology Weekly (formerly *Cancer Researcher Weekly*, also *Cancer Weekly*, *NCI Cancer Weekly*) relays news of cancer drugs in clinical trials and FDA approvals. Findings are reported from research programs at universities and government laboratories, as well as companies. This newsletter also includes summaries of articles published in scientific journals. Issued weekly by Charles W. Henderson (publisher). Complete coverage dates from December 1988 in the *IAC Newsletter Database*; selected articles also in *IAC PROMT* (January 1992–), *IAC Health & Wellness Database* (January 1991–), and *Business & Industry Database* (January 1995–).

Drug Detection Report focuses on the topic of drug analytical testing, reporting on court cases, training issues, government news, and the national laboratory certification program. Issued biweekly by Pace Publications. Complete coverage dates from April 1994 in the *IAC Newsletter Database*, with selected articles also in *IAC PROMT* (April 1994–).

Genesis Report-Dx specializes in analysis of technological advances in diagnostic medicine, with information on companies, products, business strategies, and research activities. Issued bimonthly by The Genesis Group Associates, Inc. Complete coverage from November 1991 in the *IAC Newsletter Database*; selected articles in *IAC PROMT* (January 1992–).

Genesis Report-Rx offers in-depth analysis of business implications for management dealing with the pharmaceutical industry, with a focus on product innovations, shifts in the competitive environment, and corporate strategies. Biotechnology, diagnostics, and therapeutics business areas are discussed. Issued bimonthly by The Genesis Group Associates, Inc. Complete coverage from December 1991 in the *IAC Newsletter Database*; selected articles also in *IAC PROMT* (December 1991–).

Health Industry Today is a publication intended for purchasing managers. It monitors company and product news, trade shows and exhibitions, and distribution agreements related to medical devices, medical/surgical supplies, and other health technology products. FDA regulation of marketing and advertising is among topics covered. Issued monthly by Business Word, Inc. *IAC Newsletter Database* offers complete text coverage from July 1994; selected articles can also be found in *IAC Trade & Industry Database* (1989–) and *ABI/Inform* (January 1992–).

Health Legislation & Regulation provides timely coverage of U.S. Congressional activities related to health care, including budget and appropriations updates, a running tally of new bills, and detailed summaries of major legislation and regulations. Issued 50 times/year by Faulkner & Gray, Inc. Complete coverage from February 1992 to the present in the *IAC Newsletter Database*.

Healthcare Business & Legal Strategies (formerly *Financial Ventures Report*) monitors relevant federal government agency activities and legal issues with potential impact on healthcare financing and insurance, reporting on antitrust actions, Medicare, and related news. Issued 24 times/year by Atlantic Information Services, Inc. Complete coverage from January 1993 to date in the *IAC Newsletter Database*; selected articles in *IAC PROMT* (January 1993–).

Healthcare PR & Marketing News (formerly *Healthcare PR News*) reports and analyzes business trends and government activities of interest to public relations, marketing, and advertising professionals specializing in health care. Issued biweekly by Philips Business Information. Complete coverage from November 1992 in the *IAC Newsletter Database*.

Healthcare Technology & Business Opportunities provides a directory of technologies available for license and transfer and compiles information on a broad spectrum of business opportunities, including venture capital, corporate partnerships, contract research, equipment sales and services, and distribution agreements. Issued monthly by Biomedical Business International. Complete coverage dates from January 1990 in the *IAC Newsletter Database*.

In Vivo, The Business & Medicine Report provides news summaries, commentary, and forecasts regarding medical industry developments and trends, mergers and acquisitions, sales and earnings, new products, and company directions. Issued 11 times/year by Windhover Information, Inc. Complete coverage from January 1991 to date in *IAC PROMT*.

Infectious Disease Weekly (also cited as *Infection Control Weekly*) includes abstracts from the current conference and journal literature related to infection control, etiology and transmission of infectious diseases, diagnosis, drug resistance, vaccines, and epidemiologic surveillance. Issued weekly by Charles W. Henderson (publisher). Complete text online in the *IAC Newsletter Database* from September 1994; selected articles also in *IAC PROMT* (September 1994–) and *Business & Industry Database* (January 1995–).

Marketletter reports on news affecting the worldwide pharmaceutical industry, including drug research, product launches, legislative and regulatory developments, company marketing activities, and stock market commentaries. Issued weekly by Marketletter Publications, Ltd. Complete coverage, January 1992 to date, in the *IAC Newsletter Database*; selected articles in *IAC PROMT* (January 1992–) and *Business & Industry Database* (October 1994–).

Medical Outcomes & Guidelines Alert monitors patient outcomes research and proposed, as well as published, therapeutic guidelines, with reports on managed care organizations and compliance studies. Issued 24 times/year by Faulkner & Gray, Inc. Complete coverage dates from April 1994 in the *IAC Newsletter Database*.

Medical Textiles provides a monthly review of new applications for textiles used in medicine. Issued monthly by Elsevier Advanced Technology Publications. Complete coverage from January 1988 in the *IAC Newsletter Database*.

Medicine & Health emphasizes health policy developments in the U.S. Congress, federal agencies, the courts, state legislatures, and lobbying organizations. Issued 50 times/year by Faulkner & Gray, Inc. Complete coverage from January 1992 in *IAC Newsletter Database*; selected articles also in *IAC PROMT* (February 1992–).

Membrane & Separation Technology News reports on scientific developments in microfiltration, reverse osmosis, ultrafiltration, cross filtration, gas separation, electrodialysis, and specialty chromatography, exploring potential commercial applications and business implications. Issued monthly by Business Communications Company, Inc. Complete coverage dates from December 1989 in the *IAC Newsletter Database*.

OTC News & Market Report (Europe) features product reports on European markets at the country level and includes news of new products, company mergers and acquisitions, financial performance, and advertising. Issued monthly by Nicholas Hall & Company. Complete coverage dates from January 1989 in the IAC Newsletter Database; selected articles in *IAC PROMT* (July 1989–) and *Business & Industry Database* (January 1994–).

OTC Update (formerly *OTC Market Report Update USA*) covers events in the U.S. and Canadian over-the-counter health and hygiene products marketplace. Features include company profiles, product and market reports, new product information, and statistical data compilation on market share and market size. Issued monthly by Nicholas Hall & Company. Complete coverage from May 1990 to date in the *IAC Newsletter Database*; selected articles also in *IAC PROMT* (May 1990–) and *Business & Industry Database* (January 1994–).

Pharmaceutical Business News (U.K.) reports on the latest developments in research, recent company performance, mergers, acquisitions, and joint ventures. Commentary is also included on world financial markets and important legal and regulatory affairs. Issued 24 times/year by Financial Times Business Information. Complete coverage, January 1991 to date, in the *IAC Newsletter Database*; selected articles in *IAC PROMT* (October 1991–) and *Business & Industry Database* (January 1995–).

R & D provides a timely technical review of applied research and development, surveying scientific data from all industrial areas. Issued monthly by Cahners Publishing Company. Complete text online from January 1992 forward in the *IAC Trade & Industry Database*.

Vaccine Weekly brings together relevant news on therapeutic vaccines for AIDS, cancer, and other diseases, reporting on safety and efficacy trials, product approvals, and related FDA activities. Issued weekly by Charles W. Henderson (publisher). Complete coverage dates from June 1994 in the *IAC Newsletter Database*; selected articles also in *IAC PROMT* (June 1994–) and *Business & Industry Database* (January 1995–).

Washington Health Week (formerly *Inside Healthcare Reform*) focuses on state and federal government news related to healthcare topics, such as family planning, tobacco education, AIDS drug assistance, antifraud or antitrust actions, competitive bidding for managed care and Medicaid programs, budgetary allocations, etc. Issued 45 times/year by Atlantic Information Services. Complete text online in the *IAC Newsletter Database* from July 1995.

Worldwide Biotech reports news and information on the industry from a global viewpoint, monitoring the emerging European Community marketplace, Japan's growing involvement, and international deals between companies. Issued monthly by Worldwide Videotex. Complete text online in the *IAC Newsletter Database* from March 1990.

D

Professional and Trade Associations

Familiarity with professional and trade organizations closely affiliated with a subject area is an integral part of information service. Their meetings serve as forums for communication on new developments. Many such organizations also maintain active publication programs, provide grants for research and education, and offer continuing education courses.

Organizations for Information Professionals

Special interest groups formed by full time information professionals with expertise in the pharmaceutical subject area have, for many years, been recognized as separate sections within the Special Libraries Association and Medical Library Association. Special programs for information managers have, more recently, also evolved within the Drug Information Association and the Pharmaceutical Education and Research Institute. Academic pharmacy librarians in the United States are generally affiliated with the Libraries/Educational Resources Section of the American Association of Colleges of Pharmacy (AACP), as well. Programs of the Division of Chemical Information of the American Chemical Society and other organizations listed in this section also offer excellent opportunities for professional development and networking.

American Chemical Society
Division of Chemical Information
1155 16th Street NW
Washington, DC 20036 USA
202/872-4600 Fax: 202/872-6337
http://www.lib.uchicago.edu/~atbrooks/CNIF/cinfhome.html

The Division of Chemical Information of the American Chemical Society plans its own programs within the larger American Chemical Society conferences. Online database searching, intellectual property issues, regulatory information sources, storage and retrieval of chemical data, and management of information operations are examples of the diversity of topics addressed.

Drug Information Association (DIA)
501 Office Center Drive, Suite 450
Fort Washington, PA 19034-3211 USA
215/628-2288 Fax: 215/641-1229
http://www.diahome.org

The Drug Information Association conducts workshops and sponsors seminars each year for individuals who handle drug information in government, industry, and the medical, pharmacy, and library professions. Establishing standards for technology in drug information processing and publishing is an underlying theme in many of its programs and in articles appearing in the quarterly *Drug Information Journal*. Founded in 1964, DIA today lists more than 20,000 members in its annual directory. An R&D information management group newly formed within DIA began offering annual two-day workshop meetings in 1996.

The Drug Information Association Web site provides complete descriptions of forthcoming programs serving all special interest groups within its diverse membership. Another service available to all site visitors is a *Technical Term Translation Table* that suggests corresponding terminology used in the pharmaceutical and related fields. The interface provides translation from English-language keywords into French, German, Italian, or Spanish counterparts, or vice versa. Chinese, Russian, and Japanese language capabilities are promised additions in the future.

European Association for Health Information and Libraries (EAHIL)
Pharmaceutical Information Group
Association Européenne pour l'Information et les Bibliothèques de Santé
c/o ICP-NTI
P.O. Box 23213
NL-1100 DS Amsterdam, The Netherlands
31/20 566 2095 Fax: 31/20 696 3228
http://www.med.uu.nl/eahil.html
http://www.eahil.org/pharmaceutical_information_group.htm

The Pharmaceutical Information Group was recognized as an official section of EAHIL in 1995, with a membership of information specialists working in pharmaceutical companies in any of twelve European countries. The parent organization, founded ten years earlier, includes 500 librarians and information officers from a variety of medical and health science practice settings. EAHIL's annual conference programs focus on continuing education, networking, and career development.

European Pharmaceutical Marketing Research Association (EPhMRA)
54 Sunridge Avenue
Bromley, Kent BR1 2QD UK
Fax: 44 (0) 181 466 0767
http://www.ephmra.org:80

In common with PBIRG, its sister organization in the United States, the European Pharmaceutical Marketing Research Association promotes the interests of business intelligence professionals employed in diagnostic, device, healthcare biotechnology, and drug companies. Networking, education, and liaison with other organizations sharing the same goals are primary objectives. A visit to EPhMRA's Web site shows announcements of forthcoming workshops and meetings and offers access to a *Lexicon* of marketing terms and definitions. EPhMRA's chief claim to fame is development of an anatomic/therapeutic classification (ATC) scheme used to index pharmaceutical products in several reference sources, such as *IMSworld R&D Focus Drug Updates* (15.2). Initiated by EPhMRA in 1971, the standardized, hierarchical list of codes is now maintained through an ongoing collaboration with PBIRG.

Medical Library Association (MLA)
Drug and Pharmaceutical Information Division
65 East Wacker Place, Suite 1900
Chicago, IL 60601-7298 USA
312/419-9094 Fax: 312/419-8950
http://www.mlanet.org

The 150-member Drug and Pharmaceutical Information Division of the Medical Library Association organizes two to three hours of special programs at the annual meeting of MLA and publishes its own biennial newsletter, *PDI Alert.* Membership is drawn primarily from academic pharmacy institutions and teaching hospitals, rather than pharmaceutical corporations.

Pharmaceutical Business Intelligence & Research Group (PBIRG)
P.O. Box 755
Langhorne, PA 19047 USA
215/337-9301 Fax: 215/337-9303
http://www.pbirg.com

PBIRG is a not-for-profit industry association dedicated to the advancement of global healthcare marketing research, drawing its members from pharmaceutical, biotechnology, diagnostic, and medical device companies. Annual meetings serve as a forum for professional networking and education among business intelligence professionals. PBIRG members collaborate in ongoing maintenance of the EPhMRA classification scheme.

Regulatory Affairs Professional Society (RAPS)
12300 Twinbrook Parkway, Suite 350
Rockville, MD 20852 USA
301/770-2920 Fax: 301/770-2924
http://www.raps.org

Founded in 1976, RAPS has 6,000 members working in the pharmaceutical, medical device, biologic, and biotechnology industries worldwide. The RAPS home page on the Internet features a resource center of helpful reference materials and a good collection of hotlinks to regulatory sites and related professional organizations worldwide.

Society of Competitive Intelligence Information Professionals (SCIP)
1700 Diagonal Road, Suite 600
Alexandria, VA 22314 USA
703/739-0696 Fax: 703/739-2524
http://www.scip.org

Providing educational and networking opportunities among competitive intelligence professionals has been SCIP's primary function since its formation in 1986. Programs at annual national meetings and those of numerous local chapters focus on enhancement of research, analytical, and information dissemination skills among members. The organization is also active in providing guidance on ethical issues and legal liabilities in marketing research. The quarterly journal *Competitive Intelligence Review* is published under the auspices of SCIP, whose 6,000 members include individuals employed in diverse industries and consulting firms located in any of fifty-three countries worldwide.

Special Libraries Association (SLA)
Pharmaceutical and Health Technology Division
1700 18th Street NW
Washington, DC 20009-2508 USA
202/234-4700 Fax: 202/265-9317
http://www.sla.org/division/dphm/index.htm

Now more than fifty years old, the Pharmaceutical and Health Technology Division of the Special Libraries Association is the largest professional group of library information specialists (more than 700 members) affiliated with industry or academic programs focused on pharmaceuticals, medical devices, and biotechnology. The Division publishes its own annual *Membership Directory* and a quarterly newsletter, *CapLits*. It sponsors special programs at the annual SLA meeting, including six to eight hours of invited speakers, networking breakfasts, and continuing education (CE) courses. The Division also holds separate Spring meetings featuring a variety of professional development activities. Members can participate in a closed electronic discussion group on the Internet, but the Division's new Web site, launched in February 1999, is open to all.

Pharmacy, Pharmacology, and Related Professional Associations

Organizations listed in this section serve the special interests of various groups of individuals defined by their subject interests, job functions, or employment settings.

Academy of Managed Care Pharmacy (AMCP)
100 North Pitt Street, Suite 400
Alexandria, VA 22314 USA
703/683-8416 Fax: 703/683-8417
http://www.amcp.org

The Academy of Managed Care Pharmacy is a national professional society formed to represent the interests of pharmacists working in managed care environments in the United States. Its more than 4,000 members are employed in any of 600 healthcare organizations. The Academy's official publication is *JMCP—Journal of Managed Care Pharmacy®*, the full text of which is archived for on-line access at AMCP's Web site (December 1995–).

The organization launched an *AMCP Consumer Web Page* in October, 1998. Designed to help the general public learn more about managed care pharmacy, this new site provides a series of concept papers written in everyday language on topics such as disease state management and formulary management. It also includes facts sheets about various issues often misunderstood by the lay public (e.g., generic substitution of narrow therapeutic index drugs), a list of managed care acronyms, and hyperlinks to an extensive glossary of managed healthcare terms, as well as disease-specific, general health, and drug information sites selected for their patient orientation.

Alliance for the Prudent Use of Antibiotics (APUA)
P.O. Box 1372
Boston, MA 02117-1372 USA
Fax: 617/636-3999
http://www.healthsci.tufts.edu/apua

A self-described "grassroots" organization, the Alliance for the Prudent Use of Antibiotics was founded in 1981 to promote information exchange among scientists, practitioners, and consumers about the growing problem of antibiotic resistance. APUA has succeeded in establishing local chapters in seventeen countries to support national initiatives to curb antibiotic resistance. Their objective is tailoring public health interventions to the practices and problems specific to the locale. More than ninety countries are represented in APUA's membership. Programs include sponsorship of expert speakers to participate in a health provider lecture series, development of a patient information pamphlet about appropriate antibiotic usage, and production of educational videotapes and self-study guides for healthcare professionals.

American Academy of Pharmaceutical Physicians (AAPP)
1135 Kildare Farm Road, #2008
Cary, NC 25711 USA
919/469-9906 Fax: 919/380-1098
http://www.aapp.org

The American Academy of Pharmaceutical Physicians was founded in 1994 as a forum for information exchange among MDs working in industry and directly involved in discovery, research, and development of pharmaceuticals, vaccines, medical devices, and diagnostic products. The academy sponsors a fellowship program for members new to industry. AAPP's Web site provides hotlinks to key journal and association sites on the Internet, as well as a useful page of gateways to a variety of search engines.

American Association for Clinical Chemistry (AACC)
2101 L Street NW, Suite 202
Washington, DC 20037 USA
202/857-0717 Fax: 202/887-5093
http://www.aacc.org

Clinical laboratory professionals, physicians, and research scientists located in any of ninety-three countries and working in industry, hospital labs, or independent labs make up the membership of AACC.

The association's services to its 11,000 members include monitoring legislative and regulatory affairs, providing continuing education programs, and maintaining an extensive list of publications. The journal *Clinical Chemistry* and the magazine *Clinical Laboratory News* are both produced by AACC. Other publications include the *Effects of Drugs on Clinical Laboratory Tests* (7.29) and *Abused Drugs II: A Laboratory Pocket Guide* (8.22). The association's Web site offers a *Standards Status* database organized by analyte name, enabling quick checks for accepted reference methods relevant to clinical laboratory practice.

American Association of Colleges of Pharmacy (AACP)
1426 Prince Street
Alexandria, VA 22314 USA
703/739-2330 Fax: 703/836-8962
http://www.aacp.org

The 2,200 members of AACP include the eighty-one accredited colleges of pharmacy in the United States and individuals affiliated with them, encompassing both faculty and administrative staff. The Libraries/Educational Resources Section sponsors its own programs at annual meetings of AACP. Publications of the association include the *Basic Booklist and Core Journals for Pharmaceutical Education* (5.11), the *Roster of Faculty and Professional Staff* (13.39) in colleges of pharmacy, *Graduate Programs in the Pharmaceutical Sciences* (13.41), and enrollment reports and summaries of degrees conferred, published each year in the *Profile of Pharmacy Students* (13.44). AACP's official journal is the quarterly *American Journal of Pharmaceutical Education.*

American Association of Pharmaceutical Scientists (AAPS)
1650 King Street, Suite 200
Alexandria, VA 22314-2747 USA
703/548-3000 Fax: 703/684-7349
http://www.aaps.org

Founded in 1986, the American Association of Pharmaceutical Scientists has more than 9,300 members, who are employed in academia, industry, government, and other research institutions worldwide. AAPS publishes four hardcopy journals: *Pharmaceutical Research,* the *Journal of Pharmaceutical Marketing and Management,* the *Journal of Pharmaceutical and Biomedical Analysis,* and the *Journal of Pharmaceutical Development and Technology.* An electronic journal, AAPS PharmSci™, is the latest addition to this association's prolific publication program. Members are also regular contributors to the annual series *Analytical Profiles of Drug Substances and Excipients* (11.2). The AAPS Web site provides a cumulative index of all substances covered in this series (1972–). An online *Buyer's Guide* to products and technologies, searchable by keyword, product category, and/or company name, is another service offered by AAPS to its members.

American Association of Pharmacy Technicians (AAPT)
P.O. Box 1447
Greensboro, NC 27402 USA
336/275-1700 Fax: 336/275-7222
http://www.pharmacytechnician.com

The American Association of Pharmacy Technicians provides continuing education programs and other services to help members update their skills. AAPT is also active in promoting public awareness of the role of pharmacy technicians as an integral part of the patient care team.

American Botanical Council (ABC)
P.O. Box 144345
Austin, TX 78714-4345 USA
512/926-4900 Fax: 512/926-2345
http://www.herbalgram.org

The American Botanical Council was incorporated in 1988 as a nonprofit education organization with a mission of informing the public about the benefits of herbs and plants and promoting their safe and effective use in medicine. Assistance to the media (newspapers, magazines) is a major focus, and ABC's Executive Director has appeared on numerous radio and television talk shows. Publication of *HerbalGram,* a quarterly journal produced in collaboration with the Herb Research Foundation, is another ongoing ABC project. The council was also responsible for initiation of the translation of *German Commission E Monographs* (12.4) into English. In 1996, ABS began offering accredited home study courses for pharmacists in the United States. These and other association activities are described in more detail on the council's Web site. One of the most attractive features of this site is a large, illustrated catalog of books and audiovisuals offered for sale. Both popular and professional titles are included in the impressive inventory of more than 500 sources.

American College of Apothecaries
P.O. Box 341266
Memphis, TN 38184 USA
901/383-8119

A professional society of pharmacists who own and operate ethical prescription pharmacies, the American College of Apothecaries also includes among its 1,000 members hospital pharmacists, pharmacy students, and faculty of colleges of pharmacy. Founded in 1940, today the group sponsors a fellowship program and conducts two educational conferences per year. (As of February 1999, this society is not represented on the Internet.)

American College of Clinical Pharmacology (ACCP)
3 Ellinwood Court
New Hartford, NY 13413-1105 USA
315/768-6117 Fax: 315/768-6119
http://www.accp1.org

Since its formation in 1969, ACCP has grown beyond its original MD-only membership roster to encompass nearly 1,000 professionals, 48% of whom are nonphysicians (primarily PharmDs and PhDs). Education remains ACCP's primary objective, accomplished through meetings, courses, and publications, including the *Journal of Clinical Pharmacology.*

American College of Clinical Pharmacy (ACCP)
3101 Broadway, Suite 380
Kansas City, MO 64111 USA
816/531-2177 Fax: 816/531-4990
http://www.accp.com

Advancing the practice of clinical pharmacy and interdisciplinary health care and maintaining standards in advanced training for clinical pharmacists are among the stated purposes of this group, which publishes the journal *Pharmacotherapy.* Founded in 1979, the American College of Clinical Pharmacy consists of 1,600 members.

American Council on Pharmaceutical Education (ACPE)
311 West Superior Street, Suite 512
Chicago, IL 60610 USA
312/664-3575 Fax: 312/664-4652
http://www.acpe-accredit.org

ACPE has been the accrediting agency for pre-service educational programs at colleges and schools of pharmacy in the United States since 1932. In 1975, its scope broadened to include accreditation of continuing education, as well. The council publishes *Accredited Professional Programs of Colleges or Schools of Pharmacy* (13.40) and *Approved Providers of Continuing Pharmaceutical Education* (13.42).

American Institute of the History of Pharmacy (AIHP)
Pharmacy Building
425 North Charter Street
Madison, WI 53706 USA
608/262-5378
http://www.pharmacy.wisc.edu/aihp

Founded in 1941, the American Institute of the History of Pharmacy includes both individual pharmacists and firms or organizations among its 1,100 members. Publisher of numerous monographs and bibliographies (see 12.52, 12.55, and additional sources cited at the end of Chapter Twelve), the Institute maintains biographical archives and a pharmaceutical Americana collection. It encourages contributions to scholarship dealing with historical and social aspects of the pharmaceutical field, many of which are published in the quarterly journal *Pharmacy in History* (12.53). AIHP's Web site offers a catalog of its publications.

American Pharmaceutical Association (APhA)
2215 Constitution Avenue NW
Washington, DC 20037 USA
202/628-4410 Fax: 202/783-2351
http://www.aphanet.org
http://www.pharmacyandyou.org

The APhA is the largest professional society in pharmacy, with more than 50,000 members drawn from community practice, academia, wholesale and manufacturing firms, editors and publishers, hospital pharmacists, and food and drug officials. The American Institute of Pharmacy, the Association's headquarters building in Washington, houses a library and the APhA Foundation, which is responsible for disseminating public health information and cooperating with government agencies, public and private foundations, and educational institutions.

Founded in 1852, the APhA is a prolific publisher, whose imprints include the *Handbook of Nonprescription Drugs* (6.6), *Nonprescription Products: Formulations and Features* (6.7), *The Art, Science, and Technology of Pharmaceutical Compounding* (6.43), the *Patient Counseling Handbook* (9.42), the *Ident-A-Drug Reference* (10.7), the *Handbook of Pharmaceutical Excipients* (11.19), the *Handbook of Pharmaceutical Additives* (11.20), and *Herbal Remedies* (12.12). *American Pharmacy* and the *Journal of Pharmaceutical Sciences* are other well known monthly publications of the Association.

In recent years, APhA has become active in outreach to patients, in the form of books such as the *Guide to Prescription Drugs* (9.8), the *Parents Guide to Childhood Medications* (9.9), *What Do I Take? A Consumers Guide to Nonprescription Drugs* (9.10), and the *American Pharmaceutical Association's Practical Guide to Natural Medicines* (9.20). Its latest initiative in services offered directly to consumers is the *Pharmacy and You* Web site launched in 1999 (see Chapter Nine for a description).

American Society for Clinical Pharmacology and Therapeutics (ASCPT)
117 West Ridge Pike, Suite 2
Conshohoken, PA 19428-1216 USA
610/825-3838 Fax: 610/834-8652
http://www.ascpt.org

Founded in 1900, this 2,200-member organization provides a continuing education program for practicing physicians. Most of its members are MDs (69%) or other doctoral scientists (29%). Pharmacists, nurses, research coordinators, fellows in training, and other professionals associated with the discipline of clinical pharmacology make up the remaining 2%. Numerous scientific sections within ASCPT focus on specialty areas such as biostatistics and clinical trial methodology, clinical pharmaceutical development and regulatory affairs, clinical toxicology, pharmacoepidemiology, and pediatric or geriatric pharmacology. The society has published the monthly peer reviewed journal *Clinical Pharmacology and Therapeutics* since 1960.

American Society for Pharmacology and Experimental Therapeutics (ASPET)
9650 Rockville Pike
Bethesda, MD 20814-3995 USA
301/530-7060 Fax: 301/530-7061
http://www.faseb.org/aspet

ASPET sponsors the publication of several professional journals, including *Drug Metabolism and Disposition* (bimonthly), *Journal of Pharmacology and Experimental Therapeutics* (monthly), *Molecular Pharmacology* (monthly), *Pharmacological Reviews* (quarterly), and the *Pharmacologist* (quarterly). The

4,300 members of this group include investigators in pharmacology and toxicology. Affiliated with the Federation of American Societies for Experimental Biology, ASPET meets semiannually in conjunction with FASEB.

American Society of Consultant Pharmacists (ASCP)
1321 Duke Street
Alexandria, VA 22314-3563 USA
703/739-1300 Fax: 703/739-1321
http://www.ascp.com

Members of the American Society of Consultant Pharmacists are registered pharmacists and educators involved in consultant services to nursing homes and other long-term care facilities. The term "consultant" arises from the fact that these pharmacists provide services to facilities on a contractual basis, rather than as employees of individual facilities. Founded in 1969, ASCP conducts surveys of extended care pharmacy operations, represents the interests of its constituency in Medicaid reform initiatives, and publishes *The Consultant Pharmacist* monthly journal for its 6,500 members. *Pharmacy Legislation Regulations Guidelines for Long-Term Care* (4.41) is another publication of this group.

The ASCP Web site is an excellent source of statistics related to long-term care facilities and their patients. The online directory of publications and products includes hotlinks to fact sheets full of data on nursing home demographics, medication use, and chronic conditions among the elderly in the United States. The directory also links to a bibliography on inappropriate drug use in the elderly and to two noteworthy resource pages (subject hubs) devoted, respectively, to the topics of geriatrics and immunization.

American Society of Health-System Pharmacists (ASHP)
7272 Wisconsin Avenue
Bethesda, MD 20814 USA
301/657-3000 Fax: 301/652-8278
http://www.ashp.com

One of the most respected professional societies for pharmacists, ASHP (formerly the American Society of Hospital Pharmacists) is a major publisher of drug information sources. Its output includes *AHFS Drug Information* (6.4), *Guidelines for Administration of Intravenous Medications to Pediatric Patients* (6.37), the *Handbook on Extemporaneous Formulations* (6.39), *Trissel's Stability of Compounded Medications* (6.42), the *Handbook of Basic Pharmacokinetics* (6.56), the *Handbook on Injectable Drugs* (7.31), *Practical Aspects of Intravenous Drug Administration* (7.33), the *Infusion Technology Manual* (7.34), *Medication Teaching Manual* (9.39), the *Home Care Resource Book* (9.47), *International Pharmaceutical Abstracts* in hardcopy as well as machine-readable format (14.8), *Drug Information Fulltext* (14.18) online and on CD-ROM, and an annual *Residency Directory* (13.43) of programs accredited by the society. ASHP is also well known for its professional journals, the *American Journal of Health-System Pharmacy* and *Clinical Pharmacy* (both monthly). The Society's Web page is well worth periodic visits to survey recent publications. It also provides a good pathfinder to other Internet sites.

American Society of Pharmacognosy (ASP)
P.O. Box 9558
Downers Grove, IL 60515 USA
http://www.phcog.org

The monthly *Journal of Natural Products* (formerly *Lloydia*) is a well known publication of the 1,100-member American Society of Pharmacognosy. It is issued in collaboration with the American Chemical Society and with the cooperation of the Lloyd Library and Museum. ASP was founded in 1959 for professionals engaged in the study of drugs from natural sources and for others interested in the plant sciences and natural products.

AOAC International (formerly the Association of Official Analytical Chemists)
481 North Frederick Avenue, Suite 500
Gaithersburg, MD 20877-2417 USA
301/924-7077 Fax: 301/924-7089
http://www.aoac.org

Established in 1884, AOAC International (formerly the Association of Official Analytical Chemists) is an independent organization of 4,000 scientists in the public and private sectors devoted to promoting methods validation and quality measurements in analysis techniques. Microbiologists, biochemists, toxicologists, spectroscopists, analytical chemists, and forensic scientists working in industry, academia, or government settings in any of ninety countries make up its membership. AOAC's flagship publication is the authoritative *Official Methods of Analysis* (11.4). Another important publication is the *FDA Food Additives Analytical Manual* (*FAAM,* 11.26). Numerous other AOAC titles are described on the association's Web site.

Association for the Advancement of Medical Instrumentation (AAMI)
3330 Washington Boulevard
Arlington, VA 22201-4598 USA
703/525-4890 Fax: 703/525-1424
http://www.aami.org

Founded in 1967, the Association for the Advancement of Medical Instrumentation is active in the production of standards, recommended practices, and technical information reports related to medical devices. Its 7,000 members include clinical and biomedical engineers, physicians, nurses, hospital administrators, educators, and manufacturers. AAMI conferences focus on continuing education, and the association also offers a certification program for healthcare technical specialists. *Biomedical Instrumentation & Technology* is AAMI's peer-reviewed journal, and members also have exclusive access to a *Standards Monitor Online* database linked to the association's home page on the Internet. Other recent publications have addressed important regulatory topics, such as the CE mark, the EC Medical Devices Directives, and worldwide GMP compliance. A visit to the AAMI Web site will provide full details about publications, meetings, and government news affecting the medical device industry.

Association of Clinical Research Professionals (ACRP)
1012 14th Street NW, Suite 807
Washington, DC 20005 USA
202/737-8100 Fax: 202/737-8101
http://www.acrpnet.org

The Association of Clinical Research Professionals is an international society founded in 1976 to define, promote, and maintain professional standards and best practices in the fields of clinical research and development. Its 9,000 members come from diverse backgrounds in the biotechnology, medical device, and pharmaceutical industries, as well as contract research organizations (CROs) and regulatory agencies. Annual meetings feature educational programs that address topics of interest to clinical research site managers, investigators, coordinators, auditors, independent consultants, and members of Institutional Review Boards (IRBs). Since 1992, ACRP has sponsored a certification exam for clinical research coordinators; certification of clinical research associates dates from 1995.

Association of Natural Medicine Pharmacists
P.O. Box 150727
San Rafael, CA 94915-0727 USA
415/453-3534 Fax: 415/453-4963
http://www.anmp.org

The Association of Natural Medicine Pharmacists is the group that supplies answers to herbal questions published on the natural medicine page of *Pharmacy Times* online. The association's own Web site hosts a good bookstore of botanical titles and a useful hotlinked list of herbal medicine sites on the Internet.

Board of Pharmaceutical Specialties (BPS)
2215 Constitution Avenue NW
Washington, DC 20037-2985 USA
202/429-7591 Fax: 202/783-2351
http://www.bpsweb.org

The Board of Pharmaceutical Specialties was formed in 1976 on the recommendation of the American Pharmaceutical Association. Although housed at the same address as the APhA, the Board functions autonomously to provide an objective, independent process by which pharmacists can become accredited for demonstrating an advanced level of education, experience, knowledge, and skills in selected, highly specialized areas of practice. Board specialty certification in nuclear pharmacy began in 1978, followed by nutrition support pharmacy and pharmacotherapy (both recognized as separate specialties in 1988), psychiatric pharmacy (1992–), and oncology pharmacy (1996–). The BPS Web site provides an in-depth overview of requirements for the certification process and lists organizations worldwide that have officially recognized Board Certification.

British Pharmacological Society
The Medical College
Charterhouse Square
London EC1M 6BQ UK
71/982-6171 Fax: 71/982-6173
http://www.bphs.org.uk

The British Pharmacological Society is a multinational group, with its 2,200 members drawn from industry and academia in twenty countries. It publishes the *British Journal of Clinical Pharmacology* and the *British Journal of Pharmacology* (both monthly).

Canadian Pharmacists Association (CPhA)
Association des pharmaciens du Canada (APhC)
1785 Alta Vista Drive
Ottawa, Ontario K1G 3Y6 Canada
613/523-7877 Fax: 613/523-0445
http://www.cdnpharm.ca

Formerly known as the Canadian Pharmaceutical Association, the Canadian Pharmacists Association assumed its current name in August 1997. Like the APhA in the United States, CPhA works to improve the professional image of pharmacists and the quality of healthcare services. It monitors Canadian government policies and legislation and lobbies for the interests of its 10,900 members. CPhA publishes the *Compendium of Pharmaceuticals and Specialties* (*CPS*, 10.20), the *Compendium of Nonprescription Products* (10.21), the *Nonprescription Drug Reference for Health Professionals* (9.45), *Therapeutic Choices* (6.16), and the *Canadian Pharmaceutical Journal* (monthly). The CPhA home page on the Internet offers a new drug table containing information on products slated for publication in the next annual edition of the *CPS*.

Canadian Society for Pharmaceutical Sciences (CSPS)
Société canadienne des sciences pharmaceutiques
4120 Dentistry/Pharmacy Centre
University of Alberta Campus
Edmonton, Alberta T6G 2N8 Canada
780/492-0950 Fax: 780/492-0951
http://www.ualberta.ca/%7Ecsps

Established in 1996, the Canadian Society for Pharmaceutical Sciences draws its membership not only from academia, but also government agencies and industry. Its main mission is to foster a network of pharmaceutical scientists in Canada, to which end CSPS has initiated an electronic publication, the *Journal of Pharmacy and Pharmaceutical Sciences.*

Canadian Society of Hospital Pharmacists (CSHP)
Société canadienne des pharmaciens d'hôpitaux (SCPH)
1145 Hunt Club Road, Suite 350
Ottawa, Ontario K1V 0Y3 Canada
613/736-9733 Fax: 613/736-5660
http://www.cshp.ca

The 2,400-member Canadian Society of Hospital Pharmacists focuses on promoting the interests of institutional pharmacy practice, including evaluation and accreditation of postgraduate training programs through the Canadian Hospital Pharmacy Residency Board. Its publications include *Extemporaneous Oral Liquid Dosage Preparations* (6.40) and the bimonthly *Canadian Journal of Hospital Pharmacy.*

Controlled Release Society (CRS)
1020 Milwaukee Avenue, Suite 335
Deerfield, IL 60015 USA
847/808-7071 Fax: 847/808-7073
http://www.crsadmhdq.org

The mission of the Controlled Release Society is to advance the science and technology of chemical and biological delivery systems. Individuals and companies involved in the development of controlled release of marine antifoulants from rubber and in other agrochemical applications were the prime movers behind the formation of the Society in 1973. Since that time, the subject focus has expanded to include drug delivery applications in human and animal health, along with environmental and other industrial uses. Although headquartered in the Chicago area, the Controlled Release Society is an international organization with a European office in Geneva and 3,000 members located in any of forty-three countries around the world. Two-thirds of the membership is affiliated with industry and one-third with academia or government. The *Journal of Controlled Release* is an official publication of CRS.

European Society of Clinical Pharmacy (ESCP)
International Secretariat
Theda Manshottstraat 5b
2331 JE Leiden, The Netherlands
31/71 572-2430 Fax: 31/71 572-2431
http://www.escp.nl

The European Society of Clinical Pharmacy was founded in 1979 to provide a forum for communication of new developments in clinical pharmacy and to represent the interests of the profession to other international healthcare organizations. Members include clinical pharmacy practitioners, researchers, and educators from countries throughout Europe.

Food and Drug Law Institute (FDLI)
1000 Vermont Avenue, 12th Floor
Washington, DC 20005 USA
202/371-1420 Fax: 202/371-0649
http://www.fdli.org

Manufacturers and distributors of foods, drugs, cosmetics, and medical devices, as well as law firms, are among the 500 members of the Food and Drug Law Institute (formerly the Food Law Institute), a nonprofit educational organization founded in 1949. In addition to an annual conference held in cooperation with the U.S. Food and Drug Administration each December, the Institute sponsors numerous update meetings and training workshops throughout the year. FDLI also publishes the quarterly *Food and Drug Law Journal,* sometimes cited as the *Food Drug Cosmetic Law Journal* or *FDC Law Journal.* Other publications are described in full on the FDLI home page, which also includes links to member company sites and other useful legal or regulatory sources on the Internet.

Herb Research Foundation (HRF)
1007 Pearl Street, Suite 200
Boulder, CO 80302 USA
303/449-2265 Fax: 303/449-7849
http://www.herbs.org

As its name implies, the Herb Research Foundation supports investigations into the safety and benefits of medicinal plants and into developing related agribusiness both on the supply (horticulture) and outlet (new markets) side. Press relations and promoting public awareness are major activities of HRF, as a visit to its Web site will demonstrate. The foundation collaborates with the American Botanical Council in publishing *HerbalGram,* as well as producing, in its own right, a newsletter entitled *Herb Research News* and a consumer magazine, *Herbs for Health.*

Institute for Safe Medication Practices (ISMP)
300 West Street Road
Warminster, PA 18974-3236 USA
215/956-9181 Fax: 215/956-9266
http://www.ismp.org

The Institute for Safe Medication Practices is a nonprofit organization that provides an independent review of medication errors recorded through the national, voluntary Medication Errors Reporting Program (MERP) operated by the United States Pharmacopeial Convention. Information derived from this review is shared with both the FDA and pharmaceutical companies whose products are mentioned in reports. ISMP has also established a national advisory board of practitioners for consultation and education related to adverse drug events and their prevention.

International Academy of Compounding Pharmacists (IACP)
P.O. Box 1365
Sugar Land, TX 77487 USA
713/933-8400 Fax: 281/495-0602
http://www.compassnet.com/~iacp

IACP is an association of more than 1,000 pharmacists who compound customized medications in response to physician's requests and unique patient needs. Lobbying at the state legislative, as well as federal, level is a major objective, to ensure adequate provision for extemporaneous formulations in regulations regarding drugs and dispensing. The academy provides its members with a "Universal Claim Form for Compounded Medications" to assist patients in third party reimbursement. A monthly newsletter and a quarterly case report journal, *The Compounding Pharmacist,* are additional membership benefits. IACP's Web site is a good source for background on compounding issues and laws affecting practice.

International Society for Ethnopharmacology (ISE)
c/o Ulf Nyman, Treasurer
Department of Medicinal Chemistry, Pharmacognosy Section
School of Pharmacy, Universitetsparken 2
DK-2100 Copenhagen, Denmark
http://www.dfh.dk/staff/private/ulny/ISE

One of the chief attractions of membership in the International Society for Ethnopharmacology is a significantly reduced rate for subscribing to the highly respected *Journal of Ethnopharmacology.* Published by Elsevier since 1979, this publication is the official journal of ISE.

International Society for Pharmaceutical Engineering (ISPE)
3816 West Linebaugh Avenue, Suite 412
Tampa, FL 33624 USA
813/960-2105 Fax: 813/264-2816
http://www.ispe.org

Publishers of the bimonthly journal, *Pharmaceutical Engineering,* the International Society of Pharmaceutical Engineering includes pharmaceutical, biotechnological, medical device, diagnostic, and cosmetic engineers and technicians from any of forty countries among its 5,100 members. Such individuals are responsible for designing, supervising, and maintaining process equipment, systems, and instrumentation in manufacturing facilities for healthcare materials. In recent years, ISPE has been publishing a series of *Baseline® Guides* for design of facilities that will assist companies in regulatory compliance with good manufacturing practice (GMP) regulations. Titles issued thus far are described on the society's Web site.

International Society for Pharmacoeconomics and Outcomes Research (ISPOR)
20 Nassau Street, Suite 307
Princeton, NJ 08542 USA
609/252-1305 Fax: 609/252-1306
http://www.ispor.org

Formed in 1995, the International Society for Pharmacoeconomics and Outcomes Research is dedicated to the promotion of the practice and science of health outcomes assessment for the purpose of ensuring that society allocates healthcare resources (and expenditures) wisely and efficiently. Members include physicians, pharmacists, economists, nurses, and researchers from academia, industry, government, and managed care organizations. Member services, a calendar of forthcoming subject specialty conferences, and a directory of pharmacoeconomics and outcomes research educational programs are featured at the society's Web site. The *ISPOR Lexicon*™ (5.23) is this group's first publication.

International Society for Pharmacoepidemiology (ISPE)
2000 L Street NW, Suite 200
Washington, DC 20036 USA
202/416-1641 Fax: 202/833-3843
http://www.pharmacoepi.org

Pharmacoepidemiology is defined at ISPE's Web site as the science that applies epidemiological approaches to studying the use, effectiveness, value, and safety of pharmaceuticals. The International Society for Pharmaceutical Epidemiology was established to provide a forum for sharing knowledge in this emerging discipline. Thus far, the 1,100 members represent a variety of scientific specialty areas of practice and education, including epidemiology, biostatistics, medicine, veterinary science, nursing, pharmacology, pharmacy, law, health economics, and journalism. With national chapters in Belgium, Argentina, and the Netherlands (as well as the United States), ISPE demographic data show that 36% of members are employed in industry and 41% in academia and that their addresses span the globe, encompassing at least forty-five countries. The official journal of ISPE, *Pharmacoepidemiology and Drug Safety,* is published by John Wiley.

National Association of Boards of Pharmacy (NABP)
700 Busse Highway
Park Ridge, IL 60068 USA
708/698-6227
http://www.nabp.net

Members of NABP include boards of pharmacy in the fifty states; District of Columbia; Puerto Rico; Virgin Islands; the Canadian provinces of Alberta, Ontario, and British Columbia; and the states of Victoria and New South Wales in Australia. Founded in 1904, NABP is dedicated to promoting interstate reciprocity in licensure based upon uniform minimum standards of pharmaceutical education and legislation. Its publications include the *Model State Pharmacy Act* (4.29), an annual *Survey of Pharmacy Law* (4.31), and *NABLAW®* (4.32) on CD-ROM. NABP's Web site is described in Figure 4.6.

Parenteral Drug Association (PDA)
7500 Old Georgetown Road, Suite 620
Bethesda, MD 20814 USA
301/986-0293 Fax: 301/986-0296
http://www.pda.org

More than 9,000 individuals working in research, development, or manufacture of injectable drugs are members of the Parenteral Drug Association, which was founded in 1946. In addition to sponsoring research and educational programs and operating a placement service and speakers' bureau, the Association publishes the bimonthly *Journal of Pharmaceutical Science and Technology.* PDA's home page on the Internet includes the current issue's table of contents.

Pharmaceutical Education & Research Institute (PERI)
1616 North Fort Myer Drive, Suite 1430
Arlington, VA 22209 USA
703/276-0178 Fax: 703/276-0069
http://www.peri.org

PERI was originally established by the Pharmaceutical Manufacturers Association (now the Pharmaceutical Research and Manufacturers of America) in 1989 to provide scientific and technology training for employees of member companies. Since July 1995, the Pharmaceutical Education & Research Institute has operated as an independent not-for-profit corporation, able to open its courses to all interested parties. As a visit to PERI's Web site will demonstrate, the calendar of workshops is extensive. An Information Management Professional Development Group has been fostered by PERI since 1996 and has organized its own annual symposia featuring speakers and sessions of primary interest to library information professionals associated with the pharmaceutical industry.

The Royal Pharmaceutical Society of Great Britain
1 Lambeth High Street
London SE1 7JN UK
44/171 735 9141 Fax: 44/171 735 7629
http://www.rpsgb.org.uk:80
http://www.pharmpress.com

Since its formation in 1841 under the name The Pharmaceutical Society of Great Britain, this professional association has been granted a royal charter and an official change of name, in 1988, in recognition of its patronage by reigning British monarchs since 1937. By law, the Society is required to maintain the official *Annual Register of Pharmaceutical Chemists* (individuals legally qualified to practice pharmacy, 13.29) and the *Register of Premises* (the list of recognized pharmacies). Its membership, in consequence, is large, including more than 42,000 practitioners engaged in active community or hospital pharmacy practice. Among 34,000 members employed in England, 60% work in community settings, 15% in hospitals, and 5% in industry.

The Royal Pharmaceutical Society is a prolific publisher. Its periodicals include *The Pharmaceutical Journal, Hospital Pharmacist, Industrial Pharmacist, Agricultural and Veterinary Pharmacist, The Pharmacy Assistant,* and *The International Journal of Pharmacy Practice.* Under the imprint of The Pharmaceutical Press, an equally prodigious output of books has been maintained over many years. Better known titles include *Martindale: The Extra Pharmacopoeia (6.1), Clarke's Isolation and Identification of Drugs* (8.17–8.18), *The Pharmaceutical Codex* (11.3), the *British National Formulary* (10.22), *Non-prescription Medicines* (10.23), *Drug Interactions* (7.11), *Pharmacy Law and Ethics* (4.39), *Herbal Medicines, A Guide for Healthcare Professionals* (12.10), and *The Veterinary Formulary* (12.45). The Web site for The Pharmaceutical Press, hotlinked off the Royal Society's home page, is well worth visiting at least every six months to check for new publications of potential interest.

Society for Medicinal Plant Research
Gesellschaft für Arzneipflanzenforschung
c/o Dr. B. Frank, Secretary
Kneipp-Werke
Steinbachtal 43
D-97082 Würzburg, Germany
Fax: 49/931 8002 275
http://www.uni-duesseldorf.de/WWW/GA

Publishers of the bimonthly journal, *Planta Medica,* the Society for Medicinal Plant Research includes among its 850 members scientists from any of fifty-nine countries. It was organized in 1953 to serve as a forum for international information exchange and to act as a liaison with governments, pharmacopeial commissions, and international health organizations on matters pertaining to the medicinal plant field.

Society of Infectious Diseases Pharmacists (SIDP)
P.O. Box 140046
Austin, TX 78714-0046 USA
512/452-4521 Fax: 512/452-5255
http://sidp.hosp.utmck.edu

Founded in 1990, the Society of Infectious Diseases Pharmacists is an association dedicated to promoting appropriate use of antimicrobials. Members, who include both pharmacists and other healthcare professionals, are encouraged to become actively involved in national, state, and local organizations that are likely to influence regulatory developments in prevention and management of infectious diseases. Advanced education and training are a primary focus of the Society, which sponsors its own residency program and is seeking recognition of infectious diseases pharmacy practice as a separate area of expertise to be certified by the Board of Pharmaceutical Specialties (BPS). SIDP's annual meeting is traditionally held in conjunction with the Interscience Conference on Antimicrobial Agents and Chemotherapy.

Trade, Business, and Commercial Organizations

The distinction between professional and trade associations in the pharmaceutical sciences is admittedly blurred, with both types of organizations sharing many of the same members and some of the same goals: communication, information dissemination, lobbying with government officials, and continuing education. In general, however, trade associations are founded to further the interests of commercial enterprises. As a result, they tend to contribute fewer publications of interest to nonmembers.

American Nutraceutical Association (ANA)
4647T Highway 280 East, #133
Birmingham, AL 35242 USA
215/980-5710 Fax: 205/991-9302
http://www.americanutra.com

The American Nutraceutical Association was established in 1997 to develop and provide educational materials and continuing education programs for both healthcare professionals and consumers. Its focus is on dissemination of information about nutraceutical technology.

Association of the British Pharmaceutical Industry (ABPI)
12 Whitehall
London SW1A 2DY UK
44 (0)171-930-3477 Fax: 44(0)171-747-1411
http://www.abpi.org.uk

ABPI is a trade association of one than 100 manufacturers of prescription drugs. Its Web page links to Office of Health Economics (OHE) publications, including information about a *Health Economics Evaluations Database* (HEED) on CD-ROM, developed in cooperation with the International Federation of Pharmaceutical Manufacturers Associations. ABPI pointers to other Internet sites are judiciously selected, with an emphasis on regulatory agencies, including the EMEA. This association's home page is also a good source of facts and statistics about the UK pharmaceutical industry and drug development, as well as consumption.

Association of the European Self-Medication Industry (AESGP)
7 Avenue de Tervuren
B-1040 Brussels, Belgium
32/2 735 51 30 Fax: 32/2 735 52 22
http://www.aesgp.be

The Association of the European Self-Medication Industry is an umbrella organization of twenty-four national associations for manufacturers and distributors of nonprescription drugs. Founded in 1964, AESGP represents member interests to regulatory bodies worldwide and informs its European members about relevant developments taking place outside Europe with potential impact on the EC market. A complete list of both European and non-European member associations is available at the AESGP Web site, as is a bibliography of useful publications. Two of the latter are offered free of charge for immediate display in PDF format: *OTCs in Europe—1998 Facts and Figures* and *An Economic Analysis of Self-Medication.*

BioIndustry Association
15/15 Belgrave Square
London SW1X 8PS UK
44 (171) 565-7190 Fax: 44 (171) 565-7191
http://www.bioindustry.org

The Association for the Advancement of British Biotechnology was the predecessor organization of the present BioIndustry Association, which was formed in 1989. Members include pharmaceutical, agricultural, diagnostics, bioprocessing, gene therapy, and bioremediation companies, as well as patent lawyers, investment bankers, and venture capitalists. The BioIndustry Association's primary mission is lobbying in the United Kingdom and Europe on behalf of its industry members.

Biotechnology Industry Association (BIO)
1625 K Street NW, Suite 1100
Washington, DC 20006-1604 USA
202/857-0244 Fax: 202/857-0237
http://www.bio.org

The Biotechnology Industry Association, although relatively new (founded in 1993), numbers among its members more than 800 firms employing recombinant DNA, hybridomas, and immunological technologies in areas such as human health care (drugs, biologics, and medical devices), animal husbandry, and environmental or industrial chemical production. Biotechnology equipment manufacturers and service groups, as well as academic institutions and state biotechnology centers, are also affiliated with this group. Membership spans twenty-six nations and includes related organizations in any of forty U.S. states. Thus far, the association's focus has been on public relations and on providing information pertaining to regulations, patent protection, and financing to its members. BIO publishes a *Citizens' Guide to Biotechnology* for consumers and, through its Web site, provides a hotlinked guide to professionally oriented biotechnology journals and newsletters on the Internet.

Canadian Cosmetic, Toiletry and Fragrance Association (CCTFA)
420 Britainnia Road East, Suite 102
Mississauga, Ontario L4Z 3L5 Canada
905/890-5161 Fax: 905/890-2607
http://www.cctfa.ca

CCTFA is a trade association of more than 220 companies involved in the personal care products industry in Canada. Members are manufacturers and distributors of finished products, suppliers of ingredients or raw materials, and providers of packaging or other services used in production and marketing. The association concentrates on monitoring and interpreting regulatory developments, with the purpose of keeping members well informed and ensuring that government oversight activities are competitive and internationally harmonized. The CCTFA Web site provides an annotated list of the association's own publications, as well as important documents affecting the industry issued by Canada's Health Protection Branch. CCTFA titles include *A Guide to Canadian Regulatory Requirements* and a survey of *1996/1997 Sales of Cosmetic, Toiletry and Fragrance Products in Canada.*

Canadian Wholesale Drug Association (CWDA)
5255 Yonge Street, Suite 505
Toronto, Ontario M2N 6P4 Canada
416/222-3922 Fax: 416/222-8960
http://www.cwda.com

With a focus on supply chain management and logistics, the Canadian Wholesale Drug Association was established in 1964 to assist its membership in cost effective and efficient distribution of healthcare products in Canada. CWDA represents full service drug wholesalers or distributors, pharmaceutical and consumer health products manufacturers, and related specialty organizations. The association publishes regional profiles of statistical information consolidated from diverse sources, bringing together data on the distribution and consumption of healthcare goods and services in Canada. These *CWDA Industry Trend Reports* are supplemented, on an annual basis, with another summary publication entitled *CWDA Federal and Provincial Drug Benefit Programs.* The association also issues an *Industry Directory* each year.

Consumer Healthcare Products Association: *see* Nonprescription Drug
  Manufacturers Association

Cosmetic, Toiletry and Fragrance Association (CTFA)
1101 17th Street NW, Suite 300
Washington, DC 20036-4702 USA
202/331-1770 Fax: 202/331-1969
http://www.ctfa.org

Approximately 525 manufacturers and distributors of finished cosmetics, fragrances, and personal care products, as well as suppliers of raw materials and services, form the membership of this group. The CTFA focuses on providing scientific, legal, regulatory, and legislative services and coordinating public affairs and educational activities on behalf of members. A major contribution of this organization, both to the industry and to public health, has been sponsorship of independent cosmetic ingredient reviews since the 1970s. Results are published in the *CIR Compendium* (8.37). Other association publications include the *International Cosmetic Ingredient Dictionary and Handbook* (11.29), the *CTFA International Color Handbook* (11.30), the *CTFA Compendium of Cosmetic Ingredient Composition* (11.31), an annual *Who's Who Membership Directory* (13.14), and the *CTFA International Buyers' Guide* (13.15). The CTFA home page on the Internet provides an electronic edition of the *International Buyer's Guide,* free to all, and an informative catalog of industry-related publications.

Health Industry Manufacturers Association (HIMA)
1200 G Street NW, Suite 400
Washington, DC 20005-3814 USA
202/783-8700 Fax: 202/783-8750
http://www.HIMAnet.com

With a membership of more than 800 companies, HIMA represents manufacturers of nearly 90% of the U.S. and 60% of the world's medical devices, diagnostic products, and health information systems. The association's programs center on education and advocacy related to medical technology and regulatory issues. Its home page on the Internet includes immediately displayable files on key industry topics, such as reforming the product liability system or strengthening healthcare financing and delivery. HIMA publishes the *Medical Device Submissions Handbook* and the *Emerging Market Report.*

International Federation of Pharmaceutical Manufacturers Associations (IFPMA)
30 rue de St-Jean, P.O. Box 9
1211 Geneva 18, Switzerland
41 (22) 340 1200 Fax: 41 (22) 340 1380
http://www.ifpma.org

The International Federation of Pharmaceutical Manufacturers Associations aims to be the main channel of communication between the industry and the World Health Organization, the World Intellectual Property Organization (WIPO), and various United Nations agencies. It represents the interests of both research based and other producers of prescription drugs worldwide through a membership roster that includes regional and national industry associations, rather than individual companies. A visit to IFPMA's Web site will show that its major areas of activity are patent protection, quality assurance and harmonization of standards, self regulation within the industry, and health economics advisory.

Medical Device Manufacturers Association (MDMA)
c/o Stephen Northrup
1900 K Street NW, no. 100
Washington, DC 20006 USA
202/496-7150 Fax: 202/496-7756
http://www.medicaldevices.org

MDMA is a national trade association created in 1992 to represent the interests of member companies to Washington, through lobbying in the U.S. Congress, the FDA, and other federal agencies that develop or implement policies affecting the medical device industry. Members include nearly 130 independent manufacturers of devices, diagnostic products, and healthcare information systems.

Medical Devices Canada (MEDEC)
401 The West Mall, Suite 510
Etobicoke, Ontario M9C 5J5 Canada
416/620-1595 Fax: 416/620-1595
http://www.medec.org

National advocacy is the main mission of MEDEC, an organization of more than 100 companies that was founded in 1973. The association publishes a newsletter, *MEDEC Pulse,* ten times a year to digest its legislative and lobbying activities. It also issues a *Canadian Medical Device Industry Directory* on diskette, with profiles of 931 companies and 613 product listings.

National Association of Chain Drug Stores (NACDS)
413 North Lee Street
P.O. Box 1417-D49
Alexandria, VA 22313-1480 USA
703/549-3001 Fax: 703/836-4839
http://www.nacds.org

NACDS members include more than 160 chain drug firms and 1,000 associate members involved in manufacturing, distribution, publishing, advertising, and other support services. Taken together, the membership base is responsible for the operation of more than 31,000 community retail pharmacies in the United

States. The association interprets and disseminates information regarding government agency actions affecting retail trade, covering such topics as labor laws, excise taxes, and third party payment programs. The annual *NACDS Membership Directory* (13.26) is a guide not only to member firms, but also a listing of drug trade associations, state boards of pharmacy, state pharmaceutical associations, and accredited colleges of pharmacy. The NACDS Web site is a rich repository of industry statistics and fast facts at a glance.

National Association of Pharmaceutical Manufacturers (NAPM)
320 Old Country Road
Garden City, NY 11530-1752 USA
516/741-3699 Fax: 516/741-3696
http://www.napmnet.org

This trade group represents the regulatory and legislative interests of independent generic drug manufacturers and suppliers of bulk pharmaceutical chemicals in the United States. Chartered in 1955 as the Drug and Allied Products Guild, the National Association of Pharmaceutical Manufacturers assumed its current name in 1960. Membership is open to all manufacturers and distributors of finished dosage forms, human or veterinary, as well as producers of components, raw materials, and services. Companies focusing on cosmetic products, medical foods, and dietary supplements are also included among NAPM members.

National Community Pharmacists Association (NCPA)
205 Daingerfield Road
Alexandria, VA 22314-2885 USA
703/683-8200 Fax: 703/683-3619
http://www.ncpanet.org

The National Community Pharmacists Association has undergone several changes in name since its formation 100 years ago. Known until 1988 as the National Association of Retail Druggists, then simply as NARD, NCPA today is an organization of more than 30,000 owners and managers of independent pharmacies and pharmacists employed in them.

National Wholesale Druggists' Association (NWDA)
1821 Michael Farraday Drive
Reston, VA 22190-5348 USA
703/787-0000 Fax: 703/787-6930
http://www.nwda.org

The National Wholesale Druggists' Association is a trade organization that represents pharmaceutical and related healthcare product distributors with customers in the United States, Canada, Mexico, or Central and South America. Like its Canadian counterpart (CWDA), NWDA compiles and distributes statistics, sponsors research, and provides specialized education programs. Its committees focus on topics such as sales management, government relations, human resources, and pharmaceutical, as well as consumer products, marketing. The more than 450 members include wholesalers and manufacturers of drugs, toiletries, and sundries, together with advertising agencies. The association's Web site describes its publications in detail, including the *NWDA Industry Profile & Healthcare Fact Book.*

Nonprescription Drug Manufacturers Association (NDMA)
1150 Connecticut Avenue NW
Washington, DC 20036-4193 USA
202/429-9260 Fax: 202/223-6835
http://www.ndmainfo.org

Seventy-five manufacturers of nonprescription drugs form the nucleus of this group. Approximately 150 associate members include suppliers of goods and services to the industry, such as contract packagers and advertising agencies. Known until 1989 as The Proprietary Association, the Nonprescription Drug Manufacturers Association changed its name again, as approved by its membership at a national meeting in March 1999. The new name is the Consumer Healthcare Products Association (CHPA). Throughout its history, a major activity of the association has been obtaining and disseminating regulatory information to its constituency. Until recently, its efforts were focused on the ongoing FDA OTC Review process. NDMA now also represents the interests of its members to the FDA, the Federal Trade Commission, Congress, and state legislatures as the latter turn their scrutiny on the burgeoning dietary supplement industry (hence the name change).

The association's home page on the Internet is an excellent source of background information on OTC issues, such as Rx to OTC switches, labeling, and the movement in some states toward creation of a third class of OTC drugs that would be available only in pharmacies. An "OTC Facts & Figures" section of the Web site assembles a wealth of statistical data about self medication, including the size of the U.S. market and information about costs, consumer practices and perceptions, and answers to frequently asked questions. NDMA's home page also links to an up-to-date summary of the U.S. government's OTC Review, listing final, pending, and negative monographs and ingredient and claims reviews.

Nonprescription Drug Manufacturers Association of Canada (NDMAC)
1111 Prince of Wales Drive, Suite 406
Ottawa, Ontario K2C 3TC Canada
613/723-0777 Fax: 613/723-0779
http://www.ndmac.ca

The Nonprescription Drug Manufacturers Association of Canada represents makers of over-the-counter medicines. Founded in 1896, NDMAC endorses self regulation of the industry in areas such as environmentally responsible packaging and tamper-evident or child-resistant containers. It has also encouraged its members to provide information to *POISINDEX* to ensure adequate coverage of Canadian OTCs in the information system. The association launched a Web site in June 1997 and has made its *Self-Medication Digest* newsletter available online retrospective to 1995. The Internet home page is also used to disseminate-NDMAC's policy and position papers on issues such as direct-to-consumer advertising, drug scheduling in Canada, and the regulatory framework for natural health products.

Nutraceutical Network of Canada (NNC)
34 Hennessey Drive
Winnepeg, Manitoba R3P 1P8 Canada
204/469-1105 Fax: 204/489-9831
http://www.nnoc.com

The Nutraceutical Network of Canada was established in 1996 to provide a centralized coordinating base for the industry to exchange information and influence strategic alliances among companies, research centers, and hospitals or clinics. The network aims to further the interests of producers of products variously defined as nutraceuticals, functional foods, medical foods, and foods for special dietary use. Its stated functions are to assist companies in the development and formulation of such products, in evaluating health claims, and in obtaining regulatory approval. The NNC Web site also refers to developing and maintaining specialized databases, but these do not appear to be publicly available as yet.

Pharmaceutical Manufacturers Association of Canada (PMAC)
Association canadienne de l'industrie du médicament (ACIM)
302-1111 Prince of Wales Drive
Ottawa, Ontario K2C 3T2 Canada
613/727-1380 Fax: 613/727-1407
http://www.pmac-acim.org

PMAC-ACIM is a national organization representing sixty companies whose business is research, development, production, marketing, and servicing of original brand name Rx and professional nonprescription medications. The association's Web site provides information on patent laws protecting pharmaceutical products in Canada. It also offers hotlinks to provincial fact sheets compiling statistical information about markets across the nation and to a fact sheet highlighting drug approval times and other regulatory data. The PMAC-ACIM home page on the Internet is also a direct route to the association's *Annual Review* and to a valuable 116-page summary of prevalence, consequences, and health costs of non-compliance or inappropriate use of Rx medicines in Canada, supported by a bibliography of 348 references to the literature published from 1949 through 1995.

Pharmaceutical Research and Manufacturers of America (PhRMA)
1100 15th Street NW
Washington, DC 20005 USA
202/835-3400 Fax: 202/835-3562
http://www.phrma.org

The Pharmaceutical Research and Manufacturers of America is the name adopted in 1994 for the former Pharmaceutical Manufacturers Association (PMA). The pressures of proposed healthcare reforms brought this group to re-evaluate its overall mission and organizational structure in 1993–1994. PhRMA (pronounced "pharma") bylaws were altered to permit board representation for smaller companies and affiliate or associate members involved in research and the premanufacturing stages of drug development. Membership now includes about 100 manufacturers of ethical, trademarked pharmaceutical and biological products. Industry information professionals, once an active section within the PMA, were forced to seek a new home in affiliation with other national organizations, leading to the formation of information management groups within the Drug Information Association and the Pharmaceutical Education and Research Institute.

PhRMA's primary role is as a public policy advocate, representing industry interests in the priority areas of federal and state healthcare reform, post-GATT and NAFTA intellectual property issues, the European product registration system (EMEA), domestic marketplace and reimbursement policies, and strategic alliances with physician and patient activist groups. The PhRMA home page on the Internet is an outstanding source of industry statistics (see Chapter Thirteen). It also provides a selection of consumer oriented health guides, highlighted in Chapter Nine, and a mini-database of drugs in development (cited in Chapter Fifteen). Another Web site bonus is access to the *PhRMA Studies Database System.* This service enables free searches for bibliographic information on studies, reports, and journal articles related to the pharmaceutical industry.

World Self-Medication Industry (WSMI)
15 Sydney House
Woodstock Road
London W4 1DP UK
44/181 747 8709 Fax: 44/181 747 8711
http://www.ndmainfo/worldwideMed/03_01.html
http://www.who.int/ina-ngo/ngo/ngo172.htm

Founded in 1970 under the name World Federation of Proprietary Medicine Manufacturers, the World Self-Medication Industry is a nongovernmental organization accepted into official relations with the World Health Organization since 1977. WSMI members are national and regional associations located in any of fifty-one countries worldwide that represent manufacturers of nonprescription drugs. As of February 1999, this organization does not appear to have established its own Web site. The URLs given here supply additional information about WSMI's structure and activities.

E

Practicum Exercises: Suggested Answers

Practicum exercises are designed to provide readers with material for self evaluation and review. They can be answered without actual reference to hardcopy or online sources. However, where access to a reference collection is available, educators may wish to use these, or comparable queries, in hands-on exercises. Questions represent the kinds of requests typically encountered in settings where drug and pharmacy practice information is routinely provided, and have been selected to reinforce knowledge of specific resources, unique characteristics of these resources, terminology used in pharmaceutical queries, and other concepts covered in the text. The suggested answers emphasize a systematic problem solving approach and are intended to be informative, but not definitive. In some cases, answers point ahead to titles covered later in the *Guide,* to encourage future use as pathfinders.

Practicum 1

1. calcipotriene (kal si poe' try een)
   a. type of name—nonproprietary
   b. place in development process—This type of name usually indicates that a drug is in the clinical testing phase, or beyond.
   c. reliability as an access point—5. When it is available for a given drug at the time of publication, this is the type of name preferred in indexing by most pharmaceutical information sources. The only caution: drugs can have more than one nonproprietary name. For example, *calcipotriene* is a U.S. adopted name (USAN); in sources that prefer International Nonproprietary Names (INN) or British Approved Names (BAN), the same drug is indexed under the name *calcipotriol.*

2. 112965–21–6
   a. type of name—CAS registry number
   b. place in development process—When a registry number is the starting point in a query, its use often indicates that the compound is at an early (preclinical) stage of development. Authors generally prefer to use other names, when available.
   c. reliability as an access point—2. Outside the chemical literature, CAS RNs are not a preferred form of indexing (partly because a publisher must license the right to use them from CAS, and tracking them down for application in indexing can be expensive). You will need to locate alternative names to access many hardcopy sources or to conduct thorough surveys of the literature online.

3. decaderm
   a. type of name—proprietary or brand name
   b. place in development process—Late stages (phase III or beyond). Note: a drug is often assigned a brand name prior to actual launch, so a proprietary designation is not a reliable indicator of marketing status. See Figure 13.1 for a list of sources that can be used to determine if a drug has been approved for marketing in the United States.
   c. reliability as an access point—3 or 4 in hardcopy sources, 2 online. If the name is a brand name in use in the United States, it is more likely to be used as a cross reference to the nonproprietary name preferred in most hardcopy sources than a non-U.S. brand name would be. Brand names are infrequently indexed in online databases.

4. MDL 73,945
   a. type of name—laboratory code or investigational drug number
   b. place in development process—Early, preclinical stages
   c. reliability as an access point—3 or 4. Of the three types of names used for drugs in their early stages of development (chemical names, CAS RNs, or lab codes), lab codes are usually preferred in indexing. They are easier to find in online database indexing than in hardcopy sources. Beware of possible variations in entry format (e.g., MDL 73945, MDL73,945) and in alpha-numeric placement in indexes (some hardcopy sources ignore the alphabetical portion of codes in sequencing/sorting).

5. (2) 9-[[hydroxy-1-(hydroxymethyl)ethoxy]methyl]guanine
   a. type of name—chemical
   b. place in development process—If the starting point in a query is a chemical name, the drug is probably still in the earliest stages of investigation—and may be difficult to find.
   c. reliability as an access point—1. You will need to locate alternative names

for accessing most hardcopy compendia and online resources, where chemical names are rarely preferred as index terms and can appear in a variety of formats. Authors often avoid referring to drugs by their chemical names. They are long and cumbersome to use, and they also reveal too much information about a compound (competition dictates discretion in early disclosure of study results by individuals affiliated with corporations).

6. $C_9H_{12}N_5NaO_4$
   a. type of name—molecular or empirical formula
   b. place in development process—Early
   c. reliability as an access point—2. Although many publications index formulas and include them in product descriptions, they are not necessarily unique identifiers. Alternative names are preferred starting points when initiating a literature search.

7. anxiolytic
   a. type of name—therapeutic classification or category
   b. place in development process—Not applicable; drug category terms provide no indication of developmental status.
   c. reliability as an access point—4. Many hardcopy sources index drugs by therapeutic use or indication terms. However, it may be necessary to locate synonymous terms before relevant material can be located (e.g., antianxiety agents).

8. angiotensin-converting enzyme inhibitor
   a. type of name—pharmacological action classification
   b. place in development process—not applicable (see above)
   c. reliability as an access point—4. Several hardcopy sources index drugs by their mechanism of action. This type of name is somewhat less reliable as an access point online, because not all literature indexes consistently describe drugs in this way.

9. antihypertensive
   a. type of name—therapeutic descriptor
   b. place in development process—not applicable
   c. reliability as an access point—4

10. adrenocorticoid steroid
    a. type of name—chemical classification
    b. place in development process—not applicable
    c. reliability as an access point—3. Compared to therapeutic or pharmacological classification terminology, chemical descriptive terms are less frequently used in indexing.

Practicum 2

1. Is Vitamin D ever used for topical treatment of leg ulcers? If so, what is the recommended dosage and concentration?
   a. sources (in order of priority)—*Martindale* (6.1), *AHFS Drug Information* (6.4), *DRUGDEX* (6.14), *USP DI Volume 1* (6.5), *Drug Facts and Comparisons* (6.2)
   b. rationale—The way in which the question is phrased implies that the requester is unfamiliar with this use of vitamin D. Consultation of sources that discuss both off-label (unapproved) and approved indications may, therefore, save time, and a follow-up request for background bibliography should, perhaps, be anticipated. *Martindale* is a good first choice, because of its international scope, coverage of both prescription and nonprescription products, and provision of back-up bibliography with brief abstracts. *AHFS Drug Information* and *DRUGDEX* would be second in order of priority, due to their more limited scope (fewer therapies covered, with emphasis on Rx drugs) and U.S. orientation. If this indication is, however, discussed in all three sources, *AHFS* and *DRUGDEX* are more likely to give actual dosage and concentration data. In *Martindale,* these facts may only be available through consultation of cited references, should the therapy prove to be not widely accepted. *AHFS* and *DRUGDEX* routinely provide full details regarding dosage for both off-label and approved indications, backed up with literature references (*AHFS* references omitted in the hardcopy volume are available for immediate display in its online counterpart *Drug Information Fulltext,* 14.18). Remaining sources on the candidate list cover both approved and off-label indications, but omit substantive back-up bibliography. *Drug Facts and Comparisons* has the advantage of extensive OTC product coverage, but does not always include dosage information for investigational uses.

2. Does Brand X toothpaste contain any alcohol?
   a. sources—*Nonprescription Products: Formulations and Features* (6.7), package labeling
   b. rationale—If package labeling does not indicate alcohol content, consulting *Nonprescription Products: Formulations and Features* may save a time-consuming telephone call to the manufacturer. Dentifrices are notoriously difficult subjects for ready-reference inquiries, because they may not be classified as drugs.

3. In the state of Connecticut, can syringes or injection needles be sold outside a pharmacy?
   a. sources (in order of priority)—*Pharmacy Law Digest* (4.30), state board of pharmacy
   b. rationale—*Pharmacy Law Digest* will definitely answer this question and

will not be dependent on the sometimes limited operating hours and staffing of the state board of pharmacy. Other sources of pharmacy law, such as NABP's *Survey of Pharmacy Law* (4.31) or the *USP DI Special State Supplement* (4.33) are less likely to contain detailed information of this type.

4. What is MO-911? Find the first reference to this name.
   a. sources (in order of priority)—*Unlisted Drugs* (3.8), *Martindale* (6.1), *USP Dictionary of USAN* (3.1), *Merck Index* (3.5), *Index Nominum* (3.7)
   b. rationale—Sources listed can all help identify what looks like an investigational drug number, but *Unlisted Drugs* is the only one that supplies references to where names are found and endeavors to provide the earliest listing. Among remaining titles listed, *Martindale* takes precedence for identification purposes, because of its product, versus single-entity substance, approach.

5. A community pharmacist needs to identify a U.S. source for wild cherry bark extract.
   a. sources (in order of priority)—*The Red Book* (3.15)
   b. rationale—*The Red Book* lists many ingredients likely to be required for compounding medications extemporaneously. *The Red Book*'s dictionary arrangement does, however, lack thorough cross referencing from alternative names or permutation of entries, so you may need to look under both C and W to find all available suppliers.

6. Is tolnaftate sodium soluble in alcohol?
   a. sources—*Merck Index* (3.5), *Martindale* (6.1), *Remington's Pharmaceutical Sciences* (6.52)
   b. rationale—Titles listed consistently supply solubility data, and the first two are international in scope.

7. Is paregoric a controlled substance? If so, on what schedule does it appear?
   a. sources (in order of priority)—*Drug Facts and Comparisons* (6.2), *The Red Book* (3.15)
   b. rationale—These two sources have been singled out among those that supply controlled substance data because they cover both prescription and nonprescription products. Indexing and ease of use dictate the priority accorded each. Note: By itself, paregoric is on federal schedule III; as an ingredient in combination products, many of which are sold over-the-counter, paregoric is on schedule V.

8. Has mistletoe ever been used therapeutically? Find supportive references, if possible.
   a. sources—*Martindale* (6.1)
   b. rationale—*Martindale* offers extensive coverage of herbal preparations,

past and present, and includes citations to the primary literature. Pharmacognosy resources discussed in Chapter Twelve and Fourteen could also
provide an answer, including pre-1960 editions of the *Dispensatory of the
United States.*

9. When was Brand Y reformulated?
   a. sources (in order of priority)—*American Drug Index* (3.6), *Physicians'
      Desk Reference* (6.10), *Diogenes* (16.1)
   b. rationale—A retrospective search of previous annual editions of *American
      Drug Index* will answer this question. Previous editions of the *PDR* would
      be a second choice, because the latter is more selective in its coverage of
      products on the U.S. market. *Diogenes,* an online database alluded to in
      Chapter Four and discussed in more detail in Chapter Sixteen, lists all drug
      approvals since 1938. A search in *Diogenes* for NDA authorizations asso-
      ciated with the brand name would quickly uncover the answer. If the prod-
      uct is fairly well known, reformulation would have been noted in industry
      newsletters, such as *The Pink Sheet* (4.49, 15.10).

10. What sugar-free laxatives are available? Which is the least expensive?
    a. sources (in order of priority)—*Drug Facts and Comparisons* (6.2), *Non-
       prescription Products: Formulations and Features* (6.7)
    b. rationale—*Facts and Comparisons* will answer both parts of this question,
       with its tables of Rx and OTC drugs arranged by therapeutic class, consis-
       tent identification of sugar-free preparations, and "cost index" (a relative,
       rather than actual, price indicator) feature. *Nonprescription Products: For-
       mulations and Features* is more selective in the number of products cov-
       ered and omits cost data. (Once products are located, prices could be found
       by consulting *The Red Book,* 3.15.)

11. Can a pharmacist legally fill a foreign prescription order, if it turns out to be
    for a product that is sold over-the-counter in the United States?
    a. sources—*Pharmacy Law Digest* (4.30)
    b. rationale—As was seen in question #3, answers to detailed questions re-
       lated to laws governing pharmacy practice in the United States are more
       likely to be found in *Pharmacy Law Digest* than in any other source. *The
       Digest* notes, in this case, that a pharmacist can sell the product in its origi-
       nal manufacturer's packaging, but cannot dispense and label it as in ful-
       fillment of the prescription.

12. What are some bases for hydrophilic ointments?
    a. sources (in order of priority)—*Remington's Pharmaceutical Sciences*
       (6.52)
    b. rationale—*Remington's* is a good source for traditional compounding and
       "pharmaceutical necessity" information. Web sites with compounding in-

formation, identified in Figure 6.1, could also be consulted for a choice of vehicles used in water soluble ointments.

13. Has OTC antacid Z been associated with photosensitivity reactions?

a. sources (in order of priority)—*Handbook of Clinical Drug Data* (6.19), Drug Information Handbook (6.20), *Drug Facts and Comparisons* (6.2), *The Red Book* (3.15)

b. rationale—Handbooks are designed for quick reference access to information of this type. *Drug Facts and Comparisons,* with its extensive coverage of nonprescription products, is another possible source. *The Red Book*'s Clinical Reference Section lists a selection of drugs that induce photosensitivity. (The product's package insert or labeling might also note the possibility of such a reaction.) Looking ahead to consumer oriented sources, *The Essential Guide to Prescription Drugs* (9.14) includes a table on "drug-light interactions," and *The Informed Consumer's Pharmacy* (9.29) also tabulates drugs associated with photosensitivity reactions.

14. A group of researchers need to know if their animal testing facilities are suitable for conducting preclinical investigations under contract to a pharmaceutical manufacturer preparing for an IND.

a. sources (in order of priority)—Title 21 of the *Code of Federal Regulations* (4.25), *Food Drug Cosmetic Law Reports* (4.26)

b. rationale—*21CFR* compiles all federal regulations promulgated by the FDA and will contain information on how to submit credentials for qualification, what types of test protocols are required, and other details. Because the *Code* is poorly indexed in hardcopy format, consulting *Food Drug Cosmetic Law Reports* would be helpful in locating the correct *CFR* citations. The *Reports* would also paraphrase the more formal language of *21CFR* and indicate if relevant sections have been affected by subsequent *Federal Register* (4.24) notices. Title 21 is also available in both online and CD-ROM format.

15. Where might a consumer find comparative information on diaper rash products?

a. sources (in order of priority)—*Handbook of Nonprescription Drugs* (6.6), *Nonprescription Products: Formulations and Features* (6.7), *Zimmerman's Complete Guide to Nonprescription Drugs* (9.15)

b. rationale—The latter two sources provide comparative information in chart form, but the *Handbook of Nonprescription Drugs* also includes textual discussion of product characteristics to look for and precautions involving treatment. Although intended to assist pharmacists in OTC medication counseling, the *Handbook* is easily understood by many lay readers. *Zimmerman's Guide,* to be discussed in more detail in Chapter Nine, is one of the few consumer oriented hardcopy references that focuses on OTC product comparisons.

16. Where can I find pronunciations of drug names?
    a. sources (in order of priority)—*USP Dictionary of USAN* (3.1), *American Drug Index* (3.6), *British Approved Names* (3.3), *Drug Information Handbook* (6.20), *Mosby's Nursing Drug Reference* (6.64), *Pediatric Dosage Handbook* (6.31), *Infectious Diseases Handbook* (6.46)
    b. rationale—The *USP Dictionary* will provide the most extensive listing of nonproprietary names and their pronunciation, although phonetic guidelines are included only in monographs for USAN and not for International Nonproprietary and other names indexed. *American Drug Index* would list fewer drugs, focusing on what is currently on the market (or about to be) in the United States. *British Approved Names,* also more selective in scope than the *USP Dictionary,* is issued only every four years. Remaining titles on the list offer narrower coverage, as well. Other sources with pronunciations are identified in the index and include: *USP DI Volume 2—Advice for the Patient* (9.1), *The Essential Guide to Prescription Drugs* (9.14), and *The PDR Family Guide to Prescription Drugs* (9.24).

17. A pharmacist needs to know if a scheduled drug can be sent through the U.S. postal service for intrastate delivery to the patient for whom it was prescribed.
    a. sources—*Pharmacy Law Digest* (4.30), *Survey of Pharmacy Law* (4.31), *USP DI Special State Supplement* (4.33)
    b. rationale—Regulations regarding prescription mailing are covered in pharmacy law sources.

18. A hospital pharmacist has been asked to investigate the possibility of preparing an oral preparation intended for adults in an alternative form for administration to a child, either orally or intravenously.
    a. sources (in order of priority)—*Pediatric Drug Formulations* (6.38), *Handbook on Extemporaneous Formulations* (6.39), *Extemporaneous Oral Liquid Dosage Preparations* (6.40)
    b. rationale—Since less than half of drugs marketed today are actually approved by the FDA with specific indications for use in children, preparing suitable dosage forms and dilutions is the pharmacist's responsibility. All three of the sources cited address this critical area of extemporaneous formulation, but the first is the only one that provides information on both oral and IV preparation, supported with references to stability studies. ASHP's *Handbook on Extemporaneous Formulations* and the CSHP's handbook (6.40) are limited to oral suspensions and liquids only, covering fifty-one and 139 formulations, respectively.

19. A law firm needs to find out what companies marketed Drug B in tablet form in 1980. What were the approved indications and dosage?
    a. sources—*Physicians' Desk Reference* (6.10), *American Drug Index* (3.6)

b. rationale—1980 editions of the *PDR* or *American Drug Index* would assist in answering the first part of this question; the *PDR* would be unlikely to include as complete a listing as would *ADI*, but the latter does not usually include dosage data. This question points to the need for long range planning in collection development and maintenance to support drug information service. Where space permits, retaining back volumes of selected drug compendia anticipates such inquiries; see Appendix A for a list of titles recommended for retention. Two online databases discussed later in the *Guide, IMSworld Product Monographs* (15.19) and *Diogenes* (16.1), would also be possible sources to help answer this question.

Practicum 3

1. A physician wants to know if a child will suffer ill effects from eating the contents of a four-ounce jar of vanishing cream.
   a. sources—*POISINDEX* (8.10), *Clinical Toxicology of Commercial Products* (8.8), *Martindale* (6.1)
   b. rationale—*Clinical Toxicology of Commercial Products* has a general formula section that could help answer this question, as would *POISINDEX*. Don't forget that pharmacology and therapeutics resources covered earlier in this *Guide,* such as *Martindale,* include selected poisoning information.

2. What is the LD_{50} for Drug X?
   a. sources—*RTECS* (8.33, 14.28), *POISINDEX* (8.10), *The Merck Index* (3.5)
   b. rationale—The *Registry of Toxic Effects of Chemical Substances (RTECS)* typically offers at least one LD_{50} in its entries. The Merck Index is another readily available quick-reference source for toxic values of chemical substances. Route of administration and subject (animal) population are needed when conveying an LD_{50}.

3. Will tricyclic antidepressants, Brand ABC in particular, interact with antihistamines?
   a. sources—Horn and Hansten's *Drug Interactions* (7.8), *Drug Interactions Facts* (7.10)
   b. rationale—Both sources index interactions by drug classes and selected brand names. Stockley's *Drug Interactions* (7.11) includes tables cross referencing brand and generic names, but its back-of-the-book indexing omits proprietary designations, except for combination products. *Evaluations of Drug Interactions* (7.9) does not offer brand name access.

4. Could oral amoxycillin at a dosage of two milligrams twice a day cause a false reading in a bilirubin test?

a. sources—Young's *Effects of Drugs on Clinical Laboratory Tests* (7.29), Salway's *Drug-Test Interaction Handbook* (7.30)

b. rationale—Both Young and Salway provide thoroughly researched compilations of drug-laboratory test interference data, documenting both *in vivo* and *in vitro* modifications. *Meyler's* (7.1) and other side effects/interactions sources index drug-induced test modifications more selectively.

5. Is the fruit of the weeping fig poisonous?

a. sources—*POISINDEX* (8.10), *The AMA Handbook of Poisonous and Injurious Plants* (8.49)

b. rationale—Because *POISINDEX* bases its coverage on reported incidents from poison control centers nationwide, a commonly cultivated house plant such as the weeping fig is likely to be covered. Two Web sites identified in Figure 8.2 are other possible sources: *The Canadian Poisonous Plants Information System* and the U.S. Army's *Guide to Poisonous and Toxic Plants*. This question is unusual, however, in that the weeping fig has not been documented to bear fruit in typical household or office conditions.

6. In what percentage of patients is nausea a side effect of Drug Y?

a. sources—*Drug Facts and Comparisons* (6.2), *PDR Generics* (6.8), *USP DI* (6.5)

b. rationale—*Drug Facts and Comparisons* often contains statistical data on the incidence of adverse effects, and *PDR Generics* or *USP DI* may also give this information. *Meyler's* (7.1) and *Martindale* (6.1) less frequently present data in this way.

7. A public health nurse needs to know how long syringes prepared for administration of a given medication can be stored by a home-bound patient, if cloudiness detected in the week-old preparation indicates "spoilage," and what storage conditions (temperature, light exposure) are recommended.

a. sources—*Handbook on Injectable Drugs* (7.31), *Sterile Dosage Forms* (7.32)

b. rationale—These are the kinds of inquiries Trissel's *Handbook on Injectable Drugs* is designed to answer. Turco's *Sterile Dosage Forms* is also likely to yield needed information, but its textbook format sometimes requires more time to consult.

8. Have collagen wound dressings been associated with congenital anomalies?

a. sources—*Catalog of Teratogenic Agents* (8.23), *Chemically Induced Birth Defects* (8.24)

b. rationale—Among teratogenicity sources discussed in Chapter Eight, Shepard's *Catalog* offers the most extensive coverage of nondrug substances (e.g., candle wax, cocoa powder, spray adhesives). Compared to Shepard, entries in Schardein's *Birth Defects* also tend to be much more cryptic and less immediately informative, without consultation of references cited.

9. What are the clinical signs of Brand X overdose, and how should it be treated?
   a. sources—*POISINDEX* (8.10), *Poisoning & Drug Overdose* (8.1), *Poisoning & Toxicology Handbook* (8.2), package insert, manufacturer
   b. rationale—*POISINDEX* is the most comprehensive source to answer a brand name question of this type. Where *POISINDEX* is not available, handbooks are a good place to start, along with information provided in package inserts and obtained through telephoning the manufacturer.

10. Can shoe polish (brand name unknown) cause a dermatological reaction?
    a. sources—*POISINDEX* (8.10), *Clinical Toxicology of Commercial Products* (8.8)
    b. rationale—General formulation queries can be difficult to answer, but both of the sources cited contain information of this type. However, both also focus on clinical toxicity data, and the skin reaction under scrutiny, unlikely to be an emergency situation, may not be discussed. Follow-up consultation of abstracting and indexing sources may be needed, and a search of online services would be the quickest way to accomplish this (see Chapter Fourteen). The strategy could begin with the general term "shoe polish" and be enhanced with specific ingredient terms located through general formulation indexes.

Practicum 4

1. Is there a U.S. equivalent of *Dopom* tablets, a combination OTC sleep aid last purchased in Europe by the patient?
   a. sources (in order of priority)—*Martindale* (6.1), *Unlisted Drugs* (3.8), *Drug Facts and Comparisons* (6.2), *American Drug Index* (3.6), *Nonprescription Products: Formulations and Features* (6.7)
   b. rationale—Even when a country or general locale is known, the most efficient starting point in foreign drug identification is an international, English-language source. *Martindale* is not only a worldwide product identification directory, but has the advantage of covering both prescription and nonprescription medications, both combinations and single entities. *Unlisted Drugs* is similar in the breadth of its coverage, but does not list U.S. equivalents (*Martindale* sometimes provides a starter list). Once ingredients are identified in either source, comparable products on the U.S. market can be located in *Drug Facts and Comparisons, American Drug Index,* or *Nonprescription Products: Formulations and Features.* Each covers OTC remedies, indexed by active ingredients. *Facts* is the most up-to-date

of the three (provided that the monthly looseleaf, rather than annual hardbound, edition is consulted). *Nonprescription Products* is more selective in its coverage and less frequently updated. Beyond ingredients and their relative quantities, other data that must be checked for equivalency are dosage form, strength, and OTC (versus Rx) status.

2. A patient is admitted to the hospital with white tablets, imprinted "0260" and scored on one side, in his possession. Identify the tablets.
    a. sources (in order of priority)—*IDENTIDEX* (10.1), *DrugPics* (10.2), *Ident-A-Drug Reference* (10.7), *American Drug Index* (3.6), *National Drug Code Directory* (10.9)
    b. rationale—The most extensive and up-to-date index of U.S. dosage form imprints is *IDENTIDEX*. *DrugPics* and the *Ident-A-Drug Reference* are more selective in scope. Because 0260 resembles a company identifier from the National Drug Code, checking the NDC directory in the back of the annual *American Drug Index* or consulting the *National Drug Code Directory* may be worthwhile, if other sources fail.

3. A market research company needs a list of community pharmacies in Rhode Island.
    a. sources—*The Hayes Druggist Directory* (13.22)
    b. rationale—Among retail trade directories discussed in Chapter Thirteen, *The Hayes Druggist Directory* lists all retail pharmacies in the United States, conveniently organized by state and city. Other directories distinguish between independent and chain store outlets.

4. What was the prescription volume of antihypertensive medications in the United States in 1985, 1990, and 1995?
    a. sources—The National Prescription Audit, *Drug Topics, Pharmacy Times*
    b. rationale—The National Prescription Audit (available only to subscribers) tabulates data by therapeutic class and includes time series summaries. However, the trade magazines *Drug Topics* and *Pharmacy Times* typically report Audit statistics on numbers of retail prescriptions by classes of drugs, usually published in April issues each year. Because antihypertensives are a particularly lucrative segment of the market, reports prepared by individual companies, investment analysts, or market research and consulting firms are also likely to include data needed. Searching online databases such as *Investext* (15.38) or *IAC PROMT* (15.35), discussed later in the *Guide,* will supplement trade press extracts from the National Prescription Audit, when access to the latter is not available.

5. Where can a chemist obtain sulfonyldioxide?
    a. sources—*Chem Sources* (13.5–13.7), *OPD Chemical Buyers Guide* (13.5)
    b. rationale—These directories are well known for their extensive listings of

suppliers of bulk chemicals for laboratory or industrial use. *Chem Sources* is also available online (15.27, 15.28).

6. What is the address of Tutag Pharmaceuticals?
   a. sources (in order of priority)—*Martindale* (6.1), *American Drug Index* (3.6), *The Red Book* (3.15)
   b. rationale—Consultation of an international directory will save time. Martindale includes a list of pharmaceutical companies worldwide. Because they include both Rx and OTC suppliers and many smaller U.S. generic drug manufacturers, directories in the *American Drug Index* and *The Red Book* are more extensive in scope than those in sources such as *Mosby's GenRx* (6.3) or *PDR Generics* (6.8). Although other directories are discussed in Chapter Thirteen, many standard drug identification sources offer listings sufficient for locating addresses of most manufacturers.

7. Where can I find a list of U.S. pharmacy schools and their admission requirements?
   a. sources—*Accredited Professional Programs of Colleges and Schools of Pharmacy* (13.40), *Graduate Programs in the Pharmaceutical Sciences* (13.41), *Roster of Faculty and Professional Staff* (13.39)
   b. rationale—Although all sources listed identify accredited degree providers, the AACP's directory of *Graduate Programs* also provides data for comparative analysis of schools and their admission requirements.

8. Locate a commercial source for a tablet press (machine) in the Northeast.
   a. source—*DCI Directory Issue* (13.17)
   b. rationale—*Drug and Cosmetic Industry*'s directory issue is, essentially, a catalog of equipment and supplies. It includes sources of tablet presses and punches.

9. What are the official guidelines for assaying ethylparaben?
   a. sources—*USP/NF* (11.8)
   b. rationale—Official assay guidelines applicable in this country are published in the *United States Pharmacopeia/National Formulary.*

10. What was the sales volume of prophylactics in community pharmacies each year from 1990 forward?
    a. sources—*Drug Topics*
    b. rationale—Each year the trade magazine *Drug Topics* reports consumer spending for nondrug products sold in community pharmacies. Prophylactics is one of the categories tabulated. This source is indexed in *International Pharmaceutical Abstracts* (14.8) and *IAC Trade & Industry Database* (15.36) online, access to which may be the easiest way to conduct a retrospective search for data needed. The IAC database may even include the complete text of the *Drug Topics* annual surveys.

11. Where can I find recommendations for medicines that should be on hand in the average household?

   a. sources—*Patient Drug Facts* (9.40), *Dr. Koop's Community: The Medicine Cabinet, Columbia University College of Physicians & Surgeons Complete Home Medical Guide—Chapter 34,* and APhA's *Pharmacy and You* Web site

   b. rationale—Appendices in *Patient Drug Facts* include a list of necessary household medicines. Three of the Web sites discussed in Chapter Nine and listed here also provide sections on stocking the home medicine cabinet.

12. Can you tell me which of these nonprescription products I'm considering contains ingredients that used to be available only by prescription?

   a. sources—*Zimmerman's Complete Guide to Nonprescription Drugs* (9.15)

   b. rationale—This source includes a cumulative list of ingredients switched from Rx to OTC status as a result of FDA reviews, numbering more than 400 substances as of 1992. *Diogenes* (6.1) also flags Rx to OTC switches in its product approval records online (see Figure 16.1).

13. We need to contact all academic librarians with responsibility for collections supporting pharmacy colleges.

   a. sources—*Roster of Faculty and Professional Staff* (13.39).

   b. rationale—Staff lists in AACP's annual *Roster* include both members and nonmembers and identify librarians at accredited institutions. Entries include position, degrees, and direct-dial telephone numbers.

14. Who can supply extracts from coneflowers and arnica, as well as "No leaf" and kukui nut oil, appropriate for use in cosmetic formulations?

   a. sources (in order of priority)—*DCI Directory Issue* (13.17), *Cosmetic Bench Reference* (11.32), *CTFA International Buyers' Guide* (13.15)

   b. rationale—The July *Directory* Issue of the trade journal *Drug & Cosmetic Industry* includes a raw material supplier list identifying many natural products, such as herb and plant extracts. The *Cosmetic Bench Reference* offers fewer listings for these types of ingredients. *CTFA's Buyers' Guide* is accessible free of charge on the Internet.

15. Where will I find a drug photo identification aid that is arranged by color and size, rather than product name or company?

   a. sources—*Patient Drug Facts* (9.40), *Nurses Drug Facts* (6.62), *The AMA Guide to Prescription and Over-the-Counter Drugs* (9.5), *AARP Pharmacy Service Prescription Drug Handbook* (9.6), *American Druggist's Complete Family Guide to Prescriptions, Pills, and Drugs* (9.7)

   b. rationale—These sources organize their photo identification sections by color and size, as was discussed in the photographic inserts section of Chapter Ten.

16. How many students are enrolled in doctoral programs in pharmacognosy in the United States, and how many have obtained degrees in this discipline in the past five years?

    a. sources—*Profile of Pharmacy Students* (13.44)

    b. rationale—The AACP compiles information on degrees conferred and enrollment each year in its *Profile of Pharmacy Students.*

17. In what percentage of hospitals are IV admixture programs pharmacy based? Are data available to show growth or decline in such services in the past decade?

    a. sources—*American Journal of Health-System Pharmacy* (formerly *American Journal of Hospital Pharmacy*)

    b. rationale—The ASHP conducts annual surveys of hospital pharmacy practice in the United States, gathering data on a variety of services (among which IV admixture programs may be included). Results have been published in the Society's *Journal* since 1987. Data were also published in the *Journal* from surveys conducted in 1975, 1978, 1982, and 1985. Current and retrospective indexing provided in *International Pharmaceutical Abstracts* online (14.8) would make answering this question fairly easy.

18. Where can a consumer find a discussion of nutritional supplements, with a comparison of multivitamin products?

    a. sources—*Handbook of Nonprescription Drugs* (6.6), *Nonprescription Products: Formulations and Features* (6.7), *The PDR Family Guide to Nutrition and Health* (9.26), *Drug Facts and Comparisons* (6.2)

    b. rationale—*The Handbook of Nonprescription Drugs* provides a thorough discussion of such supplements, complemented with comparison tables for multivitamins, iron, and calcium products in its companion volume *Nonprescription Products: Formulations and Features* (6.7). Although intended to assist pharmacists in medication counseling, the *Handbook*'s language and writing style are sufficiently clear to benefit many consumers. Among sources specifically developed for patient education, *The PDR Family Guide to Nutrition and Health* offers focused coverage of the topic. *Drug Facts and Comparisons* includes an extensive chart for comparison of multivitamin ingredients and relative cost, but its discussion is written for healthcare professionals. Two Internet sources highlighted in Chapter Nine would also be good choices. *MotherNature.com,* in its consumer guide and health encyclopedia sections, offers comparative information on nutritional supplements. The *E-Pharmacy by Eckerd: OTC Resource Center* also features a segment on dietary supplement selection.

19. A patient planning an extended trip to Europe wants to know equivalents of Drug X marketed abroad.

    a. sources—*Drug Facts and Comparisons* (6.2), *Mosby's GenRx* (6.3), *PDR*

Generics (6.8), *USP DI* (6.5), *Martindale* (6.1), *Index Nominum* (3.7), *Merck Index* (3.5)

b. rationale—Consultation of any of the first four sources listed is a logical first step in answering this query, in order to locate current product formulation, indications, and dosage form. The monthly looseleaf edition of *Facts* is the most up-to-date resource and lists both prescription and nonprescription products. The prescribing physician should be consulted for verification of intended indications, in case an off-label use is applicable. The next step will involve checking international compendia for possible equivalents, with *Martindale* providing the most extensive coverage. If Drug X is a single-entity (one active ingredient) product, *Index Nominum* or *Merck Index* are other possible sources. *Index Nominum* identifies countries and manufacturers, along with brand names, in its entries. *Merck* monographs simply list proprietary names (manufacturers accompany them only in indexing). However, none of these sources can be regarded as a definitive indicator of market status and equivalency. To verify availability of an approved medication with the same ingredients, indications, dosage form, and regimen in given countries, *PDR*-type publications discussed in Chapter Ten, such as *Rote Liste* (10.10) or *Dictionnaire Vidal* (10.12), can be consulted. Contacting the manufacturer of Drug X about its European marketing is another option (as is consulting the *IMSworld Product Monographs* database online; see 15.19). In general, the recommended practice for U.S. travelers abroad is to take sufficient quantities of medication with them, along with supportive documentation from a licensed physician for customs clearance and in the event of an emergency.

Practicum 5

1. Find references to the effects of bromocriptine therapy in elderly patients with both Parkinson's disease and hypertension.
   a. sources—*MEDLINE* (14.1), *EMBASE* (14.4)
   b. rationale—With its consistent indexing for a variety of age groups in humans, *MEDLINE* would be a good first choice to answer this question. *EMBASE* age tags are used for both human and animal studies, so remember to post-qualify results to human only. *International Pharmaceutical Abstracts* (14.8) and *BIOSIS Previews* (14.6) could also be used to find relevant bibliography; each identifies only two age groups: the elderly and children. Adding *BIOSIS* to the list of files to be consulted could lead to conference papers and pertinent material published in books, as well as journal articles.

2. Document the medicinal uses of yarrow, a commonly cultivated flowering perennial.

a. sources—*Natural Products Alert* (14.42), *International Pharmaceutical Abstracts* (14.8), *BIOSIS Previews* (14.6), *CAB Health* (14.16), *Allied and Alternative Medicine* (14.15), *Unlisted Drugs* (3.8), *Martindale* (6.1)

b. rationale—*NAPRALERT* is the only online resource totally dedicated to documenting the medicinal uses of plant and animal extracts. *IPA* devotes an entire section to pharmacognosy, and *BIOSIS* also provides excellent coverage of the topic. *CAB Health* includes the *Review of Aromatic and Medicinal Plants* in its coverage, and *AMED* is also likely to contribute unique bibliography. Don't forget that *Unlisted Drugs* and *Martindale,* in either hardcopy or online format, are other good sources of natural product information. The strategy should incorporate both the common and scientific names of the plant, e.g., yarrow or achillea millefolium. Also, consider checking medicinal plant and ethnobotanical databases on the Internet, discussed in Chapter Twelve.

3. What companies are investigating antibiotics for antineoplastic therapy? I'm particularly interested in topoisomerase inhibitors.

a. sources (in order of priority)—*Pharmaprojects* (15.1), *ADIS R&D Insight* (15.3), *IMSworld R&D Focus Drug Updates* (15.2), *Drug Data Report* (15.5), *NME Express* (15.4)

b. rationale—Drugs-in-development directories consistently identify therapeutic class of products under investigation, as well as originating or licensing companies. *Pharmaprojects* and *ADIS R&D Insight* take precedence in answering the second part of this question, because they routinely add pharmacological action keywords or codes to drug records. In other files, the strategy would require use of synonyms (e.g., antibiotic or anthracycline or topoisomerase).

4. I need bibliography on the comparative efficacy of two brand name products with the same active ingredients.

a. sources—*EMBASE* (14.4), *International Pharmaceutical Abstracts* (14.8)

b. rationale—These two databases both add brand name indexing to online records when products are identified by authors in the full text of primary sources cited. Both of these databases also cover journals likely to discuss bioequivalency. Other health bibliography sources, such as *MEDLINE* (14.1) or *BIOSIS Previews* (14.6), will not yield as many pertinent references, because brand names are searchable only if included by authors in their original title or abstract.

5. Find references to EC 4.1.1.33.

a. sources (in order of priority)—*MEDLINE* (14.1), CAS registry files (14.43–14.45), *EMBASE* (14.4), *BIOSIS Previews* (14.6)

b. rationale—Starting the search in *MEDLINE* would be the quickest route to relevant bibliography. Since June 1980, *MEDLINE* has added Enzyme

Commission numbers in indexing, in preference to CAS RNs, and includes a simplified (generic) name following each number in online records. In other medical bibliographic databases, EC numbers are included in indexing only when the source author cites them. Therefore, to conduct a thorough search on this enzyme in databases other than *MEDLINE,* you would need to consult one of the CAS registry files for alternate names to incorporate into a free text strategy. *EMBASE* takes precedence over *BIOSIS* in the list of possible sources, because it provides cross references from EC numbers to preferred terms in its online thesaurus.

6. Which pharmaceutical firms have FDA approval to produce generic equivalents of Zantac, and which have also launched equivalents abroad?

   a. sources—*Diogenes* (16.1), *F-D-C Reports* (15.10), *IMSworld New Product Launches* (15.18), *IMSworld Product Monographs* (15.19)

   b. rationale—Answering this question will require clarification from the requester whether equivalents of all forms and strengths of the product should be explored, or only specified presentations (e.g., 150 mg tablets). Once this additional background information has been obtained, *Diogenes* can be used to locate Zantac's original approval date in the United States and its active ingredient (ranitidine hydrochloride). The FDA home page on the Internet could also be tried, but limited retrospective data are available. Next, the nonproprietary name (and dosage form abbreviation, if desired) can be searched. This step could be accomplished in FDA drug approval files on the Internet or in *Diogenes. F-D-C Reports* also offers up-to-date coverage of ANDAs, with indexing back to January 1987. *Diogenes* has indexed the monthly list since January 1984. (If Zantac's approval date indicates that me-too products might have been introduced prior to 1984, *Diogenes* provides access to all NDAs authorized since 1938.) To find equivalents launched abroad, *IMSworld New Product Launches* will show drugs with the same active ingredient introduced in any of fifty countries from 1982 forward. Dosage form (abbreviated) and strength are also searchable. *IMSworld Product Monographs* compiles information on launches worldwide dating from 1965.

7. We've been asked to investigate a group of anti-inflammatory compounds called "antedrugs." This isn't a *MeSH* or *EMTREE* descriptor, so where would be a good place to start?

   a. sources—*MEDLINE* (14.1), *EMBASE* (14.4), *BIOSIS Previews* (14.6), *SciSearch* (14.7), *Derwent Drug File* (14.10), *InPharma* (14.11).

   b. rationale—Although newer terms such as antedrug may not yet have been adopted as part of database controlled vocabularies, keywords can, nonetheless, be searched in a free text format. Files with a high percentage of abstracted records will offer more opportunities for locating bibliography. In all of the sources listed, textual summaries accompany 55–100% of records, and each yields unique citations not found elsewhere. Because relatively few references can be anticipated, the topic is a strong candidate for a cited reference strategy in *SciSearch*. Using this capability, articles citing each reference could be located, a technique that will uncover pertinent material where the authors do not use the term antedrug. When newly coined vocabulary is the subject of inquiry, not everyone writing about the topic will use the same words. Cited reference searches are particularly effective in such cases.

8. Find toxicity data on Drug Z and on the class of compounds to which it belongs.
   a. sources (in order of priority)—CAS registry files (14.43–14.45), *MED-LINE* (14.1), *EMBASE* (14.4), *International Pharmaceutical Abstracts* (14.8)
   b. rationale—Remember that toxicity testing will have been conducted early in the product's life cycle, prior to assignment of a nonproprietary name. It will be necessary to locate names formerly used for Drug Z, such as laboratory codes, in order to survey the literature thoroughly. The starting point should be a nomenclature source, such as one of the CAS registry files. When extending the search to a class of compounds, begin in *MED-LINE,* which assists drug class searching through its *Tree Structures.* References to adverse effects or toxicity can also easily be isolated by using subheadings. *EMBASE* and *IPA* also offer drug category indexing, but with a preference for therapeutic classification and fewer mechanism of action groupings. Databases such as *TOXLINE* and *BIOSIS Previews* would cover the topic, but it would be necessary to key in individual names of specific drugs in the desired class, in order to conduct a thorough search.

9. I'm planning a prescription audit for three long-term care institutions. Where can I find articles about conducting such a survey?
   a. sources—*International Pharmaceutical Abstracts* (14.8)
   b. rationale—*IPA* is the best choice to answer questions related to the bibliography of pharmacy practice. Other potential sources, such as *Social SciSearch* or *HealthSTAR,* can be identified in the selection aids compiled in Appendix B.

10. What is the product patent for Drug Y? When does it expire?
    a. sources (in order of priority)—*Diogenes* (16.1), *IMSworld Patents International* (16.4), *IMSworld R&D Focus Drug Updates* (15.2), *Drug Data Report* (15.5)
    b. rationale—Patent databases cannot be searched directly to locate records for specific drug products, because brand or generic names are not available at the time of filing. Sources that offer access by brand and by com-

pany name and that frequently cite patent numbers are listed here, instead. If the drug was approved after the 1984 Waxman-Hatch legislation, the NDA authorization record in *Diogenes* may include a patent number and expiration date. However, be aware that if the patent term has been extended, the *Diogenes* entry may not yet reflect the extension. Like *Diogenes, IMSworld Patents International* accommodates searching by brand or generic drug names and by companies and will include expiration information, if the drug is among the 1,800 products included in its scope. If neither *Diogenes* or *Patents International* yields results, the survey can proceed to drugs-in-development directories. For products still under investigation and perhaps not yet launched worldwide, *IMSworld R&D Focus Drug Updates* and *Drug Data Report* are good sources to find patent numbers. Once Drug Y's name has been linked with a patent number, *World Patents Index* could be used to determine priority issue date and to calculate projected expiration. However, *WPI* does not include information on official extensions. The *Patent Term Extension and New Patents Docket* on the FDA's Web site is a good source for U.S. term restoration data under Waxman-Hatch legislation. The *CLAIMS/Reassignment & Reexamination* database is even better, because it is updated weekly. Finally, *INPADOC* can be checked for possible Supplementary Protection Certificates or other extensions to non-U.S. patents. Note: *Mosby's GenRx* (6.4) provides patent expiration dates from December 1986 through December 2004, but does not supply patent numbers. Monographs newly added in the eleventh or twelfth editions (1989–present) of *The Merck Index* (3.5) have begun to cite, whenever possible, U.S. product patent numbers, but lack expiration dates. *The Orange Book* (4.42) lists both patent numbers and expirations for U.S.-approved products, but its entries may not reflect recent extensions. Also, don't assume that *Orange Book* numbers are definitive answers to questions of this type (see discussion in Chapter Sixteen).

11. I've been asked to find literature references to an investigational immunosuppressant called "gusperimus trihydrochloride." When I tried searching in *MEDLINE* and *EMBASE,* there were no records that cited this name, but I was able to find a few items that used the name "gusperimus" and gave a registry number. When I showed these to the requester, she said that the registry number is incorrect, so they can't be about the same compound. What should I do next?
    a. sources (in order of priority)—CAS registry files (14.43–14.45), *Pharmaprojects* (15.1) or *IMSworld R&D Focus Drug Updates* (15.2), *ADIS R& D Insight* (15.3), *MEDLINE* (14.1), *EMBASE* (14.4), *BIOSIS Previews* (14.6), *Derwent Drug File* (14.10), *SciSearch* (14.7)
    b. rationale—*MEDLINE* frequently cites only the parent compound name

when indexing salts, so it's not unusual that adding trihydrochloride to the strategy constituted overspecification. Because of this lack of precision in nomenclature (from a chemical point of view), incorrect registry numbers are sometimes assigned. Remember that CAS RNs should not be relied upon too heavily when searching clinical databases or judging the relevance of results. The first step to overcome difficulties described here is to locate alternative nomenclature, beyond the generic name gusperimus trihydrochloride. A search of any of the CAS registry files or the larger drugs-in-development directories listed will uncover at least one lab code (in this case, four in all) and the correct registry number. A new strategy can then be constructed ORing together all of these names and used to good effect in the major bibliographic files.

12. Are statistics available on noncompliance? For example, how many people don't bother to have their initial prescription filled? Have data been compiled correlating dose regimen with incorrect use? What about types of drugs? Do certain categories show more compliance problems than others? Can you find some numeric data related to this issue?

   a. sources—*Incidence and Prevalence Database* (15.39), *International Pharmaceutical Abstracts* (14.8)

   b. rationale—Statistics related to drug use and abuse are included in the *Incidence and Prevalence Database,* along with disease morbidity and mortality data and information on surgical procedures. Noncompliance is among issues addressed, with extensive data drawn from multiple epidemiological studies compiled under one ICD-9 code. Because this is a pharmacy practice issue, *IPA* is another potential source of medication use statistics.

13. I'd like to assemble some consumer-oriented materials on the effects of herbal teas.

   a. sources (in order of priority)—*IAC Health & Wellness Database* (14.33), *MDX Health Digest* (14.34), *Allied and Alternative Medicine* (14.15)

   b. rationale—The best online sources of general (not just medication-related) consumer health information are the *IAC Health & Wellness Database* and *MDX Health Digest.* The former draws upon a much larger collection of newsletters, pamphlets, magazines, books, and other publications than does the *Health Digest* and provides the full text of many items cited. Both databases would include material on this popular topic. *Allied and Alternative Medicine* also indexes some material appropriate for lay readers and devotes considerable attention to herbal remedies. Checking some of the Internet sites discussed in Chapter Nine, such as *MotherNature.com,* could also yield relevant material.

14. I need an up-to-date list of all bronchodilators approved by the FDA in the past six months.

a. sources—The FDA home page on the Internet or *Diogenes* (16.1)

b. rationale—An important factor in this query is timeliness. FDA Web listings of recent drug approvals are more up-to-date than *Diogenes* coverage,
but will have to be accessed month by month.

15. We're interested in pharmacoeconomic evaluations of prophylactic use of
filgrastim and comparable drugs to reduce the incidence of cancer chemo-
therapy-induced neutropenia.

a. sources (in order of priority)—*PharmacoEconomics & Outcomes News*
(15.14), *ADIS LMS Drug Alerts Online* (14.12), *EMBASE* (14.4), *International Pharmaceutical Abstracts* (14.8), *CANCERLIT* (14.17)

b. rationale—References to pharmacoeconomic evaluations can be difficult
to find, especially when the therapy under scrutiny is not a highly competitive or lucrative market. *PharmacoEconomics & Outcomes News* is the
only database wholly devoted to coverage of this subject area. *ADIS LMS
Drug Alerts Online* also includes a separate section on pharmacoeconomics. *EMBASE* added pharmacoeconomics as a link qualifier for drug and
disease index terms in 1997. *International Pharmaceutical Abstracts*
adopted the term as a controlled descriptor several years earlier. Another
IPA bonus is that it is one of the few online databases with coverage of the
ADIS journal *PharmacoEconomics,* as well as the *Journal of Research in
Pharmaceutical Economics.* Because the topic is related to cancer therapy,
CANCERLIT should lead to a selection of relevant citations, but there is
no *MeSH* term, as yet, that consistently identifies the type of study requested. The subheading "economics" can be linked with the drug class
term (granulocyte colony-stimulating factor) or with the disease descriptor
neutropenia. However, a free text approach using multiple synonyms for
the economic concept will uncover additional bibliography indexed under
other terms.

16. I've been told that Company Z is investigating a new corticosteroid for
asthma. I think it's called "ciclisonide," but I can't find any references to
this name. What next? I need citations to clinical studies, if available.

a. sources (in order of priority)—*EMBASE* (14.4), *Pharmaprojects* (15.1),
IMSworld R&D FocusDrug Updates (15.2), *ADIS R&D Insight* (15.3),
IMSworld R&D Focus Drug News (15.12), bibliographic databases

b. rationale—Chances are that the drug name is spelled incorrectly. However,
if the company name and drug class are accurate, *EMBASE* would be a
good place to start, because of its manufacturer name indexing not found
in other medical literature files. The strategy could search for the company
in both the manufacturer name and author affiliation (corporate source)
fields and employ drug class *EMTREE* terms. The name, once found, will
usually be easily recognizable as a "sound alike" spelling. It should then
be searched in the *EMBASE* thesaurus online, which will list other names

also used in the literature. An alternative (more expensive) approach would be to check a pipeline directory such as *Pharmaprojects, R&D Focus Drug Updates,* or *ADIS R&D Insight,* where the company name and drug class should quickly lead to records in which the correct drug name and synonyms can be identified. Consulting *IMSworld R&D Focus Drug News* is a third option for solving the drug name problem; it is the only industry news database with controlled company name and drug category search capabilities. However, it will not provide alternative nomenclature likely to be needed to locate clinical studies in bibliographic files. After the drug has been identified and its synonyms compiled, the search can proceed in the literature files (*MEDLINE,* etc.).

17. We're looking for a drug delivery system that we can license to enable administration of our antitumor product, currently in liquid form, to be changed into a controlled release solid biodegradable implant.
    a. sources (in order of priority)—*Pharmaprojects* (15.1), *Drug News & Perspectives* (15.13), *IMSworld R&D Focus Drug News* (15.12), *IMSworld R&D Focus Drug Updates* (15.2), *IAC Newsletter Database* (15.15)
    b. rationale—*Pharmaprojects* not only routinely identifies licensing opportunities, but also provides a special classification code for formulations and drug delivery systems (category F). *Drug News & Perspectives* features a separate "Licensing Line" section and consistently singles out drug delivery options in title keywords. *R&D Focus Drug News* flags relevant records with the controlled descriptor phrase "licensing offer," but has no separate classification for drug delivery technology. *R&D Focus Drug Updates* also consistently indexes licensing opportunities, but does not provide the equivalent of category F in *Pharmaprojects.* Both *IMSworld* sources will, if used, require good free text strategies, employing multiple synonyms, to retrieve the type of delivery system desired. Several publications searchable in the *IAC Newsletter Database* are excellent current awareness sources for monitoring licensing opportunities (see Appendix C), but this full-text file will also require a strategy that anticipates alternative terminology likely to be used by authors writing in unpredictable natural language.

18. When was Drug Q recalled, and why? What tests were conducted to determine its safety and efficacy prior to its approval?
    a. sources (in order of priority)—FDA home page, *Diogenes* (16.1), *F-D-C Reports* (15.10), *IAC Newsletter Database* (15.13)
    b. rationale—If Drug Q is a top-selling drug, its recall may have been sufficiently newsworthy to be merit discussion in *F-D-C Reports.* However, regardless of the commercial or clinical significance of the recall, all sources listed index drug and device recall notices published in the weekly *FDA Enforcement Reports,* but differ in retrospective coverage offered.

The FDA Web site archives recall notices back to February, 1990. *Dioge-nes* indexes recalls dating from 1984, and *F-D-C Reports* coverage began in 1987. *Diogenes* also includes background documentation on recalls, if available, such as warning letters (1984–), and offers easy access to Summary Basis of Approval documents requested in the third part of this question. FDA coverage of warning letters began in January 1995 and of SBAs in 1997.

19. In what countries are nootropics best sellers? What brands rank highest in sales, and where?

    a. sources—*IMS World Drug Markets* (15.32)

    b. rationale—This database indexes top selling drugs on a country by country basis. It can be searched by EPhMRA classification codes or keyword equivalents, including "nootropics." Profiles for each of the seventy-six nations covered include annual sales statistics, in U.S. dollars, broken down by the ten leading therapeutic classes and listing top brand names in each class.

20. I never know how far back to go when surveying the adverse effects literature on a given drug. Are there any general guidelines for establishing retrospective delimiters in this type of online search?

    a. sources (in order of priority)—*The Merck Index* (3.5), *CA Search* (14.32) or *CA File* (14.33), *USP Dictionary of USAN* (3.1)

    b. rationale—Initial patent application date is probably the best indicator for establishing a cut-off date, before which little information will be found. *The Merck Index* often provides patent data, as could a quick search of *Chemical Abstracts* files. The date given in the *USP Dictionary* for official nonproprietary name adoption could be used for rough extrapolations of a probable timeline for toxicity testing (three to six years prior to USAN assignment).

F

Directory of Internet Resources Cited in the Guide

Academy of Managed Care Pharmacy (AMCP)
⇨http://www.amcp.org
Action plan for the provision of useful prescription drug information
⇨http://www.nyam.org/keystone
Acupuncture.com
⇨http://www.acupuncture.com
AIDS Patents Database
⇨http://app.cnidr.org
Algy's Herb Page
⇨http://www.algy.com/herb/index.html
Alliance for the Prudent Use of Antibiotics (APUA)
⇨http://www.healthsci.tufts.edu/apua
Alta Vista—Translation
⇨http://babelfish.altavista.com/cgi-bin/translate
AltVetMed—Complementary and Alternative Veterinary Medicine
⇨http://www.altmedvet.com
American Academy of Pharmaceutical Physicians (AAPP)
⇨http://www.aapp.org
American Association for Clinical Chemistry (AACC)
⇨http://www.aacc.org
American Association of Colleges of Pharmacy (AACP)
⇨http://www.aacp.org
American Association of Pharmaceutical Scientists (AAPS)
⇨http://www.aaps.org
American Association of Pharmacy Technicians (AAPT)
⇨http://www.pharmacytechnician.com
American Botanical Council (ABC)
⇨http://www.herbalgram.org

American Chemical Society Division of Chemical Information
    ⇨http://www.lib.uchicago.edu/~atbrooks/CNIF/cnifhome.html
American College of Clinical Pharmacology (ACCP)
    ⇨http://www.accp1.org
American College of Clinical Pharmacy (ACCP)
    ⇨http://www.accp.com
American Council on Pharmaceutical Education (ACPE)
    ⇨http://www.acpe-accredit.org
American Institute of the History of Pharmacy (AIHP)
    ⇨http://www.pharmacy.wisc.edu/aihp
American Nutraceutical Association (ANA)
    ⇨http://www.americanutra.com
American Pharmaceutical Association (APhA)
    ⇨http://www.aphanet.org
American Society for Clinical Pharmacology and Therapeutics (ASCPT)
    ⇨http://www.ascpt.org
American Society for Pharmacology and Experimental Therapeutics (ASPET)
    ⇨http://www.faseb.org/aspet
American Society of Consultant Pharmacists (ASCP)
    ⇨http://www.ascp.com
American Society of Health System Pharmacists (ASHP)
    ⇨http://www.ashp.com
American Society of Pharmacognosy (ASP)
    ⇨http://www.phcog.org
AOAC International (Association of Official Analytical Chemists)
    ⇨http://www.aoac.org
Association for the Advancement of Medical Instrumentation (AAMI)
    ⇨http://www.aami.org
Association of the British Pharmaceutical Industry (ABPI)
    ⇨http://www.abpi.org.uk
Association of the European Self-Medication Industry (AESGP)
    ⇨http://www.aesgp.be
Association of Clinical Research Professionals (ACRP)
    ⇨http://www.acrpnet.org
Association of Natural Medicine Pharmacists
    ⇨http://www.anmp.org
Association of the British Pharmaceutical Industry (ABPI)
    ⇨http://www.abpi.org.uk
Australian Prescription Products Guide
    ⇨http://appco.com.au/appguide/default.htm
Avoiding Food and Drug Interactions
    ⇨http://www.foodsafety.org/sf/sf162.htm

Bio Online—Biotechnology Companies and Resources
➪http://search.bio.com/search
BioIndustry Association
➪http://www.bioindustry.org
BioSpace
➪http://www.biospace.com
BioTech Chemical Acronyms Database
➪http://129.79.137.107/cfdocs/libchem/titleu.cfm
Biotech Law Web Server
➪http://www2.ari.net/foley
BioTech Life Sciences Dictionary
➪http://biotech.chem.indiana.edu/pages/dictionary.htm
Biotechnology Industry Association (BIO)
➪http://www.bio.org
Biotechnology Resources—College & Research Library News (Hart & Hart)
➪http://www.ala.org/acrl/resdec97.html
Board of Pharmaceutical Specialties (BPS)
➪http://www.bpsweb.org
Botanical Dermatology Database (BoDD)
➪http://BoDD.cf.ac.uk
Botanical Medicine Resources on the Web
➪http://cpmcnet.columbia.edu/dept/rosenthal/Botanicals.html
British Pharmacological Society
➪http://www.bphs.org.uk
British Pharmacopoeia
➪http://www.pharmacopoeia.co.uk
CAM Citation Index—National Center for Complementary and Alternative
    Medicine
➪http://altmed.od.nih.gov/nccam/resources/cam-ci
Canadian Cosmetic, Toiletry and Fragrance Association (CCTFA)
➪http://www.cctfa.ca
Canadian Pharmacists Association (CPhA, formerly Canadian Pharmaceutical
    Association)
➪http://www.cdnpharm.ca
Canadian Poisonous Plants Information System
➪http://res.agr.ca/brd/poisonpl
Canadian Society for Pharmaceutical Sciences (CSPS)
➪http://www.ualberta.ca/%7Ecsps
Canadian Society of Hospital Pharmacists (CSHP)
➪http://www.cshp.ca
Canadian Wholesale Drug Association (CWDA)
➪http://www.cwda.org

Centers for Disease Control and Prevention (CDC)
⇨http://www.cdc.gov
CenterWatch Clinical Trials Listing Service
⇨http://www.centerwatch.com
CERCLA Priority List of Hazardous Substances
⇨http://atsdr1.atsdr.cdc.gov:8080/97list.html
CHEMCYCLOPEDIA (American Chemical Society)
⇨http://pubs.acs.org/chemcy
Chemicals in the Environment: OPPT Chemical Fact Sheets
⇨http://www.epa.gov/opptintr/chemfact
ChemWeb
⇨http://chemweb.com
Clinical Pharmacology Online
⇨http://www.cponline.gsm.com
Cochrane Database of Systematic Reviews (CDSR)
⇨http://www.update-software.com/ccweb/cochrane/cdsr.htm
Columbia University College of Physicians & Surgeons Complete Home Medical
    Guide
⇨http://cpmcnet.columbia.edu/texts/guide
Compounding Formulas from the Recent Journal Literature
⇨http://www.dal.ca/~pharmwww/compound
Compounding Hotline
⇨http://members.aol.com/pharmtimes/com.html
Contemporary Compounding
⇨http://users.aol.com/mefrancom/contcmpd.html
Controlled Release Society (CRS)
⇨http://www.crsadmhdq.org
Cornell University Poisonous Plants Web Page
⇨http://www.ansci.cornell.edu/plants/plants.html
Cosmetic, Toiletry, and Fragrance Association (CTFA)
⇨http://www.ctfa.org
Criteria for assessing the quality of health information on the Internet
⇨http://www.mitrtek.org/hiti/showcase/documents/criteria.html
Current Controlled Trials
⇨http://www.controlled-trials.com
Cutaneous Drug Reaction Database
⇨gopher://gopher.Dartmouth.EDU:70/00/Research/BioSci/CDRD/README
Cyberbotanica
⇨http://biotech.chem.indiana.edu/botany
Database of Abstracts of Reviews of Effectiveness (DARE)
⇨http://nhscrd.york.ac.uk
Dictionary of Epidemiology
⇨http://www.kings.ca.ac.uk/~js229/glossary.html

Dr. Duke's Phytochemical and Ethnobotanical Databases
⇨http://www.ars-grin.gov/duke
Dr. Koop's Community: The Pharmacy and The Medicine Cabinet
⇨http://www.drkoop.com/drugstore
Drug INFONET Patient Package Inserts
⇨http://www.druginfonet.com/ppi.htm
Drug Information Association (DIA)
⇨http://www.diahome.org
Drug Information Resources for Pharmacists
⇨http://www.dal.ca/~pharmwww/druginfo
DrugBase
⇨http://www.drugbase.co.za
ECDIN (Environmental Chemical Data and Information Network)
⇨http://ecdin.etomep.net
ECPHIN (European Community Pharmaceutical Information Network)
⇨http://ecphin.etomep.net
Edmund's Home Page
⇨http://www.li.net/~edhayes/ed.html
E-Pharmacy by Eckerd: OTC Resource Center
⇨http://www.e-pharmacy.com/HTML/healthinfo/otc/index.html
EpiVetNet
⇨http://epiweb.massey.ac.nz
Essential Spanish for Pharmacists and Pharmacy Technicians
⇨http://www.pharmacyspanish.com
Ethnobotany Database
⇨http://probe.nalusda.gov:8300/cgi-bin/browse/ethnobotdb
EthnoMedicinals Home Page
⇨http://walden.mo.net/~tonytork
European Association for Health Information and Libraries (EAHIL)
⇨http://www.med.uu.nl/eahil.html
    http://www.eahil.org/pharmaceutical_information_group.htm
European Medicines Evaluation Agency (EMEA)
⇨http://www.eudra.org
European Pharmaceutical Marketing Research Association (EPhMRA)
⇨http://www.ephmra.org:80
European Scientific Cooperative on Phytotherapy (ESCOP)
⇨http://www.ex.ac.uk/phytonet/pubs.html
European Society of Clinical Pharmacy (ESCP)
⇨http://www.escp.nl
FDA Consumer Information—Drug Database
⇨http://www.fda.gov/cder/consumerinfo
FDA Home Page
⇨http://www.fda.gov

Federal Bio-Technology Transfer Directory
  ⇨http://www.bioinfo.com/biotech
Federated Drug Reference—U.S. Pharmacopeia Dispensing Information
  ⇨http://kirk.hslib.washington.edu/fdr
FEDSTATS
  ⇨http://www.fedstats.gov/search.html
First DataBank
  ⇨http://www.firstdatabank.com/drug/edi.html
Food and Drug Law Institute
  ⇨http://www.fdli.org
Gelbe Liste Online
  ⇨http://195.27.173.69/wconnect/glwin/suchen.htm
Glossary of Technical and Popular Medical Terms in Eight European Languages
  ⇨http://allserv.rug.ac.be/~rvdstich/eugloss/language.html
Glossary of Terms and Symbols Used in Pharmacology
  ⇨http://www.bumc.bu.edu/www/busm/pharmacology/Programmed/
    Framedglossary.html
Guide to Poisonous and Toxic Plants
  ⇨http://chppm-www.apgea.army.mil/ento/PLANT.HTM
Hardin Meta Directory of Pharmacy & Pharmacology
  ⇨http://www.lib.uiow.edu/hardin/md/pharm.html
HAZDAT
  ⇨http://atsdrl.atsdr.cdc.gov:8080/hazdat.html
Health-Center.com: Pharmacy
  ⇨http://www.healthguide.com/english/pharmacy
Health Economics—Places to Go
  ⇨http://www.medecon.de/healthec.htm
The Health Economics Website
  ⇨http://metz.une.edu.au/~mkortt
HealthEconomics.Com
  ⇨http://www.exit109.com/~zaweb/pjp
HealthFinder
  ⇨http://www.healthfinder.gov
Health Industry Manufacturers Association (HIMA)
  ⇨http://www.HIMAnet.com
HealthLinks: International Health and Social Statistics
  ⇨http://www.hslib.washington.edu/statistics
Health-related Web site evaluation form
  ⇨http://www.sph.emory.edu/WELLNESS/instrument.html
Health Statistics—College & Research Libraries News (Auditore & Stoklosa)
  ⇨http://www.ala.acrl/resoct97.html
Healthtouch Online Drug Information
  ⇨http://www/healthtouch.com/level1/p_dri.htm

HEALTHWEB: Pharmacy & Pharmacology
⇨http://thorplus.lin.purdue.edu/hw
HealthWeb Public Health Statistics
⇨http://www.lib.umich/hw/public.health/health.stats.html
Health WWWeb–Integrative Medicine, Natural Health and Alternative Therapies
⇨http://www.healthwwweb.com
Henriette's Herbal Homepage
⇨http://sunsite.unc.edu/herbmed
Herb Research Foundation
⇨http://www.herbs.org
The Herbal Bookworm
⇨http://www.teleport.com/~jonno/index.shtml
HerbMed
⇨http://www.amfoundation.org/herbmed.htm
HerbNET
⇨http://www.herbnet.com
HerbWeb
⇨http://www.herbweb.com
HIMA (Health Industry Manufacturers Association)
⇨http://www.himanet.com
The History of Pharmacy
⇨http://www.lindsaydrug.com/newhist.htm
History of Pharmacy: A Guide to Sources
⇨http://www.simmons.edu/~tudesco/pharmacy
The History of Pharmacy in Pictures
⇨http://barbital.phar.wsu.edu/history
HIV Clinical Trials in the United States
⇨http://hivinsite.ucsf.edu/bin/keywords
HSLS Health Statistics
⇨http://www.hsls.pitt.edu/intres/guides/statcbw.html
HSLS Pharmacy, Pharmacology & Therapeutics
⇨http://www.hsls.pitt.edu/intres/health/pharm.html
How to Read the Prescription
⇨http://www.ns.net/users/ryan/rxabrv.html
IDIN's Links (Iowa Drug Information Network)
⇨http://idin.idis.uiowa.edu/idinlink.htm
IDRAC
⇨http://www.ims-int.com/idrac
IHS Health
⇨http://www.ihshealth.com
Illustrated Buyers Guide to Veterinary Equipment and Supplies
⇨http://www.vetmedpub.com

IMS Global Services
⇨http://www.ims-global.com
INCAD
⇨http://www.incadinc.com
Incidence and Prevalence Database
⇨http://www.tdrdata.com
Infomed Drug Guide
⇨http://www.infomed.org/100drugs
Institute for Safe Medication Practices (ISMP)
⇨http://www.ismp.org
InteliHealth—U.S. Pharmacopeia Dispensing Information
⇨http://ipn.intelihealth.com/ipn
International Academy of Compounding Pharmacists (IACP)
⇨http://www.compassnet.com/~iacp
The International Bibliographic Information on Dietary Supplements Database
(IBIDS)
⇨http://www.nal.usda.gov/fnic/IBIDS
International Federation of Pharmaceutical Manufacturers Associations (IFPMA)
⇨http://www.ifpma.org
International Society for Ethnopharmacology (ISE)
⇨http://www.dfh.dk/staff/private/ulny/ISE
International Society for Pharmaceutical Engineering (ISPE)
⇨http://www.ispe.org
International Society for Pharmacoeconomics and Outcomes Research (ISPOR)
⇨http://www.ispor.org
International Society for Pharmacoepidemiology (ISPE)
⇨http://www.pharmacoepi.org
Internet Directory for Botany: Economic Botany, Ethnobotany
⇨http://www.helsinki.fi/kmus/botecon.html
Internet Health Watch
⇨http://www.reutershealth.com/ihw
Internet Mental Health
⇨http://www.mentalhealth.com
Internet resources for chemistry—College & Research Library News (Bauer)
⇨http://www.ala.org/acrl/resdec.html
Internet resources in biology—College & Research Library News (Courtois &
Goslen)
⇨http://www.ala.org/acrl/resjul96.html
InterPharma
⇨http://www.interpharma.co.uk
The Iowa Drug Information Service
⇨http://www.uiowa.edu.80/~idis

ISI Reaction Center
⇨http://www.isinet.com
Karolinska Institute Drug Therapy
⇨http://www.mic.ki.se/Diseases/e2.html
Kohler's Medizinal Pflanzen
⇨http://www.mobot.org/MOBOT/research/library/kohler
Links to Sites Related to the History of Pharmacy (AIHP)
⇨http://www.pharmacy.wisc.edu/aihp/links.html
Managed Care Digest
⇨http://www.managedcaredigest.com
Mayo Clinic Health Oasis Medicine Center
⇨http://www.mayohealth.org/usp/common/index.htm
McMaster University's Health Care Information Resources—Alternative
    Medicine
⇨http://www-hsl.mcmaster.ca/tomflem/altmed.html
Medical Device Link
⇨http://www.devicelink.com
Medical Device Manufacturers Association (MDMA)
⇨http://www.medicaldevices.org
Medical Devices Canada (MEDEC)
⇨http://www.medec.org
Medical Herbalism
⇨http://medherb.com
Medical Library Association (MLA)
⇨http://www.mlanet.org
Medical Matrix
⇨http://www.medmatrix.org
Medical Technology-Related Acronyms
⇨http://www.himanet.com/resource/acronyms.htm
Medication Info Search
⇨http://www.cheshire-med.com/services/pharm/med-form.cgi
Medicinal Plant Databases
⇨http://www.inform.umd.edu/PBIO/Medicinals/pharmacognosy.html
Medicinal Plants of North America
⇨http://probe.nalusda.gov:8300/cgi-bin/browse/mpnadb
MedicineNet—The Pharmacy
⇨http://www.medicinenet.com
Mediconsult—General Drug Information
⇨http://www.mediconsult.com/general/drugs
MediSpan Drug Information Database from The Wellness International Network
⇨http://www.stayhealth.com/medispan/index.html
MedNets Epidemiology & Public Health
⇨http://www.internets.com/epidemio.htm

Medscape Drug Search from First DataBank
⇨http://www.medscape.com/misc/formdrugs.html
Medscape Patient Information
⇨http://Patient.medscape.com/Home/Patient/PatientInfo.html
MedWeb Pharmacy and Pharmacology
⇨http://WWW.MedWeb.Emory.Edu/MedWeb/default.htm
MethodsFinder
⇨http://www.methodsfinder.org
Miller Freeman dotpharmacy
⇨http://www.dotpharmacy.co.uk/index.html
MIMS Australia
⇨http://www.mims.com.au
The Mining Company: Pharmacology
⇨http://pharmacology.miningco.com
Mosby
⇨http://www.mosby.com
Mosby's Nursing Drug Reference
⇨http://www1.mosby.com/Mosby/nursing_drug_updates
MotherNature.com (formerly Mother Nature's General Store)
⇨http://www.mothernature.com
MotherRisk
⇨http://www.motherrisk.org/publi/a_n.htm
Mrs. Grieve's A Modern Herbal
⇨http://www.botanical.com/botanical/mgmh/mgmh.html
MSDS-CCOHS on CCINFOWeb
⇨http://www.ccohs.ca
MSDS-SEARCH
⇨http://www.msdssearch.com
National Association of Boards of Pharmacy (NABP)
⇨http://www.nabp.net
National Association of Chain Drug Stores (NACDS)
⇨http://www.nacds.org
National Association of Pharmaceutical Manufacturers (NAPM)
⇨http://www.napmnet.org
National Biotechnology Information Facility Company Register
⇨http://www.nbif.org/industry/register.html
National Center for Health Statistics
⇨http://www.cdc.gov/nchswww
National Clearinghouse for Alcohol and Drug Information
⇨http://www.health.org
National Community Pharmacists Association (NCPA)
⇨http://www.ncpanet.org

National Institutes of Health
⇨http://www.nih.gov/health
National Wholesale Druggists' Association (NWDA)
⇨http://www.nwda.org
Native American Ethnobotany Database
⇨http://www.umd.umich.edu/resources/bydept2/besci/anthro/
about_ethnobot.html
Natural Health Village
⇨http://www.naturalhealthvillage.com
The NetSci Yellow Pages
⇨http://www.netsci.org/Resources/Biotech/Yellowpages/top.html
NetVet
⇨http://netvet.wustl.edu/vet.htm
NetVet: Mosby's Veterinary Guide to the Internet
⇨http://www1.mosby.com/Mosby/netvet
New Medicines in Development Database (PhRMA)
⇨http://www.phrma.org/webdb
NHS Economic Evaluation Database
⇨http://nhscrd.york.ac.uk
Nonprescription Drug Manufacturers Association (NDMA)
⇨http://www.ndmainfo.og
Nonprescription Drug Manufacturers Association of Canada (NDMAC)
⇨http://www.ndmac.ca
Nutraceutical Network of Canada (NNC)
⇨http://www.nnoc.com
Nutritional Data Resources (Physicians' Guide to Nutriceuticals)
⇨http://www.mitec.n4/~manager/index.html
Onhealth Resources
⇨http://www.onhealth.com/ch1/resource
Outcomes
⇨http://www.sph.uth.tmc.edu/www/res/outcomes/outcomes.htm
Outcomes Literature Database
⇨http://www.leeds.ac.uk/nuffield/infoservices/UKCH/chld.html
Parenteral Drug Association (PDA)
⇨http://www.pda.org
Parexel
⇨http://www.parexel.com
PDR Nurse's Handbook
⇨http://www.nursespdr.com/members/database/content.html
PediWeb
⇨http://solar.rtd.utk.edu/~esmith/pedi.html
Pharmaceutical Business Intelligence & Research Group (PBIRG)
⇨http://www.pbirg.com

Pharmaceutical Education and Research Institute (PERI)
⇨http://www.peri.org
Pharmaceutical Manufacturers Association of Canada (PMAC)
⇨http://www.pmac-acim.org
Pharmaceutical Online Regulatory and Legislative Issues Index
⇨http://news.pharmaceuticalonline.com/regulatory-articles
The Pharmaceutical Press (Royal Pharmaceutical Society of Great Britain)
⇨http://www.pharmpress.com
Pharmaceutical Research and Manufacturers of America (PhRMA)
⇨http://www.phrma.org
Pharmacy and You—American Pharmaceutical Association
⇨http://www.pharmacyandyou.org
Pharmacy Continuing Education Sites Around the World
⇨http://info.cf.ac.uk/uwcc/phrmy/WWW-WSP/PhrmCEsites.html
Pharmacy Internet Guide
⇨http://www.library.usyd.edu.au/Guides/Pharmacy/index.html
Pharmacy, Medicine and Managed Care
⇨http://members.aol.com/_ht_a/bertrx/phamedmc.htm
Pharmacy-Related Academic Institutions on the Internet
⇨http://www.pharmweb.net/pwmirror/pw8/pharmweb8.html
Pharmacy Times Callout Column
⇨http://www.pharmacytimes/callout.html
Pharmacy Times Patient Education Focus
⇨http://www.pharmacytimes.com/pated.html
Pharmacy Times—Pharmacists on the Net
⇨http://www.pharmacytimes.com/net.html
Pharmacy Times Top 200 Rx Report
⇨http://www.pharmacytimes.com/top200.html
Pharmacy Web Australia
⇨http://www.pharmacyweb.com.au
PharmaPages—Internet Issues in the Pharmaceutical Industry
⇨http://www.pjbpubs.co.uk/ppages/index2.html
PharmaVentures Links Page
⇨http://www.worldpharmaweb.com/comps.htm
PharmInfoNet DrugDB
⇨http://pharminfo.com/drugdb/
PharmInfoNet Gallery
⇨http://pharminfo.com/gallery/glly_mnu.html
PharmInfoNet Glossary
⇨http://pharminfo.com/glos_ab.html
PharmInfoNet PharmLinks
⇨http://pharminfo.com/phrmlink.html

PharmWeb
⇨http://www.pharmweb.net
Philadelphia Online—Health Philadelphia
⇨http://health.phillynews.com/pharmacy/search.asp
Physicians' Guide to Nutriceuticals
⇨http://www.mitec.n4/~manager/index.html
Phytochemical Database
⇨http://probe.nalusda.gov:8300/cgi-bin/browse/phytochemdb
PLANTOX
⇨http://vm.cfsam.fda.gov/~djw
Poisonous Plant Databases
⇨http://www.inform.umd.edu/Medicinals/harmful.html
Poisonous Plants
⇨http://hammock.ifas.ufl.edu/txt/fairs/18132
Poisonous Plants Home Page
⇨http://phl.vet.upenn.edu/~triplett/poison/index.html
QuackWatch
⇨http://www.quackwatch.com
Quality of Life Assessment in Medicine
⇨http://www.glamm.com/ql/url.htm
RAinfo
⇨http://www.medmarket.com/tenants/rainfo/rainfo.htm
Raintree
⇨http://rain-tree.com
ReCap—Signals
⇨http://www.recap.com/mainweb.nsf
Regulatory Affairs Professionals Society (RAPS)
⇨http://www.raps.org
Resources in Epidemiology
⇨http://www.pitt.edu/~epidept/resource.html
The Royal Pharmaceutical Society of Great Britain
⇨http://www.rpsgb.org.uk:80
Royal Society of Chemistry Historical Image Collection
⇨http://www.rsc.org
RxHealth.com Drug and Disease Information Service
⇨http://www.rxhealth.com
RxList
⇨http://www.rxlist.com
RxMed
⇨http://www.rxmed.com/index.html
Sanphar
⇨http://www.sanphar.ch

Sara's Pharmacy Page
  ⇨http://www.geocities.com/NapaValley/7458/pharmacy.htm
Scott-Levin
  ⇨http://www.scottlevin.com/services
Secundum Artem Index
  ⇨http://www.paddocklabs.com/SECUNDUM/secarndx.html
Selected Internet Resources for Pharmacists
  ⇨http://www.unmc.edu/library/pharm/netpharm.html
Society for Medicinal Plant Research
  ⇨http://www.uni-duesseldorf.de/WWW/GA
Society of Competitive Intelligence Information Professionals (SCIP)
  ⇨http://www.scip.org
Society of Infectious Diseases Pharmacists (SIDP)
  ⇨http://sidp.hosp.utmck.edu
South African Electronic Package Inserts
  ⇨http://home.intekom.com/pharm
Southwest School of Botanical Medicine
  ⇨http://chili.rt66.com/hrbmoore/HOMEPAGE/HomePage.html
Spanish for Pharmacists
  ⇨ http://www.nacds.org/resources/Spanish.html
Spanish for the Pharmaceutical Profession
  ⇨http://www.cpha.com
Special Libraries Association Pharmaceutical and Health Technology Division
  ⇨http://www.sla.org/division/dphm/index.htm
Sympatico HealthyWay: Health Links—Alternative Medicine Directory
  ⇨http://www1.sympatico.ca/healthyway/DIRECTORY/B1.html
TableBase
  ⇨http://www.rdsic.com
Technical Term Translation Table (DIA)
  ⇨http://www.diahome.org/tttt/TTTTMain.htm
ToxFAQs
  ⇨http://atsdrl.atsdr.cdc.gov:8080/toxfaq.html
Tufts University Nutrition Navigator
  ⇨http://navigator.tufts.edu/index.html
University of Pittsburgh—The Alternative Medicine Homepage
  ⇨http://www.pitt.edu/~cbw/altm.html
The U.S. Department of Defense Pharmacoeconomic Center
  ⇨http://www.pec.ha.osd.mil
U.S. Pharmacist
  ⇨http://www.uspharmacist.com
The U.S. Pharmacopeial Convention
  ⇨http://www.usp.org

Useful Pharmacy Links
⇨http://is.dal.ca/~pharmwww/links
Veterinary Abbreviations & Acronyms
⇨http://www.library.uiuc.edu/vex/vetdocs/abbs.htm
Veterinary Biologics Home Page (USDA)
⇨http://www.aphis.usda.gov/vs/cvb/index.html
Veterinary Emergency Drug Calculator
⇨http://www.cvmbs.colostate.edu/clinsci/wing/emdrughp.html
Virtual Drugstore—Vimy Park Pharmacy
⇨http://www.virtualdrugstore.com/druglist.html
Virtual Library: Pharmacy
⇨http://www.pharmacy.org/schools.html
The Virtual Pharmacy Center—Martindale's Health Science Guide
⇨http://www-sci.lib.uci.edu/~martindale/Pharmacy.html
Virtual Tour of the History of Pharmacy Museum—University of Arizona
⇨http://www.pharm.arizona.edu/museum/index.html
Virtual Veterinary Center—Martindale's Health Science Guide
⇨http://www-sci.lib.uci.edu/HSG/Vet.html
The Wellcome Trust Centre for the Epidemiology of Infectious Disease
⇨http://www.ceid.ox.ac.uk/Links/sql.asp
Where to Find Material Safety Data Sheets On The Internet
⇨http://www.ilpi.com/msds/index.chtml
WHO Statistical Information System (WHOSIS)
⇨http://www.who.int/whosis
The World List of Schools of Pharmacy
⇨http://info.cf.ac.uk/uwcc/phrmy/WWW-WSP/SoPListHomePage.html
World Self-Medication Industry (WSMI)
⇨http://www.who.int/ina-ngo/ngo/ngo172.htm
World-Wide Web Virtual Library: Animal Health, Well-Being, and Rights
⇨http://www.tiac.net/users/sbr/animals.html
World Wide Web Virtual Library: Epidemiology
⇨http://www.epibiostat.ucsf.edu/epidem/epidem.html
World Wide Web Virtual Library: Pharmacy
⇨http://www.pharmacy.org
Yahoo! Health: Pharmacy
⇨http://www.yahoo.com/Health/Pharmacy

G

Key to Abbreviations

Abbreviations used in the text (journal title abbreviations follow in a separate listing):

21CFR	Title 21 of the *Code of Federal Regulations* (4.25)
AACC	American Association for Clinical Chemistry
AACP	American Association of Colleges of Pharmacy
AAMI	Association for the Advancement of Medical Instrumentation
AAPP	American Academy of Pharmaceutical Physicians
AAPS	American Association of Pharmaceutical Scientists
AAPT	American Association of Pharmacy Technicians
AARP	American Association of Retired Persons
ABC	American Botanical Council
ABPI	Association of the British Pharmaceutical Industry
ACCP	American College of Clinical Pharmacology, also: American College of Clinical Pharmacy
ACD	*Available Chemicals Directory*
ACE	angiotensin-converting enzyme
ACGIH	American Conference of Governmental Industrial Hygienists
ACP	American College of Physicians
ACPE	American Council on Pharmaceutical Education
ACRP	Association of Clinical Research Professionals
ACS	American Chemical Society
ACTIS	AIDS Clinical Trial Information Service
ADE	adverse drug event or experience
ADI	*American Drug Index* (3.6)
ADR	adverse drug reaction(s)
AESGP	Association of the European Self-Medication Industry
AHFS	*American Hospital Formulary Service* (6.4)

AIDS	acquired immune deficiency syndrome
AIHP	American Institute of the History of Pharmacy
AJDC	*American Journal of Diseases of Children*
a.k.a.	also known as
AL	Alabama
AMA	American Medical Association
AMCP	Academy of Managed Care Pharmacy
AMED	*Allied and Alternative Medicine* database (14.15)
ANA	American Nutraceutical Association
ANADA	Abbreviated New Animal Drug application
ANDA	Abbreviated New Drug Application
ANEUPL	Aneuploidy, subfile in *TOXLINE* (14.27)
AOAC	Association of Official Analytical Chemists
APhA	American Pharmaceutical Association
APhC	Association des pharmaciens du Canada
	(formerly Association pharmaceutique Canadienne)
APUA	Alliance for the Prudent Use of Antibiotics
ASCII	American Standard Code for Information Interchange
ASCP	American Society of Consultant Pharmacists
ASCPT	American Society for Clinical Pharmacology and Therapeutics
ASHP	American Society of Health-System Pharmacists
	(formerly American Society of Hospital Pharmacists)
ASP	American Society of Pharmacognosy
ASPET	American Society for Pharmacology and Experimental Therapeutics
ASTM	American Society for Testing and Materials
ATC	Anatomic-Therapeutic Classification/code/category
ATSDR	Agency for Toxic Substances and Disease Registry
AZ	Arizona
AZT	azothymidine
BAN	British Approved Name
BA/RRM	*Biological Abstracts/Reports, Reviews, Meetings* (14.6)
BBI	Biomedical Business International
BBS	bulletin board service(s)
BHP	*British Herbal Pharmacopoeia* (12.6)
BIO	Biotechnology Industry Association
BIOSIS	Biosciences Information Service (14.6)
BLA	biologic license application
BMJ	*British Medical Journal*
BNF	*British National Formulary* (10.22)
BP	*British Pharmacopoeia* (11.13)
BPS	Board of Pharmaceutical Specialties
BS	Bachelor of Science

CA	California
CAB	Commonwealth Agricultural Bureaux
CABs	Conformity Assessment Bodies (under the Mutual Recognition Agreement)
CADREAC	Collaboration Agreement of Drug Regulatory Authorities in European Union Associated Countries
CANDA	Computerized New Drug Application
CAS	Chemical Abstracts Service
CBER	Center for Biologics Evaluation and Research (FDA)
CBR	*Cosmetic Bench Reference* (11.32)
CCH	Commerce Clearing House (publisher)
CCIS	Computerized Clinical Information System
CCNU	cyclohexyl chloroethylnitrosourea
CCOHS	Canadian Centre for Occupational Health and Safety
CCTFA	Canadian Cosmetic, Toiletry and Fragrance Association
CCTR	*Cochrane Controlled Trials Register* (14.24)
CD-ROM	compact disc, read-only memory
CDC	Centers for Disease Control (U.S.)
CDER	Center for Drug Evaluation and Research (FDA)
CDRH	Center for Devices and Radiological Health (FDA)
CDSR	*Cochrane Database of Systematic Reviews* (14.24)
CE	Communité Européene
CE	continuing education
CFR	*Code of Federal Regulations* (4.25)
CHPA	Consumer Healthcare Products Association
CI	Collective Index (*Chemical Abstracts*)
CIN	*Chemical Industry Notes* (Figure 15.8)
CINAHL	*Cumulative Index to Nursing and Allied Health*
CIR	Cosmetic Ingredient Review
CLAIMS/RRX	*Claims/Reassignment & Reexamination* database
CNAM	Chemical Registry Nomenclature database (14.44)
CNIDR	Center for Networked Information Discovery and Retrieval
CNP	*Compendium of Nonprescription Products* (10.21)
CNS	central nervous system
CO	Colorado
CPC	Certificat Complémentaire de Protection (French patent extension)
CPhA	Canadian Pharmacists Association (formerly Canadian Pharmaceutical Association)
CPMP	Committee for Proprietary Medical Products (European Union)
CPS	*Compendium of Pharmaceuticals and Specialties* (10.20)
CRADA	Collaborative Research and Development Agreement

CRD	Centre for Reviews and Dissemination (UK National Health Service)
CRISP	Computer Retrieval of Information on Scientific Projects, subfile in *TOXLINE* (14.27)
CRS	Controlled Release Society
CSCHE	*Chem Sources Chemical Directory* database (15.27)
CSCORP	*Chem Sources Company Directory* database (15.28)
CSHP	Canadian Society of Hospital Pharmacists
CSPS	Canadian Society for Pharmaceutical Sciences
CT	Connecticut
CTFA	Cosmetic, Toiletry and Fragrance Association
CVM	Center for Veterinary Medicine (FDA)
CWDA	Canadian Wholesale Drug Association
D&C dyes	colorants deemed safe for use in drugs and cosmetics
DARE	*Database of Abstracts of Reviews of Effectiveness* (14.24)
DART	Developmental and Reproductive Toxicology, subfile in *TOXLINE* (14.27)
DAWN	Drug Abuse Warning Network (8.43)
DC	District of Columbia
DCF	Dénomination Commune Française
DCI	*Drug & Cosmetic Industry* (13.17)
DCIT	Denominazione Commune Italiana
DCP	*Directory of Chemical Producers* (15.29–15.30)
DDF	*Derwent Drug File,* formerly *Ringdoc,* database (14.10)
DDR	*Drug Data Report* database (15.5)
DEA	Drug Enforcement Administration (U.S.)
DES	diethylstilbestrol
DESI	Drug Efficacy Study Implementation
DIA	Drug Information Association
DIC(s)	drug information center(s)
DIF	*Drug Information Fulltext* database (14.18)
DMF	Drug Master File
DNA	deoxyribonucleic acid
DNP	*Drug News & Perspectives* database (15.13)
DOD	Department of Defense (U.S.)
DOT	Department of Transportation (U.S.)
DTC	direct-to-consumer [advertising]
DUR	Drug Utilization Review
EAFUS	Everything added to food in the United States
EAHIL	European Association for Health Information and Libraries
EBM	evidence-based medicine
EC	Enzyme Commission
EC	European Community

ECDIN	Environmental Chemicals Data and Information Network
ECPHIN	European Community Pharmaceutical Information Network
ECRI	Emergency Care Research Institute
ed	editor(s) or edition
ED_{50}	effective dose for 50% of population under investigation
e.g.	*exempli gratia,* Latin "for example"
EINECS	European Inventory of Existing Commercial [Chemical] Substances
EIR	Establishment Inspection Report (FDA)
EIS	Epidemiology Information System, subfile in *TOXLINE* (14.27)
ELA	Establishment License Application
e-mail	electronic mail
EMEA	European Medicines Evaluation Agency
EMIC	Environmental Mutagen Information Center, subfile in *TOXLINE* (14.27)
EP	*European Pharmacopoeia* (11.11)
EP	European Patent
EPA	Environmental Protection Agency (U.S.)
EPAR	European Public Assessment Report
EPhMRA	European Pharmaceutical Marketing Research Association
EPI	electronic package insert
EPIDEM	Epidemiology Information System, subfile in *TOXLINE* (14.27)
EPLC	European Pharma Law Centre
EPO	European Patent Office
ESCOP	European Scientific Cooperative on Phytotherapy (12.5)
ESCP	European Society of Clinical Pharmacy
ETIC	Environmental Teratology Information Center, subfile in *TOXLINE* (14.27)
EU	European Union
Ext D&C	colors classified as safe only in externally-applied drug and cosmetic products
FAAM	*Food Additives Analytical Manual* (11.26)
FAC	fluorouracil + doxorubicin + cyclophosphamide
FAO	Food and Agriculture Organization (United Nations)
FASEB	Federation of American Societies for Experimental Biology
FAQs	frequently asked questions
Fax	telefacsimile
FCC	Federal Communications Commission (U.S. government)
FCC	*Food Chemicals Codex* (11.22)
FD&C	colors certified under the provisions of the Food Drug Cosmetic Act of 1938 and its amendments

FDA	Food and Drug Administration (U.S.)
FDAMA	Food and Drug Administration Modernization Act of 1997
FDC	Food Drug Cosmetic (Act)
FDLI	Food and Drug Law Institute
FDR	*Federated Drug Reference*
FEDRIP	*Federal Research in Progress* database
FL	Florida
FOI	Freedom of Information
FOLE	*Foodline: Current Food Legislation* database (16.3)
FOSHU	foods for specified health use
FR	*Federal Register* (4.24)
FTC	Federal Trade Commission (U.S.)
GA	Georgia
GATT	General Agreement on Tariffs and Trade
GCP	Good Clinical Practice
GLP	Good Laboratory Practice
GMP	Good Manufacturing Practice
GRAS	generally recognized as safe
GSA	General Services Administration (U.S. government)
GUI	graphical user interface
HAPAB	Health Aspects of Pesticides Abstract Bulletin, subfile in *TOXLINE* (14.27)
HBA	health and beauty aids
HCFA	Health Care Financing Administration (U.S.)
HDA	*Health Devices Alerts* database (16.2)
HDS	*Health Devices Sourcebook* database (15.25)
HEED	*Health Economics Evaluations Database*
HEEP	Health Effects of Environmental Pollutants, subfile in *TOXLINE* (14.27)
HIMA	Health Industry Manufacturers Association
HIV	human immunodeficiency virus
HMO	Health Maintenance Organization
HMR	Hoechst Marion Roussel
HMT	Hazardous Materials Technical Center, subfile in *TOXLINE* (14.27)
HND	*Health News Daily* database (15.11)
HPB	Health Protection Branch (Canada)
HPLC	high pressure liquid chromatography
HPSA	*Hospital Personal Selling Audit* (Scott-Levin)
HRF	Herb Research Foundation
HSDB	*Hazardous Substances Data Bank* (14.29)
HTML	hypertext markup language
HWD	*Health & Wellness Database* (IAC) (14.33)

IA	Iowa
IAC	Information Access Company
IACP	International Academy of Compounding Pharmacists
IARC	International Agency for Research on Cancer
IBIDS	*International Bibliographic Information on Dietary Supplements* [database]
ICD-9	*International Classification of Diseases, Ninth Revision*
ICH	International Conferences on Harmonization
ID	identification
ID	Idaho
IDdb	*Investigational Drugs Database* (15.7)
IDE	Investigational Device Exemption
IDIS	*Iowa Drug Information Service* (14.13)
i.e.	*id est,* Latin for "that is"
IEC	International Electrotechnical Commission
IFPMA	International Federation of Pharmaceutical Manufacturers Associations
IHS	Information Handling Services
IL	Illinois
ILO	International Labour Office (Figure 14.12)
IM	intramuscular
IMS	Intercontinental Medical Statistics
INCI	International Nomenclature Cosmetic Ingredient
IND	Investigational New Drug application
INN	International Nonproprietary Name
IP	intellectual property
IP	*International Pharmacopoeia* (11.12)
IP	intraperitoneal
IPA	*International Pharmaceutical Abstracts* (14.8)
IPD	*Incidence and Prevalence Database* (15.39)
IRB	Institutional Review Board
ISE	International Society for Ethnopharmacology
ISI	Institute for Scientific Information
ISMP	Institute for Safe Medication Practices
ISO	International Standards Organization
ISPE	International Society for Pharmaceutical Engineering
ISPE	International Society for Pharmacoepidemiology
ISPOR	International Society for Pharmacoeconomics and Outcomes Research
IUPAC	International Union of Pure and Applied Chemistry
IV	intravenous
IVS	*Index of Veterinary Specialties* (12.49)
JAN	Japanese Accepted Name

JMCP	*Journal of Managed Care Pharmacy*
KS	Kansas
LA	Louisiana
lab	laboratory
LC	lethal concentration
LD_{50}	lethal dose for 50% of population under investigation
LMS	*Literature Monitoring and Evaluation Service* (14.12)
LSD	lysergic acid diethylamide
MA	Massachusetts
MAC	maximum allowable concentration (of air contaminants)
MAC	maximum allowable cost
MAK	maximum arbeitplatz konzentrations (German equivalent of MEL)
MANTIS	*Manual, Alternative and Natural Therapy* database
MaPPs	Manual of Policies and Procedures (FDA)
MD	medical doctor
MD	Maryland
MEDEC	Medical Devices Canada
MDMA	Medical Device Manufacturers Association
MDR	Medical Device Report (adverse experience report)
MDX	Medical Data Exchange (14.34)
MEDDRA	Medical Dictionary of Drug Regulatory Affairs
MEDLARS	Medical Literature and Retrieval System
MEL	Maximum Exposure Level
MERP	Medication Errors Reporting Program
MeSH	*Medical Subject Headings* (14.2)
mg.	milligram
MI	Michigan
MIDAS	Multinational Integrated Data Analysis Service
MIT	Massachusetts Institute of Technology
MLA	Medical Library Association
MMWR	*Morbidity and Mortality Weekly Reports*
MN	Minnesota
MO	Missouri
MRA	Mutual Recognition Agreement
MSD	Merck, Sharp Dohme
MSDS	Material Safety Data Sheet(s)
NABP	National Association of Boards of Pharmacy
NACDS	National Association of Chain Drug Stores
NADA	New Animal Drug Application
NAFTA	North American Free Trade Agreement
NAICS	North American Industry Classification System
NAPM	National Association of Pharmaceutical Manufacturers

NAPRALERT	*Natural Products Alert* database (14.42)
NARD	National Association of Retail Druggists
NAS/NRC	National Academy of Sciences/National Research Council
N.B.	*nota bene* (note well)
NC	North Carolina
NCE	new chemical entity
NCHS	National Center for Health Statistics (U.S.)
NCPA	National Community Pharmacists Association
NDA	New Drug Application
NDC	National Drug Code
NDDF	*National Drug Data File* (First DataBank)
NDL	New Drug List
NDMA	Nonprescription Drug Manufacturers Association
NDMAC	Nonprescription Drug Manufacturers Association of Canada
NDR	*Nonprescription Drug References* (9.45)
NDR	*Nutrition Desk Reference* (7.28)
NDTI	National Disease and Therapeutic Index (IMS)
NE	Nebraska
NEJM	*New England Journal of Medicine*
NF	*National Formulary* (11.8)
NFN	Nordiska Farmacopenamden
NHS	National Health Service (U.K.)
NIH	National Institutes of Health (U.S.)
NIOSH	National Institute of Occupational Safety and Health (U.S.)
NJ	New Jersey
NLM	National Library of Medicine (U.S.)
NM	New Mexico
NME	new molecular entity
NNC	Nutraceutical Network of Canada
No.	number
NRC	National Research Council
NSAIDs	nonsteroidal anti-inflammatory drugs
NSC	National Service Center of the U.S. National Cancer Institute
NTIS	National Technical Information Service (U.S.)
NV	Nevada
NW	Northwest
NWDA	National Wholesale Druggists' Association
NY	New York
NZ	New Zealand
OBRA	Omnibus Budget Reconciliation Act, the Medicaid Drug Rebate Law
OH	Ohio
OHE	Office of Health Economics, ABPI

OHS	Occupational Health Services
OPPT	Office of Pollution Prevention and Toxins (EPA)
OR	Oregon
OSHA	Occupational Safety and Health Administration (U.S.)
OTC	over-the-counter (nonprescription)
P&T	Pharmacy and Therapeutics
PA	Pennsylvania
PAFA	Priority-Based Assessment of Food Additives (FDA)
PBIRG	Pharmaceutical Business Intelligence & Research Group
PC	personal computer
PCT	Patent Cooperation Treaty
PDA	Parenteral Drug Association
PDDA	*Physician Drug & Diagnostic Audit* (Scott-Levin)
PDF	Portable Document Format
PDMA	Prescription Drug Marketing Act of 1987
PDQ	*Physician Data Query* collection of databases (14.22, 14.35–14.36)
PDR	*Physicians' Desk Reference* (6.10)
PEL	Permissible Exposure Limit or Level
PEN	Pharmacy Equivalent Name
PEO News	*PharmacoEconomics & Outcomes News* database (15.14)
PERI	Pharmaceutical Education & Research Institute
PESTAB	Pesticides Abstracts, subfile in *TOXLINE* (14.27)
PGN	*Physicians' Guide to Nutriceuticals* (6.18)
Pharm-AID	*Pharmaceutical Activities Index-Directory* (3.10)
PharmD	Doctor of Pharmacy (academic degree)
PhD	Doctor of Philosophy (academic degree)
PhIL	Pharmaceutical Information Library (INCAD)
PHIND	*Pharmaceutical and Healthcare Industry News Database* (15.9)
photo	photograph
PhRMA	Pharmaceutical Research and Manufacturers of America (formerly PMA)
PHS	Public Health Service (U.S.)
PILs	Patient Information Leaflets
PLA	Product License Application
PMA	Pharmaceutical Manufacturers Association, now PhRMA
PMA	Premarket Application (medical device equivalent of NDA)
PMAC	Pharmaceutical Manufacturers Association of Canada
PMN	Premarket Notification (for low-risk medical devices, also known as 510k)
PNI	*Pharmaceutical News Index database* (15.17)
P.O.	Post Office

PPBIB	Poisonous Plants Bibliography, subfile in *TOXLINE* (14.27)
P.P. Guide	Australian *Prescription Products Guide* (10.25)
PPI	Patient Package Insert
ppm	parts per million
PPO	Preferred Provider Organization
PSA	*Personal Selling Audit* (Scott-Levin)
PTO	Patent and Trademark Office (U.S.)
QOL	quality of life
R&D	research and development
RAPS	Regulatory Affairs Professionals Society
RDA	recommended daily allowance
rDNA	recombinant DNA
RDS	Responsive Database Services
RFP	request for proposal
RN	registry number (Chemical Abstracts Service)
RPh	registered pharmacist (licensed pharmacy practitioner)
RPROJ	Research Projects, subfile in *TOXLINE* (14.27)
RR	related registry numbers
RSC	Royal Society of Chemistry
RTECS	*Registry of Toxic Effects of Chemical Substances* (8.33, 14.28)
RUCAM	Roussel Uclaf Causality Assessment Method
Rx	prescription (abbreviation for *recipe,* the Latin word for "take them")
SAMHSA	Substance Abuse and Mental Health Services Administration (U.S. government)
SBA	Summary Basis of Approval
SBOA	Summary Basis of Approval
SC	South Carolina
SC	subcutaneous
SCI	*Science Citation Index* (14.7)
SCIP	Society of Competitive Intelligence Professionals
SCPH	Société Canadienne des pharmaciens d'hôpitaux
SDI	selective dissemination of information
SE	substantially equivalent
SEC	Securities and Exchange Commission (U.S.)
SEMs	scanning electron microphotographs
SETS	Statistical Expert and Tabulation Systems
SH	section heading
SIC	Standard Industrial Classification
SIDP	Society of Infectious Diseases Pharmacists
SLA	Special Libraries Association
SMDA	Safe Medical Device Act
SNDA	Supplementary New Drug Application

SPA	*Source Prescription Audit* (Scott-Levin)
SPC	Summary of Product Characteristics
SPC	Supplementary Protection Certificate issued under the patent extension program of the EC
SS&E	Summary of Safety and Efficacy (equivalent of SBA for medical devices)
SSCJ	Standard Commodity Classification for Japan
STEL	Short-Term Exposure Level/Limit
TD	toxic dose
TD3	Toxicology Document and Data Depository, subfile in *TOXLINE* (14.27)
TLV	threshold limit value
TN	Tennessee
TOMES	*Toxicology, Occupational Medicine, and Environmental Series* (8.11)
TOXBIB	Toxicity Bibliography, subfile in *TOXLINE* (14.27)
TPA	tissue plasminogen activator
TPN	total parenteral nutrition
TSCA	Toxic Substances Control Act
TSCATS	Toxic Substances Control Act Test Submissions, subfile in *TOXLINE* (14.27)
TX	Texas
U.K.	United Kingdom
ULD	*Unlisted Drugs* (3.8)
URAA	Uruguay Round Agreements Act of 1994 (GATT-enabling legislation in the United States)
URL	Uniform Resource Locator (Internet address)
U.S.	United States
USA	United States of America
USAN	United States Adopted Name
USDA	United States Department of Agriculture
USP	*United States Pharmacopeia* (11.8)
USP DI	*United States Pharmacopeia Dispensing Information* (4.33, 4.43, 6.5, 9.1, 14.19, 14.33)
v.	versus (in legal case citations)
v.	volume(s) in bibliographic citations
VA	Veterans Administration (U.S.)
VA	Virginia
VPB	*Veterinary Pharmaceuticals and Biologicals* (12.44)
VT	Vermont
WA	Washington
WHO	World Health Organization
WHOSIS	World Health Information Statistical Information System

WI	Wisconsin
WIPO	World Intellectual Property Organization
WPI	*World Patents Index* database
WSMI	World Self-Medication Industry
Y2K	Year 2000

Journal title abbreviations used in chapter references and additional source bibliographies:

Acta Anaesth Scand	Acta Anaesthesiologica Scandinavica
Acta Obstet Gynecol Scand	Acta Obstetrica et Gynecologica Scandinavica
Adv Drug React Acute Poison Rev	Adverse Drug Reactions and Acute Poisoning Review
Adv Drug Reac Bull	Adverse Drug Reactions Bulletin
Adv Drug React Toxicol Rev	Adverse Drug Reactions and Toxicological Reviews
Am J Hosp Pharm	American Journal of Hospital Pharmacy
Am J Nurs	American Journal of Nursing
Am J Pharm	American Journal of Pharmacy
Am J Pharm Educ	American Journal of Pharmaceutical Education
Am Pharm	American Pharmacy
Am Demographics	American Demographics
Ann Clin Biochem	Annals of Clinical Biochemistry
Ann Intern Med	Annals of Internal Medicine
Ann Pharmacother	Annals of Pharmacotherapy
Arch Fam Med	Archives of Family Medicine
Arch Intern Med	Archives of Internal Medicine
Aust J Pharm	Australian Journal of Pharmacy
Baillieres Clin Rheumatol	Bailliere's Clinical Rheumatology
Br J Clin Pharmacol	British Journal of Clinical Pharmacology
Brit Med J	British Medical Journal
Bull Med Libr Assoc	Bulletin of the Medical Library Association
Can Med Assoc J	Canadian Medical Association Journal
Can Pharm J	Canadian Pharmaceutical Journal
Clin Exp Dermatol	Clinical and Experimental Dermatology
Clin Perinatol	Clinical Perinatology
Clin Pharm	Clinical Pharmacology
Clin Pharmacokinet	Clinical Pharmacokinetics
Coll & Res Lib News	College & Research Libraries News
Consult Pharm	Consultant Pharmacist

Contemp Pharm Pract	Contemporary Pharmacy Practice
Cosmet Toiletries	Cosmetics and Toiletries
Drexel Libr Q	Drexel Library Quarterly
Drug GMP Rep	The Drug GMP Report
Drug Inf J	Drug Information Journal
Drug Intell Clin Pharm	Drug Intelligence and Clinical Pharmacy
Drug React Toxicol Rev	Drug Reactions and Toxicology Review
Emerg Med Clin North Am	Emergency Medical Clinics of North America
Environ Health Perspect	Environmental Health Perspectives
Euro Hosp Pharm	European Hospital Pharmacy
FDA Consum	FDA Consumer
FDA Drug Bull	FDA Drug Bulletin
FDC Law J	FDC Law Journal
Food Drug Law J	Food and Drug Law Journal
Food Drug Letter	The Food & Drug Letter
Health News Rev	Health News and Review
Hosp Pharm	Hospital Pharmacy
Infor Process Manage	Information Processing and Management
Int J Epidemiol	International Journal of Epidemiology
Int J Psychiatr Med	International Journal of Psychiatry in Medicine
Int Pharm J	International Pharmacy Journal
J Affect Disord	Journal of Affective Disorders
J Am Acad Dermatol	Journal of the American Academy of Dermatology
J Am Med Inform Assoc	Journal of the American Medical Informatics Association
J Am Soc Info Sci	Journal of the American Society of Information Science
J Clin Pharmacol	Journal of Clinical Pharmacology
J Info Sci	Journal of Information Science
J Leg Med	Journal of Legal Medicine
J Pharm Technol	Journal of Pharmacy Technology
J Reprod Med	Journal of Reproductive Medicine
J Res Pharm Econ	Journal of Research in Pharmaceutical Economics
JAMA	Journal of the American Medical Association
Leg Asp Pharm Pract	Legal Aspects of Pharmacy Practice
Library J	Library Journal
Med Care	Medical Care
Med J Aust	Medical Journal of Australia

Med Lett Drugs Ther	The Medical Letter on Drugs and Therapeutics
Med Ref Serv Q	Medical Reference Services Quarterly
N Engl J Med	New England Journal of Medicine
NLM Tech Bull	NLM Technical Bulletin
Nurs Outlook	Nursing Outlook
Obstet Gynecol	Obstetrics and Gynecology
Online Rev	Online Review
Ped Clin N Amer	Pediatric Clinics of North America
Pediatr Res Commun	Pediatric Research Communications
Pharm Exec	Pharmaceutical Executive
Pharm Hist	Pharmacy in History
Pharm Int	Pharmacy International
Pharm J	Pharmaceutical Journal
Pharm Tech	Pharmaceutical Technology
Pharm Times	Pharmacy Times
Regul Toxicol Pharmacol	Regulatory Toxicology and Pharmacology
Risk Anal	Risk Analysis
Soap Perfum Cosmet	Soap, Perfumery and Cosmetics
Teratog Carcinog Mutagen	Teratogenesis, Carcinogenesis and Mutagenesis
Tex Pharm	Texas Pharmacy
Vet Hum Toxicol	Veterinary and Human Toxicology
Wash Drug Letter	Washington Drug Letter

Glossary

510k Premarket notification describing a medical device's specifications and character-istics, mandated under section 510(k) of the 1976 U.S. Medical Device Amendments. Such documents must be submitted to the FDA prior to marketing of low risk devices. Life-supporting and other higher risk devices require *PMAs* before launch.

Abstracts Concise summaries of concepts and facts discussed in primary literature sources.

Access points Elements of information by which a source is accessible, i.e., index terms. In online databases, access points are equivalent to the content of individual segments or fields that can be searched.

Accession numbers Reference numbers assigned to individual entries as they are added (accessioned) in printed indexes or online databases. Such numbers are sometimes used as cross references in hardcopy indexing, instead of page locations, to facilitate rapid location of relevant monographs.

Accreditation The process of being officially authorized or approved by a recognized group, having fulfilled its minimum standards. For example, colleges of pharmacy in the United States are not accredited unless they are approved by the American Council on Pharmaceutical Education (ACPE).

Acronym A word constructed from the initial letters of other words, that is, a pro-nounceable abbreviation, such as WHO (World Health Organization). Beware: acro-nyms tend to be ambiguous when used as search terms online and, for this reason, are rarely preferred in indexing.

Acute disease Relatively short term, often sudden and severe, single episode illness, as opposed to a chronic condition.

Acute toxicity Effects of a single dose; measure of the short term (immediate) effects of exposure.

Addiction Physical and/or psychological dependence on a drug product.

Adjuvant A drug that enhances the effect of another, but does not necessarily have a beneficial effect by itself. For example, aluminum added to certain vaccines enhances immune response (the protection given by a vaccine). Adjuvants are sometimes added to drug formulations to assist the manufacturing process; e.g., methylcellulose is an excipient that aids suspension of drug participles in a liquid.

Admixture A parenteral preparation to which other substances have been added for therapeutic purposes, to avoid multiple injection sites. Admixtures intended for intravenous administration often combine electrolytes and various drugs into a solution for infusion.

Adulterated   A drug product is said to be adulterated when foreign or inferior substances are present that render it impure, leading to unintentional or illicit contamination or decomposition of the preparation. Assays can detect adulteration.

Adverse effect   An unintended or undesirable response to a drug correctly administered within a medically accepted dosage range.

Advisory Committee/Panel   Functional unit established by the FDA to assist in assessment of data presented in new drug applications. Committee membership consists of clinical experts in the specialized therapeutic areas they will be asked to review and one consumer advocate. Members can be identified by consulting annual hardcopy editions of *NDA Pipeline* (4.20).

Agonist   Stimulant. An agonist drug bonds to a receptor, initiating or increasing a particular activity in a cell (opposite of an antagonist).

Allergen   A substance capable of producing an allergy, or one used to treat or test for allergy.

Allergy   see Hypersensitivity.

Ambulatory care   Health services delivered on an outpatient (noninstitutionalized or outside hospital) basis. If a patient visits a physician's office or surgical center, the resulting therapy is considered ambulatory care, but in-home health services are generally excluded from the definition of this term.

Anaphylactic reaction   A group of symptoms usually resulting from an overwhelming, severe allergic reaction.

ANDA   Abbreviated New Drug Application. When the patent for a drug has expired, companies other than the originator can apply to market comparable products. Manufacturers of these generic or "me-too" forms are not required to repeat the extensive testing required for new drugs, but instead may submit an Abbreviated NDA documenting the bioequivalence of their formulation to the predicate, or reference-listed, drug. This type of simplified submission is generally permitted only for products with the same active ingredients, dosage form, route of administration, strength, indication, and labeling as products already accepted as safe and effective.

ANDA Suitability Petition   Documentation submitted to the FDA requesting permission to file an Abbreviated New Drug Application (ANDA), rather than a full NDA. Such a petition is required when the generic product proposed differs in minor ways (dosage form, strength, route) from the innovator drug on which the ANDA will rely for proof of safety and efficacy.

Anodyne   A soothing medicine that relieves pain.

Antagonist   An inhibitor or blocker. An antagonist drug binds to a receptor, blocking bonds by other substances, but does not have a stimulating effect on a cell (opposite of an agonist).

Antedrug   Term coined to describe drugs that possess local anti-inflammatory activity, but which are rapidly metabolized to pharmacologically inactive compounds upon entry into blood circulation from the tissue to which they are applied, thereby resulting in no systemic toxicity. Antedrugs are converted to inactive or less active metabolites through the process of biotransformation.

Antibody   A protein produced by the body as a protective response to an antigen or foreign substance.

Antidote   A substance that counteracts the effects of a poison.

Antigen   A substance that triggers an immune response and the production of antibodies. Antigens are regulated as biologics under U.S. law.

Apothecary   The British term for pharmacist; see also Chemist.

Approvable letter   Official, written communication from the FDA to an NDA sponsor that indicates authorization to market a product, contingent upon resolution of issues listed in the letter.

Armamentarium   Arsenal or armory; in medicine, the array of therapeutic options available to practitioners.

ASCII   American Standards Code for Information Interchange, the predominant character set used in encoding computers. ASCII enables information exchange among data processing systems, data communications systems, and associated equipment worldwide. ASCII could be described as an alphabet used in machine languages.

Assay   Analysis of a drug to determine the presence, absence, or quantity of one or more components, used as a means of estimating the strength of a drug measured against a pharmacopeial (official) standard. A chemical assay quantitatively determines the amount of a specific compound present in a given sample and is sometimes used as a basis for preliminary determination of potential biological activity. A biological assay estimates the strength of a drug by using a living organism, and may involve determination of threshold or lethal dose, as well as other measurable responses indicative of drug effects.

Authority list   see Controlled vocabulary; see also Thesaurus.

Bibliographic database   A compilation of references or citations to source documents, rather than the full text of the source documents themselves.

Binder   A substance added to pharmaceutical preparations that will cause particles to adhere to one another, used as an aid to subsequent tablet compression. Synonym: adhesive.

Bioavailability   A measurement of the amount of a drug that reaches the body's general circulation and the rapidity and extent of its absorption into the bloodstream (usually expressed as a percentage of the dose given). Determinations may involve examination of drug levels in the blood at timed intervals after administration, or measuring the cumulative amount of the drug (or its breakdown products after metabolism) excreted in urine and the rate at which it accumulates in the urine. Major factors that affect a product's bioavailability are chemical and physical characteristics (formulation) of the dosage form and, if orally administered, the functional state of the digestive system of an individual who takes it.

Bioequivalence   Indicates that a drug in a given dosage form reaches the body's general circulation at the same relative rate and to the same relative extent. This type of equivalence should be distinguished from 1) chemical equivalence, indicating that two or more dosage forms contain the same quantities of a drug; 2) clinical equivalence, which occurs when the same drug from two or more dosage forms gives identical *in vivo* effects as measured by a pharmacological response or by control of a symptom or disease; and 3) therapeutic equivalence, implying that one structurally different chemical can yield the same clinical results as another chemical.

Biologics, biologicals   Products composed of, or extracted from, a living organism, defined in U.S. law (Public Health Service Act of 1944) as "any virus, therapeutic serum, toxin, antitoxin, vaccine, blood, blood component or derivative, allergenic product, or analogous product . . . applicable to the prevention, treatment, or cure of diseases, or injuries in man. . . ."

Biomaterial A substance, other than a drug, designed for use in a physiological system to supplement or replace the functions of body tissues or organs. Examples include polymers, plastics, metals, and ceramics that are biocompatible and inert.

Biometrics The statistical study of biological investigations. Biometrics often involves calculation of a dose-response curve.

Biopharmaceutics Study of the effects of formulation and physical/chemical properties of a drug product on its therapeutic efficacy and action within the body. Typical biopharmaceutics studies examine the effect of dosage form characteristics (e.g., particle size, hardness, coating) and route of administration on bioavailability, pharmacokinetics, and bioequivalence.

Biotoxins Poisonous or harmful substances found in nature (e.g., plants, animals).

Biotransformation Chemical alteration or change in a drug that occurs after its introduction into the body and as a result of the biological system's action on the externally administered therapeutic agent.

Board certified see Certification.

Bookmarks Bookmarks, also known as "Favorites" in Internet Explorer software, are URLs (Internet addresses) saved for future use in browser software for accessing the World Wide Web.

Bolus dose see Loading dose.

Boolean Logic used in online searching that employs the operators (connecting words) AND, OR, and NOT to specify relationships among terms or concept sets. Named after the mathematician George Boole.

Botanicals Medicinal preparations derived from plants (i.e., herbal drugs).

Brand name Proprietary name used in commerce (also referred to as a trade name), which is often a registered trademark.

Browser Software that can find and display data from the Internet, essentially transforming a computer screen into a window on the Web. A browser enables users to view text as it was originally formatted by its publisher, with fonts, capitalization, spacing, and hotlinks intact (accompanied by graphics and sound, in many cases). Mosaic was the first browser, launched in 1993. Netscape soon followed in 1994. Internet Explorer is another example of a popular browser software.

Buffer A chemical that resists changes in hydrogen ion concentrations, added to pharmaceutical formulations to keep pH relatively constant.

Carcinogenic Cancer causing.

CD-ROM Compact disc, read-only memory; media on which information is stored.

CE Mark The two-letter symbol affixed to products, such as medical devices, indicating that they have been designed and manufactured in compliance with European Union directives (laws). With an overall purpose of ensuring health and safety without requiring submission of evidence to regulatory authorities in individual countries, EU directives establish norms or standard specifications with which a product must conform before introduction into the European marketplace. CE is an abbreviation for Communauté Européene.

Certifiable color additives Colors whose safety for human consumption has been established and which are listed in the Code of Federal Regulations as permitted for use in foods, drugs, cosmetics, and medical devices. Before using such additives (usually derived from petroleum or coal sources), manufacturers must submit to the FDA samples from each batch produced. Agency certification is required for each batch, whereby authorization to use is based on testing validation that dyes meet established chemical specifications. See also Exempt color additives.

Certification In educational vocabulary, certification is a form of recognition by a professional, nongovernmental agency indicating that an individual has completed additional training, beyond that required for licensure to practice, and demonstrated mastery of a higher level of knowledge and skills in a given specialty. The Board of Pharmaceutical Specialties (BPS, see Appendix D) is the certification authority recognized in U.S. pharmacy practice.

CFR Code of Federal Regulations. Compilation of regulations promulgated by U.S. federal agencies under the authority of legislation. Regulations are classified by subject area for annual publication under "titles" in the *Code of Federal Regulations*. Title 21 contains most government regulations regarding drugs.

Chain drugstore One of a group of community pharmacies under common ownership and operation.

Chemist In British usage, a term referring to a provider of pharmaceutical services, i.e., a pharmacist in the United Kingdom.

Chemotherapy In its broadest and most literal sense, chemotherapy is the use of chemical agents in the treatment of disease. However, when first coined, usage of this term was originally restricted to drugs used in the treatment of infections caused by microorganisms, then later extended to include drugs used in cancer therapy. Some publications still confine coverage of chemotherapy to antimicrobials and anti-infectives; examples include *BIOSIS Previews* and *The Merck Veterinary Manual*.

Chronic Long term, persistent, or recurring; opposite of acute.

Chronic toxicity Effects of long-term exposure; chronic toxicity testing of drugs is usually six to twelve months in duration.

Chronopharmacology Study of drug action over periods of time; also, study of the effects of drugs on biorhythms or the influence of biorhythms on patient response to drugs. For example, some medications are known to achieve higher concentrations diurnally than nocturnally (during the day, versus at night).

Claims In drug or device labeling, statements made about the benefits or performance of a product. In patents, "claims" describe what applicants propose should be protected from competition, i.e., what the invention is and its unique or novel characteristics.

Class A narcotics Former name for drugs now classified as Schedule II controlled substances.

Class B narcotics Former name for drugs now classified as Schedule III controlled substances.

Classification Any systematic scheme for the arrangement of items. Document or book classification is usually according to subject. Drug classification groups together products with comparable 1) therapeutic use, 2) pharmacological action, or 3) chemical structure. When laws or regulations are classified by subject, they are said to be codified within "titles." For example, regulations affecting drugs are classified together in Title 21 of the *Code of Federal Regulations*.

Clinical Related to investigations, observations, or actual treatment of patients (usually humans), as distinct from theoretical or basic science research. The term originates from the Greek klinicos, "relating to a bed."

Community pharmacy Retail site where drugs are dispensed by a licensed pharmacist outside a hospital or institutional setting, i.e., what nonprofessionals refer to as a drugstore. It is estimated that 70% of the more than 166,240 registered pharmacists in the United States practice in a community setting, either in independent pharmacies or chain drugstores.

Compendial standards see Pharmacopeia.

Compendium A book that compiles facts in concise form; plural: compendia.

Compliance Strict adherence to a prescribed treatment plan.

Compounding The preparation, mixing, assembling, and packaging of a drug or medical device to fulfill the special requirements of a given patient. For example, in geriatric or pediatric care, the need for palatable liquid forms of medication usually administered in tablets may lead to a request for compounding. Compounding may also be called for in cases where a patient is allergic to a preservative or dye used in a commercially available product that has been prescribed.

Contraindication Any condition or disease that makes the indicated or expected treatment inadvisable (for example, pre-existing renal or liver impairment, known hypersensitivity). In prescribing literature, a contraindication is a warning that carries greater weight than a "precaution."

Control In clinical studies, controls are untreated participants or those treated using an established or previously accepted therapy. Controls are used as a standard for comparison, to verify inferences deduced from study results.

Controlled substances Substances whose distribution is regulated under anti-drug-abuse laws; see also Scheduled drugs.

Controlled vocabulary A standardized list of subject terms (descriptors) used in indexing records entered into a database to characterize the content of sources cited; also known as an authority list or database thesaurus.

Cosmetics Defined in U.S. law as products applied to the human body for the purpose of cleansing, beautifying, promoting attractiveness, or altering appearance without affecting the body's structure or function. Examples include skin creams, perfumes, deodorants, and hair dyes. Toiletries or personal care products intended to affect body structure or function, such as fluoride toothpastes, antidandruff shampoos, antiperspirants, sunscreens, or hormone creams, are regulated as drugs in the United States. Such products are sometimes referred to as cosmeticeuticals.

CRADA Cooperative research and development agreement between a U.S. government agency and collaborators in industry, academia, or another government agency. CRADAs are a means for government agencies to obtain additional money, materials, and personnel to accomplish goals. In exchange, nongovernment collaborators obtain a first option to license any patented inventions that may result from a CRADA. These partnership agreements enable participants to share ideas and costs, for the purpose of developing specific therapeutic substances or technologies for ultimate commercialization.

Cross-over trial A clinical study in which patients receive each treatment in turn, typically used when testing therapies for chronic diseases or investigating pharmacological action in healthy volunteers.

Crude drug   A nonpurified or unprocessed form of a drug, obtained from a plant or animal; sometimes used as a synonym for natural drug.

Cupping   The application of a glass cup to the surface of the skin, for the purpose of drawing blood to (or through) it by creating a partial vacuum.

Cutaneous   Of or on the skin; for example, cutaneous effects of drugs are observable skin reactions. Percutaneous action describes passing through the skin (the mechanism used in the dosage forms called transdermal patches); subcutaneous refers to injections under the skin.

Cyberspace   Popular or colloquial term for the Internet. The "space" metaphor has been extended with terms such as "Internauts," used to refer to Internet searchers or explorers in cyberspace.

Cytotoxic   Capable of killing or injuring living cells; many anticancer and antibiotic drugs use cytotoxicity to accomplish therapeutic goals.

Data sheet   Information prepared by manufacturers and intended for prescribers, to ensure safe and effective use. Comparable to a package insert or officially approved labeling.

Databank   A collection of databases accessible through a uniform command language developed by an individual online vendor.

Database   A collection of information on a common theme. Online or CD-ROM databases are in machine-readable form (magnetic tape or compact disc), accessible by computer.

Decoction   A solution containing the active constituents of crude drugs, prepared by boiling the natural drug source in water and straining the resulting solution.

Delaney Clause   Portion of the 1958 Food Additives Amendment that prohibits use in food of any substance shown to be capable of causing cancer at any dosage/exposure level in any species.

Demography   Statistical study of populations; data reflecting the pattern of occurrence of given conditions in a defined community.

Dependence   Reliance on use of a drug; includes habituation (psychological dependence) and physiological addiction.

Descriptor   A word or phrase added to a database record to describe the subject matter covered in the source document cited and to assist subsequent location and retrieval of that record.

Designer drugs   A term generally used to refer to new, illicit (not officially approved) analogs or variations on existing controlled substances, developed to duplicate or exceed their effects.

Detail man (woman)   A professionally trained manufacturer's representative who can provide detailed information to healthcare practitioners about a company's products. Also detailer.

Diagnostics   Laboratory tests used in screening, diagnosing, or monitoring a patient for disease and its progression or alleviation during the course of therapy.

Dispensing   Supplying a drug to a patient in accordance with a prescription.

Documentation   A collection of documents or references to sources, compiled to verify information on a given subject. A bibliography accompanying a drug monograph would constitute documentation of facts cited.

Dosage forms   Forms in which a drug is produced and dispensed. For example, oral dosage forms include pills, syrups, elixirs, tinctures, and emulsions. The term *pill* usually refers only to tablets that are candy-(sugar)-coated, also known in Europe and Latin America as *dragees* or *grageas*. Syrups are watery solutions of a drug with a high concentration of sugar, flavoring, and coloring. An elixir is similar to a syrup, but contains alcohol in addition to sugared flavored water. A dosage form where a drug is dissolved in water with a high concentration of alcohol is called a tincture. An emulsion is a water solution to which gum has been added to hold the drug mixture in suspension.

Dose-response curve   A graph of the relationship between the dose (drug amount administered) and the response, showing the extent or degree of the medication's effect, positive or negative.

Dosimetry   Dose range finding; determination of the appropriate quantity of a drug to administer, based on its properties and on patient characteristics such as age, gender, and body mass or surface area.

Double-blind   Drug testing where therapeutic effects are measured against a placebo, and where study participants (prescribers, dispensers, and recipients) are unaware of which patients are receiving the drug versus the placebo. The intent is to avoid bias in observations due to preconceived ideas.

Drug   Any chemical agent that affects living processes, used therapeutically. U.S. law defines drugs as "articles intended for use in the diagnosis, cure, mitigation, treatment, or prevention of disease in man . . ." and "articles (other than food) intended to affect the structure or any function of the body of man. . . ." Drug and drug product are often used interchangeably to refer to medicinals used in health care. Strictly speaking, drug refers to a single chemical entity that provokes a specific response when placed within a biological system—the active ingredient. Drug product is the manufactured dosage form (tablet, capsule, elixir) that contains the active drug intermixed with inactive ingredients to provide for convenient administration.

Drug lag   Delay in the commercial introduction of new medicines into the marketplace caused by regulatory procedures.

Drug Master File   Documentation that describes production methods (chemical synthesis and formulation) used to produce drug ingredients, including physical and chemical properties of compounds and detailed data on the manufacturing process used. A Drug Master File (DMF) already submitted to the FDA may be cited in subsequent new drug applications as a convenient way to avoid replication of information. DMFs are also a means for bulk chemical suppliers to comply with regulatory requirements of NDAs without disclosing commercially sensitive information directly to sponsors of proposed products in which their ingredients will be used.

Drug Utilization Review   A survey of drug usage. DURs are initiated to quantify the incidence of interactions, identify contraindications, gauge patient compliance (and noncompliance), evaluate prescribing patterns in terms of safety, efficacy, or economic considerations, and to uncover fraudulent practices, such as benefit use by ineligibles. The goal of Drug Utilization Review may be cost reduction through elimination of medications deemed unnecessary or inappropriate for the population studied.

Druggist   A lay (nonprofessional) term for a pharmacist in the United States. Druggist refers to a drug wholesaler in British usage (as distinct from an apothecary or chemist).

ED_{50}   Effective dose for 50% of the population under study, or, in molecular pharmacology, the dose of a drug that produces 50% of the maximum effect possible.

Efficacy   Effectiveness; product performance resulting in achieving the effects intended (treatment, cure, or prevention of the disease or symptoms). A distinction is sometimes made in the literature between efficacy, defined as effects under controlled or experimental conditions, versus effectiveness, described as efficacy under real life (uncontrolled or nonexperimental) conditions.

EIR Establishment Inspection Report, prepared by an FDA investigator to record observations from a visit to a drug manufacturing establishment or clinical investigation site; see also Form 483.

Elixir see Dosage forms.

Empirical Based on experience or observation, in contrast to theory or knowledge, resulting from controlled experiments. An empirical formula is a simplified way of noting the constituents of a compound and their proportions, but not their structural configuration.

Endogenous Originating internally, synthesized by the body; e.g., endogenous hormones or enzymes, versus those developed exogenously (outside the body).

Endpoint A measurable indicator of a drug's effect, such as pain reduction; see also Surrogate endpoints.

Enteric-coated tablet Tablets coated with a thin outer layer to prevent breakdown by stomach acid and delay release of the medication until it can be dissolved in the intestines. Synonymous with delayed-release, enteric coating is added to avoid destruction or inactivation of the drug's ingredients by gastric juices or to avoid irritation these ingredients may cause to the gastric mucosa. Enteric-coated tablets should not be crushed or chewed.

EPAR European Public Assessment Report, a document prepared by the European Medicines Evaluation Agency (EMEA) for drugs approved through the centralized registration procedure (see Chapter Four). EPARs are intended to show the scientific basis on which the product was approved and to provide background to the agency's assessment of the drug's safety, quality, and efficacy.

Epidemiology Study of the distribution and causes of disease (originally, epidemics), investigating the frequency, extent, and likelihood of occurrence (incidence and prevalence) in a specific geographic area or defined patient population, and estimating morbidity and mortality.

Ethical drugs Drugs marketed directly to physicians, hospitals, and other healthcare professional groups, as opposed to those marketed directly to the consumer. Ethical drugs can be either prescription or nonprescription products. The term originated in the early 1900s, to distinguish between drugs obtained from reputable practitioners and the less reliable "patent medicines" distributed by others.

Ethnopharmacology Scientific study of drugs traditionally used in the folk (indigenous) medicine of various cultures. Using modern pharmacological and chemical procedures, ethnopharmacologists investigate remedies derived from nature (extracted from plants, animals, marine life, fungi, etc.). Pharmacoanthropology has sometimes been used as a synonym for ethnopharmacology.

Etiology Evolution or development of a disease and study of causative agents or contributing factors.

Excipient Any component, other than the therapeutically active substance(s), intentionally added to a drug product to ensure delivery of active ingredients to the patient in the quantity and at the rate of release or bioavailability needed. Excipients are also referred to as additives, vehicles, bases, or pharmaceutical adjuvants. These ingredients are not necessarily inert or inactive. They include diluents, fillers, flavors, preservatives, binders, and lubricants.

Exempt color additives   Additives authorized by the government for use in drugs, cosmetics, medical devices, or foods without further "batch certification." Such additives are primarily derived from plant, animal, or mineral sources (other than petroleum or coal). See also Certifiable color additives.

Exempt narcotic drug   Former name for a drug that would be classified as a Schedule V controlled substance today, which could be sold without a prescription, but for which a record of sales was required.

Exogenous agents   Substances developed or originating externally (outside the body), versus endogenous chemicals.

Expiration dating   see Shelf life.

Extemporaneous   Prepared in response to a current need.

Extended-release   Pharmacopeial term for dosage forms designed to make medication available over an extended period of time. Synonyms include: prolonged-action, controlled-release, sustained-release, or repeat-action. See also Enteric-coated tablet.

Extra-label indications   see Off-label indications.

False drops   Irrelevant citations retrieved in an online search of the literature, usually resulting from ambiguity in terminology used or keywords acquiring different meanings in unanticipated contexts. Such references "drop" out (appear) in results because they match the requirements expressed in search statements entered by the user, but are inappropriate to answer the question posed. Some authors refer to these often unavoidable items as noise.

Fields   Sections or portions of an online record designated for storage of specified information; e.g., the title field or the author field in a bibliographic citation. Synonyms are paragraphs, data elements, or record elements.

File   An organized collection of information on a common theme; synonym for database.

Fine chemical   A substance sold or used in relatively small quantities (pounds or lesser units of measure), in contrast to bulk chemicals that are used or sold in quantities of more than 100 pounds. Most finished drugs are considered fine chemicals. In the context of pharmaceuticals, the term connotes quantity, rather than quality.

Folk medicine   Therapeutic or preventive practices based on the beliefs and customs traditional within a given culture.

Form 483   The form used by FDA inspectors to document objectionable or violative conditions observed during site visits to drug manufacturing facilities or clinical investigators.

Formulation   The combination of pharmacologically active and other ingredients in a given dosage form and strength (concentration), in which a medicine is presented or marketed.

Formulary   A drug compendium or list of drugs used to guide and control therapy. A positive formulary lists all drugs that may be prescribed. A negative formulary lists drugs excluded from use. State formularies have been developed to identify drugs authorized for generic substitution and/or reimbursement under sponsored medical assistance programs. A formulary developed for use within a hospital is generally the work of a pharmacy and therapeutics (P&T) committee and reflects the current clinical judgment of the medical staff. A hospital formulary provides prescribing, dispensing, and administration information about a selection of drugs on inventory in-house. See also Practice formulary.

Free text   see Natural language.

Front end   see Interface.

Full-text files   Databases that contain the complete text of documents, rather than only brief citations or bibliographic references accompanied by abstracts. Graphic (illustrative pictorial) material is generally omitted from full-text files, due to economic and technological constraints in creating and using digitized images.

Galenical   A medicinal agent prepared without the aid of chemical reactions or changes, usually involving mixing or extraction of solvents (e.g., tinctures or decoctions). The name is a reference to the formulas of Galen, a physician who practiced in Rome circa 129–200 AD. Today, galenicals are standard preparations containing organic ingredients from natural products, as contrasted with pure chemical substances.

Generic drugs   Drugs marketed under their nonproprietary name rather than a brand name.

Generic name   A simplified, nonproprietary name for a drug.

Grandfather drugs   Drugs introduced into U.S. commerce prior to passage of the 1938 Food Drug Cosmetic Act, and therefore exempt from its requirements that manufacturers submit proof of safety and efficacy prior to marketing approval.

Habituation   A form of drug dependence based upon strong psychological gratification, rather than the physical (chemical) dependence of addiction.

Half-life   The time required for one-half of an administered dose of a drug to disappear in the body (be eliminated from the bloodstream or excreted). Half-lives are plotted by measuring plasma concentrations at stated intervals after drug administration and by calculations of renal excretion. The half-life of a drug assists in determining the frequency of dosage recommended.

Hardcopy   A document in book, journal, or manuscript form, as opposed to microform or machine-readable (magnetic tape or CD-ROM) format. Not to be confused with binding: hardcopy documents may have "soft" covers.

Herb   Technically, a leafy plant without a woody stem. In pharmaceutical, rather than botanical, literature, the term *herb* is often used as a synonym for any plant.

Herbal   Related to plants (not necessarily those defined botanically as herbs). In the pharmacy literature, an herbal is also a type of book devoted to discussion of plant-derived drugs. Such publications also often contain sections on animal-derived therapeutic preparations and on minerals used medicinally (i.e., "simple" drugs, also known as *materia medica*).

Hierarchical   Arranged or classified in ranks or orders. A hierarchical classification scheme, when viewed in outline format, will usually reflect broader and narrower subject relationships among terms or codes used in indexing, and serves to bring together items that are conceptually (but perhaps not alphabetically) related.

Home page   Opening page of an Internet site (sometimes written as homepage). Information on the World Wide Web is presented in units referred to as pages. A Web site is usually a collection of pages of information, starting with an interface, or index, home page that contains hotlinks to data available at other locations in the collection.

Homeopathy   A system of medicine based on the theory that "like cures like," involving administration of minute doses of substances that, in larger doses, would produce symptoms similar to those of the disease being treated.

Hotlines Telephone answering services dedicated to answering questions within their stated scope quickly, with a minimum of referrals.

Hotlinks A software feature incorporated into the World Wide Web system for accessing the Internet whereby the user, by clicking (with a computer mouse) on highlighted words, will be connected to other pages or sites without knowing or specifying their URL address codes. Hotlinks include both hypertext and hypermedia (graphic or image) links. Hotlinks (or simply links) are essentially computer-assisted cross references instantly accessible through point-and-click software technology. URLs are the underlying mechanism of hotlinks. Creators of Web pages use Hypertext Markup Language (HTML) to enable cross references to related sources as pointers hidden behind underlined text or images "mapped" to other pages.

HTML see Hypertext.

Hydrophilic Having an affinity for water; water-loving. Opposite of hydrophobic.

Hypersensitivity Allergy, an abnormal mechanism of drug response occurring in individuals who produce injurious antibodies that react with foreign substances. Allergic reactions, which can include rash, fever, swollen glands, or jaundice, are usually attributable to a patient's immune response.

Hypertext Text that contains links to related information. Hypertext Markup Language (HTML) is the syntax used to "mark up" documents so that they can be formatted appropriately and linked to other documents on the World Wide Web. See also Hotlinks.

Iatrogenic Physician-induced.

Idiopathic Term used to describe a disease or condition of unknown cause.

Idiosyncrasy Peculiar to an individual. Idiosyncratic reactions to drugs are not a form of allergy or hypersensitivity; instead, they occur in patients with a defect in body chemistry (often hereditary) that produces an effect totally unrelated to the drug's normal pharmacological action. Examples are phenylthiourea or warfarin resistance.

Immunization Administration of a drug to induce immunity (resistance) to a disease or infection. For example, vaccines are administered to prevent the spread of infectious, communicable diseases.

Imprint In drug information, used to refer to a manufacturer's marking on dosage forms (codes, logos, monograms); in publishing, imprint equates to the publisher's name and imprint date refers to the publication date of a book.

In vitro Isolated from a living organism; artificially maintained outside the living body, as in a test tube (from the Latin *in vitro* = "in glass").

In vivo Within a living organism.

Incidence In epidemiology, a measure of the number of new cases of illness over a stated period of time in a given population. Incidence is used to describe a changing situation and gauges the occurrence of events beginning within the specified time period, in contrast with prevalence, which examines the number of cases existing at a given point in time.

Incompatibility Physical or chemical interactions between two or more therapeutic agents outside the body, before administration. The term customarily implies studies of parenteral (injectable drug) solutions and effects of their admixture for co-administration intravenously. Physical incompatibility often leads to visible, recognizable changes, such as formation of a precipitate in solutions. Incompatibility data must also address the potential effects of packaging and drug delivery system components on potency and efficacy.

IND Investigational New Drug application. Before a new drug entity can be tested in humans, U.S. drug law requires submission of information to the FDA specified as a "Notice of Claimed Investigational Exemption for a New Drug," commonly referred to as an IND. An IND includes data about the chemical composition of a drug and its manufacture; results of all preclinical testing in animals and laboratory experiments, with an analysis of their implications for human pharmacology; and proposed clinical protocols for Phase I testing, including the qualifications of investigators.

Indications Diseases or other conditions for which therapy is needed, that is, accepted medical applications or uses of a drug or device. Approved indications are those circumstances under which the drug or medical device may be safely and effectively used, as determined by government regulatory agency recommendations.

Indigenous Native to a particular place. Indigenous medicine is a synonym for folk or traditional medicine.

Informed consent Voluntary written confirmation by a patient of willingness to participate in a clinical trial. Ethical guidelines for obtaining such consent specify that prospective experimental subjects be provided with information about the study, such as its objectives, potential benefits and risks, and the patient's rights and responsibilities.

Inhibitor see Antagonist.

Institutional pharmacy The practice of pharmacy in private or government owned hospitals, HMOs, clinics, long-term care facilities, hospices, or nursing homes; differentiate from community pharmacy.

Integumentary Related to the surface or skin, sometimes used as a synonym for cutaneous or dermal.

Intellectual property Intangible property (possessions, assets) resulting from intellectual effort, i.e., copyrights, trademarks, and patents.

Interface The computer programs constructed to mediate interaction between the user and information stored in a databank; includes design of screen displays, search capabilities, context-sensitive help available, and format of output.

Internauts see Cyberspace.

Intoxication State of being poisoned (Note: not limited to the effects of alcohol overdose).

Intranets Computer networks implemented internally within companies or academic institutions that use Internet technology.

IV additives Nutrient or electrolyte solutions in which parenteral drugs are typically administered.

Labeling In drug regulations and literature, this term refers not only to information actually affixed to a container, but also to any written, printed material intended to accompany a drug product, such as a package insert.

Lag time The time period that elapses between publication of documents (journal articles, books, drug approval announcements, or notices of patent extensions) and their availability through indexing in secondary sources.

Latency period Interval from the commencement of drug administration before effects manifest themselves.

LD$_{50}$ Lethal dose for 50% of the population under study (median lethal dose). Route of administration and animal species are usually appended to this measurement or expression of toxicity.

Legend drugs   Drugs that can be purchased only when authorized by a licensed practitioner and bear the legend: "Caution: federal law prohibits dispensing without prescription."

Licensed preparations   see Registration.

Licensure   The means by which a government agency grants permission to an individual to engage in a given healthcare occupation. In the United States, licensure requirements for pharmacy are established by individual states and, at minimum, include completion of a degree program at an accredited college (see Chapter Four). Distinguish from certification.

Line extensions   Variations on previously approved products, such as new dosage forms, strengths, or indications. Line extensions are a way of prolonging the commercial life of an accepted brand.

Links   see Hotlinks.

Loading dose   Initial administration of a drug in a larger amount than usual, in order to achieve a therapeutic concentration in the bloodstream more rapidly. Synonyms: bolus dose, priming dose.

MAC (Maximum Allowable Cost)   The maximum price permitted under state or federal guidelines for reimbursement. A MAC is usually based on the lowest price charged among vendors of products accepted as bioequivalents.

Managed care   Reimbursement programs for health services that manage allocation of healthcare benefits. In contrast to indemnity insurers, which do not govern what medical services are provided as a contingency for payment, managed care firms attempt to control costs by regulating therapeutic options that may be used by participants.

Materia medica   Literally, the raw materials used in medicine; generally refers to crude drugs derived from nature.

Material Safety Data Sheet (MSDS)   A form required by the U.S. Occupational Safety and Health Administration (OSHA) for each hazardous chemical found in the workplace, describing precautionary measures to protect workers.

Medical device   An instrument, apparatus, implement, machine, implant, *in vitro* reagent, or other contrivance used in health care that is not dependent upon being metabolized to achieve its intended purpose. For example, artificial organs, wound dressings, home test kits, dental anesthetic needles, and stethoscopes are all medical devices.

MEL (Maximum Exposure Level)   Maximum concentration of an airborne substance, averaged over a reference period, to which employees may be exposed by inhalation (usually eight hours for long-term MEL or ten minutes for short term). MEL is a safety level established under British Law; comparable limits are TLV, recommended by the American Conference of Governmental Industrial Hygienists, or MAK (maximum *arbeitplatz konzentrations*), set by German authorities.

Meta-analysis   A type of literature review or survey of clinical trial reports that involves quantitative analysis of combined results drawn from independent studies, with the purpose of arriving at a synthesized conclusion or consensus in order to evaluate therapeutic efficacy or pinpoint the need for further investigation in specific areas.

Metabolite   A substance produced directly by biotransformation of a chemical. For example, phenol in urine is a metabolite of benzene and is an indicator of benzene absorption by an individual.

Me-too drug   A product intended to replicate an existing drug, with only minor chemical modifications, and offering little or no improvement in therapeutic benefit.

Monograph   Written material devoted to a single subject, e.g., a separately published book on a given topic or an entry related to a specific drug in a published compendium.

Morbidity   Incidence or prevalence of sickness or illness in a given population or locale.

Mortality   Death rate; proportion of deaths to a population.

Multisource drug products   Off-patent medications for which generic versions are approved and available on the market.

Mutagenicity   Capable of causing mutation; ability of an agent to cause alteration in genetic material that results in changes in cell reproduction.

Narcotic drug   A preparation that diminishes sensibility and relieves pain, often inducing lethargy, drowsiness, or sleep.

Natural language   Ordinary spoken or written language. Natural language searching refers to accessing databases with terms of the user's own choosing, in contrast to controlled vocabulary searching, where a user adheres to a finite list of authorized terminology known to be preferred in indexing. Synonyms for natural language searching are free-text or textword searching.

NDA   New Drug Application. To market a new drug intended for human use through interstate commerce in the United States, a manufacturer must have an approved NDA from the FDA. NDAs include documentation of the results of clinical testing sufficient to support claimed indications (efficacy) and safe use.

Neonate   Newborn, generally defined medically as up to four weeks old.

Nonproprietary   Not held under patent, trademark, or copyright by a private company or person. Nonproprietary names for drugs are synonymous with generic names.

Nootropic   Enhancing cognition (learning) or memory; nootropic agents have sometimes been called smart drugs.

Nutraceuticals   Popular term for dietary supplements; products intended to augment conventional food and marketed for ingestion in pill, capsule, tablet, or liquid form. Examples include vitamins, minerals, herbs, and other natural substances, such as fish oils, enzymes, and glandular extracts. Nutraceuticals (occasionally spelled *nutriceuticals*) usually claim some benefits to health in their labeling, although the precise wording is strictly regulated by government authorities in countries where they are marketed. Other terms for nutraceuticals are functional foods or medicinal foods.

Off-label indications   Uses or applications of a drug that are not officially approved by the government; also referred to as unlabeled, extra-label, or ex-label indications. Off-label uses are not necessarily illegal, unless directly contraindicated in labeling, but companies wishing to promote unlabeled uses of their products must comply with special FDA regulations (see Chapter Four).

Online   Interaction with a computer through a telecommunications network, in which data are transmitted and processed immediately.

Operators   In computer searching jargon, an operator is a connecting term or symbol used to indicate how words or concept sets should be logically related to one another. For example, the Boolean AND is a logical operator that, when placed between two keywords, specifies that both must be present in documents or Web pages retrieved.

Proximity operators, such as ADJ or SENTENCE, express a closer relationship (i.e., words must be next to one another or in the same sentence).

Orphan drug A drug judged by government authorities to have limited commercial value (profit potential) due to its applicability to a relatively small patient population (fewer than 200,000 people by U.S. definition, no more than 50,000 in Japan) and/or its unfavorable patent status (i.e., lacks adequate patent protection). Officially designated orphan drug status in the United States entitles drug sponsors to marketing exclusivity, tax credits, and special grants or contracts, should the product be approved.

Outcomes Results of therapy, encompassing both surgical procedures and drug use. Outcomes research examines health benefits derived from different therapies, analyzing and comparing quantifiable factors such as morbidity and mortality, as well as economic and social variables. Outcomes research adds cost considerations and quality of life measures to evaluations of clinical efficacy.

Over-the-counter (OTC) drug A medication that can be sold without a prescription. Patent medicine is sometimes used as a synonym.

Package insert Professional labeling information intended to accompany a drug product and relay information necessary for safe and effective use. Do not confuse with a patient package insert (PPI), which consists of printed instructions prepared for laypeople.

Page see Web page.

Parenteral Any route of administration other than the oral-gastrointestinal (enteral) route (e.g., injectable); general usage of the term excludes topical (surface or skin) administration. Parenteral nutrition involves the injection of nutrient solutions directly into the blood, bypassing the gastrointestinal system. Hyperalimentation is a synonym for parenteral nutrition.

Pastille A dosage form consisting of a medicated disk used to treat the mucosa of the mouth and throat. Sometimes described as a soft lozenge or *troche*.

Patent medicine see Over-the-counter drug.

PDF Portable Document Format. Documents in this format can be displayed, navigated, and printed from any computer, regardless of the fonts and software programs used to create the original. PDF enables files to be exchanged among users without modifying the format of the original document.

PEL Permissible exposure limit or level of a substance in workplace air, usually given as an average exposure during an eight-hour shift and expressed in ppm (parts per million). PELs are official standards adopted by the U.S. Occupational Safety and Health Administration (OSHA).

Pharmaceutics The study of physical pharmacy or chemistry, involving testing of pharmaceutical preparations for factors such as dissolution rates, pH, and solubility. The science of pharmaceutics focuses on determining physical and chemical attributes that influence the formulation and manufacture of drugs.

Pharmacoanthropology see Ethnopharmacology.

Pharmacodynamics The study of the biochemical and physiological effects of drugs and of their mechanisms of action, that is, the action of a drug in the body.

Pharmacoeconomics Assessment of the cost-effectiveness of drug products, which goes beyond simple comparisons of acquisition costs to incorporate outcomes research (healthcare results), cost-utility, cost-benefit, and quality of life analyses in an attempt to establish evidence of total net value among therapeutic alternatives. The focus is on providing quantitative measures of outcome in describing product performance. How do the patient, the healthcare provider, and the payer benefit from the treatment? Can, for example, fewer side effects or improved compliance be demonstrated, or can hospital stays or physicians' office visits be reduced or avoided?

Pharmacogenetics   The study of genetically inherited variations that are revealed solely by effects of drugs. Genetic aberrations in individuals result in the absence and insufficiency of specific enzyme systems, leading, for example, to an inability to taste.

Pharmacognosy   The study of drugs derived from nature (i.e., plants, animals, minerals), as well as the search for new therapeutic agents from natural sources.

Pharmacokinetics   The study of the rates of movement of a drug or its metabolites in the body and the rates of biotransformation. Kinetics information is derived from data on half-life, absorption, distribution, excretion, metabolism, and analysis of body fluid levels. These factors, coupled with dosage, determine the concentration of a drug at its intended sites of action and the intensity and timing of its effects.

Pharmacology   Study of the preparation, qualities, uses, and effects of drugs.

Pharmacopeia   A book that lists and describes medicinal substances and provides formulas for preparation, tests of purity, and strength. *Nuevo Receptario*, issued in Florence in 1498, is often cited as the first publication of this type. Today, the term generally refers to a publication that establishes official standards of identity and quality of drug preparations in the issuing or sponsoring country. It sets compendial standards for verifying drug identity and detecting products whose quality has been compromised by decomposition, degradation, or adulteration. The term *pharmacopeia*, alternatively spelled *pharmacopoeia*, is a combination of two Greek words: *pharmakon* (drug) and *poiein* (to make).

Pharmacovigilance   Literally, "watching over" drugs. The term usually refers to programs designed to monitor unexpected effects of marketed drugs. The FDA's Medwatch (adverse event reporting) program is an example of government mandated pharmacovigilance. However, pharmacovigilance generally carries the connotation of more proactive post-marketing surveillance, in which epidemiological studies are initiated and automated population databases are maintained to identify and evaluate risks.

Pharmacy   Traditionally, the art of preparing, compounding, and dispensing medications. *Pharmakon* is the Greek word for "medicine" or "drug."

Phase   A stage in clinical testing. See Chapter Four for definitions and discussion of phases in drug development.

Photosensitivity   A drug-induced change in the skin that results in a rash or exaggerated sunburn when an individual is exposed to ultraviolet light.

Phytomedicine   The therapeutic use of plants or plant-derived remedies (i.e., phytopharmaceuticals).

Phytotoxins   Toxic plants or plant parts.

Pill   see Dosage Forms.

Placebo   A "drug" that contains no pharmacologically active ingredient, e.g., starch or sugar pills. The term is derived from the Latin *placebo*, meaning "I will please." Placebos are sometimes administered to satisfy a patient's perceived psychological need for therapy and are commonly used in control group patients in clinical trials of efficacy.

PMA   Premarket Application, required for medical devices that are life supporting, implanted, or used in critical care; comparable to an NDA for new drugs.

Poisoning Harmful effects resulting from dosage beyond recommended levels of safe use.

Polypharmacy Concurrent use of several drugs; often, this term refers to situations where medications used have been prescribed separately by different physicians.

Potentiation An interaction between chemical substances in which one enhances the effect or action of another.

Practice formulary In-house inventory of frequently used products maintained by veterinarians in private practice.

Predicate device A product cited in a 510k (premarket notification) as the basis for a claim of substantial equivalence to a device on the market prior to passage of the Medical Device Amendments in 1976.

Preregistration Submission of documents required for drug approval; in the United States, synonymous with NDA submission to the Food and Drug Administration.

Prescription An order or direction authorizing use of a drug.

Prescription audit see Drug Utilization Review.

Preservative An additive that prevents microbial growth and contamination by bacteria, molds, or fungi.

Prevalence In epidemiology, a measure of the total number of cases of illness present in a given population at a particular point in time, usually stated as the number of cases per 1,000 persons. Prevalence describes the number of events existing at the time, in contrast to incidence, which refers to illnesses or related events commencing within a specified time period.

Priming dose see Loading dose.

Prodrug A biologically inactive compound that, when administered, is converted to a pharmacologically active form in the body by normal metabolic processes. For example, chloral hydrate is the inactive precursor of the active metabolite trichlorethanol, a sedative.

Prophylactic Preventive; a drug or device used to prevent a disease or condition is said to be prophylactic (e.g., a vaccine to induce immunity or a condom to prevent conception).

Proposition 65 A clause in the State of California's Safe Drinking Water and Toxic Enforcement Act of 1986 that prohibits use of more than 1/1,000th of an amount of an additive shown to have adverse developmental effects in animal testing. In addition to mandating a 1,000-fold safety factor for reproductive toxicants, Proposition 65 defines "significant risk" for carcinogens as risk resulting in more than one excess case of cancer per 100,000 people exposed during their lifetime to a chemical. Both of these provisions have been likened to controversial Delaney Clause restrictions.

Proprietary Registered to a specific manufacturer (proprietor). A proprietary name is a brand name, often registered as a trademark.

Protocol Detailed plan for investigation; procedures to be followed.

Protopharmacology The study of drugs used before the development of modern academic pharmacology (that is, pre-1849).

Proximity operators see Operators.

Quality of life Used to describe patient characteristics such as physical mobility, freedom from pain or distress, capacity for self care, and ability to engage in normal social activities, quality of life (QOL) is one measure of clinical efficacy and is used in comparing the benefits of drugs and other therapies. It is a factor often mentioned in pharmacoeconomic evaluations and outcomes research.

Receptor   A specific site on the surface of a cell.

Record   A separate entry or discrete unit of information within a database, such as a bibliographic citation or an address in a directory. A record can also be viewed as a collection of fields (searchable elements) related to a given source.

Refereed   Refereed publications are those subjected to peer review.

Reference listed drug   A drug identified by the U.S. Food and Drug Administration as the product upon which an applicant relies in seeking approval of an Abbreviated New Drug Application (ANDA), adopted as a standard against which bioequivalency will be measured. For medical devices, the counterpart is a predicate device.

Regimen   A prescribed system or regulated plan of caring for a patient. A dosage regimen consists of detailed directions for administration, including quantity, interval between doses, time of day, and relation to food intake.

Registration   Official approval by government authorities to introduce a drug into commerce; in the United States, equivalent to NDA (New Drug Application) approval by the Food and Drug Administration.

Rx   Used as a synonym for prescription; Rx is an abbreviation for *recipe*, the Latin word for "take this."

Scheduled drug   A drug whose distribution is regulated under the Comprehensive Drug Abuse Prevention Act of 1970 and its amendments, which established five schedules (lists) of controlled substances, based on their potential for abuse. The lower the schedule number, the higher the degree of control.

Scored tablet   A tablet imprinted with grooves for ease in breaking into halves or quarters.

Screening   In drug development, testing to detect compounds that will have a desired pharmacological effect. In toxicology, testing to identify substances present, using laboratory analytical techniques. Screening, when applied to literature, refers to surveys or rapid assessments to locate pertinent reference material.

Search engine   An Internet utility that enables users to search the Web for pages containing specific keywords or combinations of terms.

Shelf life   The time limit assessed for a drug product to retain its original potency and acceptable quality, when it is stored under recommended conditions (specified temperature, exposure to light). The term is sometimes used to refer to the viable commercial life of other products, such as books.

Simple drugs, simplicia   Drugs used unmixed, such as herbal remedies. Early pharmacopeias were customarily divided into two parts, one listing simplicia and the other containing directions for mixing composita (composite preparations) using simplicia.

Site   see Web site.

Smart drugs   see Nootropic.

Sorting   Sequencing or arrangement of items in a list. Entries in a dictionary are sorted alphabetically. Citations in a bibliography are often sorted by author or by publication date.

Stability   Ability of a drug to resist change in its physical/chemical properties, in order to retain product potency over time. Stability testing examines the capability of a specific drug formulation in a given container or other packaging to remain within standards established for its physical, chemical, therapeutic, and toxicological properties and is conducted to determine expiration dating and storage recommendations.

STEL   Short Term (fifteen-minute) Exposure Limit, used in the TLV List promulgated by the American Conference of Governmental Industrial Hygienists (ACGIH).

Stop words   Terms that cannot be searched in specific online systems. Stop words tend to be keywords with a high occurrence, but with little or no value in accessing the literature (e.g., of, and, by, for, from, to, the, with). The number and types of stop words vary from vendor to vendor; consult user aids to verify which terms can be searched.

Street drugs   Medications sold or obtained illicitly.

Subacute/Subchronic   Terms used to describe toxicity testing with a duration ranging from one week to three months, in contrast to acute (single dose) tests or chronic (six-to twelve-month) studies.

Subfile   A portion of a database; usually, a collection of online records related to a given subject area narrower in scope than the overall theme of the entire file.

Sunshine laws   Legislation intended to promote fuller disclosure of government activities and documents, such as the Freedom of Information Act of 1966.

Surfactant   Surface active agent, a chemical that reduces surface tension (the tendency of a fluid's surface to act as an elastic membrane), thereby enabling oil and water to form stable mixtures.

Surrogate endpoints   Endpoints are measures used to assess a drug's effectiveness. Surrogate endpoints are short-term events or markers judged to be related to the ultimate goal of drug treatment, such as blood pressure measurement as a predictor of stroke rate.

Synergistic   Used to describe an interaction of two or more substances when their combined effect is greater than the sum of their separate effects.

Systemic   Having a generalized effect throughout the body (the system, rather than a single organ or tissues). Drugs, when absorbed into the bloodstream, usually have a systemic effect.

Tentative approval   A generic drug approved by the FDA prior to the expiration of its brand name predecessor or equivalent. By completing the ANDA review process in advance, a manufacturer with a tentative approval can prepare for more rapid product introduction after the monopoly imposed by patent protection of the innovator drug ceases.

Teratogenicity   The potential for a given agent to cause congenital anomalies (e.g., birth defects). Derived from the Greek word *teras*, "monster."

Textword searching   see Natural language.

Therapeutic index   The ratio of ED_{50} to LD_{50}; also defined as the ratio of a drug's maximum tolerated dose to its minimum curative dose.

Therapeutic window   The limited dosage range or plasma concentration of a drug following administration in which the desired therapeutic effect occurs; a corollary is that the effect is absent at lower or higher concentrations. The therapeutic window is sometimes described as the range between the minimum effective dose and the highest tolerated dose.

Thesaurus   A list of subject terms or phrases preferred for use in indexing records for an online database. A thesaurus is an authority list (or controlled vocabulary) enhanced with cross references from natural language to preferred terminology and related terms.

Tincture   see Dosage Forms.

TLV   Threshold limit value, a concentration of a substance to which most workers can be exposed without adverse effect. TLVs can be expressed as a "ceiling" limit, a short-term exposure level, or a time weighted average.

Tolerance   Adaptation by the body that lessens responsiveness to a drug during prolonged or continuous administration. Development of drug tolerance is sometimes beneficial, as when side effects are reduced or eliminated after several days of administration (e.g., drowsiness and antihistamines), but tolerance can also lead to a need for increased dosage to achieve the same effect.

Topical   On the surface or site; for example, topical administration of a drug on the skin or mucous membranes for a localized effect, in contrast to administration routes intended to produce systemic effects. Topical, when applied to literature, can also refer to information "on or about a topic." For example, topical subheadings in *MEDLINE* identify recurring subject concepts, such as adverse effects.

Toxicology   The experimental study of the harmful effects of drugs and other agents on man or animals; includes studies to determine the margin of safety in dosage.

Traditional medicine   see Folk medicine.

Trivial name   A name in common usage, not necessarily authorized or sanctioned by a government agency or adhering to established standards. Brand names are sometimes referred to as trivial names in the drug literature, in contrast to official nonproprietary names, such as USAN, BAN, or INN.

Truncated   Cut off, abbreviated. In online searching, keywords are truncated to retrieve alternate endings. A special symbol is usually required to indicate truncation, such as a colon (:), dollar sign ($), question mark (?), or asterisk (*). The truncation symbol is sometimes called a wildcard character, because it enables retrieval of unspecified (and often surprising) alternate word endings. Some Internet search engines perform automatic truncation, a characteristic known as *stemming*.

Unit dose   A medication distribution system in which each individual dose is prepared beforehand and prepackaged prior to dispensing to patients.

Unlabeled indications   see Off-label indications.

URL   Uniform Resource Locator, a unique address code for connecting to a specific source (site) on the Internet. It is "uniform" in the sense that it follows an accepted format. For example, the first portion of a URL describes the application used, such as HTTP (Hypertext Transfer Protocol). What follows is the name of the host computer and its unique identifier (domain name). URLs for individual pages within a Web site (other than the home, or index, page) include additional address information following a slash. These extra characters indicate the "path" or file name on the host computer for the resource cited. For example, in the URL http://www.pjbpubs.co.uk/ppages, the last segment refers to the name assigned to the PharmaPages portion of PJB Publications' Web site.

Vaccines   Preparations derived from microorganisms (viruses, bacteria, protozoa) used to produce immunity against diseases caused by the same, or closely related, organisms. Derived from the Latin *vaccus* ("cow"), the term came into use following successful inoculation for smallpox using a preparation from cowpox.

Vehicle   In pharmaceutical parlance, a carrier or inert medium in which a medicinally active agent is formulated or administered. A vehicle assists delivery of a drug to the patient and is sometimes a solvent or diluent.

Vendors   Sellers; in the online industry, vendors are companies or organizations that provide software and/or hardware for searching one or more databases, e.g., Ovid Technologies. An online vendor may not have originally compiled the data to be searched, and thus should be distinguished from a database provider (also called a database producer or supplier, such as Elsevier or ADIS Press).

Washout period   Period of time following termination of therapy before the body rids itself of all traces of a drug.

Watching brief   A commission to remain vigilant, observe carefully and constantly, keep up-to-date and informed.

Web   see World Wide Web.

Web page   Information on the World Wide Web is presented in units referred to as pages. Individual pages on the Web vary in length from single to multiple screens. Rather than thinking of a Web page as analogous to a printed document, it's more accurate to define it as simply a compilation of data with its own unique Internet address or URL.

Web site   A Web site is usually a collection of pages of information, starting with an interface or index home page that contains hotlinks to data available at other locations in the collection.

World Wide Web   That portion of the Internet capable of supporting hypertext or hypermedia transfer from computer to computer. Hypertext Transfer Protocol (HTTP) was first released in 1991, at about the same time that restrictions on commercial use of the Internet were also lifted.

Withdrawal   Period of time and associated symptoms following cessation of drug administration; withdrawal effects often result from physical dependence.

Zoonoses   Diseases of animals capable of afflicting humans.

Zootoxins   Toxic or harmful animal extracts or excretions (such as venoms).

100 wichtige Medikamente, 181
483s, 529–531
510k, 90–91, 520, 521, 522, 523, 689
The 510(k) Register, 93
"A" documents (patents), 548
AACC. *See* American Association for Clinical Chemistry
AACP, 608–609; *Graduate Programs in the Pharmaceutical Sciences*, 381; *Pharmacy School Admission Requirements*, 381, 383; *Profile of Pharmacy Students*, 382; *Roster of Faculty and Professional Staff*, 381; Web site, 119
AAMI. *See* Association for the Advancement of Medical Instrumentation
AAPP. *See* American Academy of Pharmaceutical Physicians
AAPS. *See* American Association of Pharmaceutical Scientists
AAPT. *See* American Association of Pharmacy Technicians
AARP Pharmacy Service Prescription Drug Handbook, 241, 281, 571
Abbreviated New Drug Applications: law establishing 52–53; searching for approvals online, 510–516
abbreviations: prescription, key to, 28; regulatory, European Union, 132–133; used in this book, key to, 673–687; veterinary, key to, 353. *See also* acronyms
ABC. *See* American Botanical Council
Aberg, J.A., 167
ABI/Inform, 579, 580, 582
About Your Medicines (USP), 240
ABPI, 367, 623–624
abstracting and indexing services, 387–445
Abstracts on Hygiene and Communicable Diseases, 406
abstracts, definition, 689
Abused Drugs II: A Laboratory Pocket Guide, 218
academic programs, pharmacy, 380–382

Academy of Managed Care Pharmacy, 607
Academy of Veterinary Homeopathy, 353
access points, definition, 689
Access to Health Records Act (UK), 83
accession numbers, definition, 689
ACCP. *See* American College of Clinical Pharmacy
accreditation: definition, 689; pharmacy education, U.S., 611
Accredited Professional Programs of Colleges and Schools of Pharmacy, 381
ACD-The Available Chemicals Directory, 495
ACGIH. *See* threshold limit values
ACIM. *See* Pharmaceutical Manufacturers Association of Canada
ACPE. *See* American Council on Pharmaceutical Education
acronyms: cancer chemotherapy regimens, 29; chemical, Web database, 134; definition, 689; medical technology, Web site, 134; regulatory, 132–133. *See also* abbreviations
ACRP. *See* Association of Clinical Research Professionals
ACTIS, 536
Acupuncture.com, 264–265
acupuncturists, directories, 264
acute disease, definition, 689
acute toxicity, definition, 689
Adamovics, J.A., 218
Adams, H.R., 349
addiction, definition, 689
additives: certifiable, definition, 692–693; exempt, definition, 698; information sources, 303, 305, 309–317, 534–535, 540; toxicity sources, 198–199, 225–226, 313
ADIS: *Drug News*, 582; *Drug News and Perspectives*, 72, 478–479, 482, 487, 488; *Drugs and Disease Thesaurus*, 403, 405, 480; *InPharma*, 403, 411, 483; *LMS Drug Alerts Online*, 404–405, 411, 458; *PharmacoEconomics & Outcomes News*, 479–480, 481, 484; *R&D Insight*, 455, 458, 459–462,

472–476, 474–475, 487; *Reactions Database*, 428, 482
adjuvant, definition, 689
administration, routes, searching online, 415–417
admission requirements, pharmacy schools, 381, 383
admixture, definition, 689–690
adulterated, definition, 690
Adverse Drug Reaction System, FDA, 536
Adverse Drug Reactions: A Practical Guide, 192–193
adverse effects: definition, 690; medical devices, mandatory reporting, 91, 527–529; reference sources, 189–235, 642; searching online, 426, 427–434, 578
Adverse Reactions to Drug Formulation Agents, 198–199, 573
advertising: direct-to-consumer, 237–238; law, cosmetics and toiletries, 51
Advice for the Patient (USP DI), 239–240, 255–256, 258, 259, 260, 271, 281, 435
Advisory Committee/Panel, FDA, definition, 690
Aerzte Zeitung Online, 482
AESGP. *See* Association of the European Self-Medication Industry
African countries, drug regulation, 50
age groups, searching online, 413–414, 648
Agency for Health Care Policy and Research, *Prescription Medicines and You*, 258
Agency for Toxic Substances and Disease Registry, 433–434
aging, prescribing considerations, handbooks, 163, 168, 241
agonist, definition, 690
AGRICOLA, 342, 579, 580, 582
Agricultural and Veterinary Pharmacist, 622
AGRIS, 342, 579, 580, 582
AHFS classification, 14, 402, 405, 423
AHFS Drug Information, 145–146, 362, 407, 567, 570
Ahronheim, J.C., 163
AIDS Clinical Trials Information Service, 536–537
AIDS Database, Bureau of Hygiene and Tropical Diseases (U.K.), 406
AIDS drug assistance programs, directory, 144
AIDS Patents Database, 560
AIDS Weekly Plus, 597
AIDSDRUGS database, 536, 575, 577, 582
AIDSLINE, 406, 412
AIDSTRIALS database, 536, 577, 582
AIHP. *See* American Institute of the History of Pharmacy
Alcohol and Alcohol Problems Science Database, 577, 578, 582

alcohol-drug interactions guide, 36
alcohol-free products, list, 36
Algy's Herb Page, 264–265
Allen, L., 308
Allen, L.V., 165
allergen, definition, 690
Alliance for the Prudent Use of Antibiotics, 607–608
Allied and Alternative Medicine database, 342, 406, 436, 439
Alston, Y.R., 365
Alta Vista-Translation, 287, 288
Alternative Medicine Foundation, *HerbMed*, 341–342
alternative medicine use, statistics, 263
Alternative Medicine: Expanding Medical Horizons, 266
AltMedDex, 440
AltVetMed-Complementary and Alternative Veterinary Medicine, 352–353
AMA: Drug Evaluations, 147, 156, 569, 570, 573; *Guide to Prescription and Over-the-Counter Drugs*, 241, 281, 571; *Handbook of Poisonous and Injurious Plants*, 229, 573; *Journals Online*, 577, 578, 582; *Report on Alternative Medicine*, 266
Amazonian Ethnobotanical Dictionary, 338
ambulatory care, definition, 690
AMCP. *See* Academy of Managed Care Pharmacy
AMED, 342, 406, 436, 439
American Academy of Pediatrics: *Report of the Committee on Infectious Diseases*, 168; transfer of drugs and other chemicals into human milk, 200
American Academy of Pharmaceutical Physicians, 608
American Association for Clinical Chemistry, 608
American Association of Colleges of Pharmacy, 608–609; Web site, 119. *See also* AACP
American Association of Pharmaceutical Scientists, 609
American Association of Pharmacy Technicians, 609
American Association of Retired Persons, *Drug Handbook*, 241, 281, 571
American Botanical Council, 324, 609–610
American Chemical Society, 9, 496; Division of Chemical Information, 603–604
American College of Apothecaries, 610
American College of Clinical Pharmacology, 610
American College of Clinical Pharmacy, 610–611
American College of Physicians: *Guide for*

Adult Immunization, 166; *Journal Club*, 412; Library for Internists, 569

American Conference of Governmental Industrial Hygienists (ACGIH). *See* threshold limit values

American Council on Pharmaceutical Education, 381, 611

American Dietetic Association: *Handbook on Drug and Nutrient Interactions*, 200–201 position statement, 251

American Drug Index, 28–29, 361–362, 567, 571, 573

American Druggist, 97, 374–375; *Complete Family Guide to Prescriptions*, 241, 281, 571

American Herbal Products Association's Botanical Safety Handbook, 331

American Holistic Veterinary Medical Association, 352–353

American Hospital Association, *HealthSTAR* database, 579, 581, 587

American Hospital Formulary Service. *See* AHFS

American Indian Ethnobotany, 343

American Institute of Pharmacy, 611

American Institute of the History of Pharmacy, 354, 355, 356, 360, 611

American Journal of Health-System Pharmacy, 379, 614

American Journal of Pharmaceutical Education, 609

American Medical Association, 147, 229. *See also* AMA

American Nurses Association, *Nurses Drug Facts*, 175–176

American Nutraceutical Association, 623

American Pharmaceutical Association, 80, 148, 305, 354, 611–612; *Guide to Prescription Drugs*, 242, 281, 571; *Handbook of Pharmaceutical Additives*, 311; *Handbook of Pharmaceutical Excipients*, 310–311; *Herbal Remedies*, 328; *Pharmacy and You* consumer Web site, 262–263; *Practical Guide to Natural Medicines*, 246–247, 571

American Pharmacy, 612

American Society for Clinical Pharmacology and Therapeutics, 612

American Society for Pharmacology and Experimental Therapeutics, 612–613

American Society of Consultant Pharmacists, 84, 613

American Society of Health-System Pharmacists, 145, 379, 381, 613–614

American Society of Hospital Pharmacists. *See* American Society of Health-System Pharmacists

American Society of Pharmacognosy, 614

American Statistics Index, 378

Amerson, A.B., 569, 572

An Economic Analysis of Self-Medication, 624

ANA. *See* American Nutraceutical Association

Anabolic Steroids Control Act, 65

ANADAs, law establishing, 53

Analysis of Addictive and Misused Drugs, 218

analysis, laboratory, reference sources, 302–308, 312. *See also* analytical toxicology

Analytical Abstracts database, 437, 438

Analytical Profiles of Drug Substances and Excipients, 302

analytical toxicology, sourcebooks, 216–218

anaphylactic reaction, definition, 690

ANDA: definition, 690; law establishing 52–53; searching for approvals online, 510–516; suitability petitions, 68, 88, 690

Anderson, L.A., 328

Anderson, P.O., 158

Andrews, T., 113

Anesthesia and Critical Care Handbook, 409

Aneuploidy subfile, *TOXLINE*, 429

animal drugs. *See* veterinary drugs

Animal Pharm World Animal Health and Nutrition News, 477, 483

Annual Register of Merchants' Premises, 371

Annual Register of Pharmaceutical Chemists, 371

anodyne, definition, 690

Ansel, H.C., 308

antagonist, definition, 690

antedrug: definition, 690; searching online, 650–651

antibody, definition, 690

antidote, definition, 691

antidotes. *See* poisoning

antigen, definition, 691

Anti-inflammatory Drugs from Plants and Marine Sources, 334

Antimicrobial Therapy in the Elderly Patient, 168

Antiviral Agents Bulletin, 597

AOAC International, 614

APhA, 80, 148, 305, 354, 611–612; *Guide to Prescription Drugs*, 242, 281, 571; *Handbook of Pharmaceutical Additives*, 311; *Handbook of Pharmaceutical Excipients*, 310–311; *Herbal Remedies*, 328; *Pharmacy and You* consumer Web site, 262–263; *Practical Guide to Natural Medicines*, 246–247, 571

APhC. *See* Canadian Pharmacists Association

apothecary: definition, 691; evolution of profession, 351; symbols, key to, 28

Appelbe, G.E., 83

Applied Drug Information: Strategies for Information Management, 116–118, 569

Applied Genetics News, 597

appropriate food grade (FDA), 312
approvable letter, definition, 691
approvals, drug, information sources, 67–70, 510–516, 521–524. *See also* NDA; ANDA
approvals, FDA performance statistics, 536
approvals, medical devices, information sources, 516–524
Approved Drug Products and Legal Requirements, 88
Approved Drug Products with Therapeutic Equivalence Evaluations, 87–88, 362, 510–511, 537, 549
Approved Providers of Continuing Pharmaceutical Education, 381
APUA. *See* Alliance for the Prudent Use of Antibiotics
A-rated products, equivalence, 87
Arena, J.M., 211
armamentarium, definition, 691
Armstrong, L.L., 158
Arndt, T., 126
Aronen, J.K., 191
Aronoff, G.R., 159
The Art, Science, and Technology of Pharmaceutical Compounding, 165–166
Arzneimittel Zeitung, 482
ASCII, definition, 691
Ascione, F.J., 118
ASCP. *See* American Society of Consultant Pharmacists
ASCPT. *See* American Society for Clinical Pharmacology and Therapeutics
Ash, I., 311
Ash, M., 311
ASHP. *See* American Society of Health-System Pharmacists
Asian Business Intelligence Reports, 502
ASP. *See* American Society of Pharmacognosy
ASPET. *See* American Society for Pharmacology and Experimental Therapeutics
aspirin-free OTC product identification, 149
assay: definition, 691; compendial standards, 304–308
Association canadienne de l'industrie du médicament, 630
Association des pharmaciens du Canada, 616
Association Européenne pour l'Information et les Bibliothèques de Santé, 604–605
Association for the Advancement of British Biotechnology. *See* BioIndustry Association
Association for the Advancement of Medical Instrumentation, 614–615
Association of Clinical Research Professionals, 615
Association of Natural Medicine Pharmacists, 615
Association of Official Analytical Chemists, 614

Association of the British Pharmaceutical Industry (ABPI), 367, 623–624
Association of the European Self-Medication Industry, 624
associations, professional and trade, directory, 603–632
ASTM, 544
ATSDR, 433–434
Auditore, 506
audits, drug sales and utilization, 372–380, 651
Australia, product and pharmacy practice information resources, 125, 292–294, 350
Australian Prescription Products Guide, 292–293
author affiliation or address searching online, 423–425
authority, evaluating in reference sources, 112–113, 255
availability, U.S. products on the market, 361–362
Avis, K.E., 309
AVLINE, 406
Avoiding Food and Drug Interactions, 262

"B" publications, patents, 548
Ba, Y., 335
BA/RRM, 395
Bad Bug Book, 541
BAN, 12, 25
Banker, G.S., 309
Barbieri, E.J., 253
Barlow, S.M., 223
Barone, M.A., 160
Barrett, S., 267
Bartilucci, A.J., 297
Baseline Guides, manufacturing facility design, 620
Baselt, R.C., 217
Basic Analytical Toxicology, 217–218
Basic and Clinical Pharmacology, 172–173, 567
Basic Booklist and Core Journals for Pharmaceutical Education, 119
Basic Concepts in Teratology, 222
Basic Tests for Pharmaceutical Dosage Forms, 303–304
Basic Tests for Pharmaceutical Substances, 303
Basu, T.K., 200
Baxter, H., 332
Bazaz, M.C., 292
BBI Newsletter, 597
BCC Market Research, 502
Beaird, S.L., 569, 572
Beckett, A.H., 302
Beckstrom-Sternberg, S.M., 343
Beers, D.O., 53
Beilstein, 301, 550
Beilstein Online, 575, 576, 583

Beizer, J.L., 163
Benezra, C., 229–230
Benichou, C., 192
Benitz, W.E., 160
Bennett, P.N., 199
Bennett, W.M., 159
Bernstein, I.L., 198
Berry, M., 261
Bertram, C.T., 485
bibliographic database, definition, 691
bibliographies, annotated guides to the literature, 113–122
bibliography, compilation using online databases, 387–445
Billips, N.F., 28
binder, definition, 691
Bio Online—Biotechnology Companies and Resources, 368
BIO. *See* Biotechnology Industry Association
bioavailability, definition, 691
BioBusiness database, 396, 482
Biochemistry Abstracts, 589
BioCommerce Abstracts and Directory, 482
bioequivalence, 18, 309; definition, 691; ratings, 35, 87, 144, 150
BIOETHICSLINE, 579, 581, 583
BioIndustry Association, 624
Biological & Agricultural Index, 578, 579, 580, 583
Biological Abstracts, 395
biologicals. *See* biologics
Biologics Control Act of 1902, 41
Biologics Development: A Regulatory Overview, 47
biologics: available only from Centers for Disease Control, 143, 168; definition, 691–692; drug approvals, 69, 511; laws governing, 41–42, 57; license application, 47, 57; licensed establishments and products, directory, 540; market exclusivity under FDA Modernization Act, 57; veterinary use, 539
biomaterial, definition, 692
Biomedical Business International, 597
Biomedical Instrumentation & Technology, 615
Biomedical Market Newsletter, 597–598
Biomedical Materials, 598
Biomedical Safety & Standards, 484
Biomedical Technology Information Service, 484
biometrics, definition, 692
BioPharm, 500
biopharmaceutics: definition, 692; reference sources, 308–309
BioResearch Index, 395
BIOSIS Previews, 14, 16, 67, 395–397, 411, 423, 425, 428, 429, 430, 439
BioSpace, 368

Biotech Business, 598
BioTech Chemical Acronyms Database, 134
Biotech Equipment Update, 598
Biotech Financial Reports, 598
Biotech Law Web Server, 99, 560
BioTech Life Sciences Dictionary, 134
Biotech Patent News, 598
Biotechnology Business News, 598
The Biotechnology Directory, 365, 366
The Biotechnology Guide U.S.A., 365, 366
Biotechnology Industry Association, 624–625
Biotechnology Information Institute Web site, 488
Biotechnology Law Report, 99
Biotechnology Newswatch, 590, 598
biotechnology product registration, information sources, 48–50
Biotechnology Research Abstracts, 589
biotechnology research, online sources, 578–579
Biotechnology: A Dictionary of Terms, 133
biotoxins: definition, 692; reference sources, 229–232, 541, 642. *See also* toxicology, online searching
biotransformation, definition, 692
BioVenture View, 476–477, 483
Birth Defects and Drugs in Pregnancy, 222–223, 573
birth defects. *See* teratogenicity
Bishop, Y., 348
Bisset, N.G., 328, 329
BizInt Smart Charts, 475–476
BLA, 47, 57, 69, 511
blinding in clinical trials, 45
Blood Weekly, 598
The Blue Book, Office of Device Evaluation, FDA, 538
The Blue Sheet (CDC health information for international travel), 167
The Blue Sheet, 97, 477, 483, 488
Blumberg, M., 297
BNA Daily News from Washington, 482
BNF, 291–292
board certified. *See* certification
Board of Pharmaceutical Specialties, 615–616
Bobroff, L., 262
BoDD, 231
Bodwell, C.S., 201
book reviews, 31, 119
bookmarks: cumulative list for Web sources cited in this book, 657–671; definition, 692
Boolean, definition, 692
Booster Shots (newsletter), 154
Boschert, K., 351, 352
Boston Children's Hospital, *Manual of Pediatric Therapeutics*, 161

Boston Collaborative Drug Surveillance Program, 194
Boston Collaborative Perinatal Project, 199
Boston University, *Glossary of Terms and Symbols Used in Pharmacology*, 134
Botanical Dermatology Database, 231
Botanical Medicine Resources on the Web, 340
Botanical Safety Handbook, 331
Botanical.com, 264
Botanicals: A Phytocosmetic Desk Reference, 334–335
botanicals: definition, 692; drug information, 246–247, 287, 289, 321–347, 358–359, 653; professional and trade associations, 609, 614, 615, 618, 619, 622, 623, 630; toxicity reference sources, 229–232, 642. *See also* pharmacognosy
Bottle, R.T., 120
Bourne, D., 123, 382
Bowman, A., 132
Bowman, W.C., 132
Boylan, J.C., 317
BP. See British Pharmacopoeia
BPS. *See* Board of Pharmaceutical Specialties
Bradley, P., 326
Braithwaite, R.A., 217
brand names, 7, 12, 692; searching online, 417–420, 548–550, 649, 654–655
Brandon-Hill list, 569
B-rated products, equivalence, 87, 88
Braun, D.B., 316
breast milk, drugs excreted in, 36, 198, 199–200, 207, 222
Breckinridge, M.F., 297
Brendler, T., 328
Bricker, J.D., 216
Briggs, G.G., 199
British Approved Name (BAN), 12, 25
British Approved Names, 25
British Herbal Compendium, 326–327
British Herbal Pharmacopoeia, 326
British Journal of Clinical Pharmacology, 616
British Journal of Pharmacology, 616
British Medical Association, 292
British National Formulary, 291–292
British Pharmacological Society, 616
British Pharmacopoeia, 308
British Pharmacopoeia—Veterinary, 308
British Poisons Act, 83
British Veterinary Association, *The Veterinary Formulary*, 348–349
Brittain, H.G., 302
Brizuela, B.S., 115
Brody, T.M., 173
Brown, D., 354
Brown, E.H., 250
Brown, S.S., 217

browser (Web), definition, 692
Brumenthal, M., 324
Bruneton, J., 323, 324
Brushwood, D.B., 82
BT Catalyst, 599
Bucherl, W., 232
Buckley, E.E., 232
Budavari, S., 26
buffer, definition, 692
bulk chemicals, buyer's guides, 364, 367, 369
Burdock, G.A., 313
Bureau of Health Professions, *Factbook: Health Personnel, U.S.*, 380
Bureau of Labor Statistics, *Occupational Projections and Training Data*, 380
Burger, A., 249
Burley, D.M., 48
Business & Industry database, 482, 500
Business & Management Practices database, 580, 583
Business Communications Company, 502
Business Dateline, 481, 482
business directories and statistical data sources, 361–384
business research online, 447–508, 580–581
buyer's guides, 354, 362–367, 369, 609

CA File, 437, 559
CA Search, 67, 437–438, 559
CAB Abstracts, 577, 578, 579, 580, 583
CAB Health database, 406–407, 439
CABs, 93
CADREAC, 63
caffeine-free OTC product identification, 149
California Pharmacists Association, *Spanish for the Pharmaceutical Profession*, 288
CAM Citation Index, 341
Canada, drug information sources, 178–179, 182, 261, 271, 290–291
Canadian Cosmetic, Toiletry and Fragrance Association, 625
Canadian Journal of Hospital Pharmacy, 617
Canadian Medical Device Industry Directory, 627
Canadian Pharmaceutical Association. *See* Canadian Pharmacists Association
Canadian Pharmaceutical Journal, 616
Canadian Pharmacists Association, 291, 616
Canadian Poisonous Plants Information System, 231
Canadian Society for Pharmaceutical Sciences, 616–617
Canadian Society of Hospital Pharmacists, 617
Canadian Wholesale Drug Association, 625–626
Cancer Biotechnology Weekly, 599
The Cancer Chemotherapy Handbook, 158–159

Cancer Drug News, 480, 483
Cancer Researcher Weekly, 599
Cancer Weekly, 599
CANCERLINE, 407
CANCERLIT, 406, 407, 412
CANDAs, 59, 61
Canon Communications, *Medical Device Link* Web site, 368
Carbohydrates, Amino Acids and Peptides, 584
carcinogenic, definition, 692
carcinogens, lists, 211, 226–227
CareNotes system, Micromedex, 260
Carpenter, J.R., 131
Carriere, G., 296
CAS Registry File, 441
CAS registry numbers, 8, 10; searching online, 392, 395, 396, 402, 403, 431, 438, 441, 652–653
Casarett and Doull's Toxicology, 214–215, 567
cascaded codes online, 423
CASREACT, 576, 584
Catalog of Teratogenic Agents, 219–220, 567
categories, drugs, online searching, 420–423, 649, 651
category 1–2, OTC Review, 42, 315
category 3, OTC Review, 42–43, 244
CATLINE, 406
CBR, 315–316
CCINFOWeb, 432
CCIS, 155, 213, 278
CCTFA. *See* Canadian Cosmetic, Toiletry and Fragrance Association
CCTR, 412
CDC AIDS Weekly, 597
CDC Wonder database, 505
CDC. *See also* Centers for Disease Control and Prevention
CD-ROM, definition, 692
CDSR, 412
CE mark, 92, 93, 692
CEN/Cenelec, 544
The Center for Networked Information Discovery and Retrieval, 560
Centers for Disease Control and Prevention: biologics available from, 143, 168; *Health Information for International Travel*, 166–167, 572; *Home Page*, 437; National Center for Health Statistics, 376–378, 505. *See also* CDC
CenterWatch Clinical Trials Listing Service, 413
CERCLA Priority List of Hazardous Substances, 434
certifiable color additives, definition, 692–693
Certificat Complementaire de Protection, 558
certification: Board of Pharmaceutical Specialties, 615–616; clinical research coordinators, ACRP, 615; definition, 693

CFR. *See* Code of Federal Regulations
chain drugstore, definition, 693
chains, drug retail outlets, directories, 370–371
Chambers, J.E., 133
Chapman & Hall Chemical Database, 550, 575, 576, 578, 584
check tags, *MEDLINE*, 413
Chem Sources USA, 364–365, 494
Chem Sources-International, 364–365, 494
CHEMCYCLOPEDIA, 496
Chemical & Engineering News buying guide, 496
Chemical Abstracts online, 437–438, 441
Chemical Abstracts Service. *See* CAS
Chemical Business NewsBase, 482
Chemical Engineering and Biotechnology Abstracts, 576, 584
Chemical Industry Notes, 482
Chemical Information Sources, 120
Chemical Marketing Reporter, *OPD Chemical Buyers Guide*, 364–365
chemical names, 7–9
Chemical Registry Nomenclature database, 441
Chemical Regulation Daily, 482
Chemical Safety Newsbase, 578, 584
chemical structures, 15
Chemical Week-Buyers' Guide Issue, 367–368
Chemically Induced Birth Defects, 220–221, 567
Chemicals and Companies, 495
Chemicals in the Environment: OPPT Chemical Fact Sheets, 434
Chemicals, Formulated Products and Their Company Sources, 495
Chemist & Druggist, 500
Chemist and Druggist Directory, 279–280, 362, 371–372, 381
chemist, definition in British usage, 693
CHEMLINE, 441–442
Chemoreception Abstracts, 589
The Chemotherapy Source Book, 159, 567
chemotherapy, definition, 693
CHEMSEARCH, 441, 442
CHEMTOX Online, 431, 432
ChemWeb, 495
Cheshire Medical Center, *Medication Info Search*, 258–259
chewing, dosage forms excluded, 29, 36, 175. *See also* enteric-coated tablet
Chidmere, E.C., 50
children, prescribing considerations, handbooks, 160–162, 242, 261.
See also extemporaneous formulations, pediatric
China Academy of Traditional Chinese Medicine, 336
Chinese medicine, traditional, 264–265, 335–338

CHIROLARS, 436, 589
cholesterol-free OTC product identification, 149
CHPA. *See* Nonprescription Drug Manufacturers
  Association
chronic toxicity, definition, 693
chronic, definition, 693
chronology, IND and NDA, 69–70
chronopharmacology, definition, 693
Chudley, A.E., 222
cigarette smoking, tobacco, statistics, 228
CIN, 584
CIR Compendium, 225–226
Ciraulo, D.A., 198
CIS subfile, *TOXLINE*, 429
cited reference searching, 398, 424–425,
  650–651
Citizens' Guide to Biotechnology, 625
claims, definition, 693
CLAIMS/Reassignment & Reexamination data-
  base, 553, 556, 558, 584
CLAIMS/U.S. Patents Abstracts, 581, 584–585
Clarke, E.G., 216
Clarke, J.M., 48
Clarke's Isolation and Identification of Drugs,
  216–217, 302
Class A narcotics, 64, 693
Class B narcotics, 64, 693
Class I, II, III medical devices, 89–90
classification: definition, 693; drug, 13–14, 58–
  59, 60; online searching, 420–423, 649, 651
classifying information requests, 107–109
Clayman, C.B., 240
Clin-Alert, 193
*Clinica World Medical Device and Diagnostic
  News*, 476–477, 483
Clinical Chemistry (AACC journal), 608
*Clinical Handbook of Chinese Prepared Medi-
  cines*, 336–337
Clinical Lab Letter, 484
Clinical Laboratory News, 608
*Clinical Management of Poisoning and Drug
  Overdose*, 215–216
*Clinical Pharmacokinetics: Concepts and Appli-
  cations*, 172
Clinical Pharmacology and Therapeutics, 612
Clinical Pharmacology Online Web site,
  180–181
Clinical Pharmacy (ASHP), 614
Clinical Tools, Inc., *Health-Center.com: Phar-
  macy*, 260
Clinical Toxicology of Commercial Products,
  212, 573
clinical, definition, 694
clinical trials: database coverage, 67; online
  searching, 410–413, 536–537, 577; phases,
  45–46. *See also* pipeline, directories online
Closson, R.G., 164

Clydesdale, F.M., 312
CNIDR, 560
Cochrane Controlled Trials Register, 412
Cochrane Database of Systematic Reviews, 412
The Cochrane Library database, 412
Cochrane Review Methodology Database, 412
Code of Federal Regulations, 75–76, 315, 533,
  693
codes, DEA, 65
codes, research, 10–11; key to initial letters, 28
Collaboration Agreement of Drug Regulatory
  Authorities in European Union Associated
  Countries, 63
Collaborative Research and Development
  Agreements, 488
color additives: certifiable, definition, 692–693;
  exempt from FDA certification, 540, 698.
  See also additives, information sources
color vision screening chart, 155
Colorado State University, *Veterinary Emer-
  gency Drug Calculator*, 353
Colour Atlas of Chinese Traditional Drugs, 335
A Colour Atlas of Poisonous Plants, 229, 230
Colour Index, 313, 315, 319
*Columbia University College of Physicians &
  Surgeons Complete Home Medical Guide*,
  261, 435
combination products, in official compendia, 26
Commission E monographs, 324–325, 328, 329,
  332
Committee for Proprietary Medical Products
  (CPMP), 61, 62
Committee on Extemporaneous Formulations,
  ASHP, 164
Common Technical Document (ICH), 63
Community Pharmacy (U.K.), 500
community pharmacy: definition, 694; directories, 370–371
company codes, NDC, 29
company directories, 362–371, 490–497, 645.
  See also pipeline, directories online
compassionate INDs, 58
COMPENDEX. *See* EI COMPENDEX
compendial standards. *See* pharmacopeias
Compendium of Nonprescription Products, 290,
  291
*Compendium of Pharmaceuticals and Special-
  ties*, 281, 290–291
compendium, definition, 694
Competitive Intelligence Review (SCIP), 606
competitive intelligence, online resources, 447–
  508, 580–581
complementary medicine use, 263
*The Complete Directory for People with Chronic
  Illness*, 435
The Complete Drug Reference, 239, 240

The Complete German Commission E Monographs, 324–325

Complete Guide to Prescription and Nonprescription Drugs, 243, 571

Complete Home Medical Guide, Columbia University, 261

The Complete Medicinal Herbal, 252–253

compliance: definition, 694; statistics, 237, 238, 653

The Compounding Pharmacist, 619

Compounding Formulas from the Recent Journal Literature (Web site), 165

Compounding Hotline (Web site), 165

compounding, extemporaneous: authorized substance lists, 57, 535–536; definition, 694; ingredients for, 35, 170, 646; reference sources for, 161, 164–166, 640

Comprehensive Crime Control Act (1984), 65

Comprehensive Drug Abuse Prevention and Control Act (1970), 64

Comprehensive Environmental Response, Compensation, Liability Act, 434

Computer Retrieval of Information on Scientific Projects (CRISP), 429

computer-assisted literature research, 387–445, 476–508

Computer-Assisted New Drug Applications (CANDAs), 59, 61

Computerized Clinical Information System, 155, 213, 278

concertation, 61

conference literature, specialty databases: *Conference Papers Index*, 67, 576, 577, 578, 580, 585; *Directory of Published Proceedings*, 586; *Inside Conferences*, 588

conference papers, online coverage, 67. *See also* meeting announcements, forthcoming

Conformity Assessment Bodies, 93

congenital anomalies, drug-induced. *See* teratogenicity

Conn's Current Therapy, 156, 569, 571

Connor, C.S., 118

Consultant Pharmacist, 613

Consumer Guide to Herbs, 265

Consumer Guide to Over-the-Counter Drugs (Eckerd), 257

Consumer Health & Nutrition Index, 435

Consumer Health Information Source Book, 247, 435, 571, 572

Consumer Health USA, 247

Consumer Healthcare Products Association. *See* Nonprescription Drug Manufacturers Association

A Consumer's Guide to Medicines in Food, 252

consumers, drug information for, 237–275, 435–437, 537, 639, 653

contact dermatitis, plant-induced, reference sources, 229–230, 231, 233

containers, storage requirements, drugs, 28–29

Conte, J.E., 167

Contemporary Compounding (Web site), 165

continuing education providers, pharmacy, 381

contract research organizations (CROs), directories, 365–367, 368, 369

contraindication, definition, 694

Controlled Release Society, 617

Controlled Substance Analogue Enforcement Act, 65

The Controlled Substances Act: A Resource Manual, 65

Controlled Substances Quarterly, 65, 66

controlled substances: definition, 694; destruction, 84; lists, 65, 66, 158, 176, 218; other sources for determining schedule status, 142, 144, 150, 161, 244; under international control, 24; U.S. laws, 64–65

Controlled Trials Links Register, 413

controlled vocabulary, definition, 694

Cook, T., 49

Coombs, J., 365

Copeland Bill, 41

Copeland, R., 306

core drug information collection, 567–573

Cornell University Poisonous Plants Web Page, 353–354

corporate source, searching online, 423–425, 654–655

Cosloy, S.D., 135

Cosmetic and Toiletry Formulations, 316–317

Cosmetic Bench Reference, 315–316

Cosmetic Handbook (FDA), 540

Cosmetic Ingredient Reviews, 225–226, 315

Cosmetic, Toiletry, and Fragrance Association, 50–51, 226, 626. *See also* CTFA

Cosmetics & Toiletries, Who's Who in R&D companies directory issue, 369

Cosmetics Additives, An Industrial Guide, 316, 317

cosmetics: definition under U.S. law, 694; ingredients, information sources, 311, 313, 314–317, 334–335, 367; online information sources, 579; unwanted effects, 198

cost data, drugs. *See* pricing information

Counseling Patients on Their Medications, 273

counseling, patient: aids for, 269–273; mandated, 36, 80–81, 86

coupons, drug, government control, 86

court cases, information sources, 77–78, 81, 82, 83

Coustan, D.R., 159

Covington, T.R., 148

Cowen, D.L., 355, 356

Cox, M., 133

CPC, 558
CPhA, 291, 616
CPMP, 61, 62
CPS, 281, 291–292
CRADAs, 488, 694
Cravey, R.H., 217
CRC Ethnobotany Desk Reference, 339–340, 345
CRC Handbook of African Medicinal Plants, 338
credibility, evaluating in reference sources, 112–113, 255
Creelman, W.C., 198
CRISP subfile in *TOXLINE*, 429
CROs, directories, 365–367, 368, 369
cross-over trial, definition, 694
CRS. *See* Controlled Release Society
crude drugs, 321, 695
crushing, dosage forms excluded, 29, 36, 158, 163, 175, 176, 270. *See also* enteric-coated tablet
CSA Life Sciences Collection. *See* Life Sciences Collection
CSCHEM, 494
CSCORP, 494
CSHP. *See* Canadian Society of Hospital Pharmacists
CSPS. *See* Canadian Society for Pharmaceutical Sciences
CTFA Compendium of Cosmetic Ingredient Composition, 315
CTFA International Buyers' Guide, 367, 496
CTFA International Color Handbook, 315
CTFA International Regulatory/Resource Manual, 50–51
CTFA Labeling Manual, 50–51
CTFA List of Japanese Cosmetic Ingredients, 315
CTFA Membership Directory, 367
CTFA. *See also* Cosmetic, Toiletry, and Fragrance Association
Cunniff, P.A., 302
cupping, definition, 695
Current AIDS Literature, 406–407
current awareness sources: industry news, 476–481, 482, 597–602; regulatory, 94–98
Current Biotechnology Abstracts, 576, 577, 578, 585
Current Contents, 397
Current Contents Search, 576, 577, 578, 579, 580, 585
Current Controlled Trials Web site, 413
Current Drugs Fast-Alert, 559
Current Drugs Ltd., *IDdb*, 466, 470
Cutaneous Drug Reaction Database, 198
cutaneous, definition, 695. *See also* skin

CWDA. *See* Canadian Wholesale Drug Association
Cyberbotanica, 343
Cyberpharmacist, 130
cyberspace, definition, 695
cytotoxic, definition, 695

D&C dyes, 313
D'Amelio, F.S., 334
D'Emanuele, A., 123
Dalhousie University (Canada): *Compounding Formulas* Web site, 165; *Useful Pharmacy Links*, 123
Damage Awards Involving Prescription and Nonprescription Drugs, 78
Dangerous Aquatic Animals of the World, 230
Dangerous Marine Animals That Bite, Sting, Shock, Are Non-Edible, 230
DARE, 412, 486
DART, 223, 429
Dartmouth-Hitchcock Medical Center, *Cutaneous Drug Reaction Database*, 198
Data from the Drug Abuse Warning Network, 227–228
data sheet, definition, 695
databank, definition, 695
Database of Abstracts of Reviews of Effectiveness, 412, 486
database: definition, 695; selection aids, 575–596
database, bibliographic: definition, 691; searching online, 387–445
Datamonitor Market Research, 501, 502
Davies, R., 353
Davis, D.M., 192
Davis, E.B., 121
DAWN, 227–228, 505
DCF, 12
DCI Directory Issue, 367, 369
DCP, 495
De Groot, A.C., 198
de Wolff, F.A., 217
DEA, 64, 84; codes, 65
Decision Resources Pharmaceutical Industry Reports, 502
decoction, definition, 695
DeFelice, 252
definitions, selected terms, 689–710. *See also* dictionaries, subject specialty
Delaney Clause, 695
Deloatch, K.H., 204
DeMarco, C., 83
demographic data. *See* epidemiology
demography, definition, 695
Dental Practitioners' Formulary (U.K.), 292
dependence, definition, 695
Der Marderosian, A., 330

Derendorf, H., 171
dermatology drugs, adverse effects information, 198
dermatology, adverse effects from plants, 229–231, 233
Dermatotoxicology, 233
Derwent: *Biotechnology Abstracts*, 577, 578, 585; compilation of SPCs, 557; *DGENE*, 559; *Drug File*, 402–403, 411, 414, 423, 437; *Drug Registry*, 575, 585; *Standard Drug File*, 585; *Veterinary Drug File*, 577, 578, 579, 585; *World Patents Index*, 550, 559, 581, 592
DeSain, C., 318
descriptor, definition, 695
DESI, 42. *See also* OTC Review
Designer Drug Bill, 65
designer drugs, definition, 695
Dessing, R.P., 294
detail man/woman, definition, 695
The Development of American Pharmacology, 356
Developmental and Reproductive Toxicology (DART), 429
device. *See* medical device
Device Standards Library (IHS), 544
Devices & Diagnostics Letter, 481, 482
Devlofeu, V., 232
DGENE, 559
DIA. *See* Drug Information Association
Diagnostic Procedures Handbook, 409
diagnostics, definition, 695
Diccionario de Especialidades Farmaceuticas, 290
dictionaries, subject specialty, 130–136. *See also* translation aids
Dictionary of Antibiotic-Producing Organisms, 333–334
Dictionary of Antibiotics and Related Compounds, 584
Dictionary of Biotechnology and Genetic Engineering, 135
Dictionary of Chemical Terminology in Five Languages, 296
Dictionary of Drugs, 33–34
Dictionary of Epidemiology Web site, 134
Dictionary of Food Ingredients, 312
Dictionary of Metaphysical Healthcare, 267
Dictionary of Natural Products, 332
Dictionary of Organic Compounds, 301, 584
Dictionary of Pharmacology, 132
A Dictionary of Pharmacology and Clinical Drug Evaluation, 131
Dictionary of Pharmacy, 132
Dictionary of Plants Containing Secondary Metabolites, 334
Dictionary of Protopharmacology, 357

Dictionary of Surface Active Agents, Cosmetics, and Toiletries, 296
Dictionary of Toxicology, 133, 228–229
Dictionnaire Vidal, 286
Diet and Drug Interactions, 200–201, 573
Dietary Supplement Health and Education Act, 43–44, 252, 540
dietary supplements: industry associations, 623, 630; information sources, 157, 246–249, 251–253, 257, 263–264, 265–266, 271–272; statistics on use, 322
DIF, 407
Dighe, S.V., 309
DiGregorio, G.J., 253
Diogenes FDA Medical Devices on Cd-ROM, 93–94, 545
Diogenes, 54, 68, 72, 73, 93; 483s, 530–531; device approvals in, 518, 520–522; drug approvals in, 512, 513–516; Establishment Inspection Reports in, 530; FDA backgrounders in, 542; FDA guidelines, 534; FDA press releases, 542; FDA staff Congressional testimony, 542; FDA staff speeches, 542; FDA talk papers, 542; FDA warning letters, 532–533; MDRs, 527, 529; newsletters in, 481, 482; patent information, 549, 552, 556; product recalls, 524, 525, 526
directories: acupuncturists, 264; companies, 362–371, 490–497; drug information centers, 36, 150, 151, 293; drugs-in-development, 447–476; pharmacies, 370–372; pharmacy schools and colleges, 380–382; poison control centers, 36, 144, 150, 153, 176, 249, 263, 270, 285, 286, 293; residency programs, pharmacy, 381; state boards of pharmacy, 36, 81, 99, 151; state health departments, 166
Directory of Chemical Producers, 494
Directory of Drug Store and HBC Chains, 371
Directory of Healthcare Purchasing Organizations, 493
Directory of High Volume Independent Drug Stores, 370
Directory of Hospital Personnel, 493
Directory of Published Proceedings, 577, 578, 580, 586
direct-to-consumer advertising, 237–238, 374
DIRLINE, 580, 586
disciplinary action database, pharmacists, 99
discontinued drugs, information sources, 72–73, 153, 287, 293
Dispensatory of the United States of America, 323, 573
dispensing authority, state control, 80
Dispensing of Medication, 574
dispensing, definition, 695

Disposition of Toxic Drugs and Chemicals in Man, 217

Dixon, M.G., 77

D-List, 73

DMFs, 537–538. *See also* Drug Master Files

document types, searching online, 426

Documentation of the Threshold Limit Values and Biological Exposure Indices, 228

documentation, definition, 695

Dombrowski, S.R., 569, 573

Doody's Health Sciences Book Review Journal, 119

Dorian, A.F., 296

dosage calculation aids, 158, 176

dosage forms: definition and examples, 695–696; visual aids to identification, 281–282, 644, 646

dosage forms that should not be crushed or chewed, 29, 36, 158, 163, 175, 176. *See also* enteric-coated tablet

DOSE: The Dictionary of Substances and Their Effects, 224

dose-response curve, definition, 696

dosimetry, definition, 696

DOT shipping standards, hazardous chemicals, 213

dotpharmacy Web site, 375, 376, 503

double-blind, drug testing, definition, 696

Dowler, J.F., 233

Doyle, C., 49

DR Link reports, 502

Dr. Duke's Phytochemical and Ethnobotanical Databases, 341

Dr. Koop's Community: The Pharmacy and *The Medicine Cabinet*, 258

Dreisbach, R.H., 211

Drew, R.H., 211

drinking water standards, 215

Drug & Cosmetic Industry (DCI) Directory Issue, 367, 369

Drug & Cosmetic Industry, 500

Drug Abuse Control Amendments, 64

Drug Abuse Warning Network (DAWN), 227–228, 505

Drug Actions: Basic Principles and Therapeutic Aspects, 171

drug administration routes, searching online, 415–417

Drug and Allied Products Guild. *See* National Association of Pharmaceutical Manufacturers

drug approvals, information sources, 67–70, 510–516, 521–524. *See also* NDA; ANDA; EC marketing authorizations

drug audits, 85, 147, 651

Drug Bulletin (FDA), 482

drug coupons, government control, 86

Drug Data Report, 463–466; compared to other pipeline directories, 472–476; patent information in, 550

Drug Detection Report, 599

drug development process: related to publication sources, 7–9; U.S. regulation, 44–50, 51–61

Drug Development, 47–48

Drug Effects in Hospitalized Patients, 194, 574

Drug Efficacy Study Implementation, 42. *See also* OTC Review

Drug Enforcement Administration, 64

Drug Export Amendments (1986), 64

Drug Facts and Comparisons, 142–143, 362, 567, 568, 569, 571, 573

Drug GMP Report, 96, 481, 482

Drug Image Database, 278–279

Drug Importation Act of 1848, 40

Drug Imprint Database, 278–279

Drug INFONET Web site, 181; *Patient Package Inserts*, 260–261

Drug Information Association, 604

drug information centers, directories, 36, 150, 151, 293

Drug Information for the Health Care Professional (USP DI), 146–148, 178, 281, 407

Drug Information Fulltext, 14, 407, 442

Drug Information Handbook, 158, 409, 567

Drug Information Journal, 604

Drug Information Resources for Pharmacists, 123

Drug Interaction Facts, 195–196, 567

Drug Interactions (Stockley), 196

Drug Interactions in Psychiatry, 198

drug interactions: reference sources, 194–197, 641; searching online, 427–428

drug lag: definition, 696; laws and regulations to counteract, 51–64. *See also* FDA, performance statistics

Drug Master Files (FDA), 537–538, 696

Drug Metabolism and Disposition, 612

drug names. *See* drug nomenclature

Drug News and Perspectives, 72, 478–479, 482, 516; licensing information in, 487; line extensions in, 488

drug nomenclature: changes during drug development, 7–9; identification sources, 21–37, 440–442, 575–576; look alike/sound alike, 29, 144, 175, 270; relationship to scientific communication, 7–9; types of, 7–18

Drug Prescribing in Renal Failure, 159

Drug Price Competition and Patent Term Restoration Act, 52–53, 545

Drug Product Liability Reporter, 77–78

drug recalls: product lists, 88, 147; searching online, 524–526, 528, 655–656; statistics, 536

Drug Registration Requirements in Japan, 50

Drug Regulation in African Countries, 50
Drug Research Reports, 477
Drug Safety in Pregnancy, 222
drug samples, government regulation, 86
Drug Store Market Guide, 371
Drug Store News, 500
drug stores, directories, 370–371
Drug Topics, 97, 374, 375, 500
drug utilization review, 147, 696
drug, defined in law, 696
Drug, Device, and Diagnostic Manufacturing, 318
DrugBase Web site, 182
DRUGDEX, 150, 155–156, 569
druggist, British versus American usage of term, 696
Drug-Induced Ocular Side Effects and Drug Interactions, 197
Drug-Nutrient Interactions, 200–201, 574
DrugPics, 278
DRUG-REAX, 196
Drugs and Human Lactation, 199, 567
Drugs Available Abroad, 294–295
Drugs in Current Use and New Drugs, 574
Drugs in Litigation, 78
Drugs in Pregnancy and Lactation, 199, 567
Drugs of Choice, 574
Drugs of the Future, 466, 467–470; compared to other pipeline directories, 472–476
Drugs Under Patent, 54, 549
Drugs-Biologics Regulatory Database (INCAD), 544
Drug-Test Interactions Handbook, 202
DTC Advertising Audit, 374
DTC advertising, 237–238, 374
Duke, J.A., 333, 338, 341, 343
Dukes, M.N.G., 191, 222
Dunn, M., 125
Durgin, J.M., 297
Durham-Humphrey Amendment, 41, 79
dyes: identification of OTC products where absent, 149; subject to FDA certification, 540. *See also* additives, information sources

EAFUS database, 541
EAHIL, 604
Eastern European countries, drug approvals, 62–63
EBM Reviews database, 412
EC (Enzyme Commission) numbers, 15–16; searching online, 392, 395, 396, 649–650
EC (European Commission): marketing authorizations, 61–63; Medical Devices Directive, 92; orphan drug proposals, 55–56
ECDIN Web site, 433
Eckerd Drugs, *Consumer Guide to Over-the-Counter Drugs*, 257

economics, health, Internet sources, 481, 484–486, 623–624
ECPHIN Web site, 182–183
ECRI *Health Devices Sourcebook*, 365, 492–493
ED$_{50}$, definition, 696
Edmund's Home Page, 127–128
education, pharmacy, directories, 380–382
Effects of Drugs on Clinical Laboratory Tests, 201–202, 567, 570
efficacy, definition, 696
EI COMPENDEX, 579, 586
EINECS numbers, 315
EIRs, 529–531, 697
EIS subfile, *TOXLINE*, 429
ELA, 46–47, 57, 511
Elchisak, M.A., 128
elderly patients, prescribing considerations, handbooks, 163, 168, 241. *See also* age groups, searching online
elixir. *See* dosage forms
Elks, J., 33
Ellenhorn, M.J., 215
Ellenhorn's Medical Toxicology, 215, 568
Elsevier's Dictionary of Chemistry, 296
Elsevier's Dictionary of Pharmaceutical Science & Techniques, 296–297
Elsevier's Medical Dictionary, 295
EMBASE Alert, 586
EMBASE, 67, 192, 342, 392–395, 437; author affiliation indexing, 425; brand name searching, 417, 419, 420, 654–655; clinical trials indexing, 410–411; routes of drug administration, 415, 416; searching for adverse effects/interactions, 427; subject population indexing, 414
EMEA, 62; Web site, 99
emergencies. *See* poisoning
Emergency Care Research Institute, 493
emergency room statistics, 227–228
Emergency Scheduling Act (1984), 65
EMIC subfile, *TOXLINE*, 429
Emory University: *MedWeb*, 127; Office of Health Promotion, Web site evaluation form, 254
empirical: definition, 697; formulas, 15
EMTREE Thesaurus, 393, 422
Encyclopedia of Antibiotics, 35
Encyclopedia of Common Natural Ingredients, 331–332
Encyclopedia of Food and Color Additives, 313
Encyclopedia of Health Information Sources, 121–122
Encyclopedia of Pharmaceutical Technology, 317–318
Encyclopedia of Vitamins, Mineral and Supplements, 251

endogenous versus exogenous, 697
endpoints, 697; surrogate, 58
enteric-coated tablets: definition, 697. *See also* dosage forms that should not be crushed or chewed
Environmental Chemical Data and Information Network, 433
Environmental Mutagen Information Center, 429
Environmental Protection Agency Health Advisories, 215
Environmental Protection Agency TSCATS subfile, *TOXLINE*, 431
Environmental Teratology Information Center File, 429
Enzyme Commission numbers, 15–16; searching online, 392, 395, 396, 649–650
Enzyme Nomenclature, 37
EP (European Patent), 547
EP (European Pharmacopoeia), 306–307, 308
EPAR, 62, 99, 697
E-Pharmacy by Eckerd: OTC Resource Center, 257
EPhMRA, 14, 605
Epidemiology Information System (EIS), 429
epidemiology: definition, 697; statistics sources, 142, 150, 154, 189–191, 194, 222, 227–228, 480, 496–497
EpiVetNet, 352, 506
EPLC EC Document Database, 544–545
EPLC Update, 98, 477
EPO, 547
equivalence. *See* bioequivalence
equivalents, products, U.S. and non-U.S., identification, 283–295, 643–644, 647–648
ERA News, 97–98, 476, 477, 483
Erdman, J.W., 201
Erickson, M., 165
ESCOP Monographs on the Medicinal Uses of Plant Drugs, 325–326
ESCP. *See* European Society of Clinical Pharmacy
ESPICOM Country Healthcare Database, 497
ESPICOM Pharmaceutical & Medical Device News, 480, 483
ESPICOM Pharmaceutical and Medical Company Profiles, 490–491
The Essential Guide to Nonprescription Drugs, 244
The Essential Guide to Prescription Drugs, 244, 569, 571
The Essential Guide to Psychiatric Drugs, 245, 571
Essential Spanish for Pharmacists and Pharmacy Technicians, 288
establishment inspection reports (FDA), 77, 529–531, 697

Establishment License Application, biologics, 42, 46–47, 57, 511; directory of holders, 540
Estes, J.W., 357
Ethical and OTC Pharmaceuticals, 95
ethical drugs, 18, 697
Ethnobotany Database, 341
ethnobotany, bibliography, 335–340
EthnoMedicinals Home Page, 343
ethnopharmacology, definition, 697
ETIC, 223, 429
etiology, definition, 697
EuroBABEL, 132–133
Euromonitor Market Research, 502
European Association for Health Information and Libraries, 604–605
European Association of Hospital Pharmacists, 379
European Chemical News, 483
European Commission: marketing authorizations, 61–63; Medical Devices Directive, 92; orphan drug proposals, 55–56. *See also* European Medicines Evaluation Agency
European Community Pharmaceutical Information Network, 182–183
European Contract Research Organisations, 366–367
European Drug & Device Reports, 481, 482
European Drug Index, 294, 295
European Economic Community Standards for Quality of Herbal Remedies, 325
European Inventory of Existing Commercial Chemical Substances, 315
European Medicines Evaluation Agency (EMEA), 62; Web site, 99
European Patent Convention, 547
European Patent Office, 547
European Pharma Law Centre, 98, 544
European Pharmaceutical Marketing Research Association. *See* EPhMRA
European Pharmacopoeia, 306–307, 308
European Public Assessment Report (EPAR), 62, 99, 697
European Scientific Cooperative on Phytotherapy, 325
European Society of Clinical Pharmacy, 617–618
European Union Medical Devices Library (IHS), 544
Euro-Pharma Guide to the European Pharmaceutical Industry, 363–364
evaluating drug information sources, 107–113, 254–255
Evaluations of Drug Interactions, 195, 568
Evans, W.C., 323
EVENTLINE, 581, 586
Evidence-Based Medicine Reviews database, 412
Excerpta Medica. *See* EMBASE

excipients: adverse effects information, 198–199, 310, 311; definition, 697–698; reference sources, 305, 307, 310–317. *See also* additives
exempt color additives, definition, 698
exempt narcotic drug, definition, 697
exogenous versus endogenous agents, definition, 698
expiration dating, *SAS Drug Formulation Stability Program*, 538. *See also* shelf life
explode capability in online searching, 421–423
exports, unapproved drugs, 64
Ext D&C colors, 313
extemporaneous formulations, pediatric, information sources, 161, 164, 640. *See also* compounding, extemporaneous
Extemporaneous Ophthalmic Preparations, 164
Extemporaneous Oral Liquid Dosage Preparations, 164
extended-release, definition, 698
externship, 80
extra-label. *See* off-label
ExtraMED, 342, 577, 580, 586
eye medications, information sources, 154, 155, 164
eye, adverse effects of drugs and chemicals, 197

FAAM, 313
Factbook: Health Personnel, U.S., 380
Facts and Comparisons, 142–143, 362, 567, 568, 569, 571, 573
faculty, schools of pharmacy, directory, 381
Fairbase. *See* MediConf
false drops, definition, 698
FASEB, 613
fast track approvals of drugs, FDA Modernization Act, 57
Fazio, T., 312
FCC labeling, 312
FD&C colorants, 313
FD-483, 529–531
FDA: *Adverse Drug Reaction System*, 536; advisory committees, 68, 542, 690; backgrounders, 541–542; The Blue Book, 538; classification of drugs for priority review, 58–59, 60; classification of medical devices, database, 538; Congressional testimony, 541–542; *Cosmetic Handbook*, 540; Drug Master Files, 537–538, 696; establishment inspection reports, 77, 529–531, 697; The Green Book, 539; guidelines and guidance documents, 533–534; *Manual of Policies and Procedures*, 536; MedGuide program, 237; *Nonprescription Medicines, What's Right for You*, 257; notices of adverse findings, 531; *Pharmacy Compounding Page*, 535; pregnancy categories, 220; press releases, 542;

recalls, 524–527; Reference List (medical devices), 531; regulation of imprints on dosage forms, 282; speeches, 542; talk papers, 542; warning letters, 531–533; product approvals, searching online, 510–524; Web site, 436–437, 535–543
FDA Approved Drugs, 67–68
FDA Consumer (magazine), 436, 535, 542
FDA Consumer Information—Drug Database, 257, 436, 537
FDA Drug Bulletin, 482
FDA Enforcement Reports, 524–526, 542
FDA Food Additives Analytical Manual, 312–313
FDA Medical Bulletin, 535, 542
FDA Modernization Act, 56–57
FDA Radiological Health Bulletin, 482
FDA Veterinarian magazine, 539
FDA Week, 95
FDAMA, 56–57
FDC Act (1938), 41, 306
FDC Law Journal, 618
F-D-C Reports database, 69, 93, 477, 483, 488; patent extension requests in, 553, 556; product approvals in, 511–512, 513, 518; product recalls in, 524–525
FDLI Update, 99
FDLI. *See* Food and Drug Law Institute
feces, medications that discolor, 158, 163
Federal Bio-Technology Transfer Directory, 488
Federal Interagency Council on Statistical Policy, *FEDSTATS*, 505
Federal Register, 74–76, 488, 533, 541–542; patent extensions, 553, 554–555, 556; PMA approvals, 518–520
Federal Research in Progress database, 411, 430, 431, 577, 587
Federal versus state control, 78–79
Federated Drug Reference—U.S. Pharmacopeia Dispensing Information, 178
Federation of State Medical Boards, *Report of the Special Committee on Health Care Fraud*, 266
FEDRIP, 411, 430, 431, 577, 587
FEDSTATS, 505
Ferguson, T., 245
Ferko, A.P., 253
fetal risk. *See* pregnancy, drug use in. *See also* teratogenicity
fields, online searching, definition, 698
Fieser and Fieser's *Reagents for Organic Synthesis*, 301
file, online, definition, 698
Financial Ventures Report, 600
Fincher, J.H., 132
FIND/SVP Market Research, 501, 502
fine chemical, definition, 698

Fink, J.L., 81
Finnish Museum of Natural History, *Internet Directory for Botany*, 340
FIP database, *PharmaWeb*, 382
first aid. *See* poisoning
First DataBank, 146, 179–180, 195, 258, 260, 278
Fischer, D.S., 158
Fisher's Contact Dermatitis, 233
Fishman, D.L., 113–114
Flanagan, R.J., 217
Fleeger, C.A., 22
Flick, E.Q., 316
Florey, 302
fluoride-free OTC products identified, 149
FOI summaries, basis-of-approval documents, 522–524
Folb, P.I., 222
FOLE, 534–535
folk medicine, definition, 698. *See also* ethnobotany
Food Additive Toxicology, 225
Food Additives Handbook, 312
Food Additives: Toxicology, Regulation, and Properties, 312–313, 541
food additives, regulatory information sources, 534–535, 540–541. *See also* additives
Food and Drug Administration (Regulatory Manual Series), 48
Food and Drug Administration Modernization Act, 56–57
Food and Drug Administration. *See also* FDA
Food and Drug Law Institute, 618; Web site, 99
Food and Drug Law Journal, 99, 618
The Food & Drug Letter, 481, 482
The Food and Drug Library (IHS), 543–544
Food Chemicals Codex, 312
Food Drug Cosmetic Act (1938), 41, 89, 306
Food Drug Cosmetic Law Journal, 618
Food Drug Cosmetic Law Reports, 76
Food Law Institute. *See* Food and Drug Law Institute
Food Poisoning, Handbook of Natural Toxins, 232
Foodborne Pathogenic Microorganisms and Natural Toxins, 541
food-drug interactions guides, 36, 176, 200–201, 207–208, 262
FOODLINE: Current Food Legislation, 534–535
foreign drugs: identification sources, 283–295; importation by individuals, 64; prescriptions, legality, 79, 638. *See also* equivalents, products
forensic laboratory analysis of drugs, sources,

216–218. *See also* analysis, laboratory, reference sources
forensic. *See also* litigation, information sources
Form 483, 529–531, 698
formularies, drug, 86–87, 698. *See also* official compendia
formulas, chemical: molecular or empirical, 15; structural, 15
formulation agents, adverse effects information, 198
formulation development (manufacturing), information resources to support, 309–317
formulations, extemporaneous. *See* compounding, extemporaneous
formulations, non-disclosure, 66
FOSHU, 252
Foster, S., 331
Foy, E., 165
fragrance-free OTC products identified, 149
France, drug information sources, 286–287
Francom, M., 165
Fraser, C.M., 350
Fraunfelder, F.T., 197
Freedom of Information Act, 66
Freedonia Market Research, 502
Freeman, R.K., 199
frequently asked questions, 66–79, 108, 409–426
Fricke, U., 284
Fried, J.J., 241
Frohne, D., 229, 230
Frost & Sullivan Market Intelligence, 501, 502
Fudyma, J., 242

galenical, definition, 699
Gambertoglio, J.G., 159
Ganellin, C.R., 33
Gangolli, S., 224
Garcia, S.V., 297
Garrison, R.H., 201
GATT, 54, 545, 550
Gelbe Liste Online, 287
GEN Guides to Biotechnology Companies, 365–366
gender, online searching, 413–414
Gene Therapy Weekly, 500
General Agreement on Tariffs and Trade (GATT), 54, 545, 550
General Practitioner database, 581, 587
generally recognized as safe. *See* GRAS
Generic and Innovator Drugs: A Guide to FDA Approval Requirements, 53–54
Generic Animal Drug and Patent Term Restoration Act, 53
Generic Drug Enforcement Act, 53
Generic Drug Identification Guide, 280
generic drug scandal, 53

generic drugs: definition, 699; law, 52–53; on-line searching for comparisons with brand name products, 420; online searching for equivalents, 650; substitution, 18, 80, 86–88, 277
generic names, 11–12
Genesis Report-Dx, 599
Genesis Report-Rx, 599
Genetic Engineering News, GEN Guides to Biotechnology Companies, 365–366
Genetics Abstracts, 589
Gennaro, A.R., 170
Geriatric Dosage Handbook, 163, 409, 568
geriatric prescribing handbooks, 163, 168, 241. *See also* age groups, searching online
Germany, drug information sources, 284–286, 287, 324–325
Gfeller, R.W., 350
Ghazanfar, S.A., 338
Ghosh, M.K., 303
Gilman A.G., 169
Glamm Interactive, 485
Glasby, J.S., 35, 333, 334
Global Biotechnology Product Registration: E.U., U.S., and Japan, 49
Global Health-For-All database (WHO), 505
glossaries, 130–136, 689–710. *See also* translation aids
Glossary of Technical and Popular Medical Terms in Eight European Languages, 288
Glossary of Terms and Symbols Used in Pharmacology, 134
GLP, 47
The GMP Letter, 96, 481, 482
The Gold Sheet, 96, 481, 484
Gold Standard Multimedia, *Clinical Pharmacology Online*, 180–181
Goldfrank, L.R., 215
Goldfrank's Toxicologic Emergencies, 215, 568
Goldman, M.P., 167
Golper, T.A., 159
Good Laboratory Practice, 47
Goodman and Gilman's The Pharmacological Basis of Therapeutics, 169–170, 568, 569
Gorman, J.M., 245
Gossel, T.A., 216
Gosselin, R.E., 212
Gourley, D.R., 174
government standards: botanicals, 324; drug nomenclature, 22–26; drug substances, 304–308
Govoni & Hayes Drugs and Nursing Implications, 176
Graduate Programs in the Pharmaceutical Sciences, 381
Graef, J.W., 161
grandfather clause, 43

grandfather drugs: definition, 699; listing, 88
Grant, W.M., 197
grants (financial), news, 97
GRAS, information sources, 311, 312, 313, 332, 333, 541
Gray, L.D., 167
The Gray Sheet, 93, 477, 483, 518
Great Britain. *See* U.K.
Great Moments in Pharmacy, 355
The Green Book (*OPD Chemical Buyers Guide*), 364–365
The Green Book, FDA-approved animal drugs, 539
The Green Sheet, 97, 481, 484
Greenblatt, D.J., 194, 198
Grieve, M., 264
Griffenhagen, G., 356
Griffith, H.W., 243, 270
Gruenwald, J., 328
Guide National de Prescription des Medicaments, 286–287
Guide to Adult Immunization, 166
Guide to Drug Information, 119
A Guide to Drug Information and Literature: An Annotated Bibliography, 113
Guide to Poisonous and Toxic Plants, 231
Guide to the Literature of Pharmacy and Pharmaceutical Sciences, 113
guidelines and guidance documents, 77, 533–534
Guidelines for Administration of Intravenous Medications to Pediatric Patients, 163
guides to terminology, 130–136, 689–710
guides to the literature, 113–122

habituation, definition, 699
Haddad, L.M., 215
Hak, E.B., 163
Hale, T., 200
Hales, R.E., 245
half-life, definition, 699
Hall, D., 353
Halstead, B.W., 230
Hamilton and Hardy's Industrial Toxicology, 233
Hamner, C.E., 47
Hancock, S., 126
Handbook for Prescribing Medications During Pregnancy, 159, 568
Handbook of Antimicrobial Therapy, 168
Handbook of Arabian Medicinal Plants, 338
Handbook of Basic Pharmacokinetics, 172, 568
Handbook of Biologically Active Phytochemicals and Their Activities, 333
Handbook of Cancer Chemotherapy, 159, 568
Handbook of Clinical Drug Data, 158, 568

Handbook of Drug Therapy in Liver and Kidney Disease, 159, 160
Handbook of Federal Drug Law, 83
Handbook of Food, Drug, and Cosmetic Excipients, 311–312
Handbook of Industrial Toxicology, 211, 574
Handbook of Medical Toxicology, 209, 210
Handbook of Medicinal Herbs, 333
Handbook of Natural Toxins series, 232
Handbook of Nonprescription Drugs, 148–149, 568, 570, 571
Handbook of Over-the-Counter Drugs and Pharmacy Products, 247–248, 572
Handbook of Pharmaceutical Additives, 311
Handbook of Pharmaceutical Excipients, 310–311
Handbook of Phytochemical Constituents of GRAS Herbs and Other Economic Plants, 333
Handbook of Poisoning: Prevention, Diagnosis and Treatment, 211, 574
Handbook of Prescribing Medications for Geriatric Patients, 163
The Handbook of Psychiatric Drug Therapy for Children and Adolescents, 162
The Handbook of Psychiatric Drugs, 245, 246, 571
Handbook of Small Animal Toxicology and Poisonings, 350
Handbook of Toxic and Hazardous Chemicals and Carcinogens, 211
Handbook of Toxic Properties of Monomers and Additives, 226
Handbook of U.S. Colorants, 313–314
Handbook of Veterinary Drugs and Chemicals, 349
Handbook of Vitamins, 174
Handbook on Drug and Nutrient Interactions, 200, 201
Handbook on Extemporaneous Formulations, 164
Handbook on Injectable Drugs, 203–204, 407, 568
Handbooks and Tables in Science and Technology, 121
Hansten and Horn's Drug Interactions Analysis and Management, 194–195, 568
Hansten, P.D., 161, 194
HAPAB subfile, *TOXLINE*, 430
Harbison, R.D., 233
Harborne, J.B., 332
hardcopy, definition, 699
Hardin Meta Directory of Pharmacy and Pharmacology, 128
Hardman, J.G., 169
Hardy, H.L., 233

harmonization, drug standards, 63, 305, 306–307
The Harriet Lane Handbook, 160, 568
Harrison Narcotics Act (1915), 64
Hart, L.L., 174
Hartshorn, E.A., 273
Hartzema, A.G., 378
Harvard Medical Practice Study, 190
Hayes, E., 127
The Hayes Chain Drug Store Guide, 370
The Hayes Druggist Directory, 370
The Hayes Independent Druggist Guide, 370
hazard communication standards, OSHA, 85–86, 431, 432–433
hazard response. *See* poisoning
Hazardous Materials Technical Center File, 430
Hazardous Substances Data Bank, 431, 432
HAZDAT database, 433
Health Aspects of Pesticides Bulletin, 430
Health Care Daily (BNA), 482
Health Care Financing Administration reimbursement codes, 144
Health Devices Alerts, 524, 525, 526, 527, 528
Health Devices Sourcebook, 365, 492–493
Health Economics Evaluations Database, 486, 623
Health Economics—Places to Go Web site, 484
The Health Economics Website, 485
Health Effects of Environmental Pollutants (HEEP), 429, 430
Health Guide Series, Pharmaceutical Research and Manufacturers of America, 262
Health Industry Manufacturers Association, 626; Web site, 99, 134
Health Industry Today, 599
Health Information for International Travel, 166, 572
Health Information Technology Institute, White Paper on Web site assessment, 254
Health Legislation & Regulation (newsletter), 97, 599
Health Maintenance Organizations (HMOs), 87
Health News Daily, 96–97, 477–478, 483
Health Periodicals Database, 435
Health Planning & Administration database. *See* HealthSTAR
Health Policy and Biomedical Research, 97, 477
Health Protection Branch (Canada), 63
Health Statistics—College & Research Libraries News, 506
Health Technology Assessment Database, 486
Health WWWeb—Integrative Medicine, Natural Health and Alternative Therapies, 265–266
Health, U.S., 380
Healthcare Business & Legal Strategies, 600
Healthcare Organizations Database, 493–494
Healthcare PR & Marketing News, 600

Healthcare Technology & Business Opportunities, 600
Health-Center.com: Pharmacy, 260
HealthEconomics.Com, 481, 484
HealthFinder Web site, 254
HealthLinks: International Health and Social Statistics, 506
HealthSTAR, 579, 581, 587
Healthtouch Online Drug Information, 259
HealthWeb Public Health Statistics, 506
HEALTHWEB: Pharmacy & Pharmacology Web site, 122
Hebborn, A., 484
HEED, 486
HEEP subfile, *TOXLINE*, 430
Heilbron, 550
Heinonen, O.P., 222
Helfand, W.H., 355, 356
Helminthological Abstracts, 407
Henriette's Herbal Homepage, 344
hepatic impairment, prescribing considerations, handbook, 159
Herb Growing and Marketing Network, *Herb-NET*, 345
Herb Research Foundation, 618; Web site, 344
Herb Research News, 618
The Herbal Bookworm, 344–345
Herbal Drugs and Phytopharmaceuticals, 328–329
herbal (drugs): definition, 699; drug information, 246–247, 287, 289, 321–347, 358–359 professional and trade associations, 609, 614, 615, 618, 619, 622, 623, 630. *See also* herbal toxicity; dietary supplements
Herbal Medicine, 329
Herbal Medicines, A Guide for Healthcare Professionals, 328
Herbal Remedies, 328
herbal toxicity, reference sources, 229–232
Herbalgram, 610, 618; top ten best sellers, 345
Herbert, V., 251
Herbert, V.H., 251
HerbMed, 341
HerbNET, 345
Herbs (Eyewitness Handbook Series), 252, 253
Herbs for Health, 618
Herbs of Choice, 327–328
HerbWeb, 345
Herfindal, E.T., 174
Hesp, J.A., 115
Heymans Institute for Pharmacology, *Glossary*, 288
hierarchical, definition, 699
Higbee, M.D., 163
HIMA, 626; Web site, 99, 134
Hipple, T.F., 164
Hippocrates patient information cards, 260

Historical information, drug therapy, 640–641
history of drug regulation in the United States, 39–44
history of pharmacy, information resources, 351, 354–357, 360
History of Pharmacy: A Guide to Resources (Web site), 355
The History of Pharmacy (Web site), 355
The History of Pharmacy in Pictures (Web site), 355
HIV Clinical Trials in the United States, 413
HMO-PPO Digest (HMR), 379
HMO-PPO Directory, 493
HMOs, 87, 373, 379
HMR. *See* Hoechst Marion Roussel
HMTC subfile, *TOXLINE*, 430
Hodding, J.H., 161
Hodge, H.C., 212
Hodgson, E., 133
Hoechst Marion Roussel, *Managed Care Digest Series*, 379
Hogan, M.J., 195
Home Care Resource Book, 272
home medicine chest, recommended contents, 258, 261, 263, 270
home page, definition, 699. *See also* Web sites
Homeopathic Pharmacopoeia of the United States, 306
homeopathy: definition, 699–700; drugs, information sources, 151, 251, 265, 271, 279, 285, 289, 292, 306, 344, 353
The Honest Herbal, 246, 571
Hope, R.E., 249
Horn, J.R., 194
Hospital and Health Administration Index, 587
Hospital Literature Index, 587
Hospital Personal Selling Audit, Scott-Levin, 374
Hospital Pharmacist, 622
Hospital Pharmacy, 374
hospitals: core drug information collection, 567–570; emergency room statistics, 227–228; personnel, directory, 493; pharmacies, U.K., directory, 372
hotlinks, definition, 700
household medicines, necessary, recommendations, 258, 261, 263, 270
household products, identification, 27
How to Find Chemical Information, 120
How to Read the Prescription Web site, 263
Hoxsoll, J.F., 48
HPB, 63
HPLC Methods of Drug Analysis, 303
HPSA, 374
HRF. *See* Herb Research Foundation
HSDB, 431, 432
HSELINE, 578, 579, 587

HSLS Health Statistics Web site, 506
HSLS Pharmacy, Pharmacology & Therapeutics Web site, 124
HSTAR. *See* HealthSTAR
Hsu, H.Y., 336
HTML. *See* hypertext
Huang, K.C., 336
Hui, Y.H., 312
Human Genome Abstracts, 589
Human Pharmacology: Molecular to Clinical, 173–174
Hunter's Diseases of Occupations, 233
hypersensitivity, definition, 700
hypertext, definition, 700

IAC databases: *Health & Wellness Database*, 435, 504; *Magazine Database*, 435; *Newsletter Database*, 481, 483, 487–488, 524; *PROMT*, 481, 483, 499–500; *Trade & Industry Database*, 483, 499–500
IACP. *See* International Academy of Compounding Pharmacists
IARC Monographs on the Evaluation of Carcinogenic Risk of Chemicals, 226–227
iatrogenic, definition, 700
IBIDS, 342
IBIS, 266
ICD-9, 405, 504
ICH, 63, 542
IDdb, 466, 470
IDE, 90
Ident-A-Drug Reference, 280
IDENTIDEX, 278
identification sources, drugs: through drug nomenclature, 21–37, 283–295, 440–442, 575–576; through laboratory analysis, 216–218, 302, 308, 312; through photographs or imprint indexes, 150, 177, 277–283
IDIN's Links Web site, 126
idiopathic, definition, 700
idiosyncrasy, drug-related, definition, 700
IDIS Drug File, 405–406, 411, 417
IDRAC, 545
IEC, 544
IFI/Plenum databases: *CLAIMS/RRX* database, 553, 556, 558; *CLAIMS/U.S. Patents Abstracts*, 581, 584–585
IFPMA . *See* International Federation of Pharmaceutical Manufacturers Associations
Igoe, R.S., 312
IHS regulatory libraries, 543–544
Illustrated Buyers Guide to Veterinary Equipment and Supplies, 354
images, dosage forms and imprints, 278, 279, 281–282, 644, 646
immunization: definition, 700; guidelines sources, 29, 153, 158, 166–169, 291

Immunoclones Database, 576, 578, 588
Immunofacts: Vaccines & Immunologic Drugs, 153–154
Immunology Abstracts, 589
import laws, cosmetics and OTC drugs, 51
importation of foreign drugs by individuals, 64
imprints: definition, 700; dosage form, indexes, 150, 177, 277–283, 644, 646
IMS Global Services, 372–373, 545
IMS Marketletter, 481
IMS National Prescription Audit, 36, 373, 374–375
IMS *World Drug Market Manual*, 372. *See also* IMS/IMSworld databases
Imsmarq Pharmaceutical Trademarks in-Use, 575, 580, 588
IMSPACT audit reports, 373
IMS/IMSworld databases: *Company Directory*, 491; *New Product Launches*, 294, 372, 475, 489–490; *Patents International*, 549–550, 551–552, 556, 557; *Pharmaceutical Company Profiles*, 490; *Product Monographs* database, 72, 294, 372, 489–490; *R&D Focus Drug News*, 478, 483; *R&D Focus Drug Updates*, 453–455, 456–458, 487, 516; *R&D Meetings Diary*, 580, 588; *World Drug Market Manual*, 491, 496–497; *World Drug Markets* (countries), 496–497, 558
in vitro versus *in vivo*, definition, 700
In Vivo, The Business & Medicine Report, 600
INCAD, 544
INCI, 314
Incidence & Prevalence Database, 475, 504–505
incidence versus prevalence, definition, 700
incompatibilities, parenteral: definition, 700–701; reference sources, 202–204; searching online, 428
IND, 44–45, 701; nondisclosure, 67; Safety Report, 46. *See also* treatment INDs
independent pharmacies, retail, directories, 370–371
Index Medicus, 390
Index Nominum, 29–30, 283
Index of Veterinary Specialties (IVS), 350
Index Plantarum Medicinalium Totius Mundi Eorumque Synonymorum, 335
Index to Dental Literature, 390
India, drug product information, 292
Indian Pharmaceutical Guide, 292
Indiana University Web sites: *BioTech Chemical Acronyms Database*, 134; *Biotech Life Sciences Dictionary*, 134; *Cyberbotanica*, 343
indications, drug, definition, 701. *See also* off-label
indigenous (medicine), definition, 701. *See also* ethnobotany

Industrial Pharmacist, 622
industrial pharmacy, information needs and resources, 301–320
industrial products, identification, 27
industrial toxicology: online searching, 428–434, 578; reference sourcebooks, 233–234
Infection Control Weekly, 600
infectious disease pharmacists, society of, 622
Infectious Disease Weekly, 600
Infectious Diseases Handbook, 167, 409, 568
Infomed Drug Guide Web site, 181
Informacion de Medicamentos para el Profesional Sanitario, 146
Informacion de Medicamentos, Consejos al Paciente, 239, 240
Information Handling Services (IHS), 543–544
Information Resources in Toxicology, 120
Information Sources in Chemistry, 120
Information Sources in Pharmaceuticals, 114–115
informed consent, 701
The Informed Consumer's Pharmacy, 250
Infusion Technology Manual, 204
ingredients, non-disclosure, 66. *See also* formulation development
Ingrim, N., 158
injectable drugs, incompatibilities, reference sources, 202–204
INN, 12, 22–24
INPADOC, 550, 557–558, 588
InPharma, 403, 411, 483, 516
Inside Conferences, 576, 577, 578, 588
Inside Healthcare Reform, 601
INSPEC, 579, 588
inspections, FDA, statistics, 536. *See also* EIRs
Institute for Biotechnology Information, directory, 365, 366
Institute for Safe Medication Practices, 618–619
Institute for Scientific Information (ISI), 397–398
Institute of Chinese Materia Medica, 336
institution (author address), searching online, 423–425
Institution of Electrical Engineers (U.K.), *INSPEC* database, 588
Institutional Digest (HMR), 379
institutional pharmacy, definition, 701
Instructions for Patients, 270, 569
Integrated Health Systems Digest (HMR), 379
Integrative Body Mind Information System, 266
integumentary, definition, 701. *See also* skin
InteliHealth—U.S. Pharmacopeia Dispensing Information, 178, 256
intellectual property, definition, 701. *See also* patents; trademarks
Intercontinental Medical Statistics (IMS), 372
interface (computer), definition, 701

Interim Rule Subpart E, 58, 59
International Academy of Compounding Pharmacists, 619
International Agency for Research on Cancer (IARC), 226–227
The International Bibliographic Information on Dietary Supplements Database, 342
International Biological Reference Preparation, 24
International Biological Standard, 24
International Chemical Reference Preparation, 24
International Classification of Diseases, 405, 504
International Conferences on Harmonization (ICH), 63, 542
International Cosmetic Ingredient Dictionary and Handbook, 314–315, 402
The International Directory of Chemical Companies, 492
The International Directory of Pharmaceutical Companies, 492
The International Directory of Pharmaceutical Personnel, 492
International Electrotechnical Commission, 544
International Encyclopedia of Cosmetic Material Trade Names, 315–316
International Federation of Pharmaceutical Manufacturers Associations, 626–627
International Federation of the Societies of Cosmetic Chemists, *KOSMET* database, 589
The International Journal of Pharmacy Practice, 622
International Labour Office CIS subfile, *TOXLINE*, 429
International Nomenclature Cosmetic Ingredient (INCI), 314
International Nonproprietary Name, 12, 22–24
International Nonproprietary Names (INN) for Pharmaceutical Substances: Cumulative List, 24, 295
International Nursing Index, 390
International Pharmaceutical Abstracts, 14, 356, 375, 399–402, 412, 414, 437, 439; brand name searching, 417–418; drug category searching, 422–423; searching routes of drug administration, 416–417
International Pharmaceutical Federation database, 382
International Pharmaceutical Services, 84
International Pharmacopoeia, 307
International Society for Ethnopharmacology, 619
International Society for Pharmaceutical Engineering, 619–620
International Society for Pharmacoeconomics and Outcomes Research, 620

International Society for Pharmacoepidemiology, 620
International Standards Organization reference name, 24, 34
International Standards Organization, medical device compliance, 92, 93, 544
International Union of Pure and Applied Chemistry, 9, 15–16
Internet Directory for Botany: Economic Botany, Ethnobotany, 340
Internet Mental Health Web site, 182
Internet: criteria for inclusion, 5; directory of sources cited in this book, 657–671; evaluating health information on, 254–255; news and reviews, 130; pathfinders (pharmacy subject hubs), 122–130; value in drug information, 117. *See also* Web sites
InterPharma, 368
interstate commerce and drug law, 79
intoxication, definition, 701. *See also* poisoning
Intranets, definition, 701
intravenous drugs, incompatibilities, 202–204
Introduction to Reference Sources in the Health Sciences, 114
Investext, 373, 501, 502, 503, 558
Investigational Device Exemption (IDE), 90
investigational drug codes, 10–11; key to initial letters, 28
Investigational Drug Patents Fast-Alert, 470, 559–560, 561
Investigational Drugs Database, 466, 470
Investigational New Drug Application, 44–45. *See also* IND
Iowa Drug Information Network, *IDIN's Links* Web site, 126
Iowa Drug Information Service, 405–406, 411, 417
IP. See International Pharmacopoeia
IPA subfile, *TOXLINE*, 428, 430
IPA Thesaurus and Frequency List, 402, 437
IPA, 399–402. *See also* International Pharmaceutical Abstracts
Isada, C.M., 167
ISE. See International Society for Ethnopharmacology
ISI Reaction Center, 439
ISMP. See Institute for Safe Medication Practices
ISO, medical device compliance, 92, 93, 544
ISO, reference name, 24
Isolation and Identification of Drugs, 216–217, 302, 574
ISPE. *See* International Society for Pharmaceutical Engineering.
See also International Society for Pharmacoepidemiology
ISPOR LEXICON, 132

ISPOR. *See* International Society for Pharmacoeconomics and Outcomes Research
Italy, drug information sources, 289–290
Ito, S., 200
IUPAC. *See* International Union of Pure and Applied Chemistry
IV additives, definition, 701. *See also* intravenous drugs, incompatibilities
IVS-Index of Veterinary Specialties, 350
Iwu, M.M., 338

Jabbari, D., 49
Jaeger, R.W., 247
Jaenicke, C., 328
James, K., 569, 572
JAN, 12, 25
Japan Drug Guide, 287, 289
Japan Drug Index, 289
Japan Pharmaceutical Reference, 287
Japan: cosmetic ingredients, CTFA list of, 315; medical device regulations, 94; orphan drug legislation, 55–56
Japanese Accepted Names for Pharmaceuticals, 25
Japanese Pharma-Devices Update (IHS), 544
The Japanese Standards for Herbal Medicines, 287, 289
Jellin, J., 280
Jepson, M.H., 116
JMCP—Journal of Managed Care Pharmacy, 607
John, G., 253
Johns Hopkins Encyclopedia, 256
Johns Hopkins Hospital, *The Harriet Lane Handbook*, 160
Johnson, T., 339, 345
Journal of Clinical Pharmacology, 610
Journal of Controlled Release, 617
Journal of Ethnopharmacology, 619
Journal of Managed Care Pharmacy, 607
Journal of Natural Products, 614
Journal of Pharmaceutical and Biomedical Analysis, 609
Journal of Pharmaceutical Development and Technology, 609
Journal of Pharmaceutical Marketing and Management, 609
Journal of Pharmaceutical Science and Technology, 621
Journal of Pharmaceutical Sciences (APhA), 612
Journal of Pharmacology and Experimental Therapeutics, 612
Journal Watch database, 577, 589
JPR, 287, 289
Julia, A.M., 297

Kafader, D., 100
Karig, A.W., 273
Karolinska Institute Drug Therapy Web site, 127
Kasten, B.L., 167
Katzung, B.G., 172
Kauffman, R.E., 200
Kefauver-Harris Amendments, 42, 89
Keli, P., 335
KEMI subfile, *TOXLINE*, 430
Keyguide to Information Sources in Pharmacy, 116
kidney disease, prescribing considerations, handbooks, 159
Killion, V., 122
Kindscher, K., 339
Kingsbury, J.N., 229
Kirk-Othmer Encyclopedia of Chemical Technology Online, 575, 576, 589
Kirsch-Volders, M., 223
Klaassen, C.D., 214
Klaus, W., 284
Klein, E.G., 132
Knoben, J.E., 158
Knodel, L.C., 148
Kohler, H.A., 345
Kohler's Medizinal Pflanzen, 345
Kolb, V.M., 223
Kommission E. *See* Commission E
Koren, G., 222
Kortt, M., 485
KOSMET, 576, 577, 578, 579, 581, 589
Kraus, D.M., 161
Kremer's and Urdang's History of Pharmacy, 354, 356
Kress, H., 344
Kryt, D., 296

L'Informatore Farmaceutico, 289
labeling: definition, 701; requirements, cosmetics and OTC drugs, 51; requirements, foods, 534–535
laboratory analysis of drugs: sourcebooks, 216–218, 302–308, 312; *Standards Status* database, 608
laboratory codes, 10–11; key to initial letters, 28
laboratory research methods and techniques, 439
Laboratory Test Handbook, 409
laboratory test modifications by drugs, 201–202, 428
Lachant, N., 159
Lachman, L., 309
lactation, drug effects, information sources, 36, 198, 199–200, 207, 222
lactose-free OTC product identification, 149
Lacy, C., 158
lag time, definition, 701. *See also* drug lag; timelines, IND and DNA

Lampe, K.F., 229
Lance, L.L., 158
language equivalents, multilingual guides, 288, 295–298, 299, 604
Language Guide for the Clinical Pharmacist, 297
LaNier, M., 228
Larner, J., 173
Lasagna, L., 48
latency period, definition, 701
Laurence, D.R., 131
Law for Retailers (U.K.), 280
The Lawrence Review of Natural Products, 330–331
laws and regulations, background on, 39–105. *See also* legal information
lay people, drug information for, 237–275, 435–437, 537
LD_{50}:
    definition, 702; quick reference sources, 641
Le Vidal Therapeutique, 286
Leatherhead Food Research Association (U.K.), *FOODLINE*, 534
Leber, M.R., 247
Leff, R.D., 204
legal information, online sources, 581. *See also* litigation; regulatory information
legend drugs, definition, 702. *See also* prescription drugs
legislation versus regulation, 73–74
legislation, food, 534–535
LEGSTAT, 558, 589
Lehrbuch der Phytotherapie, 329
Leikin, J.B., 209, 210
Letner, A., 130
letters, FDA, 531–533, 691
Leung, A.Y., 331
Lewis, D.A., 334
Lewis, R.A., 133
Lewis, R.J., 212, 312
Lewis, R.L., 221
Lewis' Dictionary of Toxicology, 133
Lexi-Comp Clinical Reference Collection, 408–409
Lexicon Plantarum Medicinalium, 335
LEXIS, 77
Liberti, L., 330
Library for Internists, 569
license, establishment (biologics), 42, 57
license, pharmacy, probation, suspension, revocation, 99
license, product (biologics), 41. *See also* BLA, ELA, PLA
licensed establishments, biologics, directory, 540
licensing: applications, biologics, 46–47, 57; government-owned inventions, news, 97; op-

portunities, searching for online, 486–488, 655
licensure: definition, 702; requirements, pharmacy, 36, 80, 351; statistics, pharmacists, 380
Lieberman, H.A., 309
Life Sciences Collection database, 576, 577, 578, 579, 580, 589
Limbird, L.E., 169
Lindley, C.M., 204
Lindsay Drug Company, *The History of Pharmacy* Web site, 355
line extensions, 71–72, 488–490, 650, 702
link terms, *EMBASE*, 394
Links to Sites Related to the History of Pharmacy (AIHP), 355
Lipkowitz, M.A., 251
Literature Monitoring and Evaluation Service (LMS), 404–405
litigation, information sources, 77–78, 81, 82, 83. *See also* forensic laboratory analysis of drugs
Litt, J.Z., 198
liver impairment, prescribing considerations, handbook, 159
Lloydia, 614
LMS Drug Alerts Online, 404–405, 411, 458
loading dose, definition, 702
Long, J.W., 244
Long, P.W., 182
long-term care facilities, pharmacy regulations, 84–85
look alike drug names, 29, 144, 175, 270
Lubinieki, A.S., 49
Lund, E., 302

M1 ICH initiative, 63
MAC, 144; definition, 702
Machlin, L.J., 174
Maciocia, G., 337
Maga, J.A., 225
Maibach, H.I., 233
Mailman, R.B., 133
Maizell, R.E., 120
MAK. *See* MEL
Managed Care Digest Series, 376, 379
managed care, definition, 702
Mangum, O.B., 161
Manifold, C.C., 118
manpower, pharmacy, statistics sources, 379–380, 382
MANTIS, 342, 436, 577, 578, 580, 589
Manual de Enseñanze de Medicamentos en Español, 269–270
Manual of Antibiotics and Infectious Diseases, 167, 568
Manual of Pediatric Therapeutics, 161, 568

Manual of Policies and Procedures, FDA, 536
Manual, Alternative and Natural Therapy. *See* MANTIS
manufacturer names, online searching, 654–655. *See also* company directories
Manufacturing Chemist, 500
manufacturing, pharmaceutical: facility design, *Baseline Guides*, 620; information needs and resources, 301–320
MaPPs, 536
market exclusivity: biologics, FDA Modernization Act, 57; list of drugs that qualify, 88; pediatric drugs, FDA Modernization Act, 56–57; Waxman-Hatch law, 52–53, 549
market research sources, 372–380, 447–508, 580–581
Marketletter, 481, 483, 600
MarketLine International, 581, 589
Markush DARC, 559
Markush Pharmsearch, 575, 581, 590
Marler, E.E.J., 34
Marmion, D.M., 313
MARPAT, 559
Marquardt, K.W., 81
Martin, L., 113
Martindale Online, 442, 590
Martindale: The Extra Pharmacopoeia, 139–141, 283, 362, 568, 573
Martindale's Health Science Guide—The Virtual Pharmacy Center, 124
Martindale's Health Science Guide—Virtual Veterinary Center, 352
Marzulli, F.N., 233
Mason, P., 271
Massachusetts Medical Society, *Journal Watch* database, 589
Massey University (New Zealand), *EpiVetNet*, 352, 506
materia medica, definition, 702
Material Safety Data Sheets, 85–86, 432–433, 702
maternal-fetal risk. *See* pregnancy, drug use in. *See also* teratogenicity
Maternal-Fetal Toxicology: A Clinician's Guide, 222
Mathieu, M., 47, 49
Matsutani, Y., 94
maximum allowable cost (MAC), 144; definition, 702
maximum exposure level. *See* MEL
Maxmen, J.S., 162
Mayo Clinic Health Letter, 260
Mayo Clinic Health Oasis Medicine Center Web site, 259–260
McCann, M.A., 229
McCrea, J., 164

McGraw-Hill Publications Online, 578, 581, 590
McMaster University's Health Care Information Resources—Alternative Medicine, 267
MDCA News, 480, 483
MDIS. *See* ESPICOM
MDMA. *See* Medical Device Manufacturers Association
MDRs, 91–92, 527, 529
MDX Health Digest database, 435–436
MedAxon, 146
MEDDRA, 63
MEDEC. *See* Medical Devices Canada
MedGuide program, FDA, 237
Median, J., 286
MEDICAID Drug Rebate Law, 84
MEDICAID information, 36
Medical Database Limited, *InterPharma* Web site, 368
Medical Device & Diagnostic Industry, 368
Medical Device Amendments, 89–92
Medical Device Companies Analysis, 490
Medical Device Link Web site, 368
Medical Device Manufacturers Association, 627
Medical Device Register, 365, 492
Medical Device Regulations in Japan, 94
Medical Device Reports (MDRs), 91–92, 527, 529
Medical Device Submissions Handbook (HIMA), 626
Medical Device Technology, buyers guide and resource directory issue, 369
medical devices: definition in law, 702; government regulation, 88–94; *Standards Monitor Online* database, 615; year 2000 compliance status information, 542
Medical Devices Canada (association), 627
Medical Devices, Diagnostics, and Instrumentation Reports, 93, 477
Medical Dictionary for Regulatory Affairs, 63
Medical Group Practice Digest (HMR), 379
Medical Herbalism, 345–346
The Medical Letter on Drugs and Therapeutics, 156–157, 168
Medical Library Association, Drug and Pharmaceutical Information Division, 605
Medical Malpractice Pharmacy Law, 82
Medical Marketing & Media, Pharmaceutical Marketers Directory, 364
Medical Matrix Web site, 125–126
Medical Outcomes & Guidelines Alert, 600
Medical School of the College of Philadelphia, 351
Medical Subject Headings. *See* MeSH
Medical Subject Headings—Annotated Alphabetic List, 390. *See also* MeSH

Medical Subject Headings—Tree Structures, 390. *See also* Trees
Medical Technology-Related Acronyms Web site, 134
Medical Textiles, 600
Medicare-Medicaid AntiFraud and Abuse Amendments, 84
Medication Errors Reporting Program, 619
Medication Guide Plan, FDA, 237
Medication Info Search Web site, 258–259
Medication Teaching Manual: The Guide to Patient Drug Information, 269–270, 272, 568, 570, 571, 572
Medications and Mother's Milk, 200
Medicinal Plant Databases Web site, 340–341
medicinal plants. *See* botanicals
Medicinal Plants in China, 335, 336
Medicinal Plants in Vietnam, 338
Medicinal Plants of North America, 342, 343
Medicinal Plants of the Desert and Canyon West, 339
Medicinal Plants of the World, 329–330
Medicinal Wild Plants of the Prairie, 339
Medicine & Health, 601
MedicineNet—The Pharmacy Web site, 256–257
Medicines Act of 1968 (U.K.), 83
MediConf (Fairbase), 581, 590
Mediconsult—General Drug Information Web site, 258
MediSpan: *Drug Image Database*, 278–279; *Drug Imprint Database*, 278–279; *Drug Information Database*, 259
MediStat News, 480, 483
Medizinal Pflanzen, 345
MEDLINE, 14, 16, 67, 341, 342, 389–392, 406, 407; author affiliations or addresses, 425; brand name searching, 417, 419, 420; drug category searching, 421–422; indexing of clinical trials 410; publication type indexing, 426; searching for adverse effects/drug interactions, 427; searching routes of drug administration, 415–416; subject population indexing, 413–414; TOXBIB subfile, 430, 431
MedNets Epidemiology & Public Health, 506
Medscape: *Drug Search from First DataBank*, 179–180; *Patient Information*, 260
MedWeb Pharmacy and Pharmacology, 127
meeting announcements, forthcoming: *EVENT-LINE*, 586; *IMSworld R&D Meetings Diary*, 588; *MediConf (Fairbase)*, 590
meeting papers, online coverage, 67. *See also* conference literature, specialty databases
MEL, definition, 702
Membrane & Separation Technology News, 601
Merck Index, 14, 26–28, 281, 550, 568
The Merck Index Online, 442, 590

Merck Manual of Diagnosis and Therapy, 146, 153
The Merck Veterinary Manual, 350, 353
MERP. *See* Medication Errors Reporting Program
MeSH Tree Structures, 14, 390, 421–422
MeSH, 396, 407, 421
Messonnier, S.P., 350
meta Register of Controlled Trials, 413
meta-analysis, definition, 702
metabolite, definition, 702–703
MetaMaps databases, 412–413
MethodsFinder, 439
me-too products: defined, 703; law governing approval, 52–53; searching online, 650
Mexico, drug information sources, 290
Meyler's Side Effects of Drugs, 191–192, 568, 573
MIDAS sales audits, 372
milk, human. *See* lactation
Millares, M., 116, 569
Miller Freeman, *dotpharmacy* Web site, 375, 376, 503
Miller, R.R., 194
MIMS Australia, 293
MIMS Disease Index, 293–294
MIMS *Index of Veterinary Specialties*, 350
MIMS Magazine, 587
MIMS OTC, 293
minimum ready-reference collection, 567–570
The Mining Company: Pharmacology Web site, 128
Ministerio de Sanidad y Consume de Espana, 146
Minneman, K.P., 173
Misuse of Drugs Act (U.K.), 83, 280
MLA. *See* Medical Library Association
MMWR, 505
Mochizuki, T.K., 159
Model List of Essential Drugs (WHO), 303, 319
Model State Pharmacy Act, 80
Modell's *Drugs in Current Use and New Drugs*, 574
Modern Drug Encyclopedia & Therapeutic Index, 574
Moerman, D.E., 343
Moffatt, A.C., 216
Molderman, J., 312
molecular formulas, 15
Molecular Pharmacology, 612
monograph, as defined in drug literature, 21, 703
Moore, M., 339, 346
Moores, K., 126
Morbidity and Mortality Weekly Reports, 505
morbidity, definition, 703
Morrison, G., 159

mortality: definition, 703; statistics, drug abuse, 227–228. *See also* epidemiology
Mosby's GenRx, 144–145, 146, 177, 179, 281, 362, 374, 568, 570, 571, 572, 574
Mosby's Medical, Nursing, and Allied Health Dictionary, 435
Mosby's Nursing Drug Reference, 176, 568
Mosby's Patient GenRx, 242
Mosby's Veterinary Guide to the Internet, Net-Vet, 351
MotherNature.com, 265
MotherRisk Web site, 198
The Mount Sinai School of Medicine Complete Book of Nutrition, 251
MRA, 92
mRCT, 413
Mrs. Grieve's A Modern Herbal, 264
MSDS, 85–86
MSDS-CCOHS database, 432
MSDS-OHS database, 432
MSDS-SEARCH, 433
Mueller, L., 345
Muller, N.F., 294
Mullins, C.D., 378
Multilingual Dictionary of Narcotic Drugs and Psychotropic Substances under International Control, 296
multilingual guides (translation aids), 288, 295–298, 299, 604
Multinational Integrated Data Analysis Service (MIDAS), 372
multisource drug products, definition, 703. *See also* generic drugs
Munro, D., 231
Munson, P.L., 171
Murphy, G.R., 370
Mutagenicity, Carcinogenicity, and Teratogenicity of Industrial Pollutants, 223
mutagenicity, definition, 703. *See also* teratogenicity
Mutschler, E., 171
Mutual Recognition Agreement (medical devices), 92
mutual recognition (European drug approvals), 62

NABLAW, 82
NABP, 80, 99, 570, 620–621
NACDS, 627–628; *Membership Directory*, 370; *Spanish for Pharmacists*, 288; Web site, 375, 376, 380, 503
NADA, 53. *See also* New Animal Drug Application
NAFTA, 51
Nahata, M.C., 164
NAICS indexing, 499, 500, 501

NAPM. *See* National Association of Pharmaceutical Manufacturers
NAPRALERT, 346, 439–440
narcotic drugs: definitions, 697, 703; law (U.S.), 64–65; under international control, 24
NARD. *See* National Community Pharmacists Association
NAS/NRC, 42
Nater, J.P., 198
Nathan, A., 292
National Ambulatory Medical Care Survey, 376–377
National Association of Boards of Pharmacy, 80, 99, 570, 620–621
National Association of Chain Drug Stores. *See* NACDS
National Association of Pharmaceutical Manufacturers, 628
National Association of Retail Druggists. *See* National Community Pharmacists Association
National Biotechnology Information Facility Company Register, 368
National Cancer Institute (U.S.). *See* NCI
National Center for Complementary and Alternative Medicine, 341
National Center for Health Statistics, 376–378, 380, 505
National Clearinghouse for Alcohol and Drug Information Web site, 228
National Community Pharmacists Association, 628
National Council Against Health Fraud, 267
National Council for Patient Information and Education, *Prescription Medicines and You,* 258
National Detailing Audit (IMS), 373
National Disease and Therapeutic Index (IMS), 373
National Drug Code Directory, 280, 537, 538
National Drug Code, 16. *See also* NDC
National Drug Data File (*NDDF*), 146, 179–180, 260, 278
National Eye Institute, 260
National Fire Protection Association hazardous class codes, 210
The National Formulary (U.S.), 304–306, 310
National Health Service (U.K.), 83
National Hospital Ambulatory Medical Care Survey, 377–378
National Household Survey on Drug Abuse, 228, 505
National Institute of Mental Health, 260
National Institutes of Health. *See* NIH
National Journal Audit (IMS), 373
National Mail Audit (IMS), 373

National Pharmaceutical Association (U.K.), patient information leaflets, 262
National Prescription Audit (IMS), 36, 373, 374–375
National Primary Drinking Water Standards, 215
National Registry of Drug-Induced Ocular Side Effects, 197
National Technical Information Service, 430, 488
National Wholesale Druggists' Association, 628–629
Native American Ethnobotany Database, 342–343
Natural Health Village Web site, 266
Natural HealthLine newsletter, 266
natural language (searching): definition, 703; example, 650–651
Natural Product Medicine, 330
Natural Products Alert, 439–440
natural remedies, information sources, 246–247, 321–347, 358–359, 439–440. *See also* botanicals
Nature-Biotechnology Directory, 366
Navarra, T., 251
NCAHF Newsletter, 267
NCHS, 376–378, 380, 505
NCI Cancer Weekly, 599
NCI, *Survey of Compounds Which Have Been Tested for Carcinogenic Activity,* 227
NCPA. *See* National Community Pharmacists Association
NDA, 8, 41, 46, 703; approvals, searching online, 510–516, 521–524; filing, nondisclosure, 67
The NDA Book, 67
NDA Days, 61
NDA Pipeline, 14, 68, 470–472; compared to other pipeline directories, 472–476
NDC company code designations, 29, 280. *See also* National Drug Code
NDDF, 146, 179–180, 260, 278
NDMA. *See* Nonprescription Drug Manufacturers Association
NDMAC. *See* Nonprescription Drug Manufacturers Association of Canada
NDR, 271, 572
NDTI, 373
Negwer, M., 34
Neilsen, J.R., 83
Neofax: A Manual of Drugs Used in Neonatal Care, 161
neonate, definition, 703. *See also* lactation
The NetSci Yellow Pages, 368
NetVet, 351, 352
Neue Arzneimittel, 284–285
New Animal Drug Application, 53, 511, 523, 539

New Drug Application. *See* NDA
New Drug Development: A Regulatory Overview, 47
New England Journal of Medicine database, 577, 590
New Medicines in Development Database, PhRMA, 472
New Medicines in Development Series, PhRMA, 262
Newall, C.A., 328
news sources: online, 476–481, 482–484, 597–602; regulatory, 94–98
NF, 304–306, 310
NFN, 12
Nies, A.S., 569, 572
NIH: clinical trials databases, 57; research grants, news, 97; *Unconventional Cancer Treatments*, 266
NIOSHTIC, 578, 590
NME Express, 458, 462–463; compared to other pipeline directories, 472–476; patent information in, 550
NNC. *See* Nutraceuticals Network of Canada
nomenclature. *See* drug nomenclature
noncompliance with treatment plan, statistics, 237, 238, 630, 653
Nonprescription Drug Manufacturers Association of Canada, 629–630
Nonprescription Drug Manufacturers Association, 544, 629
Nonprescription Drug References for Health Professionals, 271
nonprescription drugs. *See* OTC drugs
Non-prescription Medicines, 292
Nonprescription Medicines, What's Right for You, 257
Nonprescription Pharmaceuticals and Nutritionals, 96, 477
Nonprescription Products: Formulations and Features, 148, 149, 568, 571
nonproprietary names, 7–8, 11–12, 703
nootropic, definition, 703
normal laboratory values, 28, 143, 158, 175, 176, 270
Norman, D.C., 168
North American Free Trade Agreement, 51
North American Industry Classification System, 499, 500, 501
Notice of Claimed Investigational Exemption for a New Drug, 45
notices of adverse findings, FDA, 531
Novartis Pharmacy Benefit Report, 379
NSC, 11
NTIS database, 488, 577, 581, 590
NTIS subfile, *TOXLINE*, 430
Nurse Prescribers' List (U.K.), 292
Nurses Drug Facts, 175–176, 281, 568

The Nurse's Drug Handbook, 176
nurses, drug compendia designed for, 174–177, 179
nursing homes, pharmacy regulations, 84
nursing mother/infant, drug effects. *See* lactation
Nutraceutical Network of Canada, 630
nutraceuticals: definition, 703; information sources, 157, 252. *See also* dietary supplements
Nutrient Interactions, 201
Nutrition Abstracts & Reviews, 407
Nutrition and Dietary Advice in the Pharmacy, 271–272
The Nutrition Desk Reference, 201, 572
Nutrition Labeling and Education Act (1990), 252
nutrition, information resources, 201, 251–252, 265, 271–272. *See also* dietary supplements
Nutritional Data Resources (company) Web site, 157
NWDA. *See* National Wholesale Druggists' Association

O'Reilly, J.T., 48
Oak Ridge National Laboratory subfiles in *TOXLINE*, 429
OBRA, 81–82, 84, 86, 163, 270, 570
Occupational Projections and Training Data, 380
Occupational Safety and Health database. *See* NIOSHTIC
occupational toxicology reference sources, 233–234. *See also* toxicology, online searching
ocular adverse effects, drugs and chemicals, 197
ocular drugs, reference sources, 154, 155, 164
Ody, P., 252
Office of Dietary Supplements (NIH) Web site, 342
official (government) compendia: botanicals, 324; drug nomenclature, 22–26; drug standards, 304–308
Official Methods of Analysis of AOAC International, 302–303
off-label (drug) uses: definition, 703; law governing information dissemination, 57, 70–71; quick-reference sources, 140, 143, 144, 145, 146, 150, 154, 155, 156, 159, 163, 177, 179
Okabe, H., 49
Olson, K.R., 209
Omnibus Budget Reconciliation Act (OBRA), 81–82, 84, 86, 570
oncology drugs, handbooks, 159
Onhealth Resources Web site, 256
online resources, 387–563, 575–602
online vendors, database availability guide, 592–596

OPD Chemical Buyers Guide, 364–365
operators (computer searching), definition, 703–704
ophthalmic adverse effects, drugs and chemicals, 197
ophthalmic. *See also* ocular drugs, reference sources
Ophthalmic Drug Facts, 154, 155
OPPT Chemical Fact Sheets, 434
Orange Book, 87–88, 362, 510–511, 537, 549
organic name reactions, 28
Organic-Chemical Drugs and Their Synonyms (Negwer), 34
organizations, directory, 603–632
Oriental Materia Medica, 336, 337
Orphan Drug Act, 55–56
orphan drugs: definition, 704; listings, 68, 88, 143, 175
Orphan Drugs—Your Complete Guide to Effective, Tested Medications Outside the U.S. and Their Availability, 294
OSHA: hazard communication standards, 85–86; *Registry of Toxic Effects of Chemical Substances*, 224, 431, 432. *See also* permissible exposure limits; material safety data sheets
OTC drugs: coverage in literature, 17; labeling, changes under FDA Modernization Act, 67; monographs for personal care products, 51; sources of comparative information, 148–149, 244, 639. *See also* OTC products
OTC Electronic Library (INCAD), 544
OTC Market Report Update USA, 601
OTC News & Market Report, 601
OTC products: industry associations, 624, 625, 626, 629, 631; information sources, 148–149, 151, 240, 242, 243, 244, 246, 247, 250, 251, 257, 265, 271, 291, 292, 314–317, 544. *See also* OTC drugs
OTC Review (DESI), 42–43, 244–245, 629; *Ingredient Status Report*, 536
OTC Update, 601
OTCs in Europe—1998 Facts and Figures, 624
Outcomes Activities Database, 485
Outcomes Database of Structured Abstracts, 485
Outcomes Literature Database, 485
outcomes research and health economics, Web sites, 481, 484–486, 620
Outcomes, 484
out-of-state prescriptions, 79
Overall Evaluations of Carcinogenicity (IARC), 226–227
overdose. *See* poisoning
over-the-counter drugs, definition, 704. *See also* OTC drugs
Over-the-Counter Pharmaceutical Formulations, 316

P.P. Guide (Australia), 292–293
package insert, definition, 704
Packaged Facts, FIND/SVP, 502
packaging: liabilities, 84; potential toxicity, 226
Paddock Laboratories, *Secundum Artem Index*, 165
PAFA database, 313, 541
Pagliaro, A.M., 161
Pagliaro, L.A., 161
Paloucek, F.P., 209, 210
paper NDAs, 53
parallel track testing, 58
Parascandola, J., 356
Parent's Guide to Childhood Medications, 242, 571
Parenteral Drug Association, 621
parenteral: definition, 704; incompatibilities, 202–204, 428
Parenti, M.A., 118
Parexel publications: Home Page, 50; *Pharmaceutical R&D Statistical Sourcebook*, 378; *Worldwide Pharmaceutical Regulation Series*, 50
Paris Convention of 1883, 547
PASCAL database, 342, 577, 578, 580, 591
Pashos, C.L., 132
pastille, definition, 704
The Patent Cooperation Treaty, 547
patent medicines, 148. *See also* OTC drugs
patents: background on law, 546–548; expirations, 36, 88, 550–558, 651–652; licensing, news sources, 486–488, 558; term extensions, Waxman-Hatch law, 52–53, 88, 538, 545–546, 549–558, 651–652; terms, GATT adjustments, 54, 550
patient confidentiality under Freedom of Information provisions, 66
Patient Counseling Handbook, 270
patient counseling: aids for, 269–273; mandated, 36, 80–81, 86. *See also* patients, drug information for
Patient Dosage Instructions: A Guide for Pharmacists, 297
Patient Drug Facts, 270, 281, 568, 571, 572
Patient Education Leaflets, USP DI, 256, 271
Patient Information Leaflet (PIL), European mutual recognition, 62
patient package inserts, 237, 238, 291
patients, drug information for, 217–275, 434–437, 537, 639, 653
Patterson, R.M., 78
Patti People's Health Economics Resource Page, 484
PBIRG, 605
PCA News, 480, 483
PCT, 547
PDA. *See* Parenteral Drug Association

PDDA, 373
PDF, definition, 704
PDMA, 86
PDQ databases, 409, 437–437
The PDR Companion Guide, 196–197
The PDR Family Guide to Nutrition and Health, 248–249, 281, 572
The PDR Family Guide to Prescription Drugs, 248, 281, 572
The PDR Family Guide to Women's Health and Prescription Drugs, 248, 281, 572
PDR for Herbal Medicines, 328, 571
PDR for Nonprescription Drugs, 151, 281, 362, 569, 570, 572
PDR for Ophthalmology, 154–155
PDR Generics, 150, 281, 362, 568, 572
PDR Nurse's Handbook, 177, 179, 281
PDR, 151–153, 238–239, 281, 362, 568, 570, 574
PDUFA, 56; FDA progress reports, 536
Pediatric Dosage Handbook, 161–162, 409
Pediatric Drug Formulations, 164
The Pediatric Drug Handbook, 160, 568
pediatric drugs, market exclusivity under FDA Modernization Act, 56–57
PediWeb, 261
Peirce, A., 242, 246
PEL. *See* permissible exposure limits
Pelikan, E.W., 134
PEN names, 26
Penso, G., 335
The People's Book of Medical Tests, 435
PERI. *See* Pharmaceutical Education & Research Institute
permissible exposure limits, industrial chemicals: definition, 704; sources of, 211, 213, 215, 225, 228
Perry, M.C., 159
Persaud, T.V.N., 222
Personal Selling Audit (PSA), Scott-Levin, 374
Pesticides Abstracts (PESTAB), 430
Peter, G., 168
Peterson, G.R., 49
Petska, S., 241
Pfeiffer, D., 352
Pharma Japan, 484, 500
PharmaBiomed database, 483
PharmaBusiness, 500
Pharmaceutical Activities Index-Directory, 31
Pharmaceutical and Healthcare Industry News Database, 476–477, 483
Pharmaceutical Approvals Monthly, 68–69, 477, 483, 511–512; patent extension notices, 553, 556
Pharmaceutical Bioequivalence, 309
Pharmaceutical Business Intelligence & Research Group, 605–606

Pharmaceutical Business News (U.K.), 601
Pharmaceutical Chartbook, 378–379
The Pharmaceutical Codex, 303
Pharmaceutical Companies Analysis, 490
Pharmaceutical Company Image reports, 373
Pharmaceutical Dosage Forms and Drug Delivery Systems, 308
Pharmaceutical Dosage Forms: Disperse Systems, 309
Pharmaceutical Dosage Forms: Parenteral Medications, 309
Pharmaceutical Dosage Forms: Tablets, 309
Pharmaceutical Education and Research Institute, 621
Pharmaceutical Engineering, 619
Pharmaceutical Executive, 500
Pharmaceutical Historian, 356
Pharmaceutical Industry Weekly, 500
Pharmaceutical Information Library (INCAD), 544
Pharmaceutical Journal, 380, 622
Pharmaceutical Manufacturers Association of Canada, 630–631
Pharmaceutical Manufacturers Association. *See* Pharmaceutical Research and Manufacturers of America
Pharmaceutical Manufacturing Encyclopedia, 317
Pharmaceutical Manufacturing Review, 500
Pharmaceutical Marketers Directory, 354
Pharmaceutical Markets, Drugstores (IMS audit), 373
Pharmaceutical Markets, Hospitals (IMS audit), 373
Pharmaceutical Medicine, 48
Pharmaceutical News Index, 480–481, 484
Pharmaceutical Online Regulatory and Legislative Issues Index, 100
Pharmaceutical Research and Manufacturers Association of America, 631; Web site, 262, 367, 375–376, 472
Pharmaceutical Society of Great Britain, 310. *See also* Royal Pharmaceutical Society
Pharmaceutical Technology (USA), directory issue, 369
Pharmaceutical Technology International, global resource directory issue, 369
pharmaceutical technology: online sources, 437–439, 576; sourcebooks, 317–318
Pharmaceuticals Biotechnology & The Law, 49
pharmaceutics: definition, 704; information needs and resources, 301–320, 437–439, 576
pharmacies, directories, 370–372
Pharmacist and Pharmacy Achievement and Discipline Database, 99
The Pharmacist and the Law, 83
pharmacodynamics, definition, 704

PharmacoEconomics & Outcomes News, 479–480, 481, 484

pharmacoeconomics: definition, 704–705; Internet sources, 481, 484–486, 620; searching online, 654

Pharmacoepidemiology and Drug Safety, 620

pharmacogenetics, 170, 705

Pharmacognosy and Pharmacobiotechnology, 323–324

pharmacognosy: definition, 705; information sources, 321–347, 358–359; online access to literature, 439–440, 580, 648–649; professional and trade associations, 609, 614, 615, 618, 619, 622, 623, 630

Pharmacognosy, Phytochemistry, Medicinal Plants, 323, 324

pharmacokinetics: definition, 705; reference sources, 172

Pharmacological and Chemical Synonyms (Marler), 34–35, 192

pharmacological categories, searching online, 420–423, 649, 651

Pharmacological Reviews, 612

Pharmacologist, 612

pharmacology and therapeutics reference sources, 139–186.

See also bibliography, compilation using online databases

The Pharmacology of Chinese Herbs, 336

Pharmacontacts, 487, 491–492

Pharmacopeial Discussion Group, 63

Pharmacopeial Forum, 24, 304, 305

pharmacopeias: definition, 705; misconceptions about, 21; official compendial standards, 304–308

Pharmacor series, Decision Resources, 502

PharmacoResources, 479

Pharmacotherapy, 611

pharmacovigilance, definition, 705

pharmacy: calculations, tables, 36, 158, 176; history, information sources, 351, 354–357, 360; law, 80–88; licensure, 36, 80, 99, 351; practice, online information sources, 579–580; schools and colleges, directories, 380–382; services and operations, statistics, 379–380; symbols (apothecary), key to, 28; technician education and training programs, 381

Pharmacy and the Law, 83

pharmacy and therapeutics committee, hospital, 87

Pharmacy and You—American Pharmaceutical Association Web site, 262–263

The Pharmacy Assistant, 622

Pharmacy Continuing Education Sites Around the World, 382

Pharmacy Equivalent Name, 26

Pharmacy Guild of Australia, *Pharmacy Web Australia*, 125

Pharmacy in History, 356

Pharmacy Internet Guide, University of Sydney, 125

Pharmacy Law and Ethics, 83–84

Pharmacy Law Cases and Materials, 83

Pharmacy Law Digest, 81

Pharmacy Legislation Regulations Guidelines for Long-Term Care, 84–85

Pharmacy Museums and Historical Collections, 356

Pharmacy School Admission Requirements, 381, 383

Pharmacy Times: Callout column, 100; *Compounding Hotline*, 165; drug sales and utilization statistics, 374; *Patient Education Focus*, 263; *Pharmacists on the Net* column, 130

Pharmacy Today, 500

Pharmacy Web Australia, 125

Pharmacy, An Illustrated History, 356

Pharmacy, Medicine and Managed Care, 485

Pharmacy-Related Academic Institutions on the Internet, 382

Pharm-AID, index to *Unlisted Drugs*, 31–32

PharmaPages Web site, 130, 134

Pharmaprojects, 14, 448–453; compared to other pipeline directories, 472–476; patent information, 550; searching for drug registrations in, 516; as source of drug names, 442, 474; as source of licensing opportunities, 487, 655

PharmaVentures Links Page, 368

Pharmeuropa newsletter, 307

PharmInfoNet DrugDB Web site, 182

PharmInfoNet Gallery, 355

PharmInfoNet Glossary Web site, 134

PharmInfoNet PharmLinks Web site, 124–125

Pharm-Line, 409

Pharmsearch, 559. *See also* Markush Pharmsearch

PharmWeb, 123–124, 382

PharmWeb—Patient Information, 262

phase IV, 59

phases in drug development, 45–46. *See also* pipeline, directories online

Phelps, S.J., 163

phenylalanine-containing OTC products identified, 149

PhIL (INCAD), 544

Philadelphia College of Pharmacy founded, 354

Philadelphia Online—Health Philadelphia Web site, 259

Phillipson, J.D., 328

PHIND, 476–477, 483

photographs, dosage forms, 281–282

photosensitivity: definition, 705; list of drugs that induce, 36, 158, 244, 250
PhRMA, 631; Web site, 262, 367, 375–376, 472
PHS-149, 227
physical/chemical properties, sources of data, 27, 216–217, 302–317, 576
Physician Data Query Directory File, 436
Physician Data Query Patient Information File, 436
Physician Data Query Protocol File, 409
Physician Drug & Diagnosis Audit (PDDA), 373
Physicians' Desk Reference for Nonprescription Drugs, 151, 281, 362, 570, 572
Physicians' Desk Reference for Ophthalmology, 154–155
Physicians' Desk Reference, 151–153, 238–239, 281, 362, 568, 570, 574
Physicians' Generix, 573
Physicians' GenRx, 144, 573
Physicians' Guide to Nutriceuticals, 157
Phytochemical Database, 343
Phytochemical Dictionary, 332–333
phytomedicine, definition, 705. *See also* phytotherapeutics
Phytopharm Consulting, 328
phytotherapeutics, literature of, 321–347, 358–359, 439–440. *See also* plants, medicinal use
phytotoxins: definition, 705; reference sources, 229–232, 333, 338, 642. *See also* toxicology, online searching
Pickering, W.R., 114
PIL, 62
The Pill Book, 250–251, 281, 572
The Pink Sheet, 95, 477, 483, 511
pipeline, directories online, 447–476, 649, 654–655
PLA, 46–47, 511
placebo, definition, 705
Plant Contact Dermatitis, 229–230, 574
Planta Medica, 622
PLANTOX Web site, 231–232
plants, medicinal use: information sources, 246–247, 287, 289, 321–347, 358–359, 439–440; professional and trade associations, 609, 614, 615, 618, 619, 622, 623, 630
plants, toxicity reference sources, 229–232, 333, 642. *See also* toxicology, online searching
Plunkett, E.R., 211
PMA (Pharmaceutical Manufacturers Association). *See* Pharmaceutical Research and Manufacturers of America
PMA (premarket application, medical devices), 90, 705
PMA approvals, online sources, 516–520, 521, 523–524
PMAC. *See* Pharmaceutical Manufacturers Association of Canada

PMEA-Rx Link, 374
PMN, 90. *See also* 510k
PNI, 480
Pocket Guide to Injectable Drugs, 204
points to consider, FDA guidelines, 533
POISINDEX, 212–214, 568, 569
Poison Act (U.K.), 280
poison antidote chart, 36
poison control center directories, 36, 144, 150, 153, 176, 249, 263, 270, 285, 286, 293
Poison Prevention Packaging Act, 88, 277
Poisoning & Drug Overdose, 209–210, 568
Poisoning & Toxicology Handbook, 209–210, 409, 568
poisoning: definition, 706; information sources, 209–235, 350, 353. *See also* toxicology, online searching
Poisoning: Toxicology, Symptoms, Treatments, 211, 574
Poisonous and Venomous Marine Animals of the World, 230
Poisonous Plant Databases (Web site), 232
Poisonous Plants Bibliography, *TOXLINE*, 430
Poisonous Plants Home Page, University of Pennsylvania, 353
Poisonous Plants of the United States and Canada, 229, 574
Poisonous Plants, University of Florida Web site, 353
polypharmacy, definition, 706
Popovich, N.G., 308
Poppenga, R., 353
population characteristics, searching online, 413–414, 648
post-marketing surveillance (phase IV), 59; medical devices, 91–92
potentiation, definition, 706
Powell, R.H., 121
PPAD, 99
PPBIB, 232, 430
PPIs, 237, 238
PPOs, 87, 379
Practical Aspects of Intravenous Drug Administration, 204
Practical Exercises in Pharmacy Law and Ethics, 84
Practical Pharmaceutical Chemistry, 302
practice formulary, veterinary, 348, 706
practice guidelines, searching online, 426
The Practice of Chinese Medicine, 337–338
practicum exercises, 20, 187–188, 236, 385–386, 564–565; suggested answers, 633–656
practicum, prerequisite to pharmacy licensure, 80
preceptorship, 80
preclinical: studies, online access to, 576–577;

testing, drugs, 45. *See also* pipeline, directories online
predicate device, 91, 706
pre-explosions, *MEDLINE*, 414
Preferred Provider Organizations (PPOs), 87
pregnancy, drug use during, handbooks, 159, 199. *See also* teratogenicity.
Premarket Application (PMA), medical devices, 90. *See also* PMA approvals
Premarket Notification (PMN), medical devices, 90–91, 93. *See also* 510k
pre-registration, 8, 706. *See also* pipeline, directories online
prescription: audit. *See* drug utilization review; authority, who may prescribe, 79; drug status, federal versus state control, 79; drugs, coverage in literature, 17; drugs, first defined by law, 41; notations, key to, 28; statistics, sources, 372–379, 644, 656
Prescription and OTC Pharmaceuticals, 95
Prescription Drug Marketing Act (1987), 86
Prescription Drug User Fee Act, 56; FDA progress reports, 536
Prescription Medicines and You, 258
Prescription Pharmaceuticals and Biotechnology, 95
preservatives: definition, 706; identification of OTC products where absent, 149
press releases, FDA, 542
prevalence data. *See* epidemiology
prevalence versus incidence, definition, 706
pricing information, 35, 142, 144, 150, 156, 162, 287, 362, 489, 493
primary sources, 109
Principles of Clinical Toxicology, 216
Principles of Drug Information and Scientific Literature Evaluation, 118
Principles of Drug Information Services, 118–119
Principles of Pharmacology: Basic Concepts and Clinical Applications, 171
priority 1 and 2 journals, *MEDLINE*, 425
priority review, FDA classification, 58–59, 60
Priority-Based Assessment of Food Additives (PAFA) database, 313, 541
Problems in Pediatric Drug Therapy, 161
prodrug, definition, 706
Product Liability Daily (BNA), 482
product liability litigation, information sources, 77–78
Product License Application (PLA), biologics, 41, 46–47, 511
production, pharmaceuticals, information needs and resources, 301–320
Professional's Guide to Patient Drug Facts for Improved Patient Counseling, 270
Profile of Pharmacy Students (AACP), 382

PROMT database, 481, 483, 499–500
pronunciations of drug names, 23, 25, 28, 158, 161, 167, 176, 244, 248
Proposition 65, 706
The Proprietary Association. *See* Nonprescription Drug Manufacturers Association
proprietary names, 12. *See also* brand names
protocol (clinical trials) locator services online, 409, 413, 536–537
protopharmacology, dictionary, 357
Protozoological Abstracts, 407
Prous databases, 458, 462–466, 478–479; compared to other pipeline files, 472–476
psychiatric drugs, quick reference handbooks, 162, 245–246
Psychotropic Drugs: Fast Facts, 162
PsycINFO, 342
PTO, 553
Public Health Services Act (1944), 41–42
public libraries, recommended core collection, 570–572
publication types, 109–110; searching online, 426
Purdue University, *HEALTHWEB*, 122
Pure Foods and Drug Act (1906), 40, 304
purine-free OTC product identification, 149

Quality Assurance for Biopharmaceuticals, 48–49
Quality Control Reports, 96, 481, 484
quality control, pharmaceutical manufacturing, resources, 302–308
Quality of Life Assessment in Medicine, 484–485
quality of life, definition, 706–707
questions typically encountered, 108, 409–426; regulatory hot topics, 66–79
Quick Reference to Discontinued Drugs, 73

R&D (newsletter), 601
R&D Focus Drug News (IMSworld), 478, 483
R&D Focus Drug Updates (IMSworld), 453–455, 456–458; compared to other pipeline directories, 472–476; licensing information in, 487; searching for drug registrations, 516
R&D Insight (ADIS), 455, 458, 459–462; compared to other pipeline directories, 472–476; as source of licensing info, 487
R&D pipeline: intelligence sources online, 447–476. *See also* drug development process; pipeline, directories online
R&D statistics, 375–376, 378
Radiological Health Bulletin (FDA), 482
Radiology & Imaging Newsletter, 484
Raffle, P.A., 233
Rainbow Series, 376–378
RAinfo Web site, 100

Raintree Web site, 346
RAJ-Devices, 98
Rakel, R.E., 156
rapporteur, 61, 62
RAPS, 606; Web site, 100
Raso, J., 267
RDA charts/lists, 251, 252
Reactions (newsletter), 193
Reactions Database, 428, 482
reactions. *See also* adverse effects
reactions, organic name, key to, 28
Reagents for Organic Synthesis, 301
recalls: drug product lists, 88, 147; searching on-
    line, 524–526, 528, 655–656; statistics, 536
ReCap—Signals, 368
receptor, definition, 707
Recombinant Capital, Web database, 368
record (online), definition, 707
The Red Book (American Academy of Pediat-
    rics), 168
The Red Book, 35–36, 281, 362
Rees, A.M., 247, 572
refereed, definition, 707
reference listed drug, 707
regimen, definition, 707
registration, 8, 46, 510–521, 707. *See also* drug
    approvals
registry numbers. *See* CAS registry numbers
*Registry of Toxic Effects of Chemical Sub-
    stances*, 224, 431, 432
regulations, drug and device, background on,
    39–105, 282. *See also* regulatory informa-
    tion
The Regulatory Affairs Journal, 97–98
Regulatory Affairs Professional Society, 606;
    Web site, 100
regulatory hot topics, 66–79
regulatory information, searching online, 509–
    563, 581
regulatory news sources, 94–98
*Regulatory Practice for Biopharmaceutical Pro-
    duction*, 49
Reid, B.J., 116
Remington's Pharmaceutical Sciences, 170–
    171, 568, 569
renal disease, prescribing considerations, hand-
    books, 159
repackaging, pharmacist liabilities, 84
Repertorio Farmaceutico Italiano, 289, 290
Report of the Committee on Infectious Disease,
    American Academy of Pediatrics, 168
*Report of the Special Committee on Health Care
    Fraud*, 266
Report on Alternative Medicine (AMA), 266
reprint address, searching online, 423–425
reproductive effects. *See* teratogenicity

Reproductive Hazards of Industrial Chemicals,
    223
Reproductively Active Chemicals, 221
REPRORISK, 219
Research Centers and Services Directory, 581,
    591
*Research Guidelines for Evaluating the Safety
    and Efficacy of Herbal Medicines*, 327
Residency Directory (ASHP), 381–382
Resources in Epidemiology Web site, 506
retention, older reference sources, 573–574
Review of Aromatic and Medicinal Plants, 407,
    439
Review of Medical and Veterinary Entomology,
    407
Review of Medical and Veterinary Mycology,
    407
Reynolds, J.E.F., 139
Reynolds, L., 164
RFPs, news, 97
Richardson, M.L., 224
Rieger, M.M., 309
Rietschel, R.L., 233
RINGDOC, 402
Ringer, D.L., 157
Ritschel, W.A., 172
RN. *See* CAS registry numbers
Robbers, J.E., 323, 327
Roberts, R.J., 204
Robertson, W.O., 211
Roe, D.A., 200
Rogers, K., 165
The Rose Sheet, 96, 477, 483
Rosenberg, J.M., 569, 572
Rosenthal Center for Complementary and Alter-
    native Medicine, 340
Ross, I.A., 329
Rossoff, I.S., 349
Rote Liste, 284–285
Roussel Uclaf Causality Assessment Method,
    193
routes of administration, searching online,
    415–417
Rowland, J.F.B., 120
Rowland, M., 172
Royal Pharmaceutical Society of Great Britain,
    380, 621–622
Royal Society of Chemistry: *Analytical Ab-
    stracts*, 437, 438; *Chemical Engineering and
    Biotechnology Abstracts*, 576, 584; *Chemi-
    cal Safety Newsbase*, 578, 584; *Chemicals
    and Companies*, 495; *Current Biotechnology
    Abstracts*, 576, 577, 578, 585; *DOSE: The
    Dictionary of Substances and Their Effects*,
    224; *Historical Image Collection* Web site,
    355
RPROJ, 429, 430